Epilepsy

NEUROLOGICAL DISEASE AND THERAPY

Advisory Board

Epilepsy

Scientific Foundations of Clinical Practice

edited by

Jong M. Rho

University of California at Irvine College of Medicine
Irvine, California, U.S.A.

Raman Sankar

University of California, Los Angeles
Los Angeles, California, U.S.A.

José E. Cavazos

University of Texas Health Science Center at San Antonio
San Antonio, Texas, U.S.A.

MARCEL DEKKER, INC.   NEW YORK · BASEL

Library of Congress Cataloging-in-Publication Data
A catalog record for this book is available from the Library of Congress.

ISBN: 0-8247-5043-8

This book is printed on acid-free paper.

Headquarters
Marcel Dekker, Inc., 270 Madison Avenue, New York, NY 10016, U.S.A.
tel: 212-696-9000; fax: 212-685-4540

Distribution and Customer Service
Marcel Dekker, Inc., Cimarron Road, Monticello, New York 12701, U.S.A.
tel: 800-228-1160; fax: 845-796-1772

Eastern Hemisphere Distribution
Marcel Dekker AG, Hutgasse 4, Postfach 812, CH-4001 Basel, Switzerland
tel: 41-61-260-6300; fax: 41-61-260-6333

World Wide Web
http://www.dekker.com

The publisher offers discounts on this book when ordered in bulk quantities. For more information, write to Special Sales/Professional Marketing at the headquarters address above.

Current printing (last digit):
10 9 8 7 6 5 4 3 2 1

PRINTED IN THE UNITED STATES OF AMERICA

Preface

Epilepsy is an episodic neurological disorder that has afflicted humankind throughout most the span of recorded history, yet throughout the millenia, it has never properly been acknowledged as a disease with a biological basis. In ancient times, epilepsy was referred somewhat ironically as the "sacred disease", as it was imbued with negative references to the supernatural, and later believed to represent a form of demonic possession, and thus, leading to social eschewal and persecution. It was only late in the 19th century that epilepsy began its long and arduous journey to being justly recognized as a physical illness with complex pathophysiological substrates. Even today, the public is not fully apprised of the true nature of the epilepsies (as they are now considered), and efforts to expand awareness of this condition have been thwarted in large measure by the deeply rooted preconceptions promulgated through the ages.

Within the last half century, great progress has been made in our basic understanding of the epileptic brain, and significant advances in drug development and in surgical techniques, and the emergence of innovative approaches such as electrical stimulation of the nervous system, have led to a substantial reduction in the morbidity and mortality of epileptic patients (both children and adults). At the same time, we have been witness to remarkable developments in the basic neurosciences, and our current understanding of brain structure and function is at ever-finer levels of molecular, cellular, and genetic detail.

The intrinsic complexities associated with understanding normal brain structure and function are at the heart of the challenges investigators face in deciphering the epileptic brain. The development of universally effective therapeutic approaches for epileptic patients has been the elusive goal of clinicians and researchers since the early 20th century. Yet, despite the availability of many new pharmacological agents within the last generation, a third of the epileptic patients (estimated to represent 1% of the population) remain refractory to medical therapy, and only a small minority of these individuals are suitable candidates for epilepsy surgery. It is this last frustrating reality that has been the focus of many professionals in the epilepsy field.

Within the research arena, there has been increasing focus on "translational" research (i.e., that which bridges the gap between the patient beside and the laboratory); effective communication and interchange between clinicians and basic researchers has been difficult to achieve on a broad basis. It is clear that such activity is paramount in the development of novel treatments based on a detailed knowledge of fundamental mechanisms.

The co-editors, representing only a small handful of clinicians motivated to pursue important clinical questions in the laboratory, were inspired by the founders and leaders of the epilepsy field to pursue academic careers. Reflective of this goal is the current volume, which is aimed at clinicians and scientists alike. We wish to collectively thank our mentors (Jerome "Pete" Engel, Philip A. Schwartzkroin, Claude Wasterlain, Michael A. Rogawski, Thomas P. Sutula, Thomas V. Dunwiddie, W. Donald Shields, D. Alan Shewmon, Harry T. Chugani, and Tallie Z. Baram, among others), colleagues, students, and most of all, our patients and their families, for providing the inspiration and encouragement to help facilitate this "translational" dialogue. Additionally, we thank the publisher and our families for the support they have given us throughout this project.

Jong M. Rho, M.D.
Raman Sankar, M.D., Ph.D.
José E. Cavazos, M.D., Ph.D.

Contents

Part III: Epilepsy Surgery

Part IV: Alternative Therapies

Part V: Other Modulators of the Epileptic State

Part VI: The Future of Epilepsy Therapy

Contributors

Massoud Akhtari Huntington Medical Research Institutes and Epilepsy and Brain Mapping Program, Pasadena, California, and Department of Physics and Astronomy, University of New Mexico, Albuquerque, New Mexico, U.S.A.

Gail D. Anderson Department of Pharmacy, University of Washington, Seattle, Washington, U.S.A.

Deborah Arthur Huntington Medical Research Institutes, Pasadena, California, U.S.A.

Jacquelyn L. Bainbridge Neurosciences Center, University of Colorado Health Sciences Center, Denver, Colorado, U.S.A.

Gregory K. Bergey Department of Neurology, The Johns Hopkins University School of Medicine, Baltimore, Maryland, U.S.A.

Edward H. Bertram Department of Neurology, University of Virginia, Charlottesville, Virginia, U.S.A.

Kristopher J. Bough Department of Pharmacology, Emory University, Atlanta, Georgia, U.S.A.

Rochelle Caplan Director of Pediatric Neuropsychiatry Program, Department of Psychiatry and Behavioral Sciences, UCLA Neuropsychiatric Institute, Los Angeles, California, U.S.A.

José E. Cavazos Department of Medicine (Neurology) and Pharmacology, University of Texas Health Science Center at San Antonio, San Antonio, Texas, U.S.A.

Edward C. Cooper Department of Neurology, University of Pennsylvania, Philadelphia, Pennsylvania, U.S.A.

Ara J. Deukemedjian Department of Neurosurgery, and McKnight Brain Institute, University of Florida, Gainesville, Florida, U.S.A.

F. Edward Dudek Anatomy and Neurobiology Section, Department of Biomedical Sciences, Colorado State University, Fort Collins, Colorado, U.S.A.

Ross Eto Departments of Neurology, Neurosurgery and Radiology, Huntington Hospital, Pasadena, California, U.S.A.

Edward Flynn   Department of Physics and Astronomy, University of New Mexico, Albuquerque, and Los Alamos National Laboratory, Los Alamos, New Mexico, U.S.A.

Piotr J. Franaszczuk   Department of Neurology, Epilepsy Research Laboratory, Johns Hopkins Epilepsy Center, The Johns Hopkins University School of Medicine, Baltimore, Maryland, U.S.A.

William A. Friedman   Department of Neurosurgery, and McKnight Brain Institute, University of Florida, Gainesville, Florida, U.S.A.

Tracy A. Glauser   Children's Comprehensive Epilepsy Program, Department of Neurology, Cincinnati Children's Hospital Medical Center, Cincinnati, Ohio, U.S.A.

Paul T. Golumbek   Department of Neurology, Washington University School of Medicine, St. Louis, Missouri, U.S.A.

Michael M. Haglund   Division of Neurosurgery, Duke University Medical Center, Durham, North Carolina, U.S.A.

Janina Z.P. Janes   Neurosciences Center, University of Colorado Health Sciences Center, Denver, Colorado, U.S.A.

Christophe Jouny   Department of Neurology, Epilepsy Research Laboratory, Johns Hopkins Epilepsy Center, The Johns Hopkins University School of Medicine, Baltimore, Maryland, U.S.A.

Jaideep Kapur   Department of Neurology, University of Virginia, Charlottesville, Virginia, U.S.A.

Richard B. Kim   Surgical Director, The Epilepsy Center of Hoag and Children's Hospitals, Newport Beach, California, U.S.A.

Pavel Klein   Director, Epilepsy Chair, Clinical Neuroendocrinology Unit, Department of Neurology, Georgetown University Hospital, Washington, D.C., U.S.A.

Robert C. Knowlton   Epilepsy Center, Department of Neurology, University of Alabama at Birmingham, Birmingham, Alabama, U.S.A.

Richard Leahy   Signal Imaging Processing Institute, University of Southern California, Los Angeles, California, U.S.A.

Kenneth M. Little   Division of Neurosurgery, Department of Surgery, and Department of Neurobiology, Duke University Medical Center, Durham, North Carolina, U.S.A.

Nancy Lopez   Epilepsy and Brain Mapping Program, Pasadena, California, U.S.A.

Adam N. Mamelak   Huntington Medical Research Institutes, Epilepsy and Brain Mapping Program, and Departments of Neurology, Neurosurgery and Radiology, Huntington Hospital, Pasadena, and City of Hope Medical Center, Durate, California, U.S.A.

Warren Merrifield   Huntington Medical Research Institutes, Pasadena, and Department of Psychology, Loma Linda University, Loma Linda, California, U.S.A.

John Mosher   Los Alamos National Laboratory, Los Alamos, New Mexico, and Signal Imaging Processing Institute, University of Southern California, Los Angeles, California, U.S.A.

Dean K. Naritoku   Department of Neurology and Pharmacology, Director, Office of Therapeutics Research, Director, Center for Epilepsy, Southern Illinois University, Springfield, Illinois, U.S.A.

Jeri E. Nichols   Epilepsy and Brain Mapping Program, Pasadena, California, U.S.A.

Rachelle Padilla   Epilepsy and Brain Mapping Program, and Departments of Neurology, Neurosurgery and Radiology, Huntington Hospital, Pasadena, California, U.S.A.

D. Scott Pollock   Neurosciences Center, University of Colorado Health Sciences Center, Denver, Colorado, U.S.A.

Mark Quigg   Department of Neurology, University of Virginia, Charlottesville, Virginia, U.S.A.

Doodipala S. Reddy   Department of Molecular Biomedical Sciences, North Carolina State University College of Veterinary Medicine, Raleigh, North Carolina, U.S.A.

Jong M. Rho   Department of Pediatrics, University of California at College of Medicine, Irvine, California, U.S.A.

Michael A. Rogawski   Chief, Epilepsy Research Section, National Institute of Neurological Disorders and Stroke, National Institutes of Health, Bethesda, Maryland, U.S.A.

Steven N. Roper   Department of Neurosurgery, and McKnight Brain Institute, University of Florida, and Gainesville VA Medical Center, Gainesville, Florida, U.D.A.

Russell Sanchez   Department of Medicine (Neurology) and Pharmacology, University of Texas Health Science Center at San Antonio, San Antonio, Texas, U.S.A.

Raman Sankar   Mattel Children's Hospital at UCLA, University of California, Los Angeles, California, U.S.A.

Joy Sarafian   Epilepsy and Brain Mapping Program, Pasadena, California, U.S.A.

Philip A. Schwartzkroin   Department of Neurological Surgery, University of California, Davis, California, U.S.A.

Carl E. Stafstrom   Department of Neurology, University of Wisconsin, Madison, Wisconsin, U.S.A.

William W. Sutherling   Huntington Medical Research Institutes, Epilepsy and Brain Mapping Program, and Departments of Neurology, Neurosurgery and Radiology, Huntington Hospital, Pasadena, California, U.S.A.

James W. Wheless Department of Neurology and Pediatrics, and Director, Pediatric Epilepsy Services and Texas Comprehensive Epilepsy Program, University of Texas–Houston, Houston, Texas, U.S.A.

H. Steve White Anticonvulsant Screening Project, Department of Pharmacology and Toxicology, University of Utah, Salt Lake City, Utah, U.S.A.

Epilepsy

1
Introduction

Jong M. Rho
University of California at Irvine College of Medicine
Irvine, California, U.S.A.

Raman Sankar
University of California, Los Angeles
Los Angeles, California, U.S.A.

José E. Cavazos
University of Texas Health Science Center at San Antonio
San Antonio, Texas, U.S.A.

Epilepsy is a common episodic neurological condition that is heterogeneous in clinical presentation, yet characterized at a more fundamental level by the common denominators of neuronal hyperexcitability and hypersynchrony. Our understanding of epilepsy has advanced significantly over the past several decades, and the treatment options (both medical and surgical) have expanded greatly as well. Progress in the basic neurosciences has translated to yet ever-growing observations of molecular and cellular changes that are associated with the epileptic condition, and some of which may be critical to the processes of epileptogenesis—i.e., the pathological changes that ensue over a latent period, ultimately resulting in spontaneous recurrent seizures and their attendant negative consequences. Further, within the past decade, advances in molecular genetics have defined not only more clearly the role of seizure susceptibility genes and multi-gene influences, but genetic mutations that are specifically linked to certain, albeit rare epileptic syndromes.

Nevertheless, despite such exciting developments, the clinical practice of epilepsy remains largely empiric, and few insights from the research bench have had meaningful clinical impact. The relative dearth of true translational (i.e., clinic to bench and back to clinic) research has hampered our ability to move beyond the limited trial-and-error approach of anticonvulsant drug therapy, to one that is based on a detailed understanding of how specific molecular changes might dictate truly rational and targeted pharmacotherapy. Yet despite this, and even as the mainstay of epilepsy therapy continues to be represented by anticonvulsant medications, there are other novel drug approaches and nonpharmacological (e.g., deep brain stimulation) considerations that clinicians have brought forth to the treatment armamentarium, including innovative surgical interventions.

There are many books dealing with the subject of epilepsy, with some focusing on clinical diagnosis and treatments, while others explore the pathological substrates of the various epilepsies. And there are some noteworthy volumes that provide comprehensive overviews and discussions about both basic science and clinical topics in the field of epilepsy. However, we perceived a need for a volume that attempts to integrate the most relevant research developments with that of clinical issues that impact directly on therapeutics. Such a translational research book would attempt to define the scientific basis of clinical practice, and pose a set of challenging questions and considerations that could help shape not only the future of clinical research, but also provide novel insights and avenues into more fundamental investigations that would yet again make us go "back to the bench, and return to the clinic." The thoughtful clinicians, who can appreciate insights drawn from the fundamental neurosciences, can and should take a more rational approach toward the treatment of epileptic patients. Incorporating the exciting research developments in the field into their knowledge base will empower them to "think outside the box," and to test clinical hypotheses derived from implications of basic research findings.

This volume is divided into five sections. The first section begins with a general treatment of the basic anatomic and functional substrates of seizure genesis. This is followed by a mechanistic discussion of advances in our understanding of drug resistance and status epilepticus, and concludes with a detailed review of the paradigm shift we have undergone in the past decade—viewing certain epilepsies as channelopathies, i.e., disorders arising from mutations in genes encoding ion channels, which are the essential currency of neuronal excitability.

The second section includes novel concepts related to antiepileptic drug therapy, including the impact of ontogeny of molecular targets of antiepileptic drugs (AEDs) on drug choice, and the possibility that certain AEDs may exert effects on the disease process itself (rather than simply quench recurrent seizures). Other considerations in the use of AEDs, both clinically available and investigational, include an appreciation for non-synaptic mechanisms yielding potent anticonvulsant effects (e.g., those mediated by certain diuretics), pharmacokinetic and pharmaco-dynamic effects, and the ever important concern for toxicities—especially those of the serious, idiosyncratic variety. However, with a better understanding of drug interactions and toxicities, beyond what can be established as mechanisms explaining clinical efficacy, the clinician can undoubtedly optimize the long-term care of patients suffering from epilepsy.

The third section highlights advances in the fields of structural and functional neuroimaging, which have helped enormously in the selection of epilepsy surgery candidates and improving post-surgical outcomes. At the same time, there are emerging non-surgical methods for ablation of epileptic tissue.

The fourth section reviews the variety of non-traditional treatment options, many which have established efficacy in the treatment of medically refractory epilepsies (such as the ketogenic diet and the vagus nerve stimulator), but others whose particular clinical niches remain to be defined (immunomodulators, neurosteroids, etc.). Section five deals with neuroendocrine and biobehavioral factors that influence seizure susceptibility, information which should be incorporated into the design of treatment algorithms on an individualized basis.

Finally, the last section of this book gives a glimpse of what future epilepsy therapies might look like, from novel mechanisms of drug delivery, to deep brain stimulation, and seizure detection which provides the pretext for highly targeted and early preventative intervention. Along these lines, the final chapter provides an overview of what has become the holy grail of epilepsy therapeutics over the past several years—the goal of preventing epilepsy itself by first identifying populations at risk, and perhaps more importantly, the critical mediators and influences that in a causal manner produce an enduring epileptic condition. Such knowledge would then be employed to intervene during critical windows of disease ontogeny, as well as during brain development.

The idea for this book was inspired by our collective desire to promote bridging of the so-called "translational divide"—i.e., covering innovative treatment strategies based on scientific principles that have yet to be tested rigorously in the clinical setting, but yet may provide practitioners with new approaches toward epilepsy therapeutics. It is in this spirit that we earnestly hope that the reader will benefit from exploration of this volume.

2
Pathophysiology of Seizures and Epilepsy

José E. Cavazos and Russell Sanchez
University of Texas Health Science Center at San Antonio
San Antonio, Texas, U.S.A.

INTRODUCTION

Epileptic seizures are paroxysmal clinical events arising from neuronal hyperexcitability and hypersynchrony of the cerebral cortex, either locally or simultaneously in both hemispheres. A seizure occurs when there is a sudden imbalance between the excitatory and inhibitory inputs to a network of neurons such that there is overall excessive excitability. The behavioral manifestations of a seizure depend on the area of the cerebral cortex that is involved—directly, in the seizure focus, or indirectly, through recruitment and propagation of this abnormal paroxysmal neuronal activity. Convulsions are defined as seizures that include motor manifestations such as repeated and rhythmic jerking of the limbs, most often due to involvement of the motor cortex. Anticonvulsant drugs are medications that attempt to compensate for this abnormal cellular hyperexcitability by shifting the delicate balance back toward its normal state. Epilepsy is a chronic disorder characterized by recurrent unprovoked seizures, and is associated with a variety of medical conditions and neurological diseases. Antiepileptic medications attempt to treat this chronic seizure propensity, and, by definition, antiepileptogenic drugs aim to prevent the natural history of the epileptic disease.

For several decades, experimental animal models of convulsions have been employed in screening for effective medications to treat epileptic seizures from tens of thousands of investigational compounds. This drug development approach led to the discovery of medications that are very effective in preventing recurrent primary or secondarily generalized tonic-clonic seizures (anticonvulsants) but that appear less effective against other seizure types. This observation is likely due to the fundamental differences in the mechanisms that underlie the various seizure types. It is believed that the mechanisms underlying recruitment of other regions of the cerebral cortex by secondary propagation away from the epileptic focus are different from the mechanisms underlying the initial development of cellular hyperexcitability within the epileptic focus. In this chapter, we will broadly review the basic mechanisms of epilepsy and seizures, and we shall also indicate steps in the pathophysiological cascades of seizures and epilepsy where available anticonvulsant medications may intervene.

The pathophysiological mechanisms that underlie partial-onset seizures differ considerably from those that underlie generalized-onset seizures. In both cases, there is an overall net increase in synchronized cortical excitability, but it appears that the mechanisms that lead to neuronal synchronization are significantly different from each other, and thus, these will be discussed in separate sections.

PATHOPHYSIOLOGY OF PARTIAL-ONSET SEIZURES AND EPILEPSY

The neurophysiological hallmark of partial-onset seizures is the focal interictal epileptiform spike or sharp wave recorded in the electroencephalogram (EEG), electrocorticogram (ECoG), or depth electrode recordings near the seizure focus (Fig. 1). The intracellular correlate of the interictal epileptiform discharge is the

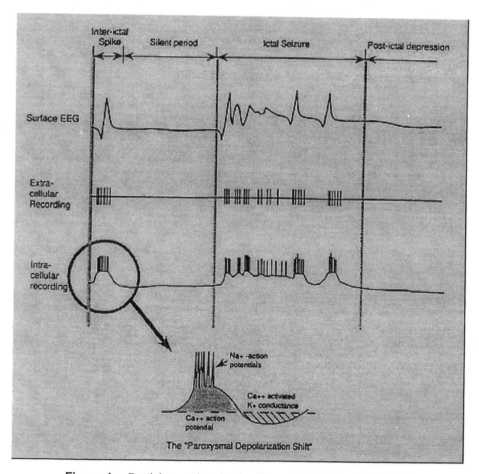

Figure 1. Partial-onset interictal spike and PDS. (From Ref. 44.)

paroxysmal depolarization shift (PDS). The PDS is characterized by a prolonged calcium-dependent conductance that depolarizes the neuronal membrane to a degree beyond the threshold for activation of voltage-gated sodium channels. This causes multiple sodium-dependent action potentials to be fired during the prolonged depolarization phase of the PDS, and which is followed by a prominent after-hyperpolarization (AHP) mediated by a calcium-activated potassium current. The temporal and spatial summation of multiple synchronous PDSs within the abnormally activated cortical circuitry results in an interictal spike observed in the scalp EEG. It has been calculated that several million neurons firing synchronous PDS discharges are needed over a time span of 30–75 msec, and from an area of at least about $6\,cm^2$ of cerebral cortex, to generate an interictal spike detectable with scalp electrodes in the EEG (1).

There are several factors that may be associated with the transition from an interictal spike to an epileptic seizure. It is presumed that when any of the mechanisms responsible for an acute seizure become enduring, patients develop the propensity for spontaneous recurrent seizures that characterize the epileptic state. Mechanisms leading to hyperexcitability have been demonstrated at multiple levels of brain structure and function, including abnormalities of the (1) neuronal circuitry; (2) neurons; (3) glia and the extracellular milieu; (4) subcellular regions; (5) receptor composition, distribution, or biophysical properties; (6) signal transduction; (7) genetic code; and (8) posttranslational regulation. Pathological alterations in structure and/or function at any or all of these levels can involve changes that affect intrinsic neuronal properties or their synaptic excitability, leading to cellular hyperexcitability, which might become permanent. Multiple combinations of these alterations might coexist to explain the heterogeneity of the epilepsies and the unpredictability of epileptic seizures.

MECHANISMS LEADING TO DECREASED INHIBITION

Defective GABA$_A$ Receptor-Mediated Inhibition

Gamma-aminobutyric acid (GABA) is the main inhibitory neurotransmitter in the brain. GABA binds to two major classes of receptors: the GABA$_A$ and the GABA$_B$ receptors. GABA$_A$ receptors mediate fast inhibition while the onset and duration of the effects of GABA$_B$ receptor activation are on a much longer timescale (Fig. 2). GABA$_A$ receptors are ligand-gated anion channels that are permeable to Cl^- and HCO_3^-. Among GABA receptors, they are the main target of modulation by currently available anticonvulsants. The reversal potential of GABA$_A$ channels in mature neurons typically is near the resting membrane potential, and therefore, they contribute little to changes in membrane potential in neurons at rest. However, GABA$_A$ receptors become more important upon synaptic excitation, as they oppose the summation of excitatory postsynaptic potentials (EPSPs) through both electrical shunting of the membrane (decreasing membrane resistance) and promoting membrane hyperpolarization back toward the resting membrane potential. In this manner, GABA$_A$ receptor activation makes it more difficult to achieve the threshold membrane potential necessary for generation of an action potential.

GABA$_A$ receptor channels are heteropentamers composed of different molecular subunits designated $\alpha1–6$, $\beta1–4$, $\gamma1–3$, δ, $\rho1–3$, ε, π, and θ (for reviews,

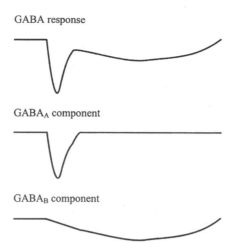

GABA response

GABA$_A$ component

GABA$_B$ component

Figure 2. The inhibitory postsynaptic potential (IPSP) induced by GABA: GABA response; GABA$_A$ component; and GABA$_B$ component.

see 2–4). Diversity among GABA$_A$ receptors—in their affinity for GABA, single-channel conductance and kinetics, and pharmacological sensitivities—arises from different combinations of these subunits (5). Given the number of known GABA$_A$ receptor subunits, the number of possible random combinations for a pentameric receptor is enormous. However, only ~20 of the possible combinations have been found in the normal mammalian brain. Native GABA$_A$ receptors typically contain at least one each of α, β, and γ subunits, with δ and ε subunits able to substitute for a γ subunit (6). Recombinant GABA$_A$ receptors comprised of only α and β subunits form functional channels that have all of the physiological characteristics of native GABA$_A$ receptors, except that they are completely insensitive to modulation by benzodiazepines—unless a γ subunit is included (7).

Some of the epilepsies might be due to mutations or abnormal expression of specific GABA$_A$ receptor subunits. For example, deletions in chromosome 15 (e.g., as seen with Angelman syndrome) results in the loss of genes for the α5, β3, and γ3 GABA$_A$ receptor subunits (8) and a resultant severe epileptic phenotype (9). Two naturally occurring mutations involving the γ2 subunit gene also have been found to be associated with febrile seizures and absence epilepsy (10,11). When recombinant receptors are expressed with α1 and β2 subunits, one of these γ2 mutations results in decreased whole-cell current responses to GABA (10), and the other leads to decreased benzodiazepine sensitivity (11).

Experimentally, changes in the expression of GABA$_A$ receptor subunits also have been observed in several animal models of partial epilepsy such as electrical kindling (12,13), chemical kindling (14), kainate-induced status epilepticus (15), and pilocarpine-induced status epilepticus (16,17). In this last model, decreases in the concentration for mRNA for the α5 subunit of the surviving interneurons in the CA1 region of the rat hippocampus have been reported (16). Additionally, granule cells of the dentate gyrus appear to undergo various changes in their GABA$_A$ receptor subunit expression, exhibiting decreased mRNA for α1 relative to α4, decreased β1 relative to β3, and increased δ relative to γ2 (17). These molecular changes appear to be associated with functional $GABA_A$ receptors that produce less effective inhibition, thus promoting neuronal hyperexcitability in the principal neurons. For example, a decrease in $\alpha1$-containing $GABA_A$ receptors in favor of $\alpha4$-containing receptors would be expected to render the receptors more sensitive to inhibition by synaptically released zinc, thus promoting depression of inhibition during increased synaptic activity, and also less sensitivity to augmentation by benzodiazepines (18).

The functional properties of $GABA_A$ receptor channels can be modulated clinically by benzodiazepines (i.e., diazepam, lorazepam, clonazepam, etc.), barbiturates (i.e., phenobarbital, pentobarbital, etc.), topiramate, and felbamate. Benzodiazepines increase the *frequency* of $GABA_A$ receptor channel openings, whereas barbiturates increase the mean *duration* of channel openings. Macroscopically, both of these effects augment GABA-mediated inhibition. Topiramate also increases the frequency of channel openings, but does so by binding to a site on the $GABA_A$ receptor that is distinct from the benzodiazepine recognition site (19). Although topiramate does not alter ligand binding at the benzodiazepine or barbiturate binding sites (20), it is yet unknown whether combining topiramate with either benzodiazepines or barbiturates would further increase GABA-mediated currents. Felbamate, a broad-spectrum anticonvulsant similar in profile to topiramate, appears to enhance GABA-mediated inhibition through barbituratelike actions (21).

Ion channels additionally are subject to modulation via posttranslational mechanisms, such as protein phosphorylation, and such changes alter the conformational state of the receptor ionophore. The $GABA_A$ receptor channel has several phosphorylation sites, one of which might be modulated by topiramate (22). Phosphorylation of $GABA_A$ receptors can induce a variety of effects on channel function and cell surface receptor expression depending on the particular molecular composition of the receptor (23), and these can have opposing consequences for macroscopic inhibition. For example, in studies of recombinant $GABA_A$ receptors, protein kinase A–mediated phosphorylation of β subunits resulted in decreased responses to GABA mediated by $\alpha1\beta1$-containing receptors (24), but increased GABA responses mediated by $\alpha1\beta3$-containing receptors (25). Clearly, the macroscopic effects of drugs that alter the phosphorylation states of $GABA_A$ receptors depend critically on the molecular composition of the receptors affected.

In summary, the behavior of individual $GABA_A$ receptor channels summate to generate a largely chloride-mediated membrane hyperpolarization that counterbalances the depolarization created by the summation of excitatory postsynaptic potentials (EPSPs). Defective $GABA_A$ receptor-mediated inhibition can result in seizures and epilepsy, whereas augmentation of this inhibition can be anticonvulsant and antiepileptic.

Defective $GABA_B$ Inhibition

Postsynaptic $GABA_B$ receptors are coupled to voltage-gated potassium channels, and yield a current of relatively long duration as compared to that evoked by activation of the $GABA_A$ receptor. Because of this, it is believed that the $GABA_B$ receptor may play a major role in the transition between the interictal state and the onset of a partial seizure. The molecular structure of the $GABA_B$ receptor is that of a heterodimer—i.e., two subunits, each possessing seven membrane-spanning domains. The coupling to ion channels is mediated by G-proteins, which may account for the prolonged latency and long duration of the hyperpolarization. $GABA_B$ receptors are also localized to presynaptic terminals, where they may suppress synaptic neurotransmitter release by decreasing voltage-gated calcium currents. The release of GABA from the interneuron terminal would then inhibit the post-synaptic neuron via two mechanisms: (1) directly by inducing a fast ($GABA_A$ receptor-mediated) and slow ($GABA_B$ receptor-mediated) postsynaptic IPSP; and (2) by $GABA_B$ receptor-mediated inhibition of the release of excitatory neurotransmitter in the presynaptic afferent projection. Alterations or mutations in the different $GABA_B$ subunits, or in the molecules that regulate their function or distribution, might impact seizure threshold or a propensity for recurrent seizures. Clinically, $GABA_B$ receptors are indirectly modulated by increasing the GABA concentration in the synaptic cleft such as by increasing the overall production of GABA (i.e., gabapentin) or blockade of the synaptic reuptake mechanisms (i.e., tiagabine).

Defective Activation of GABA-ergic Neurons

GABAergic neurons in hippocampus are activated via feed-forward and feedback projections of excitatory neurons (Fig. 3). These two types of inhibition within the neuronal network are defined on the basis of the time of activation of the GABA-ergic interneuron relative to the principal neuron that is the output of the network, such as the hippocampal pyramidal CA1 neuron. In feed-forward inhibition, the GABA-ergic interneuron receives a collateral projection from the main excitatory afferent projection that activates hippocampal pyramidal CA1 neurons, in this particular case, the Schaffer collateral axons from the CA3 pyramidal neurons. The feed-forward projection activates the somata of GABA-ergic interneurons prior to, or simultaneously with, the activation of the apical dendrites of the CA1 pyramidal neurons. Therefore, the activation of the GABA-ergic interneurons would result in an IPSP that inhibits the soma or axon hillock of the CA1 pyramidal neurons almost simultaneously with the passive propagation of the excitatory potential (EPSP) from the apical dendrites to the axon hillock. In this manner, the feed-forward projection primes the inhibitory system in a manner that allows it to make it difficult for the pyramidal cell to depolarize and fire an action potential.

Feedback inhibition is another system that allows control of repetitive firing in principal neurons such as pyramidal cells and inhibition of the surrounding pyramidal cells. Recurrent collaterals from the pyramidal neurons activate the GABA-ergic neurons once the pyramidal neurons have fired an action potential once. Over the past few years, experimental evidence has indicated that some other kind of interneuron might function as a gate between the principal neurons and the GABA-ergic interneurons. In the dentate gyrus, the mossy cells of the hilar polymorphic region appear to gate the inhibitory tone and activate the GABA-ergic neurons. The mossy cells receive both feedback and feed-forward excitation, which they convey to the GABA-ergic interneurons (Fig. 4). However, in certain circumstances they appear highly vulnerable to seizure-related neuronal loss. Once some of the mossy cells are lost, the activation of the GABA-ergic interneurons is impaired (26).

Synaptic reorganization is a form of brain plasticity induced by neuronal loss (27). The formation of new circuits that include excitatory and inhibitory cells

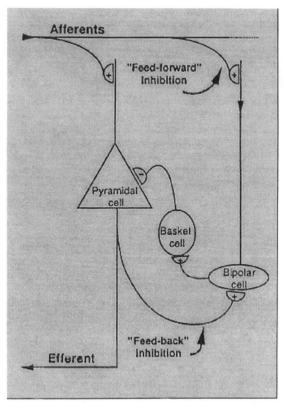

Figure 3. Schematic representation of the inhibitory circuitry. (From American Epilepsy Society, http://www.aesnet.org/edu_pub/med_edu_residents.cfm.)

has been demonstrated in several animal models and in humans with intractable temporal lobe epilepsy. Insufficient sprouting that attempts to restore inhibition might alter the balance between excitatory and inhibitory tone in the neural network. High doses of phenobarbital, at peak concentrations associated with lethargy and stupor, can prevent the loss of hilar interneurons and the development of mossy fiber synaptic reorganization induced in the rat kainic acid model (28). In this particular model, phenobarbital-treated rats appeared less susceptible to further seizures as demonstrated by the normalization of the rate at which generalized convulsive kindled seizures develop (also known as the kindling rate). Recent preliminary observations with topiramate after the onset of status epilepticus induced by kainic acid suggest that it has similar neuroprotective properties (29). In this setting, these neuroprotective drugs may be antiepileptogenic by preventing the synaptic reorganization that is triggered by the initial cell loss.

Defective Intracellular Buffering of Calcium

Recurrent seizures induced by a variety of methods result in a pattern of interneuron loss in the hilar polymorphic region in rodents, with a striking loss of the neurons that lack the calcium-binding proteins parvalbumin and calbindin. In rat hippocampal

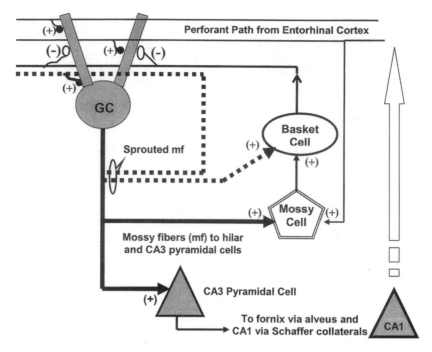

Figure 4. Schematic representation of the Epileptic Dentate Gyrus circuitry. Granule cells receive their major input via the perforant path. The perforant path also stimulates hilar interneurons (such as mossy cells and basket cells) to provide *feed-forward inhibition* of the granule cells. Granule cell axons, the mossy fibers, make synaptic contact with CA3 pyramidal cells. Mossy fiber collaterals innervate the hilar interneurons such as the mossy cell shown in the diagram. Mossy cells are excitatory to GABAergic basket cells which provide *feedback inhibition* to the granule cell. Sprouting of mossy fibers (in response to seizure-induced loss of CA3 pyramidal cells and hilar mossy cells) can result in enhanced excitation by forming autapses (an axon sprout synapsing with the dendrites of the same cell) and can augment synchronization by stimulating neighboring granule cells (not shown), thus contributing to epileptogenicity. It has also been suggested that the sprouted mossy fibers may restore inhibition lost after seizure-induced death of hilar mossy cells by direct stimulation of de-afferented (i.e., "dormant") basket cells. (From Ref. 45.)

slices, these interneurons demonstrate a progressive inability to maintain a hyperpolarized resting membrane potential; eventually, those neurons die. In an experiment using microelectrodes containing the calcium chelator BAPTA, a reversal of the deterioration in the membrane potential was observed as the calcium chelator was allowed to diffuse into the interneuron, thus demonstrating the critical role for calcium-binding proteins (30). It is possible that a contributing factor to medical intractability in some patients is an abnormally low concentration or defective function in one or more of these calcium-binding proteins, resulting in a premature loss of interneurons, which would alter inhibitory tone in the local neuronal network in favor of net excitation. Valproate, lamotrigine, levetiracetam, topiramate, and zonisamide are modulators of various voltage-gated calcium channels and thus exert some influence on intracellular calcium concentrations.

Defective Intrinsic Membrane Properties of Principal Neurons

The h-current (I_h) is a slowly activating inward cationic current that plays a major role in shaping the intrinsic membrane properties of neurons. This depolarizing current is activated by membrane hyperpolarization, has a time course of activation in the range of several hundred milliseconds, does not inactivate, and is carried primarily by sodium and potassium ions. In hippocampal CA1 pyramidal neurons, these channels are mainly localized to the proximal dendrites. Although I_h slightly depolarizes the neuronal membrane potential, it also decreases the membrane resistance, and thus prevents further depolarization from summation of EPSPs.

Changes in the hippocampal expression of genes that encode I_h channels (dubbed HCNs for hyperpolarization-activated, cyclic nucleotide-gated channels) have been observed following hyperthermia-induced seizures in immature (P10) rats, particularly in neurons within the CA1 pyramidal cell layer (31). These neurons in the immature hippocampus normally express multiple HCN isoforms, and hyperthermia-induced seizures resulted in a decrease in HCN1 mRNA with a concomitant increase in HCN2 mRNA expression (31). Concurrent with these changes, the I_h in CA1 pyramidal neurons was observed to exhibit a rightward shift in the voltage dependence of activation such that the current is increased at membrane potentials near rest (32). The functional consequences of this shift in CA1 pyramidal neurons are complex, but increased I_h activation by bursts of IPSPs was observed to increase the likelihood of a rebound action potential upon depolarization, thus translating what would appear to be enhanced inhibitory activity into a mechanism of hyperexcitability (32) and, possibly, epileptogenesis.

Recently, lamotrigine (33) and gabapentin (34) have been shown to increase the amplitude of I_h in hippocampal CA1 pyramidal neurons and, in so doing, *decrease* intrinsic and synaptic excitability. Although at first glance these results might appear to contradict the observations of Chen et al. (32), the net effect of pathological I_h modulation will ultimately depend on its complex interactions with other variables (e.g., enhanced synaptic inhibition) that may be additionally altered by recurrent seizures and epileptogenesis. Nonetheless, pathophysiological alterations of the biophysical properties of I_h channels might contribute to predisposing the brain to recurrent seizures under certain conditions, and these might be amenable to further pharmacological manipulation.

MECHANISMS LEADING TO INCREASED EXCITATION

The excitatory postsynaptic potentials (EPSPs) constitute the main form of communication between neurons, and they are produced by the release of the excitatory amino acid glutamate from presynaptic terminals. The postsynaptic effects of glutamate are mediated through three ionotropic glutamate receptor subtypes—NMDA, AMPA, and kainate—and several metabotropic glutamate receptors, which are coupled via different mechanisms to ion channels yielding depolarizing currents. The AMPA and kainate receptors mediate fast glutamatergic neurotransmission while the activation of the NMDA receptor results in a slower depolarization (Fig. 5). The excitatory effect of glutamatergic neurotransmission is

Glutamate response

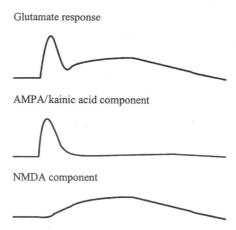

AMPA/kainic acid component

NMDA component

Figure 5. The excitatory postsynaptic potential (EPSP) induced by glutamate: glutamate response; AMPA/kainic acid component; and NMDA component.

tempered by the inhibitory postsynaptic potentials (IPSPs), and it is enhanced by the activation of depolarizing voltage-gated sodium and calcium channels.

Defective Ion Channel Modulation

Voltage-gated sodium channels exist in one of three functional states: open, closed, and inactivated. The study of the transitions between these functional states is known as channel kinetics. The open configuration allows the passage of sodium ions, creating an electrical current that is the major determinant for membrane depolarization. Once some sodium ions cross the pore of the channel, the channel becomes inactivated for a period of time, the so-called absolute refractory period; the channel is unable to open again during this period. After some period of time, the channel is no longer inactivated (it becomes "de-inactivated") and joins the pool of channels that is available to open again upon depolarization (i.e., the closed state). It is possible that genetic differences may contribute to slightly faster or longer channel kinetics. Clinically, a prolongation of the inactivated state is considered to be the primary mechanism of action for phenytoin and carbamazepine, and a major mechanism that contributes to the pharmacological action of other drugs such as lamotrigine and topiramate. Of interest is that the effect of topiramate in spontaneously bursting neurons occurs only in about one-third of the cortical neurons, but its effect persists beyond the washout of the drug from the experimental preparation suggesting a mechanism mediated by receptor phosphorylation (22).

Another important consequence of sodium and calcium channel blockers is that they diminish the extent of depolarization in the excitatory presynaptic terminal and thus decrease the synaptic release of glutamate. However, they can also attenuate the activation of inhibitory neurotransmitters and neuromodulators. It is presumed that lamotrigine decreases the release of glutamate by blocking presynaptic release of glutamate. This pharmacological property is not unique to lamotrigine, as other drugs (such as phenytoin, carbamazepine, and topiramate) can do the same thing.

Increased Activation of Glutamate Receptors

Glutamate is the major excitatory neurotransmitter in the mammalian brain. Fast neurotransmission is achieved through faster biophysical activation of AMPA and kainate receptors, whereas slow excitation is mediated through NMDA receptors. In contrast, the metabotropic glutamate receptors alter cellular excitability via second messenger systems with delayed onset but prolonged duration. The major functional difference between the fast receptor types is that AMPA and kainate receptor channels, for the most part, allow passage of monovalent cations (i.e., sodium and potassium) whereas NMDA receptor channels additionally allow passage of some divalent cations (i.e., calcium). Calcium is a catalyst for many intracellular reactions that lead to changes in phosphorylation and gene expression. Thus, it is in itself a second messenger. The activation of NMDA receptors is increased in several animal models of epilepsy such as kindling, and kainic acid- or pilocarpine-induced status epilepticus (35). It is possible that some patients with epilepsy may have an inherited predisposition for faster or longer-lasting activation of glutamate receptors resulting in an alteration of seizure threshold.

The glutamate receptors are composed of multiple subunits, with different biophysical properties. The differential expression of some of those subunits might increase the relative frequency of some combinations that are more likely to promote hyperexcitability. For example, AMPA receptors that lack a GluR2 subunit are highly permeable to calcium, and the absence of this critical subunit may underlie an important pathophysiological alteration in hippocampal pyramidal neurons that normally express GluR2-containing, and hence calcium-impermeable, AMPA receptors. In support of this, decreased GluR2 expression by hippocampal CA1 pyramidal neurons has been observed following seizures induced by global hypoxia (36) and following kainate-induced status epilepticus (37), raising this as a possible mechanism of epileptogenic plasticity or neurodegeneration. Further, transient knockdown of hippocampal GluR2 expression was observed to induce both spontaneous seizures and hippocampal cell loss (38).

Other possible alterations leading to persistent hyperexcitability might include differences in phosphorylation states or in the physical location of those receptors within the dendritic and somatic structure. Glutamate-activated channels located in dendritic spines with a long spine neck have a lesser contribution in excitability than a similar ionophore located near the main dendritic shaft or the cell soma. Furthermore, the functional ability of subcellular structures might impact the ability to buffer calcium ions in some locations, whereas in others locations they might activate signal transduction pathways more effectively. Although these latter mechanisms remain speculative, there are theoretical reasons to suggest that they may play a significant role in cellular hyperexcitability and neuronal vulnerability to seizure genesis.

Increased Synchrony Between Neurons
Due to Ephaptic Interactions

The electrical fields created by synchronous activation of pyramidal neurons in laminar structures such as the hippocampus may further increase the excitability of neighboring neurons through nonsynaptic interactions, otherwise known as *ephaptic* interactions. Other possible nonsynaptic interactions include electrotonic coupling through gap junctions or changes in extracellular ionic concentrations of potassium and calcium. No clinical studies are available, but theoretically it could be suggested that the acute use of hyperosmolar substances such as mannitol, or diuretics such as furosemide, would have a significant impact in nonsynaptic interactions. It is unclear whether some of the anticonvulsant effects of acetazolamide, topiramate, and zonisamide are mediated by alterations in nonsynaptic interactions related to their inhibition of carbonic anhydrase activity.

Increased Synchrony and/or Activation Due to Recurrent Excitatory Collaterals

Neuropathologic studies of patients with intractable partial-onset epilepsy have revealed characteristic abnormalities within limbic structures, particularly within the hippocampal formation. A common lesion is hippocampal sclerosis, which consists of a pattern of gliosis and neuronal loss primarily in the hilar polymorphic region and CA1 pyramidal region with relative sparing of the CA2 pyramidal region, and an intermediate lesion in the CA3 pyramidal region and dentate granule cells. Prominent hippocampal sclerosis is found in about two-thirds of patients with intractable temporal lobe epilepsy. Experimentally, animal models of status epilepticus are able to replicate this pattern of injury. Even brief repetitive seizures such as those induced by kindling can yield a similar pattern (27). A more subtle and apparently more prevalent neuropathological feature of intractable temporal lobe epilepsy is the presence of mossy fiber sprouting (39). The mossy fibers are the axons of the dentate granule cells and typically project into the hilar polymorphic region and the CA3 pyramidal neurons (see Fig. 5). As neurons in the hilar polymorphic region are lost, their feedback projection into the dentate granule cells also degenerates. The denervation by the loss of the hilar projection induces sprouting of the neighboring mossy fiber axons. Sprouting of recurrent excitatory synapses is a putative mechanism explaining, at least in part, the cellular hyperexcitability of dentate granule cells observed in intractable partial-onset epilepsy.

Computer modeling of this abnormally connected circuitry demonstrate that even small increases (from 1% to 5%) in the number of recurrent excitatory collaterals in the dentate gyrus due to sprouted mossy fibers are sufficient to cause persistent cellular hyperexcitability (40). The net consequence of this phenomenon is the formation of recurrent excitatory loops that recruit additional dentate granule neurons for the generation of epileptiform discharges. In one sense, the sprouted circuitry becomes a dysfunctional amplifier, and its surgical removal may eliminate the recurrent seizures but perhaps not the true generator. This concept suggests that most patients with intractable temporal lobe epilepsy treated with an anterior temporal lobectomy should remain on at least low doses of one anticonvulsant, but preferably an antiepileptogenic drug should one become available, or if evidence emerges that a currently available anticonvulsant possesses antiepileptogenic activity.

The mechanisms discussed above likely operate in combination to cause partial-onset seizures. If the mechanisms leading to increased neuronal excitability become permanent, patients may experience medically refractory partial-onset epilepsy. The current anticonvulsant medications were developed in acute seizure models and are better at blocking the propagation of seizures (i.e., secondarily generalized tonic-clonic seizures) rather than abolishing seizure onset within the epileptic foci (i.e., simple partial seizures). Further understanding into the mechanisms that permanently increase net excitability may lead to the development of antiepileptogenic drugs, which would be designed to alter the natural history of epilepsy.

PATHOPHYSIOLOGY OF PRIMARILY GENERALIZED-ONSET EPILEPSY

The best-understood example of mechanisms of primarily generalized-onset epilepsy is the thalamocortical interactions that underlie typical or classic absence seizures. The thalamocortical circuit subserves normal oscillatory rhythms characterized by alternating periods of relatively increased excitation and periods of relatively increased inhibition. This circuit generates the oscillations seen, for example, in sleep spindles. The circuitry includes the pyramidal neurons of the neocortex, the thalamic relay neurons, and the neurons in the nucleus reticularis of the thalamus (NRT). Pathological alterations in thalamocortical rhythms may result in primarily generalized-onset seizures.

The thalamic relay neurons receive ascending inputs from the spinal cord and project to the neocortical pyramidal neurons. The circuitry responds prominently to regulatory input from cholinergic pathways arising from the forebrain as well as the ascending serotonergic, noradrenergic, and cholinergic pathways originating in the brainstem (41). The thalamic relay neurons are capable of oscillations in their resting membrane potential that result in a higher probability of synchronous activation of the neocortical pyramidal neurons during the period of depolarization, and a significantly lower probability of activating the neocortex during the relative period of hyperpolarization.

A critical substrate necessary for the oscillatory properties of thalamic relay neurons is the presence of a transient low voltage-activated calcium current, also known as T-type calcium current (I_t). In experimental animals, the activity of thalamic relay neurons is controlled by inhibitory GABA-ergic inputs from the NRT. The NRT neurons regulate the activation of I_t channels in thalamic relay neurons because these channels require membrane hyperpolarization to remove steady-state inactivation and allow them to synchronously open for a brief period of time.

I_t channels have three functional states: open, closed, and inactivated. Calcium enters the cells when the channels are open. Immediately after closing, the channel is unable to open again, reaching a state of inactivation. The thalamic relay neurons have $GABA_B$ receptors in their cell soma which receive tonic GABA-ergic activation from the NRT neurons. Once the thalamic relay neuron is hyperpolarized, the inactivation state of the I_t channels is removed, but they remain nonconducting. This is the closed state in which the channel is potentially able to open (i.e., activate) if adequate membrane depolarization occurs. As the membrane hyperpolarizations during oscillations are considerably longer than the depolarizations, essentially all of the channels are in the closed state during hyperpolarization, thus permitting the synchronous opening of a large population to the I_t channels every 100 msec or so.

Several animal models of absence seizures, such as the *lethargic* mouse, demonstrate that $GABA_B$ receptor antagonists suppress absence seizures, while agonists worsen them (42). The traditional anticonvulsants that prevent absence seizures (such as ethosuximide and valproic acid) are thought to act in part by inhibiting T-type calcium currents, although there remains controversy surrounding this concept. These two medications, along with lamotrigine, another antiabsence agent, block rhythmic bursting in thalamic relay neurons (43). Antagonism of the T-type calcium currents can explain this effect in the thalamicocortical network; however, lamotrigine does not block T-type calcium currents, and its mechanism to block rhythmic thalamic bursting remains elusive. However, the recently demonstrated effect of LTG on h-currents on hippocampal neurons might be a potential mechanism, but it remains to be tested in thalamic neurons. Additionally, some anticonvulsants that increase GABA levels, such as gabapentin, tiagabine, and vigabatrin, can be associated with exacerbation of absence seizures under certain conditions. It is possible that increases in GABA allow for a higher degree of synchronization of the thalamocortical circuit and allow a larger pool of I_t channels to be available for activation.

REFERENCES

1. Goldensohn ES, Salazar AM. Temporal and spatial distribution of intracellular potentials during generation and spread of epileptogenic discharges. Adv Neurol 1986; 44:559–582.
2. Hevers W, Luddëns H. The diversity of $GABA_A$ receptors. Mol Neurobiol 1998; 18:35–86.
3. Mehta AK, Ticku MK. An update on $GABA_A$ receptors. Brain Res Rev 1999; 29:196–217.
4. Sieghart W, Fuchs K, Tretter V, Ebert V, Jechlinger M, Hoger H, Adamiker D. Structure and subunit composition of $GABA_A$ receptors. Neurochem Int 1999; 34:379–385.
5. Barnard EA, Skolnick P, Olsen RW, Mohler H, Sieghart W, Biggio G, Braestrup C, Bateson AN, Langer SZ. International Union of Pharmacology. XV. Subtypes of γ-aminobutyric acid$_A$ receptors: classification on the basis of subunit structure and receptor function. Pharmacol Rev 1998; 50:291–313.
6. McKernan RM, Whiting PJ. Which $GABA_A$ receptor subtypes really occur in the brain? Trends Neurosci 1996; 19:139–143.
7. Wieland HA, Luddens H. Four amino acid exchanges convert a diazepam-insensitive, inverse agonist-preferring $GABA_A$ receptor into a diazepam-preferring $GABA_A$ receptor. J Med Chem 1994; 37:4576–4580.
8. Greger V, Knoll JH, Woolf E, Glatt K, Tyndale RF, DeLorey TM, Olsen RW, Tobin AJ, Sikela JM, Nakatsu Y. The gamma-aminobutyric acid receptor gamma 3 subunit gene (GABRG3) is tightly linked to the alpha 5 subunit gene (GABRA5) on human chromosome 15q11-q13 and is transcribed in the same orientation. Genomics 1995; 20: 258–264.
9. Lossie AC, Whitney MM, Amidon D, Dong HJ, Chen P, Theriaque D, Hutson A, Nicholls RD, Zori RT, Williams CA, Driscoll DJ. Distinct phenotypes distinguish the molecular classes of Angelman syndrome. J Med Genet 2001; 38:834–845.
10. Baulac S, Huberfeld G, Gourfinkel-An I, Mitropoulou G, Beranger A, Prud'homme JF, Baulac M, Brice A, Bruzzone R, LeGuern E. First genetic evidence of $GABA_A$ receptor dysfunction in epilepsy: a mutation in the γ2-subunit gene. Nat Genet 2001; 28:46–48.
11. Wallace RH, Marini C, Petrou S, Harkin LA, Bowser DN, Panchal RG, Williams DA, Sutherland GR, Mulley JC, Scheffer IE, Berkovic SF. Mutant $GABA_A$ receptor γ2-subunit in childhood absence epilepsy and febrile seizures. Nat Genet 2001; 28:49–52.

12. Clark M, Massenburg GS, Weiss SRB, Post RM. Analysis of the hippocampal GABA$_A$ receptor system in kindled rats by autoradiographic and in situ hybridization techniques: contingent tolerance to carbamazepine. Mol Brain Res 1994; 26:309–319.

13. Poulter MO, Brown LA, Tynan S, Willick G, William R, McIntyre DC. Differential expression of alpha1, alpha2, alpha3, and alpha5 GABA$_A$ receptor subunits in seizure-prone and seizure-resistant rat models of temporal lobe epilepsy. J Neurosci 1999; 19:4654–4661.

14. Lewin E, Bleck V, Dildy-Mayfield JE, Harris RA. GABA$_A$ and glutamate receptor subunit mRNAs in cortex of mice chemically kindled with FG 7142. Mol Brain Res 1994; 22:320–322.

15. Schwarzer C, Tsunashima K, Wanzenbock C, Fuchs K, Sieghart W, Sperk G. GABA$_A$ receptor subunits in the rat hippocampus. II. Altered distribution in kainic acid-induced temporal lobe epilepsy. Neuroscience 1997; 80:1001–1017.

16. Houser C, Esclapez M. Vulnerability and plasticity of the GABA system in the pilocarpine model of spontaneous recurrent seizures. Epilepsy Res 1996; 26:207–218.

17. Brooks-Kayal AR, Shumate MD, Jin H, Rikhter TY, Coulter DA. Selective changes in single cell GABA$_A$ receptor subunit expression and function in temporal lobe epilepsy. Nat Med 1998; 4:1166–1172.

18. Coulter DA. Epilepsy-associated plasticity in gamma-aminobutryic acid receptor expression, function, and inhibitory synaptic properties. Int Rev Neurobiol 2001; 45:237–252.

19. White HS, Brown SD, Woodhead JH, Skeen GA, Wolf HH. Topiramate enhances GABA-mediated chloride flux and GABA-evoked chloride currents in murine brain neurons and increases seizure threshold. Epilepsy Res 1997; 28:167–179.

20. Shank RP, Gardocki JF, Vaught JL, Davis CB, Schupsky JJ, Raffa RB, Dodgson SJ, Nortey SO, Maryanoff, BE. Topiramate: preclinical evaluation of a structurally novel anticonvulsant. Epilepsia 1994; 35:450–460.

21. Rho JM, Donevan SD, Rogawski MA. Barbiturate-like actions of the propanediol dicarbamates felbamate and meprobamate. J Pharmacol Exp Ther 280:1383–1391, 1997.

22. Shank RP, Gardocki JF, Streeter AJ, Maryanoff BE. An overview of the preclinical aspects of topiramate: pharmacology, pharmacokinetics, and mechanism of action. Epilepsia 2000; 41(suppl 1):S3–S9.

23. Brandon NJ, Jovanovic JN, Moss SJ. Multiple roles of protein kinases in the modulation of γ-aminobutyric acid$_A$ receptor function and cell surface expression. Pharmacol Ther 2002; 94:113–122.

24. Moss SJ, Smart TG, Blackstone CD, Huganir RL. Functional modulation of GABA$_A$ receptors by cAMP-dependent protein phosphorylation. Science 1992; 257:661–665.

25. McDonald BJ, Amato A, Connolly CN, Benke D, Moss SJ, Smart TG. Adjacent phosphorylation sites on GABA$_A$ receptor beta subunits determine regulation by cAMP-dependent protein kinase. Nat Neurosci 1998; 1:23–28.

26. Sloviter RS. Status epilepticus-induced neuronal injury and network reorganization. Epilepsia 1999; 40(suppl 1):S34–S41.

27. Cavazos JE, Das I, Sutula TP. Neuronal loss induced in limbic pathways by kindling: evidence for induction of hippocampal sclerosis by repeated brief seizures. J Neurosci 1994; 14:3106–3121.

28. Sutula TP, Cavazos J, Golarai G. Alteration of long-lasting structural and functional effects of kainic acid in the hippocampus by brief treatment with phenobarbital. J Neurosci 1992; 12:4173–4187.

29. Cavazos J, Kanske J, Perez J, Garcia M. Neuroprotective effects of topiramate in the kainic acid model of status epilepticus. Epilepsia 2002; 43(suppl 7):15.

30. Scharfman H, Schwartzkroin PA. Protection of dentate hilar cells from prolonged stimulation by intracellular calcium chelation. Science 1989; 246:257–260.

31. Brewster A, Bender RA, Chen Y, Dube C, Eghbal-Ahmadi M, Baram TZ. Developmental febrile seizures modulate hippocampal gene expression of hyperpolarization-activated channels in an isoform- and cell-specific manner. J Neurosci 2002; 22:4591–4599.

32. Chen K, Aradi I, Thon N, Eghbal-Ahmadi M, Baram TZ, Soltesz I. Persistently modified h-channels after complex febrile seizures convert the seizure-induced enhancement of inhibition to hyperexcitability. Nat Med 2001; 7:331–337.

33. Poolos NP, Migliore M, Johnston D. Pharmacological upregulation of h-channels reduces the excitability of pyramidal neuron dendrites. Nat Neurosci 2002; 5:767–774.

34. Surges R, Freiman TM, Feuerstein TJ. Gabapentin increases the hyperpolarization-activated cation current Ih in rat CA1 pyramidal cells. Epilepsia 2003; 44:150–156.

35. Holmes GL. Seizure-induced neuronal injury: animal data. Neurology 2002; 59(suppl 5):S3–S6.

36. Sanchez RM, Koh S, Rio C, Wang C, Lamperti ED, Sharma D, Corfas C, Jensen FE. Decreased glutamate receptor 2 expression and enhanced epileptogenesis in immature rat hippocampus after perinatal hypoxia-induced seizures. J Neurosci 2001; 21:8154–8163.

37. Friedman LK, Pellegrini-Giampietro DE, Sperber EF, Bennett MVL, Moshe SL, Zukin RS. Kainate-induced status epilepticus alters glutamate and GABA$_A$ receptor gene expression in adult rat hippocampus: an in situ hybridization study. J Neurosci 1994; 14:2697–2707.

38. Friedman LK, Koudinov AR. Unilateral GluR2(B) hippocampal knockdown: a novel partial seizure model in the developing rat. J Neurosci 1999; 19:9412–9425.

39. Sutula TP, He XX, Cavazos J, Scott G. Synaptic reorganization in the hippocampus induced by abnormal functional activity. Science 1988; 239:1147–1150.

40. Lytton WW, Hellman KM, Sutula TP. Computer models of hippocampal circuit changes of the kindling model of epilepsy. Artif Intell Med 1998; 13:81–97.

41. McCormick DA. Cortical and subcortical generators of normal and abnormal rhythmicity. Int Rev Neurobiol 2002; 49:99–114.

42. Hosford DA, Clark S, Cao Z, Wilson WA Jr, Lin FH, Morrisett RA, Huin A. The role of GABAB receptor activation in absence seizures of lethargic (lh/lh) mice. Science 1992; 257:398–401.

43. Gibbs JW 3rd, Zhang YF, Ahmed HS, Coulter DA. Anticonvulsant actions of lamotrigine on spontaneous thalamocortical rhythms. Epilepsia 2002; 43:342–349.

44. Ayala et al. Brain Res 1973; 52:1–17.

45. Menks JH, Sankar R. Paroxysmal disorders. In: Menks JH, Sarnat HB, eds. Child Neurology, 6th ed. New York: Lippincott Williams & Wilking, 2002:919–1024.

3
Drug Resistance in Epilepsy and Status Epilepticus

Jaideep Kapur and Edward H. Bertram
University of Virginia
Charlottesville, Virginia, U.S.A.

INTRODUCTION

Resistance to pharmacotherapy is a common occurrence among patients with chronic epilepsy and during prolonged status epilepticus. It is estimated that about one-third of patients with epilepsy will be resistant to pharmacotherapy (1). For patients with the prolonged seizures of status epilepticus, the numbers are more difficult to determine, as resistance is tied to the duration of the seizures as well as the etiology, but about one-third to one-half of patients in status epilepticus will not respond to the first lines of treatment (2,3).

Why do some patients respond, while others fail at all attempts to control the seizures? It is a question that has plagued patients and their physicians since the first effective therapies appeared in the latter part of the 19th century. In this chapter, we will discuss what is meant by resistance and what the underlying mechanisms might be. Because the mechanisms behind resistance are likely different in chronic epilepsy and in status epilepticus, we will discuss the two conditions separately. However, it is also likely that there is at least some overlap in the causes of pharmacoresistance in these two conditions, so one should keep in mind that the mechanisms discussed in the chronic epilepsy section could apply to status epilepticus, and similarly the mechanisms for resistance in status epilepticus could contribute to resistance in epilepsy. One should also keep in mind that many of the mechanisms discussed are hypothetically valid, but most, especially in chronic epilepsy, have not been proven as contributing to therapy resistance. In the following sections, we will define resistance and some broad possible causes for the condition, and then we will discuss what is known for each of these possible causes.

RESISTANCE AND ITS CAUSES

Although physicians treating patients with seizures and epilepsy have a general concept of what drug resistance is, it is our common experience that there are many gradations of this condition and, likely, different factors that contribute to resistance. The simplest definition for resistance could be "failure of the drug to control seizures completely." This definition implies resistance to a single compound, which does occur, but a common experience is that a patient who is resistant to a single compound is resistant to multiple drugs. Although the mechanisms underlying resistance to a single compound and multiple-drug resistance may be similar, we will focus on multidrug resistance, as single-drug resistance is not a significant clinical problem over the long term.

Under the definition of resistance there are several additional concepts that need further evaluation, as there are subcategories of this condition that are worth considering. The first is *complete drug resistance*. Under this category are the patients that do not respond in any way to any pharmacological therapy. Their seizure frequencies, clinical severity, and duration are unaffected by the available drugs. This condition, despite the lack of good epidemiological studies to ascertain the actual incidence, is probably quite rare. The second and likely more common category of resistance is *partial drug resistance*, which implies that some feature(s) of the condition respond to therapy but not completely. Under this category there are several additional divisions. The first is *frequency reduction*, which can be defined as treatment that prevents some but not all seizures. The second is *severity reduction*. In this situation, the seizures have the same frequency, but the duration or the clinical severity is less than in the untreated state. A common example would be the patient with secondarily generalized seizures that are reduced to partial complex or partial simple seizures. Another category of pharmacoresistance is *intolerable side effects*. In this situation the patient has seizures that were or would be suppressed, but side effects resulted in the reduction of the dose into a subtherapeutic range, or the complete removal of the only therapy that controlled the seizures.

Finally, resistance may result from drug *tolerance*. After a variable period of exposure to a particular drug, the brain gradually alters the receptors or channels in a way that makes that drug less effective. With the exception of the benzodiazepines, for which tolerance is a well-described phenomenon, the role of tolerance in therapy resistance is unclear. Patients have experienced "honeymoon" periods during which they will respond to a new drug well, only for resistance to appear later. After the seizures recur, the patients typically fall into one of the categories above. How resistance might develop after a period of successful treatment for most of the antiepileptic drugs is a matter of speculation, as is the issue of how many patients actually have this pattern of transient response. The mechanisms for these different types of treatment failure are probably quite different, and we will speculate about these possible causes in subsequent sections.

One form of clinical resistance that we will not discuss is the resistance that results from the use of the wrong medicine. It is a common experience that patients with some form of generalized epilepsy are initially prescribed a medication that is better suited for focal seizure disorders. Their seizures are readily controlled when the appropriate medication is prescribed. Although these patients may be considered therapy resistant, the underlying problem is one of correct diagnosis and treatment.

Why are patients resistant to therapy, specifically to multiple drugs? At the moment we have no good answers, especially for patients with chronic epilepsy. In status epilepticus, there is more known about how alterations in receptor function may alter the responsiveness of the condition to specific treatments, but the same is not true for chronic epilepsy. Possible mechanisms for resistance in epilepsy can be broadly divided into four categories: (1) wrong molecular target (i.e., channel or receptor); (2) exclusion of therapeutic concentrations from the brain; (3) maldistribution of the drug within the brain so that it does not reach its targets; and (4) induced tolerance so that a specific compound has reduced efficacy. There is some overlap in the middle two in concept and mechanism, but they are sufficiently different to warrant separate discussion. In the following sections, we will discuss the possible basis for each of these mechanisms, the evidence that exists at the moment, and at the end of this chapter, possible research directions that will allow for a better understanding of drug resistance and ways that we might overcome it.

ACHIEVING A BALANCE

One concept we will emphasize is the balance between side effects and therapeutic efficacy, not so much from the mechanisms of side effects, but rather from what this relationship might tell us about some of the sources of resistance. This relationship is well known to any physician treating patients with epilepsy: toxic side effects such as dizziness, sedation, or double vision appear before the seizures are controlled. This common difficulty in the therapy of epilepsy should be expected because we treat with drugs that are designed to affect the central nervous system but which, we hope, will affect seizures before they have a significant effect on normal function. For the majority of patients successfully treated with the current antiepileptic compounds, this relationship is true. For the remaining third, the relationship is reversed. The reasons are unclear, but the hypothetical causes can give us some directions for investigating the mechanisms that underlie therapeutic resistance in general. The basis for the breakdown in the therapeutic/toxic balance could lie in several areas: (1) in the nature of the blood–brain barrier and selective permeability; (2) in the regional affinity of receptor and channel subtypes for a particular drug; (3) the relative potency of the compound at the different receptor and channel subtypes; and (4) the possible regional variation in the sequestration of a compound that prevents achieving therapeutic levels at the target, whereas toxic levels are achieved at other regions at the same time. Resolving this issue will depend, as we will discuss later, on a better understanding of the function of the blood–brain barrier and the pharmacology of the relevant channels. Some of these problems in brain pharmacokinetics and dynamics may be altered further in the epileptic condition, which is associated with many structural abnormalities.

RECEPTORS, CHANNELS, AND RESISTANCE

One of the problems in understanding why drugs are not completely effective is that we do not have a good understanding of how they work to prevent seizures. Although many possible mechanisms are ascribed to them, most commonly the blockade of voltage-gated sodium channels and the enhancement of GABA-ergic function (pre- or postsynaptically) have been associated with the compounds used to treat epilepsy. Other purported mechanisms include the inhibition of the low-threshold T-type calcium currents (for antiabsence therapy) and the diminished release of excitatory neurotransmitters (4). For a few drugs, a mechanism of action has not been determined. All of these mechanisms could represent important means for suppressing seizure activity, but it is also possible that the real basis for AED efficacy is completely unrelated to any of these demonstrated mechanisms. There are many other mechanisms involving neuromodulatory systems that could be targets for therapy.

Part of the difficulty in determining the site of action for these compounds is that the true mechanisms underlying epilepsy, especially the mechanisms underlying the initiation of a seizure, are unknown. However, there have been a number of studies using animal models of epilepsy that have shown changes in the physiology and pharmacology of specific channels and receptors. These observations are important for several reasons that concern pharmacotherapy. First, the studies clearly indicate that there is more than one change in the brain that can predispose to hyperexcitability. Second, the pharmacology of these altered receptors and channels is likely to be or has already been shown to be quite different from the native state. These changes could have significant implications for the relative efficacy and potency of the current group of antiepileptic drugs, most of which were developed on normal nervous systems using acute seizure models. Finally, the changes are not uniform throughout the presumed seizure circuit, which raises the possibility that the antiepileptic drugs will have differing potency at different points in the circuit, depending on which channel or receptor is expressed.

The changes that occur in the seizure circuit have been described best in limbic epilepsy (also known as mesial temporal lobe epilepsy) for which there are a number of animal models. Most of the work has focused on the hippocampus, and changes have been described in the GABA receptor, the NMDA receptor, the AMPA receptor, and the sodium and calcium channels. The GABA-ergic system in the hippocampus has been studied most extensively, and within this region alone there are a number of changes that have occurred in the subunit composition, as has been determined by anatomical, physiological, and pharmacological, studies. Although we will not describe the changes in detail, there are several key findings across the studies. First, as determined by mRNA expression and immunocytochemical staining methods, there are significant changes in the subunit composition of the GABA receptor (5–8). Second, the GABA-induced inhibitory potentials are altered, with many having significantly reduced duration, resulting in epileptiform-evoked responses (9–11). Third, the response of the GABA currents to a variety of neuromodulators is significantly altered, so that compounds that are quite effective in neurons from normal animals have greatly reduced potency in neurons from epileptic animals (9–13). Finally, the changes are not uniform throughout the hippocampus, which complicates the development of pharmacotherapy that is selective and effective for the epileptic condition (14). There are some preliminary reports that changes in GABA-induced responses are also found in other limbic sites involved in seizures such as the amygdala (15). Whether changes also occur in the entorhinal cortex or other limbic sites is less clear.

There is growing evidence for changes in voltage-gated sodium channels in limbic epilepsy. In one study, increased expression of type II and III alpha isoforms of the sodium channel were found in the dentate gyrus and CA1 pyramidal cells following an episode of experimental status epilepticus in rats. This change persisted after the animals developed spontaneous seizures (16). A follow-up study examining the sodium currents in these neurons demonstrated a significant change associated with chronic epilepsy with lower thresholds for activation and an increase in the

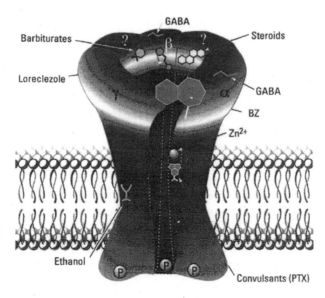

Figure 1. Schematic representation of the GABA-A receptor. The GABA-A receptor is a heteropentameric, ligand-gated ion channel that is selectively permeable to chloride ions. The precise subunit composition of native GABA-A receptors has yet to be identified, it is thought that most functional GABA-A receptors contain either α and β, or α, β, and γ subunits with uncertain stoichiometry. Binding sites for the endogenous ligand GABA and receptor modulators are assigned to their respective subunits (or, in the case of the benzodiazepine binding site, the juxtaposition of an α and β subunit). (From Ref. 74.)

overall sodium currents (17). These changes were region specific, as has been seen with the GABA receptor, with clear changes in CA1 but no such changes in the dentate granule cells. Sodium channel mutations have also been described in several of the familial epilepsy syndromes (18–21). At least one of these mutations has been created in a transgenic mouse, and these animals have had documented spontaneous seizures (22). Reconstitution of these mutated channels in heterologous expression systems has shown that the resultant sodium currents are greater than wild-type controls, with slowed inactivation. Although these findings are important in our quest to understand the pathophysiology of epilepsy, they may also be important in our attempts to determine the basis for drug resistance. Because many of the drugs that we use to treat epilepsy are sodium channel blockers, there is a real possibility that the drugs that have been developed in normal animals may not be so effective in the mutated channels. It is also possible that the current drugs will also work at the altered channels, but at a lower potency, so that these drugs have a much greater effect at the normal channels, a situation in which toxicity may appear before seizure efficacy. In the future, it will be important to identify the changes that are associated with and are possibly contributory to the epileptic condition. With this information in hand, we will be able to design compounds that are specific to the channels so that the seizures can be prevented and the toxicity avoided.

Changes have also been described for the glutamate receptor family, specifically AMPA and NMDA receptors, either by anatomic demonstration of altered subunit expression or physiologically by showing that prolonged depolarizations can be significantly reduced through channel blockade (8,23,24). At this time, little is known about the biophysical regulation of these receptors. Although some attempts have been made to use the glycine modulatory site on the NMDA receptor as a target for seizure control, in general, attempts to affect seizures through direct inhibition of these receptors have been plagued by significant psychomimetic side effects that have limited the potential clinical usefulness of this approach. Until more selective approaches to modulation of excitatory neurotransmission are developed, this path to treatment may not be as fruitful as others, but it may be possible, as with sodium channels and GABA receptors, to identify the specific changes associated with epilepsy such that those changes can be targeted pharmacologically, with the ultimate goal of defining therapy that is specific to the epileptogenic receptors and regions, while leaving the uninvolved and unchanged regions unaffected. With this approach we may be able to avoid resistance that results from neurotoxicity appearing before clinical efficacy.

MULTIPLE DRUG-RESISTANT PROTEINS

Until recently, multiple drug-resistant (MDR) proteins were largely an issue of concern to cancer research. However, there are increasing reports that these proteins are somehow connected to intractable and drug-resistant epilepsy. These observations, together with work done in animal models, have raised the question about the potential role of these proteins in epilepsy drug resistance. At present, there are no clear answers, but, because of the potential relevance for chronic intractable epilepsy, it is an area that demands further exploration. In the following paragraphs, we will explore what these proteins are, where they are located, how they might function in the development of drug resistance, and whether they really have the potential to limit the efficacy of drugs. It is far beyond the scope of this chapter to explore MDR proteins in any depth. For the interested reader, there are several recent reviews on the subject that greatly expand on the points raised here (25–27).

What are MDR proteins? The evolution of our understanding of these proteins began with the initial observations of proteins that were capable of transporting compounds across membranes against their concentration gradients. This function required energy in the form of ATP, and, with time, this class of proteins became known as the ABC (ATP-binding cassette) family of membrane transporters. The first one described in association with drug resistance, and the one of possibly greatest relevance for epilepsy, was P-glycoprotein (P-gp), which is also known as multidrug-resistant protein, or MDR1. More recently a series of additional proteins have also been identified in various normal and neoplastic tissues. The largest group is the multidrug resistance-associated proteins (MRP1-7) and mitoxantrone resistance protein (MXR) (there are other nomenclature systems that are used, but these appear to be most commonly employed) (25). Each of these proteins has specific substrates, activators, and inhibitors, and there are cell lines and tissue types that each is most commonly associated with. MDR1 is the protein that is most commonly associated with the brain, and one that has been associated with tissue taken from patients with intractable epilepsy, with increased expression in neurons and astrocytes. In normal brain, MDR1 is typically seen at the level of the capillary epithelium, which comprises in part the blood–brain barrier, which restricts compounds to the extracellular space (25,28–30). MRP1, although not normally expressed in brain, has been found in the neurons and astrocytes of dysplastic tissue. It is quite likely that there are other, yet undiscovered or known proteins that may play roles in this process as well.

There has been a steady evaluation of those compounds that may be subject to transport and those compounds that are not. Within the family of these proteins, multiple compounds, endogenous and exogenous, are transported, but the proteins are selective in what each will transport (25–27). Although there is some overlap in substrate compounds, some substances can only be transported by a specific protein, a situation in which some cells may be resistant to the effects of a particular drug, and others may not because they lack the protein that is specific for that drug. This selectiveness is of some importance in epilepsy because not all antiepileptic drugs are substrates for MDR1. Phenytoin has been well described as one compound that is a substrate for MDR1 (31–33). There are conflicting reports about carbamazepine, and there is no information about the other antiepileptic drugs (34,35). Inhibitors of these transporter proteins have been shown to cause an increase in the concentrations of phenytoin and carbamazepine in the brain (31,35), but it is not known whether the increase was the specific result of inhibition of these proteins, nor is it known if such increases would be of therapeutic benefit.

The importance of being a substrate for transport by one of these proteins varies for several reasons that depend, in part, on where the drug has its primary site of action. Because the proteins predominantly pump the compounds from the intracellular to the extracellular space, they will have the greatest effect if the compounds work at intracellular sites, which is clearly relevant for many of the cancer drugs but is less certain for the antiepileptic drugs. Similarly, if a compound does not readily diffuse into a cell, the proteins will have less of an effect. If, on the other hand, the drug rapidly diffuses into a cell, its inward diffusion rate may far exceed the maximum rate that can be achieved through active transport through the protein. The calcium channel blocker verapamil is a good example of the difficulties associated in determining the net effect. Verapamil is a known blocker of MDR1. However, it is a very potent activator of ATPase, a feature that is essential for transport to occur. Finally, this compound is a fast diffuser, so that it returns to the interior of the cell as fast as it is pumped out, with the overall result that there is no net flux (25).

However, verapamil, when given with other compounds that are potential substrates for MDR1, is associated with increased intracellular accumulations of the other compounds (25). In the brain, the issue is further complicated by the role of the blood–brain barrier in allowing access to the brain extracellular space. The role that the drug resistant proteins play in this activity is unknown. There are several reports that inhibition of these proteins with verapamil and several other compounds results in an increase in the amount of recoverable phenytoin as measured by microdialysis (31,35). Whether this observation is the result of inhibition of the protein and improved diffusion of phenytoin into the brain or the results are secondary to some other effect (e.g., alterations in protein binding; shift of phenytoin from the intracellular space to the extracellular space) is not known. For the moment, we can only say that there are pharmacological manipulations that may affect the extracellular concentration of antiepileptic drugs in the brain.

There is substantial evidence for increased expression of several of these proteins associated with chronic epilepsy. Examination of tissue taken from patients with epilepsy at the time of therapeutic surgery has revealed a significant upregulation of MDR1 and MRP1 in the brain. MDR1 has been associated with the endothelium of the cerebrovasculature in normal tissue, but in presumed epileptogenic regions from patients with intractable epilepsy, there is significant expression in neurons and reactive astrocytes (28–30). Further, MRP1, which is not normally expressed in the brain, is found in neurons and astrocytes as well (28). To some extent, the degree of expression depends on the nature of the abnormality (e.g., cortical dysplasia, dysembryoplastic neuroepithelioma or hippocampal sclerosis). Similar findings have been reported in several animal models of pharmacoresistant epilepsy, at least one of which has shown a decreased sensitivity to the seizure suppressant effects of phenytoin (32). There are concerns that some of the findings associated with chronic epilepsy may be the result of induction of the protein by the antiepileptic drugs, but there is at least one report suggesting that the increased expression of these proteins in cortical dysplasias may precede the use of antiepileptic drugs (33).

The primary question remains unanswered: "Does the presence of MDR proteins cause drug resistance in chronic epilepsy?" There are a number of correlations that suggest that they may play a role, but for the moment, causality has not been established. There are a number of issues that must be clarified, including determining which of the antiepileptic drugs are substrates for these proteins. Further, does the presence of these proteins result in lower concentrations of the drugs at the critical sites for drug action? And, finally, can blocking the action of these proteins alter the levels of the drugs in the brain parenchyma and subsequently have a demonstrable effect on seizure control? These are important questions that must be addressed in our quest for a solution to drug resistance.

DRUG MALDISTRIBUTION

Steering a drug to the right target in the CNS is the key to successful therapy, but this has always been complicated by the presence of the blood–brain barrier, which is well known for its ability to exclude a variety of potentially useful compounds. The general assumption has been that once a compound crosses the blood–brain barrier, it is evenly distributed throughout the brain. Is this assumption correct, or is the blood–brain barrier regionally selective, allowing drugs through more effectively in some areas than others? These questions are important because, if there is nonuniform distribution, a potentially effective compound may go to an area outside of the therapeutic target in far greater concentrations. Such a scenario could be responsible for the observation of significant neurological side effects in the absence of clinical efficacy. What is the evidence that such a maldistribution occurs? There are only a few reports concerning this issue, and they have not really been linked to any clinical phenomenon, but the findings are important for their illustrative value.

In a series of experiments that used microdialysis to determine the relative concentrations of antiepileptic drugs in the frontal cortex and the hippocampus, investigators found that some of the drugs were relatively evenly distributed (levetiracetam, lamotrigine) (36,37), whereas others (phenytoin, vigabatrin) (38,39) were not. In the latter group, phenytoin had an increased area under the concentration curve in the hippocampus compared to the frontal lobe, whereas vigabatrin had significantly higher concentrations (as well as concomitant GABA concentrations) in the frontal lobe than in the hippocampus. These findings emphasize the potential for regional variation in the distribution of a drug in the brain, and that this variable distribution may be drug dependent.

Another study examined the distribution of phenytoin in the whole rat brain, with the intent of defining specific phenytoin receptors (40). Radiolabeled phenytoin was given intravenously to rats, and it was also exposed to ex vivo brain slices. This slice-binding study showed a fairly even distribution of binding that was nonspecific throughout the gray matter. However, when given intravenously to active rats, the phenytoin at steady state was found overwhelmingly in the white matter. This study revealed several key points about the distribution of phenytoin in the brain. First, the distribution of a drug in vivo may not be in any way similar to the binding studies that are performed on slices, emphasizing that there are active processes in the living brain that may have a great influence over drug distribution. Second, the drug may have a preferential distribution (in this case white matter) that is presumably quite different from the target (in this case the gray matter, or, better, a specific region in the gray matter such as the hippocampus).

Taken together, the microdialysis studies and the phenytoin distribution study emphasize that the drug concentrations can vary considerably across the brain in a drug-specific manner. Although we have no supportive evidence at this time, there is a very real possibility that resistance is, at least in part, related to a drug's failing to reach the appropriate target. The issue of drug distribution in the epileptic brain is further complicated by the overexpression of multidrug-resistant proteins that may alter the relative distribution of the drug in the central nervous system. Proof of this concept, that the maldistribution of a drug contributes to pharmacoresistance, is much further away, because one must first define the regional localization of a drug, determine the existence of drug resistance, and then show that the resistance is significantly ameliorated by providing the drug greater access to the epileptogenic sites.

TOLERANCE

Another possible contributor to the refractoriness of seizures is development of tolerance to the anticonvulsant effect of the drugs. While tolerance may develop to many classes of anticonvulsants, it is most consistently observed with benzodiazepines such as clonazepam, diazepam, and nitrazepam. Some clinical studies suggest that diazepam loses its antiepileptic effect in as many as 40% of patients, within 4–6 months of initiating treatment. Tolerance to anticonvulsant action of benzodiazepines appears to develop in both partial and generalized epilepsies. The development of tolerance to benzodiazepines is functional and not metabolic since the serum benzodiazepine levels do not decrease during long-term treatment (41).

Tolerance to the anticonvulsant effect of benzodiazepines is not only observed in humans but also in laboratory animals (42,43). Mechanisms of benzodiazepine tolerance have been investigated intensively in experimental animals. Benzodiazepines potentiate fast, γ-aminobutyric acid (GABA)-mediated inhibitory neurotransmission (44) by binding to an allosteric site on GABA-A receptors and increasing their affinity for GABA. A dysfunction of the GABA-A receptor appears to underlie benzodiazepine anticonvulsant tolerance (45). GABA-A receptors are composed of various combinations of five subunit proteins, derived from multiple families with multiple variants. The nature of the GABA-A receptor dysfunction that is central to benzodiazepine tolerance remains uncertain. Several studies suggest that changes in subunit gene expression underlie a fundamental change in GABA-A receptor subunit composition, whereas others indicate that a posttranslational mechanism mediates a change in GABA-A receptor function. For example, changes in specific GABA-A receptor subunit mRNA and protein expression localized to specific regions occur after chronic benzodiazepine treatments that result in anticonvulsant tolerance (46,47). In contrast, other laboratories have demonstrated that exposure to the benzodiazepine antagonist flumazenil can rapidly reverse some of the functional and biochemical changes associated with chronic diazepam treatment (48). These findings suggest that a conformational or other posttranslational change may play a key role in mediating tolerance.

At present, it is uncertain whether tolerance to the effects of other antiepileptic drugs contributes to therapy resistance. The phenomenon of a drug "honeymoon," during which time a patient has a transient benefit from a particular compound after which the seizures return to pretreatment frequency, is a common observation by physicians who treat epilepsy. It is unknown whether this phenomenon represents the development of tolerance, so that the drug induces another mechanism (such as a drug-resistant protein) that reduces its efficacy, or a progression of the underlying disorder. Further, wihle the honeymoon phenomenon is well accepted, it is unclear how many patients actually experience this. Perhaps only after a full examination of the true nature of pharmacoresistance in epilepsy can a greater understanding of the drug honeymoon be achieved. Although human epidemiological studies are necessary, the use of realistic animal models may also better define the nature and patterns of drug resistance.

DRUG RESISTANCE IN STATUS EPILEPTICUS

Prolonged, self-sustaining seizures are commonly referred to as status epilepticus. Status epilepticus is often refractory to currently used first- and second-line agents in humans and experimental animals. Studies on experimental animals provide many insights into the mechanisms of refractoriness, and suggest novel treatments for refractory status epilepticus.

There are at least 126,000–195,000 episodes of status epilepticus associated with 22,000–42,000 deaths each year in the United States (49). Results of two prospective, randomized double-blind clinical trails suggest that as many as 35–50% of patients with generalized convulsive status epilepticus are refractory to benzodiazepines, the first-line agents for treatment of status epilepticus (2,3). When benzodiazepines fail to control status epilepticus, it is commonly treated with one of the second-line agents: phenytoin, fosphenytoin, or phenobarbital. Additionally, data from the Veterans Administration cooperative study suggest that only a small fraction of patients refractory to the first agent are likely to respond to a second.

In addition to convulsive status epilepticus, there exists a subtle or non-convulsive form of status epilepticus. These patients are comatose and have subtle facial or eye movements and ictal discharges on EEG. The Veterans Administration cooperative study and others suggest that 80–90% of the patients with subtle status epilepticus are refractory to first- and second-line agents. A retrospective analysis of patients in convulsive and subtle status epilepticus in a large academic hospital found that 31% of seizures were refractory to a combination of a benzodiazepine and a second-line agent—phenytoin, fosphenytoin, or phenobarbital (50). If the rate of refractory status epilepticus is conservatively estimated at 30% of all episodes, then there are 38,000–54,500 episodes of refractory status epilepticus in the United States each year.

CLINICAL FACTORS THAT CONTRIBUTE TO THERAPY RESISTANCE IN STATUS EPILEPTICUS

Refractoriness of status epilepticus may relate to the underlying cause. There has been no systematic study of the relationship of the cause of status epilepticus and the responsiveness to treatment. However, causes of status epilepticus that do respond to first-line treatment can be compared with the causes in patients who require more aggressive therapy such as continuous intravenous infusion with propofol, midazolam, or pentobarbital for refractory status epilepticus. Anticonvulsant withdrawal, remote neurological insult, and stroke are common causes of status epilepticus overall (49). In contrast, the most common conditions associated with refractory status epilepticus include encephalitis, toxic metabolic encephalopathy, and intracerebral hemorrhage (51).

It is a common clinical observation that status epilepticus appears to become refractory the longer it lasts. Studies have shown that the likelihood of a patient responding to first-line therapy declines as the time between the onset of seizures and treatment initiation increases (52). In the Veterans Administration cooperative study, patients in subtle status epilepticus were enrolled 5.2 h after onset and were refractory to treatment, while patients in overt status epilepticus were enrolled 2.8 h after onset and responded more often to therapy. It is uncertain whether the delay in treatment or the underlying cause in patients with subtle seizures contributed to the difficulties in seizure control. For the moment, however, the relationships among underlying cause, patient's condition, the duration of status epilepticus, and the ability to control the seizure activity remain unclear. Some of these issues will be explored in the discussion of animal studies.

Pharmacological Basis of Treatment and Refractoriness

To understand the mechanism of drug refractoriness in status epilepticus, it is important to recognize that current treatment of status epilepticus largely focuses on a single mechanism—enhancement of GABA-mediated inhibition. Benzodiazepines, lorazepam, and diazepam are commonly used first-line agents for the treatment of status epilepticus. The therapeutic doses of these agents enhance GABA-A receptor-mediated inhibition (53). Barbiturates used to treat status epilepticus, phenobarbital, and pentobarbital, and other agents like propofol, primarily exert their effects by enhancing GABA-A receptor-mediated inhibition (44) as well. Only two agents used regularly to treat status epilepticus, phenytoin, and fosphenytoin, have a distinct mechanism of action on the sodium channel (4). Clearly, the current treatment of status epilepticus strongly emphasizes enhancement of GABA-A receptor-mediated inhibition.

Mechanisms of Refractory Status Epilepticus: Animal Models

It is not possible to study the mechanisms of refractory status epilepticus in humans. However, key features of status epilepticus can be replicated in experimental models. The salient features of animal models of status epilepticus have been discussed in detail in other reviews (54,55). Walton and Treiman first demonstrated drug refractoriness in an experimental model of status epilepticus (56). In lithium-pilocarpine-induced status epilepticus, the pattern of electrographic seizures changes progressively over time. Initially, EEG recordings show discrete electrographic seizures, followed by waxing and waning seizures. Later, electrographic seizures become continuous. Discrete seizures occurred in the first 5 min of status epilepticus; 10 and 20 min after the onset, waxing and waning seizures were present; continuous seizures were present in all rats 45 min after onset. Rats in each of the three groups were treated with diazepam. Diazepam stopped all seizures in all rats that showed discrete seizure patterns on EEG. In contrast, seizures were controlled in only 17% of rats that showed a continuous seizure pattern on EEG. This study clearly demonstrated that status epilepticus becomes rapidly refractory to benzodiazepines. Several groups have confirmed the findings of this study in lithium-pilocarpine and other models. One study demonstrated that, with passage of time, there was a substantial reduction of diazepam potency for termination of the seizures (57). However, time-dependent resistance to anticonvulsants is not restricted to benzodiazepines. In experimental animals the seizures of status epilepticus become progressively resistant to treatment with phenobarbital over a relatively short period of time (58).

In addition to GABA-ergic agents, during the course of status epilepticus, resistance to phenytoin also develops. In an electrical stimulation model of status epilepticus, phenytoin became less effective with the passage of time (59). Phenytoin was effective when administered 10 min after the onset of status epilepticus but not when administered 40 min after the onset of status epilepticus. Clearly, the first-line agents diazepam, phenytoin, and lorazepam are quite effective in terminating early status epilepticus. However, when seizures last 45–60 min, and the EEG pattern shows continuous ictal discharge, first- and second-line agents both fail.

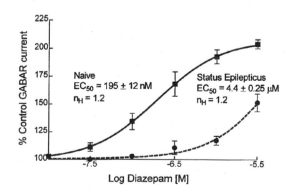

Figure 2. Diazepam concentration-response curves for isolated dentate granule cells taken from control animals (solid line) and from animals undergoing status epilepticus (dashed line). Compared to naive controls, GABA-A receptor currents from rats undergoing status epilepticus were less sensitive to diazepam. (From Ref. 75.)

The cellular and molecular mechanisms of refractory status epilepticus are explored in the following sections. In theory, status epilepticus could become refractory to current treatments, if GABA-mediated inhibition collapses or if seizures are sustained by other mechanisms such as excitatory neurotransmission. There is evidence from studies in experimental models of status epilepticus for both loss of GABA-mediated inhibition, and seizures sustained by excitatory transmission.

THE GABA HYPOTHESIS OF RESISTANT STATUS EPILEPTICUS

The structures involved in the genesis of status epilepticus have been delineated by use of the ^{14}C-2-deoxy-glucose mapping technique combined with EEG recordings in experimental animals. In the late stages of status epilepticus, the hippocampal formation, subiculum, entorhinal cortex, amygdala, pyriform cortex, substantia nigra, and midline thalamic nuclei show increased glucose utilization in a bilateral symmetrical fashion (60,61). Other studies indicate that sustained seizures of status epilepticus can be maintained in a combined entorhinal cortex–hippocampal slice preparation (62). These studies suggest that the hippocampus is an attractive site to study the mechanisms of refractory status epilepticus.

GABA-mediated inhibition in the CA1 region and dentate gyrus of the hippocampus plays a critical role in the pathogenesis of refractoriness of status epilepticus. In many experimental models of status epilepticus, a loss of GABA-ergic inhibition has been documented. Early studies used paired-pulse inhibition technique to study the relationship of GABA-mediated paired-pulse inhibition in the CA1 region of hippocampus and evolution of status epilepticus (63,64). After measurement of GABA-mediated inhibition in the CA1 region, status epilepticus was induced by electrical stimulation of the hippocampus. Those stimulated animals, which developed hippocampal status epilepticus had a loss of paired-pulse inhibition. The remaining animals showed a mild reduction of paired pulse inhibition after stimulation and did not develop self-sustaining status epilepticus. A similar reduction of paired-pulse inhibition was demonstrated in cholinergic models (64). Paired-pulse inhibition in the CA1 region of the hippocampus could be reduced by diminished release of GABA or diminished postsynaptic GABA-A receptor responsiveness. While the release of GABA from neurons during status epilepticus has not been studied, there is growing evidence that responsiveness of GABA-A receptors to GABA is diminished during status epilepticus.

GABA-A receptor function was investigated by measuring chloride currents from CA1 pyramidal neurons acutely isolated from rats experiencing status epilepticus. These experiments demonstrated that during status epilepticus, GABA-A receptor currents were reduced owing to reduction of both conductance and changes in chloride reversal potential. These findings suggested that the GABA-A receptor is modified during an episode of status epilepticus (65), and this modification may contribute to the development of resistance to pharmacotherapy. The finding that the number of GABA-A receptors available for binding GABA is reduced during partial status epilepticus further supported these results (66). GABA-A receptor function during status epilepticus was also studied in dentate granule cells of the hippocampus. Whole-cell GABA-A receptor currents were obtained from hippocampal dentate granule cells isolated acutely from control rats and from rats undergoing status epilepticus. GABA-A receptor properties were characterized by determining GABA sensitivity, and the sensitivity of GABA-A receptors to regulation by benzodiazepines, barbiturates, and Zn^{2+}. When compared to those from naive controls, GABA-A receptor currents from rats undergoing status epilepticus were less sensitive to diazepam and Zn^{2+} but retained their sensitivity to GABA and pentobarbital (57). These findings suggested that the prolonged seizures of status epilepticus rapidly altered the benzodiazepine sensitivity of GABA-A receptor on hippocampal dentate granule cells. More recent studies have shown that the molecular structure of GABA-A receptors expressed by dentate granule cells is altered by status epilepticus (7).

Role of Excitatory Transmission in Status Epilepticus

In addition to loss of inhibition, there is growing evidence that excitatory neurotransmission is enhanced in the self-sustaining phase of status epilepticus. Several recent studies have demonstrated that prolonged status epilepticus—refractory to benzodiazepines and phenobarbital—is effectively controlled by NMDA receptor antagonists (67–69). NMDA receptor antagonists can prevent the neuropathology and delayed development of epilepsy-associated status epilepticus. Finally, neuropeptides such as galanin and substance P can modulate prolonged, refractory status epilepticus. They are known to exert their cellular effects on excitatory transmission.

A growing number of studies demonstrate the effectiveness of NMDA receptor antagonists in the treatment of refractory status epilepticus. In the perforant path stimulation model of status epilepticus, seizures that rapidly become refractory to benzodiazepines were controlled by NMDA receptor antagonists (67). Another study found that the NMDA receptor antagonist ketamine did not control seizures when administered in the early phase of status epilepticus but was effective after prolonged seizures (58,68). Other studies indicate that NMDA receptor antagonist MK-801 prevents development of refractoriness to diazepam in the lithium-pilocarpine model of status epilepticus (69).

Neuropeptides in Status Epilepticus

Neuropeptides have emerged as candidates for termination of refractory status epilepticus. Neuropeptide Y suppresses epileptiform activity in rat hippocampal slices (70) and mice lacking neuropeptide Y have uncontrollable seizures in response to the excitotoxin kainic acid, with 93% progressing to death while death was rare in wild-type littermates. Intracerebroventricular neuropeptide Y prevented kainic acid seizure-induced death (71). Taken together, these studies suggest a critical role for neuropeptide Y in seizure termination.

Galanin is a 29- or 30-amino acid residue neuropeptide present in the septal projections to the hippocampus and has an inhibitory effect on the hippocampus by inhibiting excitatory neurotransmission. Galanin immunoreactivity in the hippocampus is diminished following limbic status epilepticus (72). Injection of galanin into the hippocampal dentate hilus prevents onset of limbic status epilepticus and can stop established limbic status epilepticus (73). It appears that galanin can act as an endogenous anticonvulsant stopping status epilepticus.

In status epilepticus, it is clear that a number of acute changes occur that limit the response to standard therapy. Experimental models can help discover new therapies for some forms of status epilepticus, but they cannot help (for the moment) with some forms that are associated with specific conditions such as encephalitis. For now, the studies emphasize the need to treat early and aggressively so that the patients do not have a chance to develop a refractory condition. It is unclear whether certain causes of status epilepticus are resistant because of the duration of the seizure activity or because of the underlying cause. It is an area that needs more investigation. Perhaps the best approach would be to assure that all patients are treated aggressively if seizures last >5–7 min.

MOVING TOWARD A SOLUTION

How do we get beyond the problem of pharmacotherapy resistance in epilepsy and status epilepticus? The first, obvious answer is to understand the pathophysiology associated with the many causes of the two conditions. Because the basis for these conditions is multifactorial and involves complex neural circuits, and because (in status epilepticus, at least) the pathophysiology is constantly evolving, it is unlikely that we will arrive at that understanding in the near future. For this reason, we have to be much more empiric in our approach, while recognizing the many caveats that may adversely affect a promising drug's performance in vivo. The issues that need to be addressed in this process are what we described above.

Are the compounds that we are testing appropriate for the receptors and channels that we are targeting? The changes in these membrane proteins are well described, with many more yet to be described. It is essential that drugs are designed for the specific channels that play important roles in seizure initiation and evolution, so that the drugs are maximally effective at these channels while simultaneously much less potent at related channels. Solving this problem may also resolve the problem of clinical side effects before clinical efficacy.

Are the drugs reaching the appropriate targets? This issue may be influenced by the drug resistance proteins and the blood–brain barrier, which may, in some cases, have resulted in regional variation in the distribution of the drugs. Compounds should be designed with these issues in mind, so that they actually reach the intended targets, preferably with reduced distribution to other sites.

Do effective drugs lose their efficacy over time? Tolerance is the most difficult issue to identify and to design for, especially in the preclinical phase. The benzodiazepines are known for the rapid development of tolerance, an issue that limits the utility of an otherwise very effective drug. Whether loss of efficacy over time for the other drugs is the result of tolerance is unknown, but there are anecdotes to suggest that this process may occur in some patients. Designing studies to determine whether tolerance develops in the course of treatment is an important step. This information will let us know to avoid certain mechanisms of drug action that may be prone to the induction of tolerance or to develop a method for preventing tolerance.

How do we resolve these seemingly insurmountable problems? The first step is, as it is for so many challenges, awareness of what the problems are. One problem lies in the methods that have been used to identify antiepileptic drugs. In general, the process has depended on normal animals that experienced acute seizures induced by some exogenous stimulus (as opposed to the natural state of spontaneous seizures that occur in an abnormal brain region). It is unknown whether the models used at present will identify compounds that will be effective in altering spontaneous seizures, especially the critical seizure initiation phase that can be determined only in models with spontaneous seizures. It is unclear whether the distribution of the drugs in these normal brains approximates the distribution in an epileptic brain that has alterations in glia, upregulation of drug-resistant proteins, and possible changes in blood–brain barrier function. Because the receptors and channels are altered in many of the epileptic models that have been examined, it is not known whether the mechanisms identified in the acute models are the most efficacious or are even relevant for epilepsy. Perhaps the first step in resolving this issue is to start using models that are as realistic as possible at some point in the drug discovery process. Such models may simultaneously test for efficacy of mechanism and appropriate targeting. The downside to this approach is that, for most of the realistic models, the spontaneity of seizures makes timing of the drug application in relation to seizure onset problematic, especially in animals that have rapid metabolic turnover of the compounds. The beauty of the acute models is that they are predictable in response and the timing of the seizure and drug administration can be precisely and consistently coordinated. The practicality of screening large numbers of compounds will dictate the maintenance of the some of the older models, but at some point the more realistic models must be incorporated.

In summary, there are a number of ways a drug can fail in controlling seizures, and the real reasons continue to elude us. There are now some definable and testable hypotheses about mechanisms that may have considerable impact on our understanding of drug resistance. The first step in resolving the issue is to start investigating drug resistance in status epilepticus and chronic epilepsy as a specific phenomenon using appropriate models. Only then can we begin to make true advances in this area.

REFERENCES

1. Jacobs MP, Fischbach GD, Davis MR, Dichter MA, Dingledine R, Lowenstein DH, Morrell MJ, Noebels JL, Rogawski MA, Spencer SS, Theodore WH. Future directions for epilepsy research. Neurology 2001; 57:1536–1542.
2. Alldredge BK, Gelb AM, Isaacs SM, Corry MD, Allen F, Ulrich S, Gottwald MD, O'Neil N, Neuhaus JM, Segal MR, Lowenstein DH. A comparison of lorazepam, diazepam, and placebo for the treatment of out-of-hospital status epilepticus. N Engl J Med 2001; 345:631–637.
3. Treiman DM, Meyers PD, Walton NY, Collins JF, Colling C, Rowan AJ, Handforth A, Faught E, Calabrese VP, Uthman BM, Ramsay RE, Mamdani MB. A comparison of four treatments for generalized convulsive status epilepticus. N Engl J Med 1998; 339:792–798.
4. Macdonald RL, Kelly KM. Antiepileptic drug mechanisms of action. Epilepsia 1995; 36(suppl 2):S2–S12.
5. Schwarzer C, Tsunashima K, Wanzenbock C, Fuchs K, Sieghart W, Sperk G. GABA(A) receptor subunits in the rat hippocampus. II. Altered distribution in kainic acid-induced temporal lobe epilepsy. Neuroscience 1997; 80:1001–1017.
6. Tsunashima K, Schwarzer C, Kirchmair E, Sieghart W, Sperk G. GABA(A) receptor subunits in the rat hippocampus. III: Altered messenger RNA expression in kainic acid-induced epilepsy. Neuroscience 1997; 80:1019–1032.

7. Brooks-Kayal AR, Shumate MD, Jin H, Rikhter TY, Coulter DA. Selective changes in single cell GABA(A) receptor subunit expression and function in temporal lobe epilepsy. Nat Med 1998; 4:1166–1172.

8. Mathern GW, Bertram EH, Babb TL, Pretorius JK, Kuhlman PA, Spradlin S, Mendoza D. In contrast to kindled seizures, the frequency of spontaneous epilepsy in the limbic status model correlates with greater fascia dentata excitatory and inhibitory axon sprouting, and increased staining for NMDA, AMPA and GABA-A receptors. Neuroscience 1997; 1003–1019.

9. Gibbs JW, Shumate MD, Coulter DA. Differential epilepsy associated alterations in postsynaptic GABA-A receptor function in dentate granule and CA1 neurons. J Neurophysiol 1997; 77:1924–1938.

10. Mangan PS, Rempe DA, Lothman EW. Changes in inhibitory neurotransmission in the CA1 region and dentate gyrus in a chronic model of temporal lobe epilepsy. J Neurophysiol 1995; 74:829–840.

11. Mangan PS, Lothman EW. Profound disturbances of pre- and post synaptic GABA$_B$ receptor-mediated processes in region CA1 in a chronic model of temporal lobe epilepsy. J Neurophysiol 1996; 76:1282–1296.

12. Shumate MD, Lin DD, Gibbs JW, Holloway KL, Coulter DA. GABA-A receptor function in epileptic human dentate granule cells: comparison to epileptic and control rat. Epilepsy Res 1998; 32:114–128.

13. Mtchedlishvili Z, Bertram EH, Kapur J. Diminished allopregnanolone enhancement of GABA$_A$ receptor currents in a rat model of chronic temporal lobe epilepsy. J Physiol 2001; 537:453–465.

14. Rempe DA, Mangan PS, Lothman EW. Regional heterogeneity of pathophysiological alterations in CA1 and dentate gyrus in a chronic model of temporal lobe epilepsy. J Neurophysiol 1995; 74:816–828.

15. Mangan PS, Scott C, Williamson JM, Bertram EH. Aberrant neuronal physiology in the basal nucleus of the amygdala in a model of chronic limbic epilepsy. Neuroscience 2000; 101:377–391.

16. Aronica E, Yankaya B, Troost D, van Vliet EA, Lopes da Silva FH, Gorter JA. Induction of neonatal sodium channel II and III alpha-isoform mRNAs in neurons and microglia after status epilepticus in the rat hippocampus. Eur J Neurosci 2001; 13:1261–1266.

17. Ketelaars SO, Gorter JA, van Vliet EA, Lopes da Silva FH, Wadman WJ. Sodium currents in isolated rat CA1 pyramidal and dentate granule neurones in the post–status epilepticus model of epilepsy. Neuroscience 2001; 105:109–120.

18. Escayg A, Heils A, MacDonald BT, Haug K, Sander T, Meisler MH. A novel SCN1A mutation associated with generalized epilepsy with febrile seizures plus—and prevalence of variants in patients with epilepsy. Am J Hum Genet 2001; 68:866–873.

19. Lerche H, Jurkat-Rott K, Lehmann-Horn F. Ion channels and epilepsy. Am J Med Genet 2001; 106:146–159.

20. Steinlein OK. Genes and mutations in idiopathic epilepsy. Am J Med Genet 2001; 106:139–145.

21. Wallace RH, Scheffer IE, Barnett S, Richards M, Dibbens L, Desai RR, Lerman-Sagie T, Lev D, Mazarib A, Brand N, Ben-Zeev B, Goikhman I, Singh R, Kremmidiotis G, Gardner A, Sutherland GR, George AL Jr, Mulley JC, Berkovic SF. Neuronal sodium-channel alpha1-subunit mutations in generalized epilepsy with febrile seizures plus. Am J Hum Genet 2001; 68:859–865.

22. Kearney JA, Plummer NW, Smith MR, Kapur J, Cummins TR, Waxman SG, Goldin AL, Meisler MH. A gain-of-function mutation in the sodium channel gene Scn2a results in seizures and behavioral abnormalities. Neuroscience 2001; 102:307–317.

23. Lothman EW, Rempe DA, Mangan PS. Changes in excitatory neurotransmission in the CA1 region and dentate gyrus in a chronic model of temporal lobe epilepsy. J Neurophysiol 1995; 74:841–848.

24. Aronica E, van Vliet EA, Mayboroda OA, Troost D, da Silva FH, Gorter JA. Upregulation of metabotropic glutamate receptor subtype mGluR3 and mGluR5 in reactive astrocytes in a rat model of mesial temporal lobe epilepsy. Eur J Neurosci 2000; 12:2333–2344.

25. Litman T, Druley TE, Stein WD, Bates SE. From MDR to MXR: new understanding of multidrug resistance systems, their properties and clinical significance. Cell Mol Life Sci 2001; 58:931–959.

26. Matheny CJ, Lamb MW, Brouwer KR, Pollack GM. Pharmacokinetic and pharmaco-dynamic implications of P-glycoprotein modulation. Pharmacotherapy 2001; 21:778–796.

27. Tanigawara Y. Role of P-glycoprotein in drug disposition. Ther Drug Monit 2000; 22:137–140.

28. Sisodiya SM, Lin WR, Harding BN, Squier MV, Thom M. Drug resistance in epilepsy: expression of drug resistance proteins in common causes of refractory epilepsy. Brain 2002; 125:22–31.

29. Sisodiya SM, Heffernan J, Squier MV. Over-expression of P-glycoprotein in malforma-tions of cortical development. Neuroreport 1999; 10:3437–3441.

30. Tishler DM, Weinberg KI, Hinton DR, Barbaro N, Annett GM, Raffel C. MDR1 gene expression in brain of patients with medically intractable epilepsy. Epilepsia 1995; 36:1–6.

31. Potschka H, Loescher W. In vivo evidence for P-glycoprotein-mediated transport of phenytoin at the blood-brain barrier of rats. Epilepsia 2001; 42:1231–1240.

32. Potschka H, Loescher W. Multidrug resistance-associated protein is involved in the regulation of extracellular levels of phenytoin in the brain. Neuroreport 2001; 12:2387–2389.

33. Rizzi M, Caccia S, Guiso G, Richichi C, Gorter JA, Aronica E, Aliprandi M, Bagnati R, Fanelli R, D'Incalci M, Samanin R, Vezzani A. Limbic seizures induce P-glycoprotein in rodent brain: functional implications for pharmacoresistance. J Neurosci 2002; 22:5833–5839.

34. Owen A, Pirmohamed M, Tettey JN, Morgan P, Chadwick D, Park BK. Carbamazepine is not a substrate for P-glycoprotein. Br J Clin Pharmacol 2001; 51:345–349.

35. Potschka H, Fedrowitz M, Löscher W. P-Glycoprotein and multidrug resistance-associated protein are involved in the regulation of extracellular levels of the major antiepileptic drug carbamazepine in the brain. Neuroreport 2001; 12:3557–3560.

36. Tong X, Patsalos PN. A microdialysis study of the novel antiepileptic drug levetiracetam: extracellular pharmacokinetics and effect on taurine in rat brain. Br J Pharmacol 2001; 133:867–874.

37. Walker MC, Tong X, Perry H, Alavijeh MS, Patsalos PN. Comparison of serum, cerebrospinal fluid and brain extracellular fluid pharmacokinetics of lamotrigine. Br J Pharmacol 2000; 2:242–248.

38. Walker MC, Alavijeh MS, Shorvon SD, Patsalos PN. Microdialysis study of the neuropharmacokinetics of phenytoin in rat hippocampus and frontal cortex. Epilepsia 1996; 37:421–427.

39. Tong X, O'Connell MT, Ratnaraj N, Patsalos PN. Vigabatrin and GABA concentration inter-relationship in rat extracellular fluid (ECF) from frontal cortex and hippocampus. Epilepsia 2000; 41(suppl Florence):9.

40. Geary WA, Wooten GF, Perlin JB, Lothman EW. In vitro and in vivo distribution and binding of phenytoin to rat brain. J Pharmacol Exp Ther 1987; 241:704–713.

41. Schmidt D. Benzodiazepines: diazepam. In: Levy RH et al, eds. Antiepileptic Drugs. New York: Raven Press, 1989:735–764.

42. Rosenberg HC, Tietz EI, Chiu TH. Tolerance to the anticonvulsant action of benzodiazepines. Relationship to decreased receptor density. Neuropharmacology 1985; 24:639–644.

43. Rosenberg HC, Tietz EI, TH Chiu. Tolerance to anticonvulsant effects of diazepam, clonazepam, and clobazam in amygdala-kindled rats. Epilepsia 1989; 30:276–285.

44. Macdonald RL, Olsen RW. GABAA receptor channels. Ann Rev Neurosci 1994; 17:569–602.

45. Poisbeau P, Williams SR, Mody I. Silent GABAA synapses during flurazepam withdrawal are region-specific in the hippocampal formation. J Neurosci 1997; 17:3467–3475.

46. Pesold C, Caruncho HJ, Impagnatiello F, Berg MJ, Fritschy JM, Guidotti A, Costa E. Tolerance to diazepam and changes in GABA(A) receptor subunit expression in rat neocortical areas. Neuroscience 1997; 79:477–487.

47. Tietz EI, Zeng XJ, Chen S, Lilly SM, Rosenberg HC, Kometiani P. Antagonist-induced reversal of functional and structural measures of hippocampal benzodiazepine tolerance. J Pharmacol Exp Ther 1999; 291:932–942.

48. Primus RJ, Yu J, Xu J, Hartnett C, Meyyappan M, Kostas C, Ramabhadran TV, Gallager DW. Allosteric uncoupling after chronic benzodiazepine exposure of recombinant gamma-aminobutyric acid(A) receptors expressed in Sf9 cells: ligand efficacy and subtype selectivity. J Pharmacol Exp Ther 1996; 276:882–890.

49. DeLorenzo RJ, Hauser WA, Towne AR, Boggs JG, Pellock JM, Penberthy L, Garnett L, Ko D. A prospective, population-based epidemiologic study of status epilepticus in Richmond, Virginia. Neurology 1996, 46.1029–1035.

50. Mayer SA, Claassen J, Lokin J, Mendelsohn F, Dennis LJ, Fitzsimmons BF. Refractory status epilepticus: frequency, risk factors, and impact on outcome. Arch Neurol 2002; 59:205–210.

51. Prasad A, Worrall BB, Bertram EH, Bleck TP. Propofol and midazolam in the treatment of refractory status epilepticus. Epilepsia 2001; 42:380–386.

52. Lowenstein DH, Alldredge BK. Status epilepticus at an urban public hospital in the 1980s. Neurology 1993; 43:483–488.

53. Treiman DM. The role of benzodiazepines in the management of status epilepticus. Neurology 1990; 40:32–42.

54. Fountain NB, Lothman EW. Pathophysiology of status epilepticus. J Clin Neurophysiol 1995; 12:326–342.

55. Kapur J, Macdonald RL. Status epilepticus: a proposed pathophysiology. In: Shorvon S et al, eds. The Treatment of Epilepsy. Oxford: Blackwell Science, 1996:258–268.

56. Walton NY, Treiman DM. Response of status epilepticus induced by lithium and pilocarpine to treatment with diazepam. Exp Neurol 1988; 101:267–275.

57. Kapur J, Macdonald RL. Rapid seizure-induced reduction of benzodiazepine and Zn^{2+} sensitivity of hippocampal dentate granule cell GABAA receptors. J Neurosci 1997; 17:7532–7540.

58. Borris DJ, Bertram EH, Kapur J. Ketamine controls prolonged status epilepticus. Epilepsy Res 2000; 42:117–122.

59. Mazarati AM, Baldwin RA, Sankar R, Wasterlain CG. Time-dependent decrease in the effectiveness of antiepileptic drugs during the course of self-sustaining status epilepticus. Brain Res 1998; 814:179–185.

60. Lothman EW, Bertram EH, Stringer JL. Functional anatomy of hippocampal seizures. Prog Neurobiol 1991; 37:1–82.

61. Van Landingham KE, Lothman EW. Self-sustaining limbic status epilepticus. I. Acute and chronic cerebral metabolic studies: limbic hypermetabolism and neocortical hypometabolism. Neurology 1991; 41:1942–1949.

62. Rafiq A, DeLorenzo RJ, Coulter DA. Generation and propagation of epileptiform discharges in a combined entorhinal cortex/hippocampal slice. J Neurophysiol 1993; 70:1962–1974.

63. Kapur J, Lothman EW. Loss of inhibition precedes delayed spontaneous seizures in the hippocampus after tetanic electrical stimulation. J Neurophysiol 1989; 61:427–434.

64. Michelson HB, Kapur J, Lothman EW. Reduction of paired pulse inhibition in the CA1 region of the hippocampus by pilocarpine in naive and in amygdala-kindled rats. Exp Neurol 1989; 104:264–271.

65. Kapur J, Coulter DA. Experimental status epilepticus alters GABA$_A$ receptor function in CA1 pyramidal neurons. Ann Neurol 1995; 38:893–900.

66. Kapur J, Lothman EW, DeLorenzo RJ. Loss of GABA$_A$ receptors during partial status epilepticus. Neurology 1994; 4:2407–2408.

67. Mazarati AM, Wasterlain CG. N-methyl-D-asparate receptor antagonists abolish the maintenance phase of self-sustaining status epilepticus in rat. Neurosci Lett 1999; 265:187–190.

68. Bertram EH, Lothman EW. NMDA receptor antagonists and limbic status epilepticus: a comparison with standard anticonvulsants. Epilepsy Res 1990; 5:177–184.

69. Rice AC, DeLorenzo RJ. N-methyl-D-aspartate receptor activation regulates refractoriness of status epilepticus to diazepam. Neuroscience 1999; 93:117–123.

70. Klapstein GJ, Colmers WF. Neuropeptide Y suppresses epileptiform activity in rat hippocampus in vitro. J Neurophysiol 1997; 78:1651–1661.

71. Baraban SC, Hollopeter G, Erickson JC, Schwartzkroin PA, Palmiter RD. Knock-out mice reveal a critical antiepileptic role for neuropeptide Y. Neuroscience 1997; 17:8927–8936.

72. Mazarati AM, Liu HT, Soomets U, Sankar R, Shin D, Katsumori H, Langel U, Wasterlain CG. Galanin modulation of seizures and seizure modulation of hippocampal galanin in animal models of status epilepticus. J Neurosci 1998; 18:10070–10077.

73. Mazarati AM, Hohmann JG, Bacon A, Liu H, Sankar R, Steiner RA, Wynick D, Wasterlain CG. Modulation of hippocampal excitability and seizures by galanin. J Neurosci 2000; 20:6276–6281.

74. McKernan RM, Whiting PJ. Which GABAA-receptor subtypes really occur in the brain? Trends Neurosci 1996; 19(4):139–143.

4

Genetics of Human Epilepsy—Epilepsy as a Channelopathy

Edward C. Cooper

University of Pennsylvania
Philadelphia, Pennsylvania, U.S.A.

INTRODUCTION

During a seizure, normal patterns of neuronal excitation are replaced by pathological rhythms that are excessively synchronized, prominent, and widespread. The capacity for seizure activity is latent in normal brain—for example, seizures can be provoked in anyone as a symptom of simple metabolic disturbances such as hypoglycemia, hypocalcemia, or uremia. What is intrinsically different about the brains of people with epilepsy, who exhibit seizures without such provocations?

One approach in answering this key question is studying their underlying genetics. Human genetic studies usually involve comparing the genes groups of people with a particular trait with individuals lacking that trait in order to identify the differences that may be responsible. Genetic research can lead to the identification of responsible gene (or genes), even when no other biological information about the cause of a disorder is available. So a successful genetic study offers the potential to "think outside the box" by identifying factors previously completely unknown or unsuspected of being involved with a particular disease process.

Over the past two decades, increasing efforts have been made to identify families in which epilepsy occurred in patterns suggesting Mendelian inheritance— that is, in patterns suggesting that the epileptic trait resulted from mutations in a single gene. Over the past 5 years, aided by tools derived from the Human Genome Project, investigators have discovered many such mutations. With occasional exceptions (1), the mutations causing idiopathic epilepsy discovered so far lie in genes encoding ion channels.

What are ion channels? Ion channels are membrane proteins, tiny molecular machines about 10 nm in size, that allow ions to enter or leave the cell interior at high rates—usually 10^6–10^7 ions per second per channel (2). These ion fluxes through individual channels cause transient, local changes in neuronal membrane potentials—the smallest units of brain excitation. All neurons possess different classes of channels that are selectively permeable to the cations Na^+, K^+, and Ca^{2+} or the anion Cl^-. Owing to the activity of ATP-consuming pumps and cotransporters, Na^+, Ca^{2+}, and Cl^- are usually more concentrated extracellularly, and K^+ more concentrated intracellularly. As a result, when channels permeable to Na^+ or Ca^{2+} open, these ions enter the cell, depolarizing the membrane potential. When channels selective for K^+ or Cl^- open, the membrane is made more hyperpolarized, owing to K^+ leaving, or Cl^- entering, the cell interior. So, at the simplest level, Na^+ and Ca^{2+} channel activity leads to increased excitation, and K^+ and Cl^- channel activity reduces excitation.

However, channels also underlie more complex, dynamic changes in the membrane potential—oscillations and rhythmic activity in neurons and neuronal networks. Grouping two channels capable of causing opposing changes in the membrane potential together in a neuronal membrane creates a mechanism for generating membrane potential oscillations. The propagated action potential, mediated by sequential opening of voltage-gated Na^+ channels (the depolarizing phase) and potassium channels (the hyperpolarizing phase) grouped along nerve axons, is the best-studied example of such signaling. We now know, however, that other channel groupings occur everywhere in nervous tissue—on neuronal dendrites and their spines; on cell bodies; at the somatic origin (hillock), branch points, and presynaptic terminals of axons; and on glia.

Indeed, vertebrate nervous systems, from worms to flies to mammals, possess a large set of ion channels types, several hundred in number, that differ in key functional properties such as opening and closing rates (*kinetics*), the type of ions passed (*ion selectivity*), and the signals that bring about channel opening and closing (*gating* and *modulation*). This diversity allows particular channels to be deployed at specific locations, for specialized purposes. Thus, different neurons express distinct subsets of ion channels, and the different channel types expressed by each neuron are localized at specific sites in the cell membrane with great precision. For example, some channels are specifically expressed on dendrites, but others are found on axons or at presynaptic terminals. Some channels are preferentially expressed on inhibitory or excitatory neurons within a brain region, or on glia. These cell-specific differences in ion channel expression give each cell a particular electrical "personality," enabling neurons to perform distinctive functions in local networks, and contributing to the differences between the network properties of different brain regions.

So, when we learn that an ion channel mutation causes seizures, this leads to questions at several levels. At the level of the channel molecule, we seek to learn how the mutation alters intrinsic channel properties such as kinetics, selectivity, gating, and modulation. At the cellular level, we want to know how the mutation affects channel abundance and distribution. At the local network level, we need to know how the mutation alters the rhythmic properties and synchronization of firing occurring in networks of neurons in particular brain regions, since it is at this level that the seizure phenotype is manifest.

During the past few years, we have learned much about the consequences of the epilepsy channel mutations at the molecular level—that is, the effects of mutations on channel intrinsic properties. However, much remains to be learned, especially the consequences of mutations for cellular and network properties. In the discussion that follows, we will try to identify both the key areas of progress made and the unanswered questions remaining for future investigation.

A first expectation, based on earlier studies of channel defects in hyperexcitability disorders of skeletal muscle (e.g., myotonia) and heart (longed QT syndrome), would be that channel mutations leading to epilepsy would be associated with increases in Na^+ and/or Ca^{2+} channel activity (since such activity leads to membrane depolarization) or with reductions in K^+ or Cl^- channel activity (since these currents prevent membrane depolarization). Initial studies show that this expectation is often, but not always, fulfilled. To facilitate further reading, we have provided the listing for each disorder in the National Library of Medicine's online Mendelian Inheritance in Man database (http://www.ncbi.nlm.nih.gov/omim/).

HEREDITARY EPILEPSIES DUE TO CHANNEL GENE MUTATIONS

Autosomal-Dominant Frontal Lobe Epilepsy (ADNFLE; MIM #600513)

In 1994, Sheffer et al. described a new epilepsy syndrome characterized by clusters of brief nocturnal motor seizures (3,4). The attacks began in childhood (median age, 8 years) and persisted throughout life, often misdiagnosed as night terrors, nightmares, hysteria, or paroxysmal nocturnal dystonia. Video-EEG telemetry revealed that the nocturnal attacks were epileptic seizures heralded by frontally predominant sharp and slow-wave activity (4), usually arising from stage 2 non-REM sleep. Pedigree analysis suggested autosomal dominant inheritance with incomplete (~70%) penetrance, thus the name autosomal dominant nocturnal frontal lobe epilepsy or ADNFLE. Subsequent molecular genetic studies revealed mutations in genes for two subunits of neuronal nicotinic acetylcholine receptors (nAchRs), *CHRNA4* on chromosome 20q and *CNRNB2* on chromosome 1 in affected individuals (5–8). Phillips et al. (9) mapped a third ADNFLE locus to chromosome 15q24, near genes for three additional nAchRs, but mutations at this locus remain to be identified.

Central nAchRs are pentameric cation channels, closely related to the well-studied nAchRs at skeletal muscle endplates, but are composed of α and β subunits expressed only (or at least, primarily) by neurons (Fig. 1). Acetylcholine binding to recognition sites on α subunits (Fig. 1C) results in channel opening and membrane depolarization. Although there are distinct genes for seven neuronal nAchR α subunits and three β subunits, heteromeric channels formed by coassembly of α4 and β2 subunits appear to be the most abundant form expressed in brain. The subunits share a common basic structure, with a large, extracellular amino-terminal domain and four transmembrane α-helices (Fig. 1B). The second (M2) helix lines the transmembrane ion pathway (Fig. 1A,B) and is believed to undergo a twisting conformational change after acetylcholine binding that allows ions to flow.

The ADNFLE mutations described so far all result in single amino acid changes at key positions within the α4 or β2 pore-lining helices, and might therefore be expected to cause changes in gating or ion conductance properties. Indeed, cellular electrophysiological experiments using the mutant subunits expressed in experimental cells such as *Xenopus* oocytes or mammalian cultured cells have revealed marked, albeit complex, changes in these properties (6,10,11). The α4 S248F mutant AchR responses showed faster desensitization, slower recovery from desensitization, less inward rectification, and virtually no Ca^{2+} permeability as

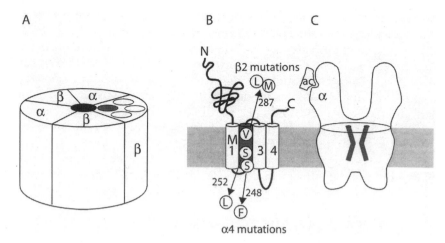

Figure 1. Mutations in neuronal nicotinic acetylcholine receptor subunits associated with autosomal-dominant nocturnal frontal lobe epilepsy (ADNFLE) are located on the pore-lining M2 section. (A) Schematic indicating that each channel is composed of five subunits (two α, three non-α) arranged around the central ion pore. (B) Each subunit polypeptide traverses the membrane four times (termed M1, M2, M3, M4). The amino-terminal region (containing the acetylcholine-binding domain) and carboxy-terminal region are both extracellular. Positions of mutations that introduce single amino acid substitutions in M2 are labeled. (C) Cut-through view of a receptor, showing the extracellular binding of acetylcholine (ac) and the position of the M2 transmembrane sections lining the ion pore.

compared with wild-type α4 beta2 AChRs (11). Although these effects would all tend to reduce channel activity, this mutation also caused use-dependent upregulation of activity and was more strongly activated by low levels of agonist, effects that might result in enhanced activity in vivo. Studies of the two known CHRNB2 mutants show differing effects: The V287M mutation shows normal kinetics but 10-fold increased ACh sensitivity (8), whereas the V287L mutation shows normal ACh sensitivity but 30-fold slower kinetics (7).

Immunolocalization studies show that the α4 subunit is widely expressed and is localized on neuronal somata and dendrites in cortical and subcortical structures, and is particularly highly expressed by dopaminergic neurons in the substantia nigra (12). Labarca et al. generated CHRNA mutant mice harboring a point mutation in the pore near the position of the ADNFLE mutations (13). This mutation caused 30-fold increased ACh sensitivity and was partially activated by choline at levels that are normally present in cerebrospinal fluid. Mice exhibited early lethality and loss of nigral dopaminergic neurons.

Acetylcholine is thought to be an important neuromodulator in the thalamocortical circuits that regulate transitions between sleep and wakefulness (14); a disruption of cholinergic function in this circuit by altered nAChR activity could explain why seizures occur in sleep. The frontal lobe predominance of the epileptic discharge in ADNFLE patients is not explained by the distribution pattern of the receptors, which is widespread, and this aspect of the clinical phenotype remains to be clarified.

Episodic Ataxia with Myokymia (and Partial Epilepsy)
(EA-1; MIM 160120)

EA-1 is a dominantly inherited disorder involving both the brain and peripheral nerves (15–17). Patients experience recurrent attacks of unsteady gait and loss of limb coordination lasting minutes to hours. This phenotype suggests an intermittent derangement of cerebellar function. In some cases, transient cognitive deficits accompany the motor symptoms. Attacks may be provoked by a sudden stress or startle. Myokymia is continuously present in many EA-1 patients. This myokymia is unaffected by pharmacological block at the proximal portion of peripheral nerves, but is reduced by distal nerve block and abolished by inhibition of neuromuscular transmission. This observation suggests that, unlike myotonia or epilepsy, myokymia results from abnormal hyperactivity in the peripheral nerve. However, patients with EA-1 have about a 10-fold greater risk of epileptic seizures compared to the general population (15,18).

In 1994, Litt and colleagues (17) linked EA-1 to missense mutations in *KCNA1*, a voltage-gated potassium channel gene. *KCNA1* is a mammalian homolog of the fruit fly *Drosophila* gene Shaker. Adult Shaker flies exhibit abnormal limb shaking when anesthetized with ether. Shaker larvae showed abnormal hyperexcitability of the motor nerve terminals (19).

Extensive further work, including physiological studies of the mutant channels, anatomical studies of KCNA1 channel localization in the central nervous system and peripheral nerve, and knockout mouse studies, gives useful clues for understanding the basis of the EA-1 phenotype in the brain and peripheral nerve (20). Studies in *Xenopus* oocytes indicate that the mutations causing EA-1 result in reductions in KCNA1 expression and current magnitude (18,21,22). In some cases, EA-1 mutant channels in heterologous cells exhibit clear "dominant negative" effects, interacting with coexpressed normal channels and preventing them from functioning normally or trafficking to the cell surface. Other EA-1 mutants exhibit simple loss-of-function properties in vitro. Tempel and colleagues generated knockout mice lacking the murine homologue of *KCNA1* (that is, *Kcna1*, which encodes the potassium channel delayed rectifier protein Kv1.1) as a useful animal model for EA-1 (23). Interestingly, mice heterozygous for the knockout allele appear normal; this is in contrast to the dominantly inherited effects of EA-1 mutations in humans. Mice that are homozygous for the knockout allele have subtle defects in cerebellar function (24), but the most obvious aspects of their phenotype are very frequent generalized epileptic seizures believed to be of limbic origin, and associated premature death (23). It has proved difficult to identify the alterations in cellular physiology that cause frequent spontaneous seizures in the Kv1.1 knockout mice—hippocampal slices prepared from the knockouts exhibit remarkably normal intrinsic neuronal and synaptic properties (23). This is likely because channels containing the subunit are localized to small axons and terminals of excitatory neurons which are difficult to study directly using available physiological methods (25). An interesting clue to the pathophysiology of EA-1 may be the responsiveness of the condition in some but not all pedigrees to treatment with the carbonic anhydrase inhibitor acetazolamide (26).

As a larger number of patients with EA-1 have been identified, it has become clear that a they differ in the severity of their symptoms over a broad spectrum, and

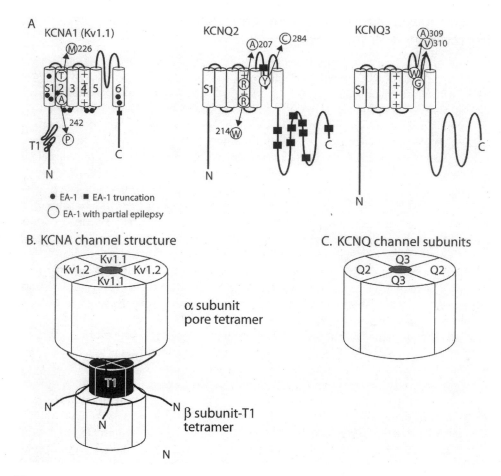

Figure 2. Mutations in neuronal KCNA1 and KCNQ potassium channel subunits associated with EA-1, EA-1 and epilepsy, and BFNC. (A) Cartoons showing the transmembrane topology of the KCNA1 (also known as Kv1.1), KCNQ2, and KCNQ3. The subunits have intracellular amino- and carboxy-terminal regions and six transmembrane segments (S1–S6). The amino terminal region of KCNA1 includes a domain (T1) involved in channel assembly. Positions of amino acid substitution (circles) and truncation mutations (rectangles) associated with disease are indicated. Missense mutations associated with epilepsy are also labeled with the position number in the amino acid sequence. (B) Schematic indicating the tetrameric structure of the KCNA1 channel. The transmembrane portion of the channel contains a central ion pore; the intracellular T1 domains interact tightly with each other and with accessory subunits, termed β subunits. (C) KCNQ channels are tetramers of membrane spanning subunits; in brain, some channels contain a combination of KCNQ2 and KCNQ3 subunits (however, the subunit stoicheometry within these channels is not known).

that more severe forms of the disorder are often associated with epilepsy. Zuberi et al. described a family containing five patients with episodic ataxia and myokymia, two of whom additionally had complex partial seizures (18). Eunson et al. described a second family with this combination of symptoms, as well as families with severe and acetazolamide-resistant ataxia, or isolated myokymia (27). When studied in heterologous cells, the mutations associated with severe ataxia and epilepsy caused severe reductions in channel activity (28). In some cases, the EA-1 plus epilepsy mutant subunits were capable of dominant-negative interactions with wild-type subunits; that is, they were capable of coassembling with the wild types, but the resulting channels were hypofunctional owing to failure of intracellular trafficking or lack of intrinsic channel activity (28). Trafficking defects are likely to be particularly critical in neurons, because the KCNA1 channel proteins are normally localized to sites along myelinated and nonmyelinated axons and at presynaptic terminals, which are very distant from their sites of translation and assembly in the endoplasmic reticulum (25,29,30).

Benign Familial Neonatal Convulsions (BFNC; MIM 121200)

Benign familial neonatal convulsions (BFNC) is an idiopathic generalized epilepsy characterized by recurrent, brief, generalized seizures that begin on about the fourth day of life and remit after 1–3 months (31). Infants otherwise grow and develop normally. However, affected persons carry a 10–16% risk of experiencing seizures again later in life. When seizures occur after infancy, they are in many instances provoked by sudden emotional stress or startle (31). In 1989, Leppert and colleagues found linkage of the disease gene to chromosome 20 (32). Later, Lewis et al. (33) and Steinlein and colleagues (34) identified two families in which the BFNC syndrome was linked not to chromosome 20 but to chromosome 8.

The two BFNC genes on chromosomes 20 and 8 encode highly homologous potassium channel subunits, KCNQ2 and KCNQ3 (35–37). Expression of either gene alone in *Xenopus* oocytes results in only small currents, but expression of the two genes together results in currents that are 10–50 times larger (38,39). Some disease causing missense mutations in KCNQ2 and KCNQ3 are associated with only modest reductions (20–30%) in current magnitude (38). This finding suggests that the epileptic syndrome can result from simple loss of function and does not require a toxic gain of function or dominant-negative activity. This implies the critical dependence of neuronal excitability on the absolute magnitude of KCNQ2/KCNQ3 potassium channel activity, especially during the neonatal period. It is noteworthy that KCNQ2 and KCNQ3 are relatives of a cardiac channel, KCNQ1, which previously was shown to be mutated in both dominantly and recessively inherited forms of the long QT syndrome (40,41).

Heteromeric KCNQ2/KCNQ3 channels (Fig. 2c) underlie an extensively studied potassium channel found in central and autonomic neurons, known as the M channel (42). M channels are important effectors for acetylcholine and other neurotransmitters that activate intracellular G proteins (43). M channels open occasionally at the resting membrane potential and are slowly activated by membrane depolarization. Because of such slow kinetics, M channel activation causes a delayed membrane hyperpolarization after a cell receives excitatory input, or slow inhibitory postsynaptic potential (IPSP). As a result, sympathetic neurons expressing large amounts of M channels tend to fire one action potential after receiving excitatory input, then become transiently quiescent. Inhibition of the M channel causes these neurons to become slightly depolarized and to fire multiple action potentials rhythmically after receiving excitatory inputs. Thus, M channels may serve as a general brake on excess neuronal excitation that can be selectively removed when they are inhibited by neurotransmitters such as acetylcholine.

Consistent with this, KCNQ2 subunits are widely expressed in circuits implicated in generation of epileptic seizures (44). Interestingly, some of the highest levels of KCNQ2 expression are in inhibitory neurons important for synchronization of the firing of excitatory neurons, including the thalamic reticular neurons and several populations of interneurons in the hippocampus and cortex.

Retigabine, a novel anticonvulsant initially identified by the anticonvulsant drug screening program (sponsored by the National Institutes of Health), is effective in preventing seizures induced by electrical shock or by a broad range of chemical convulsants (pentylenetetrazole, NMDA, 4-aminopyridine, picrotoxin, but not bicuculline or strychnine) (45). BMS-204352 is another drug initially developed as a potential therapy for acute stroke (46). Remarkably, recent studies have revealed that both these agents are potent activators of neuronal KCNQ channels (47–49). In addition, drugs that block M channels directly, and thereby mimic some of the central actions of acetylcholine, have been evaluated as potential treatments for Alzheimer's disease (50). Although these agents have not yet been shown to be of clinical usefulness, it is clear that the cloning of the KCNQ channels has revealed an important potential new target for drug screening studies.

Generalized Epilepsy with Febrile Seizures Plus (GEFS+; MIM 604233) and Severe Myoclonic Epilepsy of Infancy (SMEI; MIM 607208)

Febrile seizures occur in 3–5% of all children. When febrile seizures occur in isolation, between the ages of 6 months and 6 years, in children who are otherwise developing normally, the risk of later epilepsy is low. For a minority of cases, however, febrile seizures herald epilepsy comprising a variety of forms and degrees of severity.

In a seminal clinical study, Scheffer and Berkovic (1997) described a large multigenerational family in which typical febrile seizures were common, but a variety of nonfebrile seizure types also occurred (50a). This spectrum of other seizure types represented in the pedigree included nonfebrile convulsions, absences, myoclonic seizures, atonic seizures, and severe myoclonic-astatic epilepsy with developmental delay. Scheffer and Berkovic argued that this heterogeneity represented variable phenotypes associated with the dominantly inherited trait, and introduced the term Generalized Epilepsy with Febrile Seizures Plus (GEFS+) to describe the new seizure syndrome. They further noted that such phenotypic heterogeneity would make this syndrome difficult to detect in isolated cases, obscuring its frequency in the clinic. They concluded that molecular studies of large pedigrees such as the one described might reveal the underlying genetic mechanism(s). Follow-up studies by the authors and others have confirmed all of these predictions.

Mutations in four channel genes have thus far been identified in families with GEFS+. These include the genes for subunits of voltage-gated Na^+ channels (*SCN1A*, *SCN2A*, and *SCN1B*) and GABA receptors (*GABRG2*). *SCN1A* and *SCN2A* encode two widely expressed neuronal isoforms of the large, pore-forming sodium channel α subunit. *SCN1B* encodes a single-transmembrane β subunit.

The single mutation in *SCN1B*, C121W, has been described in two Anglo-Australian pedigrees (51,52). C121 is located in the extracellular domain of the encoded β1 subunit, where it forms a disulfide bridge that plays a critical role in the proper assembly of the extracellular domain into an immunoglobulin-like folding pattern (53). Sodium channel β1 subunits have multiple roles, enhancing surface expression of the pore-forming α subunits, participating in protein-protein interactions with extracellular proteins that are important for channel clustering at key sites such as the nodes of Ranvier, and enhancing rates of channel inactivation (54). Evidence from expression studies in cultured mammalian cells and *Xenopus* oocytes suggests that the C121W mutants retain the ability to promote channel surface expression, but lose the ability to enhance channel inactivation, resulting in prolonged sodium currents and excessive membrane depolarization (51,55).

The discovery of a second GEFS+ locus on chromosome 2q (56,57), a region that harbors a cluster of three genes encoding sodium channel α subunits, led to a search for mutations within these genes in GEFS+ pedigrees. Recent studies have revealed nine different mutations in *SCN1A* and a single mutation in *SCN2A*, all resulting in single amino acid substitutions (missense mutations) in the resulting α subunit polypeptides (58–62). Interestingly, these additional family studies have revealed a high frequency of partial seizures in members of some pedigrees that otherwise fit the original GEFS+ profile (52,61,62). Although the electrophysiological properties of these mutant α subunits have only begun to be studied in heterologous cells, initial results suggest that defective inactivation mechanisms may be involved, as previously observed in studies of the C121W mutation in β1 discussed above.

Lossin et al. (63) studied two mutations (T875M, R1648H) that lead to changes in amino acids in the S4 voltage sensors of *SCN1A*, and a third mutation (W1204M) located in an intracellular linker domain (Fig. 3A). In each case, the mutant channels exhibited a persistent current during prolonged depolarizations due to an apparent failure of inactivation gating. Conflicting results were obtained by Alekov et al. (64), and additional studies are needed. For now, it appears that, similar to the effects of the *SCN1B* mutation, missense mutations in *SCN1A* properties would be expected to enhance cellular excitability under most circumstances in vivo. Thus, epilepsy may result from mutations in sodium channel α or β subunits that enhance channel activity, similar to the mutations in heart and skeletal muscle Na$^+$ channels that cause disorders of hyperexcitability and excessive synchrony (myotonia, long QT syndrome) in those tissues (65,66).

This notion is further illuminated by recent genetic and clinical evidence that an additional epilepsy syndrome, Severe Myoclonic Epilepsy of Infancy (SMEI), represents a severe form of the GEFS+ spectrum (67–69). SMEI, first described by Dravet in 1978, is a progressive syndrome of refractory seizures and cognitive decline (69a). After a normal early infancy, patients present with prolonged generalized or unilateral febrile seizures at 5–12 months of age. Other seizure types, including myoclonic, absence, partial, and atonic seizures, begin between 1 and 4 years of age. Psychomotor slowing becomes apparent during the second year of life, and the patient may also experience obtunded states associated with myoclonus and develop ataxia, pyramidal dysfunction, and refractory generalized tonic-clonic and partial seizures. Intellectual outcome is generally poor.

Although a family history of epilepsy had been previously recognized as common in SMEI, the nature of the seizure disorder in family members had not been systematically explored until recently. Singh et al. (2001) presented 12 SMEI

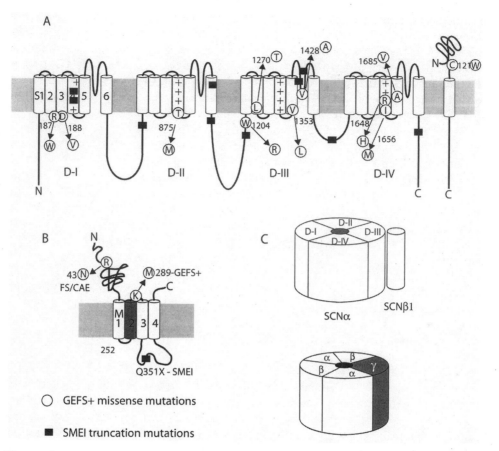

Figure 3. Sodium channel and GABA-A receptor subunit mutations in Generalized Epilepsy with Febrile Seizures Plus (GEFS+) and Severe Myoclonic Epilepsy of Infancy (SMEI). (A) Membrane topology of large α subunit and small β1 subunit of the voltage-gated sodium channel. The α subunit has four homologous domain (D-I through D-IV) that each contain six transmembrane subunits (S1 through S6). Positions of amino acid substitution mutations associated with GEFS+ (open circles, number indicates position in sequence) and of truncations associated with SMEI (filled rectangles) are shown. (B) Membrane topology of GABA-A receptor γ2 subunit and mutations associated with forms of epilepsy. Mutations are labeled as in A. (FS/CAE, febrile seizures and childhood absence epilepsy.) (C) Schematic illustrating the arrangement of homology domains of sodium channel and subunits of pentameric GABA-A receptor within the membrane.

pedigrees within which other family members exhibited forms of epilepsy consistent with the GEFS+ spectrum. Independently, two groups screened SMEI patients for mutations in *SCN1A* mutations and discovered a total of 17 new mutations (Fig. 3) (68,69). Remarkably, 16 of the mutations were frame-shift, nonsense, or splice-donor mutations predicted to result in markedly aberrant, truncated forms of the channel protein. In contrast to the modest changes in gating seen with GEFS+ mutations causing single amino acid changes, the SMEI truncations would be expected to produce proteins incapable of conducting ions.

These clinical and genetic observations are provocative and lead to many questions concerning genotype-phenotype relations in the GEFS+/SMEI patients. It is notable that SCN1A is widely expressed by excitatory and inhibitory neurons and exhibits a perisomatic distribution; SCN2A underlies the sodium currents at axon initial segments, nodes of Ranvier, and along unmyelinated fibres (70). It is not immediately apparent that loss of Na^+ channel activity at these sites would lead to hyperexcitability and epilepsy. The distinctive developmental profile associated with FS, GEFS+, and SMEI may hold some clues, perhaps indicating that the brain responds in stereotyped and developmentally regulated ways to the loss or gain of Na^+ channel activity associated with the various mutations, leading to epilepsy and sometimes other disabilities. Alternatively, could some of the mutant channels have toxic gain-of-function properties, not yet discovered, resulting from impaired intracellular trafficking or other protein-protein interactions? These issues may be clarified by additional studies in vitro and with transgenic mouse models. Such studies have recently begun with the SCN2A gene: transgenic mice expressing a gain-of-function SCN2A mutant exhibit a progressive phenotype of focal seizures, hippocampal sclerosis, generalized seizures, and premature death (71); mice homozygous for a knockout of *SCN2A* die soon after birth and exhibit widespread neuronal apoptosis (72).

Screening of large clinical populations suggests, however, that mutations in *SCN1A*, *SCN2A*, and *SCN1B* account for only ~20% of familial cases of GEFS+ and a far lower percentage of cases of idiopathic generalized epilepsy (59,60). This implies that other genes are involved, and the search has begun. Very recently, mutations in *GABRG2* that encodes the γ_2 subunit of GABA-A receptor subunit were also identified as causes of GEFS+ (73). GABA-A receptors are ligand-gated Cl^- channels (74). GABA released at inhibitory synapses binds to sites on the extracellular side of the channel, leading to channel opening, Cl^- influx, and generating a fast inhibitory postsynaptic potential (IPSP). There are 16 human genes for subunits of GABA receptors; α_{1-6}, β_{1-4}, γ_{1-3}, δ, ε, and θ.

Each GABA receptor is pentameric complexes, consisting of two α subunits, two β subunits and single subunit of class γ, δ, ε, or θ. Although receptors containing a variety of different subunit combinations are represented in vivo, the most abundant and widely distributed form of the receptor is formed by α_1, β_2, and γ_2 subunits. The three known γ_2 subunit mutations range widely in the severity of their effects on channel function and the associated clinical phenotype. One mutation (R43N), found in a pedigree with a relatively mild seizure phenotypes (febrile seizures and childhood absence epilepsy), introduces a point mutation in the site for channel modulation by benzodiazepines such as diazepam and lorazepam (75). R43N mutant channels expressed in *Xenopus* oocytes exhibited only 10% reductions in GABA current amplitudes, though responsiveness to benzodiazepines was abolished completely. A second missense mutation (K289M) in an extracellular loop between the M2 and M3 transmembrane segments was associated with a ~90% reduction in GABA currents, and a more severe phenotype of febrile seizures and afebrile generalized tonic-clonic seizures (73). Finally, a truncation mutation in GABRG2 was found in a patient with SMEI within a branch of a large GEFS+ pedigree with bilineal inheritance of epilepsy (76). When expressed in oocytes or cultured mammalian cells, this truncation mutation (Q351) acted as a potent dominant negative, coassembling with normal GABA receptor subunits and preventing them from leaving the endoplasmic reticulum (76). Although the genetic evidence linking this truncation mutation to SMEI was weak because only three individuals carried the mutation in the pedigree studied, the findings are provocative in view of the previous discussion of SCN1A truncations in SMEI.

Juvenile Myoclonic Epilepsy (JME; MIM 606904)

Juvenile Myoclonic Epilepsy is characterized by the onset—usually during adolescence—of bilateral single or repetitive myoclonic jerks, occurring most commonly upon morning awakening (77). A majority of patients have at least one generalized tonic-clonic seizure, and ~15% have absences. A characteristic EEG finding is frontally predominant bilateral 4–6 Hz polyspike-wave discharges. JME is not uncommon, and represents ~4–6% of all patients with epilepsy (77). Nevertheless, identifying genes for JME has been particularly difficult, likely owing to the genetic heterogeneity and complexity underlying the syndrome. Recently, Cossette et al. ascertained that a familial form of epilepsy, with clinical and electroencephalographic features of common JME, was inherited in an autosomal-dominant pattern (78). The locus was mapped to chromosome 5q34, which contains a cluster of GABA-A receptor genes. A missense mutation was found in *GABRA1*, resulting in an A322D change in a conserved site in the third transmembrane helix of the GABAα1 subunit (Fig. 4). Two α subunits are present in each pentameric GABA receptor; each of these subunits contributes to both a binding site for GABA and the transmembrane pore (Fig. 4B). Peak currents mediated by receptors including the A322D GABAα1 mutants were only 10% of those of wild-type receptors, and this

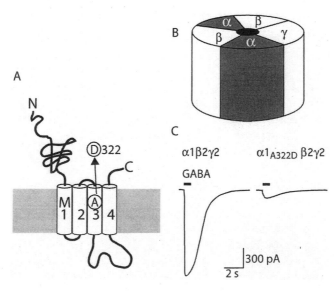

Figure 4. GABA-A receptor α1 mutation in dominantly inherited Juvenile Myoclonic Epilepsy (JME). (A) Membrane topology of the subunit and position of the mutation in the M3 transmembrane segment. (B) Schematic illustrating that each tetrameric receptor contains two α subunits. (C) Receptor containing the mutant subunit exhibit markedly reduced responsiveness to GABA (s, seconds; pA, picoamperes of channel current).

weak response required 200-fold higher concentrations of GABA (Fig. 4C). Accordingly, the epileptic phenotype would be expected to be associated with reduced responsiveness to inhibitory neurotransmission. It is unclear why this mutation results in epilepsy of the JME type, and this question is ripe for further examination.

Voltage-Gated Calcium Channels and Absence Seizures in Mouse and Man

Understanding how human single-gene mutations contribute to complex phenotypes in vivo can often be aided by studies in model animals including mice. Although the generation of mutant mice harboring human epilepsy mutations has only recently begun, a number of distinct *spontaneously arising* lines of mutant mice that exhibited seizures similar to human absence epilepsy were discovered beginning in the 1960s, and have been extensively investigated (79–81). Mouse lines called tottering (*tg*), lethargic (*lh*), stargazer (*stg*), mocha (*mh*), ducky (*du*), and slow-wave epilepsy (*swe*) exhibit spike-wave encephalographic seizures associated with transient interruption of behavior. Recent studies have demonstrated that in four of these lines, mutations are present in genes encoding components of neuronal high voltage activated (HVA) calcium channels.

The neuronal HVA calcium channels are heterotetramers comprised of pore-forming $\alpha 1$ subunits and auxiliary $\alpha 2\delta$, β, and γ subunits. Multiple genes encode isoforms of each subunit type, and 10 $\alpha 1$, four β, eight γ, and three $\alpha 2\delta$ have been cloned in mammals. Tottering alleles are mutations in the pore-forming $\alpha 1a$ subunit (82); other mouse epilepsy mutations are found in the auxiliary subunits $\beta 4$ (lethargic), $\alpha 2\delta 2$ (ducky), and $\gamma 2$ (stargazer) (83–85).

Anatomical and physiological investigations of these models have begun to help us to understand the complexity of the links between a particular molecular defect and the associated phenotypes. For example, initial studies of the lethargic mutation in $\beta 4$ revealed that this mutation abolished interactions with $\alpha 1$ subunits, causing reduced calcium currents in heterologous cells (83). However, recordings of lethargic Purkinje neurons revealed normal calcium current amplitudes (86). This is because lethargic mice exhibit increased association between $\alpha 1$ subunits and the remaining $\beta 1$–3 subunits, without associated increases in $\beta 1$–3 subunit mRNA. Thus, a process of "subunit shuffling" occurs posttranscriptionally in lethargic mice, leading to a complex change in the composition of expressed channels (86). The phenotype may result from a combination of loss of function (in cells where insufficient $\beta 1$–3 is expressed to compensate for the loss of $\beta 4$) and gain of function (from the increase in incorporation of $\beta 1$–3 subunits with distinctive properties, in cells that express mRNA for these subunits).

Physiological studies of thalamic neurons from lethargic, stargazer, and tottering mice indicate that these mutations result in increases in the amplitude of the low voltage–activated (LVA) or T-type calcium channels that are important for thalamic rhythmicity (87). The mechanisms through which these mutations cause increases in LVA currents are currently under intense investigation. These studies of mouse models of epilepsy involving calcium channel genes strongly suggest that mechanisms underlying human epilepsy associated with channel mutations are likely to be more multifaceted and complex than previously expected.

Paralleling studies of mutant calcium channel subunits in mice, efforts to identify human families with epilepsy and mutations in these genes have as yet revealed only a single case in which an α1a mutation was associated with epilepsy, episodic and progressive ataxia, and cognitive delay (88). It is expected that additional studies will more fully reveal the potential of alterations in these genes as causes of human epilepsy.

CONCLUSIONS AND IMPLICATIONS FOR THERAPEUTICS

Although the first identification of a channel gene mutation in epilepsy occurred only in 1994, many such mutations have now been identified in ten different channel subunits (Fig. 5). What do these efforts reveal about the causes of epilepsy and potential for novel treatments? One remarkable result is that many of the mutations have been found in subunits of voltage-dependent Na^+ channels and GABA-A receptors, important targets of the majority of currently approved drugs, all developed through in vivo pharmacological screening. Many (if perhaps not all) Na^+ channel mutations in GEFS+, for example, result in increased Na^+ channel activity; in contrast, drugs like phenytoin, carbamazepine, and lamotrigine act by blocking Na^+ channel activity. Similarly, in autosomal-dominant JME and some cases of GEFS+, mutations in GABA GABA-A receptor subunits that reduce activity are implicated, whereas benzodiazepines and barbiturates normally potentiate GABA receptor activity.

All of this is satisfying, but is also potentially a cause for concern. If genetics were only to lead us back to the targets we know about, it would be of little utility. In this regard, the story of the identification of the KCNQ channel mutations in Benign Familial Neonatal Convulsions is an exciting and potentially reassuring counter-example. The neuronal KCNQ channels were unknown before these mutations led to the cloning of the channel genes. It seems possible that a new class of KCNQ opener drugs may be developed, with patterns of clinical usefulness that are quite different from available agents. It is my view that the Na^+ channel and GABA-A subunit mutations should be regarded as "positive controls" that suggest that the

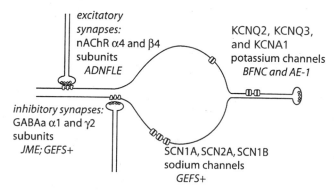

Figure 5. Summary illustration of the variety of channel mutations associated with human epilepsy. Epilepsy is associated with changes in excitatory and inhibitory neurotransmission, generation of action potentials, and neuromodulation. For abbreviations, see text.

identification of mutations underlying hereditary forms of idiopathic epilepsy will be of utility in pinpointing molecular targets for anticonvulsant drug development. One hopes that additional genetic studies will reveal additional novel targets for drug screening.

Many aspects of genotype-phenotype relationships remain poorly understood. For example, in GEFS+ families, it is not known whether the variable phenotype seen within pedigrees may reflect differences in genetic background among individuals, environmental exposures, or both. The spectrum of phenotypes associated with SCN1A mutations, ranging from normal gene carriers or patients with only FS in GEFS+ pedigrees to SMEI patients with severe refractory seizures and progressive motor and cognitive decline, is impressive and requires further study. It is unclear whether the more severe phenotypes in GEFS+ pedigrees and SMEI should be seen as a part of the GEFS+ spectrum, since they are almost certainly associated with changes in brain structure and function (e.g., cell death, network reorganization, changes in the levels of expression of other channels and signaling proteins) that do not occur in mildly affected individuals. Analyzing these and other unforeseen questions arising with the identification of novel epilepsy mutations should prove extremely fruitful toward a better understanding of basic mechanisms underlying seizures and epileptogenesis and especially for drug development.

REFERENCES

1. Kalachikov S, Evgrafov O, Ross B, Winawer M, Barker-Cummings C, Boneschi FM, Choi C, Morozov P, Das K, Teplitskaya E, Yu A, Cayanis E, Penchaszadeh G, Kottmann AH, Pedley TA, Hauser WA, Ottman R, Gilliam TC. Mutations in LGI1 cause autosomal-dominant partial epilepsy with auditory features. Nat Genet 2002; 30:335–341.
2. Hille B. Ionic Channels of Excitable Membranes, 3rd ed. Sunderland, MA: Sinauer, 2001.
3. Scheffer EI, Bhatia KP, Lopes-Cendes, I, Fish DR, Marsden CD, Andermann F, Andermann E, Desbiens R, Cendes F, Manson JI. Autosomal dominant frontal epilepsy misdiagnosed as sleep disorder. Lancet 1994; 343:515–517.
4. Scheffer IE, Bhatia KP, Lopes-Cendes I, Fish DR, Marsden CD, Andermann E, Andermann F, Desbiens R, Keene D, Cendes F. Autosomal dominant nocturnal frontal lobe epilepsy. A distinctive clinical disorder. Brain 1995; 118(Pt 1):61–73.
5. Steinlein OK, Mulley JC, Propping P, Wallace RH, Phillips HA, Sutherland GR, Scheffer IE, Berkovic SF. A missense mutation in the neuronal nicotinic acetylcholine receptor alpha 4 subunit is associated with autosomal dominant nocturnal frontal lobe epilepsy. Nat Genet 1995; 11:201–203.
6. Steinlein OK, Magnusson A, Stoodt J, Bertrand S, Weiland S, Berkovic SF, Nakken KO, Propping P, Bertrand D. An insertion mutation of the CHRNA4 gene in a family with autosomal dominant nocturnal frontal lobe epilepsy. Hum Mol Genet 1997; 6:943–947.
7. De Fusco M, Becchetti A, Patrignani A, Annesi G, Gambardella A, Quattrone A, Ballabio A, Wanke E, Casari G. The nicotinic receptor beta 2 subunit is mutant in nocturnal frontal lobe epilepsy. Nat Genet 2000; 26:275–276.
8. Phillips HA, Favre I, Kirkpatrick M, Zuberi SM, Goudie D, Heron SE, Scheffer IE, Sutherland GR, Berkovic SF, Bertrand D, Mulley JC. CHRNB2 is the second acetylcholine receptor subunit associated with autosomal dominant nocturnal frontal lobe epilepsy. Am J Hum Genet 2001; 68:225–231.
9. Phillips HA, Scheffer IE, Crossland KM, Bhatia KP, Fish DR, Marsden CD, Howell SJ, Stephenson JB, Tolmie J, Plazzi G, Eeg-Olofsson O, Singh R, Lopes-Cendes I, Andermann E, Andermann F, Berkovic SF, Mulley JC. Autosomal dominant nocturnal

frontal-lobe epilepsy: genetic heterogeneity and evidence for a second locus at 15q24. Am J Hum Genet 1998; 63:1108–1116.

10. Bertrand S, Weiland S, Berkovic SF, Steinlein OK, Bertrand D. Properties of neuronal nicotinic acetylcholine receptor mutants from humans suffering from autosomal dominant nocturnal frontal lobe epilepsy. Br J Pharmacol 1998; 125:751–760.

11. Kuryatov A, Gerzanich V, Nelson M, Olale F, Lindstrom J. Mutation causing autosomal dominant nocturnal frontal lobe epilepsy alters Ca^{2+} permeability, conductance, and gating of human alpha4beta2 nicotinic acetylcholine receptors. J Neurosci 1997; 17:9035–9047.

12. Arroyo-Jiminez MM, Bourgeois JP, Marubio LM, Le Sourd AM, Ottersen OP, Rinvik E, Fairen A, Changeux JP. Ultrastructural localization of the alpha4-subunit of the neuronal acetylcholine nicotinic receptor in the rat substantia nigra. J Neurosci 1999; 19:6475–6487.

13. Labarca C, Schwarz J, Deshpande P, Schwarz S, Nowak MW, Fonck C, Nashmi R, Kofuji P, Dang H, Shi W, Fidan M, Khakh BS, Chen Z, Bowers BJ, Boulter J, Wehner JM, Lester HA. Point mutant mice with hypersensitive alpha 4 nicotinic receptors show dopaminergic deficits and increased anxiety. Proc Natl Acad Sci USA 2001; 98:2786–2791.

14. McCormick DA, Bal T. Sleep and arousal: thalamocortical mechanisms. Annu Rev Neurosci 1997; 20:185–215.

15. Van Dyke DH, Griggs RC, Murphy MJ, Goldstein MN. Hereditary myokymia and periodic ataxia. J Neurol Sci 1975; 25:109–118.

16. Gancher ST, Nutt JG. Autosomal dominant episodic ataxia: a heterogeneous syndrome. Mov Disord 1986; 1:239–253.

17. Browne DL, Gancher ST, Nutt JG, Brunt ER, Smith EA, Kramer P, Litt M. Episodic ataxia/myokymia syndrome is associated with point mutations in the human potassium channel gene, KCNA1 [see comments]. Nat Genet 1994; 8:136–140.

18. Zuberi SM, Eunson LH, Spauschus A, De Silva R, Tolmie J, Wood NW, McWilliam RC, Stephenson JP, Kullmann DM, Hanna MG. A novel mutation in the human voltage-gated potassium channel gene (Kv1.1) associates with episodic ataxia type 1 and sometimes with partial epilepsy. Brain 1999; 122:817–825.

19. Jan YN, Jan LY, Dennis MJ. Two mutations of synaptic transmission in *Drosophila*. Proc R Soc Lond Ser B: Biol Sci 1977; 198:87–108.

20. Cooper EC, Jan LY. Ion channel genes and human neurological disease: recent progress, prospects, and challenges. Proc Natl Acad Sci USA 1999; 96:4759–4766.

21. Adelman JP, Bond CT, Pessia M, Maylie J. Episodic ataxia results from voltage-dependent potassium channels with altered functions. Neuron 1995; 15:1449–1454.

22. Zerr P, Adelman JP, Maylie J. Episodic ataxia mutations in Kv1.1 alter potassium channel function by dominant negative effects or haploinsufficiency. J Neurosci 1998; 18:2842–2848.

23. Smart S, Lopantsev V, Zhang CL, Robbins C, Wand H, Chiu SY, Schwartzkroin PA, Messing A, Tempel B. Deletion of the Kv1.1 potassium channel causes epilepsy in mice. Neuron 1998; 20:809–820.

24. Zhang CL, Messing A, Chiu SY. Specific alteration of spontaneous GABAergic inhibition in cerebellar purkinje cells in mice lacking the potassium channel Kv1. 1. J Neurosci 1999; 19:2852–2864.

25. Cooper EC, Milroy A, Jan YN, Jan LY, Lowenstein DH. Presynaptic localization of Kv1.4-containing A-type potassium channels near excitatory synapses in the hippocampus. J Neurosci 1998; 18:965–974.

26. Lubbers WJ, Brunt ER, Scheffer H, Litt M, Stulp R, Browne DL, Van Weerden TW. Hereditary myokymia and paroxysmal ataxia linked to chromosome 12 is responsive to acetazolamide. J Neurol Neurosurg Psychiatry 1995; 59:400–405.

27. Eunson LH, Rea R, Zuberi SM, Youroukos S, Panayiotopoulos CP, Liguori R, Avoni P, McWilliam RC, Stephenson JB, Hanna MG, Kullmann DM, Spauschus A. Clinical, genetic, and expression studies of mutations in the potassium channel gene KCNA1 reveal new phenotypic variability. Ann Neurol 2000; 48:647–656.

28. Rea R, Spauschus A, Eunson LH, Hanna MG, Kullmann DM. Variable K(+) channel subunit dysfunction in inherited mutations of KCNA1. J Physiol 2002; 538:5–23.

29. Rhodes KJ, Keilbaugh SA, Barrezueta NX, Lopez KL, Trimmer JS. Association and colocalization of K$^+$ channel alpha- and beta-subunit polypeptides in rat brain. J Neurosci 1995; 15:5360–5371.

30. Laube G, Roper J, Pitt JC, Sewing S, Kistner U, Garner CC, Pongs O, Veh RW. Ultrastructural localization of Shaker-related potassium channel subunits and synapse-associated protein 90 to septate-like junctions in rat cerebellar pinceaux. Brain Res Mol Brain Res 1996; 42:51–61.

31. Ronen GM, Rosales TO, Connolly M, Anderson VE, Leppert M. Seizure characteristics in chromosome 20 benign familial neonatal convulsions. Neurology 1993; 43:1355–1360.

32. Leppert M, Anderson VE, Quattlebaum T, Stauffer D, O'Connell P, Nakamura Y, Lalouel JM, White R. Benign familial neonatal convulsions linked to genetic markers on chromosome 20. Nature 1989; 337:647–648.

33. Lewis TB, Leach RJ, Ward K, O'Connell P, Ryan SG. Genetic heterogeneity in benign familial neonatal convulsions: identification of a new locus on chromosome 8q. Am J Hum Genet 1993; 53:670–675.

34. Steinlein O, Schuster V, Fischer C, Haussler M. Benign familial neonatal convulsions: confirmation of genetic heterogeneity and further evidence for a second locus on chromosome 8q. Hum Genet 1995; 95:411–415.

35. Singh NA, Charlier C, Stauffer D, DuPont BR, Leach RJ, Melis R, Ronen GM, Bjerre I, Quattlebaum T, Murphy JV, McHarg ML, Gagnon D, Rosales TO, Peiffer A, Anderson VE, Leppert M. A novel potassium channel gene, KCNQ2, is mutated in an inherited epilepsy of newborns [see comments]. Nat Genet 1998; 18:25–29.

36. Charlier C, Singh NA, Ryan SG, Lewis TB, Reus BE, Leach RJ, Leppert M. A pore mutation in a novel KQT-like potassium channel gene in an idiopathic epilepsy family [see comments]. Nat Genet 1998; 18:53–55.

37. Biervert C, Schroeder BC, Kubisch C, Berkovic SF, Propping P, Jentsch TJ, Steinlein OK. A potassium channel mutation in neonatal human epilepsy. Science 1998; 279:403–406.

38. Schroeder BC, Kubisch C, Stein V, Jentsch TJ. Moderate loss of function of cyclic-AMP-modulated KCNQ2/KCNQ3 K channels causes epilepsy. Nature 1998; 396:687–690.

39. Yang WP, Levesque PC, Little WA, Conder ML, Ramakrishnan P, Neubauer MG, Blanar MA. Functional expression of two KvLQT1-related potassium channels responsible for an inherited idiopathic epilepsy. J Biol Chem 1998; 273:19419–19423.

40. Neyroud N, Tesson F, Denjoy I, Leibovici M, Donger C, Barhanin J, Faure S, Gary F, Coumel P, Petit C, Schwartz K, Guicheney P. A novel mutation in the potassium channel gene KVLQT1 causes the Jervell and Lange-Nielsen cardioauditory syndrome [see comments]. Nat Genet 1997; 15:186–189.

41. Wang Q, Curran ME, Splawski I, Burn TC, Millholland JM, VanRaay TJ, Shen J, Timothy KW, Vincent GM, de Jager T, Schwartz PJ, Toubin JA, Moss AJ, Atkinson DL, Landes GM, Connors TD, Keating MT. Positional cloning of a novel potassium channel gene: KVLQT1 mutations cause cardiac arrhythmias. Nat Genet 1996; 12:17–23.

42. Wang H-S, Pan Z, Shi W, Brown BS, Wymore RS, Cohen IS, Dixon JE, McKinnon D. KCNQ2 and KCNQ3 potassium channel subunits: molecular correlates of the M-channel. Science 1998; 282:1890–1893.

43. Brown D. M-currents: an update. Trends Neurosci 1988; 11:294–299.

44. Cooper EC, Harrington E, Jan YN, Jan LY. M-channel KCNQ2 subunits are localized to key sites for control of neuronal network oscillations and synchronization in mouse brain. J Neurosci 2001; 21:9529–9540.

45. Rostock A, Tober C, Rundfeldt C, Bartsch R, Engel J, Polymeropoulos EE, Kutscher B, Löscher W, Hönack D, White HS, Wolf HH. D-23129: a new anticonvulsant with a broad spectrum activity in animal models of epileptic seizures. Epilepsy Res 1996; 23:211–223.

46. Gribkoff VK, Starrett JE Jr, Dworetzky SI, Hewawasam P, Boissard CG, Cook DA, Frantz SW, Heman K, Hibbard JR, Huston K, Johnson G, Krishnan BS, Kinney GG, Lombardo LA, Meanwell NA, Molinoff PB, Myers RA, Moon SL, Ortiz A, Pajor L, Pieschl RL, Post-Munson DJ, Signor LJ, Srinivas N, Taber MT, Thalody G, Trojnacki JT, Wiener H, Yeleswaram K, Yeola SW. Targeting acute ischemic stroke with a calcium-sensitive opener of maxi-K potassium channels. Nat Med 2001; 7:471–477.

47. Schroder RL, Jespersen T, Christophersen P, Strobaek D, Jensen BS, Olesen SP. KCNQ4 channel activation by BMS-204352 and retigabine. Neuropharmacology 2001; 40:888–898.

48. Wickenden AD, Yu W, Zou A, Jegla T, Wagoner PK. Retigabine, a novel anticonvulsant, enhances activation of KCNQ2/Q3 potassium channels. Mol Pharmacol 2000; 58:591–600.

49. Main MJ, Cryan JE, Dupere JR, Cox B, Clare JJ, Burbidge SA. Modulation of KCNQ2/3 potassium channels by the novel anticonvulsant retigabine. Mol Pharmacol 2000; 58:253–262.

50. Rockwood K, Beattie BL, Eastwood MR, Feldman H, Mohr E, Pryse-Phillips W, Gauthier S. A randomized, controlled trial of linopirdine in the treatment of Alzheimer's disease. Can J Neurol Sci 1997; 24:140–145.

50a. Scheffer IE, Berkovic SF. Generalized epilepsy with febrile seizures plus. A genetic disorder with heterogeneous clinical phenotypes. Brain 1997; 120:479–490.

51. Wallace RH, Wang DW, Singh R, Scheffer IE, George AL Jr, Phillips HA, Saar K, Reis A, Johnson EW, Sutherland GR, Berkovic SF, Mulley JC. Febrile seizures and generalized epilepsy associated with a mutation in the Na$^+$-channel beta1 subunit gene SCN1B. Nat Genet 1998; 19:366–370.

52. Wallace RH, Scheffer IE, Parasivam G, Barnett S, Wallace GB, Sutherland GR, Berkovic SF, Mulley JC. Generalized epilepsy with febrile seizures plus: mutation of the sodium channel subunit SCN1B. Neurology 2002; 58:1426–1429.

53. McCormick KA, Isom LL, Ragsdale D, Smith D, Scheuer T, Catterall WA. Molecular determinants of Na$^+$ channel function in the extracellular domain of the beta1 subunit. J Biol Chem 1998; 273:3954–3962.

54. Isom LL. Sodium channel beta subunits: anything but auxiliary. Neuroscientist 2001; 7:42–54.

55. Tammaro P, Conti F, Moran O. Modulation of sodium current in mammalian cells by an epilepsy-correlated beta 1-subunit mutation. Biochem Biophys Res Commun 2002; 291:1095–1101.

56. Baulac S, Gourfinkel-An I, Picard F, Rosenberg-Bourgin M, Prudhomme JF, Baulac M, Brice A, LeGuern E. A second locus for familial generalized epilepsy with febrile seizures plus maps to chromosome 2q21–q33. Am J Hum Genet 1999; 65:1078–1085.

57. Moulard B, Guipponi M, Chaigne D, Mouthon D, Buresi C, Malafosse A. Identification of a new locus for generalized epilepsy with febrile seizures plus (GEFS+) on chromosome 2q24–q33. Am J Hum Genet 1999; 65:1396–1400.

58. Escayg A, MacDonald BT, Meisler MH, Baulac S, Huberfeld G, An-Gourfinkel I, Brice A, LeGuern E, Moulard B, Chaigne D, Buresi C, Malafosse A. Mutations of SCN1A, encoding a neuronal sodium channel, in two families with GEFS+2. Nat Genet 2000; 24:343–345.

59. Wallace RH, Scheffer IE, Barnett S, Richards M, Dibbens L, Desai RR, Lerman-Sagie T, Lev D, Mazarib A, Brand N, Ben-Zeev B, Goikhman I, Singh R, Kremmidiotis G, Gardner A, Sutherland GR, George AL Jr, Mulley JC, Berkovic SF. Neuronal sodium-channel alpha1-subunit mutations in generalized epilepsy with febrile seizures plus. Am J Hum Genet 2001; 68:859–865.

60. Escayg A, Heils A, MacDonald BT, Haug K, Sander T, Meisler MH. A novel SCN1A mutation associated with generalized epilepsy with febrile seizures plus—and prevalence of variants in patients with epilepsy. Am J Hum Genet 2001; 68:866–873.

61. Abou-Khalil B, Ge Q, Desai R, Ryther R, Bazyk A, Bailey R, Haines JL, Sutcliffe JS, George AL Jr. Partial and generalized epilepsy with febrile seizures plus and a novel SCN1A mutation. Neurology 2001; 57:2265–2272.

62. Sugawara T, Mazaki-Miyazaki E, Ito M, Nagafuji H, Fukuma G, Mitsudome A, Wada K, Kaneko S, Hirose S, Yamakawa K. Nav1.1 mutations cause febrile seizures associated with afebrile partial seizures. Neurology 2001; 57:703–705.

63. Lossin C, Wang DW, Rhodes TH, Vanoye CG, George AL Jr. Molecular basis of an inherited epilepsy. Neuron 2002; 34:877 884.

64. Alekov AK, Rahman MM, Mitrovic N, Lehmann-Horn F, Lerche H. Enhanced inactivation and acceleration of activation of the sodium channel associated with epilepsy in man. Eur J Neurosci 2001; 13:2171–2176.

65. Bennett PB, Yazawa K, Makita N, George AL Jr. Molecular mechanism for an inherited cardiac arrhythmia [see comments]. Nature 1995; 376:683–685.

66. Cannon SC, Brown RH Jr, Corey DP. A sodium channel defect in hyperkalemic periodic paralysis: potassium-induced failure of inactivation. Neuron 1991; 6:619–626.

67. Singh R, Andermann E, Whitehouse WP, Harvey AS, Keene DL, Seni MH, Crossland KM, Andermann F, Berkovic SF, Scheffer IE. Severe myoclonic epilepsy of infancy: extended spectrum of GEFS+? Epilepsia 2001; 42:837–844.

68. Claes L, Del-Favero J, Ceulemans B, Lagae L, Van Broeckhoven C, De Jonghe P. De novo mutations in the sodium-channel gene SCN1A cause severe myoclonic epilepsy of infancy. Am J Hum Genet 2001; 68:1327–1332.

69. Sugawara T, Mazaki-Miyazaki E, Fukushima K, Shimomura J, Fujiwara T, Hamano S, Inoue Y, Yamakawa K. Frequent mutations of SCN1A in severe myoclonic epilepsy in infancy. Neurology 2002; 58:1122–1124.

69a. Dravet C. Les epilepsies graves de l'enfant. Vie Med 1978; 8:543–548.

70. Westenbroek RE, Merrick DK, Catterall WA. Differential subcellular localization of the RI and RII Na$^+$ channel subtypes in central neurons. Neuron 1989; 3:695–704.

71. Kearney JA, Plummer NW, Smith MR, Kapur J, Cummins TR, Waxman SG, Goldin AL, Meisler MH. A gain-of-function mutation in the sodium channel gene Scn2a results in seizures and behavioral abnormalities. Neuroscience 2001; 102:307–317.

72. Planells-Cases R, Caprini M, Zhang J, Rockenstein EM, Rivera RR, Murre C, Masliah E, Montal, M. Neuronal death and perinatal lethality in voltage-gated sodium channel alpha(II)-deficient mice. Biophys J 2000; 78:2878–2891.

73. Baulac S, Huberfeld G, Gourfinkel-An I, Mitropoulou G, Beranger A, Prud'homme JF, Baulac M, Brice A, Bruzzone R, LeGuern E. First genetic evidence of GABA(A) receptor dysfunction in epilepsy: a mutation in the gamma2-subunit gene. Nat Genet 2001; 28:46–48.

74. Moss SJ, Smart TG. Constructing inhibitory synapses. Nat Rev Neurosci 2001; 2:240–250.

75. Wallace RH, Marini C, Petrou S, Harkin LA, Bowser DN, Panchal RG, Williams DA, Sutherland GR, Mulley JC, Scheffer IE, Berkovic SF. Mutant GABA(A) receptor gamma2-subunit in childhood absence epilepsy and febrile seizures. Nat Genet 2001; 28:49–52.

76. Harkin LA, Bowser DN, Dibbens LM, Singh R, Phillips F, Wallace RH, Richards MC, Williams DA, Mulley JC, Berkovic SF, Scheffer IE, Petrou S. Truncation of the GABA(A)-receptor gamma2 subunit in a family with generalized epilepsy with febrile seizures plus. Am J Hum Genet 2002; 70:530–536.

77. Janz D. Epilepsy with impulsive petit mal (juvenile myoclonic epilepsy). Acta Neurol Scand 1985; 72:449–459.

78. Cossette P, Liu L, Brisebois K, Dong H, Lortie A, Vanasse M, Saint-Hilaire JM, Carmant L, Verner A, Lu WY, Wang YT, Rouleau GA. Mutation of GABRA1 in an autosomal dominant form of juvenile myoclonic epilepsy. Nat Genet 2002; 31:184–189.

79. Barclay J, Rees M. Mouse models of spike-wave epilepsy. Epilepsia 1999; 40(suppl 3):17–22.

80. Burgess DL, Noebels JL. Single gene defects in mice: the role of voltage-dependent calcium channels in absence models. Epilepsy Res 1999; 36:111–122.

81. Noebels JL, Sidman RL. Inherited epilepsy: spike-wave and focal motor seizures in the mutant mouse tottering. Science 1979; 204:1334–1336.

82. Fletcher CF, Lutz CM, O'Sullivan TN, Shaughnessy JD Jr, Hawkes R, Frankel WN, Copeland NG, Jenkins NA. Absence epilepsy in tottering mutant mice is associated with calcium channel defects. Cell 1996; 87:607–617.

83. Burgess DL, Jones JM, Meisler MH, Noebels JL. Mutation of the Ca^{2+} channel beta subunit gene Cchb4 is associated with ataxia and seizures in the lethargic (lh) mouse. Cell 1997; 88:385–392.

84. Letts VA, Felix R, Biddlecome GH, Arikkath J, Mahaffey CL, Valenzuela A, Bartlett FS 2nd, Mori Y, Campbell KP, Frankel WN. The mouse stargazer gene encodes a neuronal Ca^{2+}-channel gamma subunit. Nat Genet 1998; 19:340–347.

85. Barclay J, Balaguero N, Mione M, Ackerman SL, Letts VA, Brodbeck J, Canti C, Meir A, Page KM, Kusumi K, Perez-Reyes E, Lander ES, Frankel WN, Gardiner RM, Dolphin AC, Rees M. Ducky mouse phenotype of epilepsy and ataxia is associated with mutations in the Cacna2d2 gene and decreased calcium channel current in cerebellar Purkinje cells. J Neurosci 2001; 21:6095–6104.

86. Burgess DL, Biddlecome GH, McDonough SI, Diaz ME, Zilinski CA, Bean BP, Campbell KP, Noebels JL. beta subunit reshuffling modifies N- and P/Q-type Ca^{2+} channel subunit compositions in lethargic mouse brain. Mol Cell Neurosci 1999; 13:293–311.

87. Zhang Y, Mori M, Burgess DL, Noebels JL. Mutations in high-voltage-activated calcium channel genes stimulate low-voltage-activated currents in mouse thalamic relay neurons. J Neurosci 2002; 22:6362–6371.

88. Jouvenceau A, Eunson LH, Spauschus A, Ramesh V, Zuberi SM, Kullmann DM, Hanna MG. Human epilepsy associated with dysfunction of the brain P/Q-type calcium channel. Lancet 2001; 358:801–807.

5
Ontogeny of Molecular Targets of Antiepileptic Drugs: Impact on Drug Choice

Raman Sankar
University of California, Los Angeles
Los Angeles, California, U.S.A.

Jong M. Rho
University of California at Irvine College of Medicine
Irvine, California, U.S.A

INTRODUCTION

Since the introduction of phenobarbital as an antiepileptic drug (AED) in 1912, many thousands of investigational compounds have been screened in acute seizure models. However, only a small fraction of these agents have made it to human clinical trials, and only several dozen such drugs have ultimately been approved for clinical use (1). Most of the AEDs currently used in the epilepsies are believed to regulate ion channels in synaptic terminals of the brain, leading to a net decrease in membrane excitability (2).

Most clinically significant AEDs exert their principal effects on voltage-gated ion channels or those associated with postsynaptic receptors for γ-aminobutyric acid (GABA) or glutamate. Theses sites include: (1) GABA-A receptors; (2) glutamate receptors, including N-methyl-D-aspartate (NMDA) and α-amino-3-hydroxy-5-methyl-4-isoxazoleproprionic acid (AMPA), and kainate receptors; (3) voltage-dependent sodium channels; and (4) voltage-dependent calcium channels. Prominent examples include use-dependent blockade of voltage-gated sodium channels by phenytoin (PHT) and carbamazepine (CBZ), and augmentation of inhibitory GABA-A receptors by benzodiazepines and barbiturates. That the putative molecular targets of currently available AEDs are largely limited to a few membrane-bound ion channels and enzymes affecting neurotransmitter metabolism underscores the need for identifying newer (and perhaps more important) targets for intervention.

Recent research attempting to reveal the mechanisms of action of AEDs have focused on what appears to be a growing multiplicity of molecular targets, whereas investigations aimed at elucidating changes associated with the epileptic condition have revealed subunit rearrangements and differential expression of targets such as GABA-A and glutamate receptors (3,4). However, there is virtually no published information regarding how the ontogeny of molecular targets, whether associated with brain development or involved in the pathogenesis of epilepsy, predicts pharmacodynamic effects and ultimately clinical efficacy. In this chapter, we review recent studies that address the question of whether truly rational drug choice must take into account developmental and pathophysiological differences in the receptor targets of AEDs.

GLUTAMATE RECEPTOR ANTAGONISTS

What have we learned mechanistically about novel AEDs that have become available in the past 7 years? There are two examples worthy of mention: felbamate (FBM) and topiramate (TPM). FBM is a broad-spectrum AED that exerts dual and opposing actions on NMDA and GABA-A receptors, the first agent exhibiting such activity in the same clinically relevant concentration range (5). It is now well established that there is a marked surge in glutamate receptor expression early in brain development (concurrent with the period of intense synaptogenesis), and that early-onset seizures may arise in part due to overactivation of these receptors (6). Thus, inhibition of glutamate receptors may represent one important mechanism of AED action particularly relevant to the developing brain. Recently, it was demonstrated that FBM exhibits some selectivity for NMDA receptors composed of NR1A and NR2B subunits, the latter of which is found more abundantly than other NR2 subunits in the immature brain (7). This finding may in part account for FBM's clinical utility in pediatric epileptic disorders such as the Lennox-Gastaut syndrome (8).

While FBM was shown to antagonize NMDA-mediated Ca^{2+} currents, TPM antagonizes Na^+ currents mediated by the action of glutamate on non-NMDA receptors, which are sensitive to kainic acid (KA) or AMPA. It has been demonstrated that a single dose of TPM administered prior to global hypoxia-ischemia in rats at P10 (roughly equivalent to a human term newborn) not only suppressed acute seizures, but decreased later susceptibility to kainate-induced seizures and seizure-induced neuronal injury (9). In a study that subjected weanling rats to status epilepticus (SE) and then treated them with TPM for 4 weeks, TPM provided a moderate degree of neuroprotection, with TPM-treated rats performing better in the water maze than rats receiving saline (10). These authors demonstrated that chronic treatment with TPM following SE improved cognitive function. Further, this study showed that long-term administration of TPM in the normal developing rat brain did not impair spatial learning and memory as tested by the Morris water maze.

One may argue that the multiple mechanisms of action described for TPM could contribute to the observed protective effect. However, this is unlikely, since as discussed later in this review, GABA-ergic agonists have been shown to produce neuronal apoptosis at this developmental stage (11,12). Such an effect is also known to occur with blockers of voltage-gated Na^+ channels (12). The effect of TPM on voltage-gated Na^+ channels is very gradual (unlike that of phenytoin and lamotrigine) and is not exhibited by all neurons (13). It should also be mentioned that the neuroprotective and potential antiepileptogenic effect of TPM is reminiscent of the effect of 6-nitro-7-sulfamoylbenzo(f)quinoxaline-2,3-dione (NBQX), a selective antagonist of AMPA-sensitive glutamate receptors (14).

Another interesting aspect of developmental pharmacology pertaining to AEDs deserves mention here. While blockade of the action of glutamate at AMPA- and kainate-sensitive sites is associated with neuroprotective and potential anti-epileptogenic actions in the immature brain, such is not the case for antagonism of NMDA-sensitive sites. Even though the NMDA receptor remains an important target for the design of antagonists calculated to provide neuroprotection in the mature brain, open-channel blockers of the NMDA receptor (such as phencyclidine, MK-801) actually produce widespread neuronal apoptosis in the immature brain (15,16).

In the absence of human data, it is difficult to state with confidence what the clinical implications are for treating infants with glutamate receptor antagonists. Nevertheless, the animal data suggest that topiramate could ultimately find a distinctive niche for clinical use in the very young. The authors believe it is extremely important to initiate clinical trials to evaluate this possibility. On the other hand, the safety of FBM in the very immature brain cannot be readily taken for granted, given its action on multiple sites (blockade of voltage-gated Na^+ channels and calcium flux through NMDA receptors, as well as potentiation of GABA-A receptor-mediated Cl^- currents), all of which have been connected to neuronal injury in immature rodents.

GABA-ERGIC MODULATION

The heteropentameric GABA-A receptor is coupled to a chloride channel, and has an agonist site for GABA and several allosteric modulatory recognition sites for barbiturates, benzodiazepines (BZD), and neurosteroids, among others. There are several features of interest regarding the ontogeny of GABA-ergic function. In the immature brain, GABA has been demonstrated to function as an excitatory neuro-transmitter (17) at postsynaptic sites. As development progresses, the function of "fast" or early depolarization mediated by GABA is replaced by glutamatergic action at AMPA-sensitive sites. This action results in the depolarization that removes the voltage-dependent Mg^{2+} block of the NMDA-sensitive Ca^{2+} channel to provide for the "late" phase of sustained depolarization. The depolarization mediated by GABA is a consequence of the embryonic expression of the Na^+-K^+-$2Cl^-$ cotransporter NKCC1, which is inwardly directed and thus accumulates Cl^- within cells (18,19).

In the rat, this transformation of the role of GABA from excitatory to inhibitory neurotransmission is estimated to occur around postnatal day 5 (P5), which in human terms corresponds to a stage somewhat earlier than that of a term newborn. A P7–P10 rat pup is considered to be roughly equivalent to a term newborn human, but we do not know exactly when such a transformation from GABA-ergic depolarization to hyperpolarization is completed. However, we do know that this phenomenon correlates well with the dramatic increase of expression after the first postnatal week of the K^+-Cl^- cotransporter KCC2, which extrudes Cl^- from the cell (19–21).

Current data support the view that the properties of embryonic or early postnatal GABA-A receptor isoforms differ markedly from those expressed in the adult brain (22). The ontogeny of the expression of the subunits that contribute to the GABA receptor has been studied in the marmoset monkey by Hornung and Fritschy (23). The BZD-sensitive $\alpha1$ subunit begins to be expressed shortly before birth, and dramatically replaces the $\alpha2$ after birth. The $\beta2$ and $\beta3$ subunits, also important for BZD action, were ubiquitous at every age examined. Nevertheless, Kapur and Macdonald (24) showed that the sensitivity to diazepam was increased in granule cells isolated from P28–35 rats more than fourfold compared to that in cells obtained from P7–14 rat pups. By P45–52, the sensitivity to BZD increased to >25-fold compared to P7–14. Such an increase in sensitivity to BZD was attributed to the gradual *disappearance* of the $\beta1$ subunit. These data, when cautiously extended to the human, would suggest that the BZD sensitivity of GABA receptors develops mainly postnatally, and increases through childhood and adolescence to young adulthood.

In terms of practical application to clinical situations, the pharmacokinetic changes with development impact on the selection of AED doses as well. However, the data described above raise some concerns about whether BZD are reasonable choices in the extremely immature brain. Over and beyond the excitatory versus inhibitory role of GABA and the questionable sensitivity of the extremely immature GABA-A receptor to BZD, there is another concern regarding the application of GABA-ergic medications to the immature brain. A variety of GABA-A agonists, including ethanol, barbiturates, and BZD, cause widespread neuronal apoptosis in the immature brain (11,12). In the rodent, this toxicity disappears before P21.

Felbamate (FBM) was demonstrated to possess actions on both NMDA and GABA-A receptors (5). The GABA-ergic action of FBM could not be demonstrated in receptors containing the $\beta1$ subunit along with the $\alpha1$ and the $\gamma2$ subunits (Simeone et al. unpublished observations). However, receptors containing either the $\beta2$ or the $\beta3$ subunits in combination with the $\alpha1$ and the $\gamma2$ subunits were able to exhibit enhancement of GABA-mediated chloride currents. The sensitivity of a heteromeric receptor containing $\beta1$ subunit in combination with a $\beta2$ or $\beta3$ subunit is not known. As described earlier, there is a switch from $\alpha2$ to $\alpha1$ in the postnatal brain.

Topiramate is another novel broad-spectrum agent that enhances GABA-A receptor-mediated chloride flux (25) and, among additional actions, blocks kainate-activated currents (26,27). GABA-A receptor subunit expression in the central nervous system is differentially regulated. In single dentate granule cells from epileptic hippocampi, selective changes in GABA-A receptor subunit expression have been identified, with the $\alpha4$ subunit being prominently coexpressed (3). Interestingly, TPM was recently found to be a potent allosteric modulator of GABA-A receptors containing the $\alpha4$ subunit (28), suggesting that this mechanism may account for its efficacy against partial seizures of temporal lobe origin.

Studies that have evaluated the expression of GABA-A receptor subunits as a function of development, or as a consequence of epilepsy, have been limited largely by the methods employed. Specifically, these experimental approaches were not sensitive enough to determine the subcellular localization of these receptors. In spite of the recent dramatic advances in molecular biology, the functioning of the nervous system cannot be adequately described without detailed anatomic specifications. Recent data suggest that $\alpha4$-containing GABA-A receptors are predominantly *extrasynaptic* and may have their principal role in mediating *tonic* inhibition, rather than the better-understood *phasic* inhibition resulting from presynaptice release of GABA which then acts on postsynaptic receptors containing the α1 subunit (29). Further, because these extrasynaptic receptors, which also tend to contain the δ subunit, exhibit much higher affinity for GABA than those that mediate synaptic inhibition (and also do not inactivate rapidly like the latter), drugs that increase brain GABA may disproportionately increase tonic inhibition.

Thus, a case can also be made that enhanced expression of α4-containing GABA-A receptors, which are extrasynaptic, may promote synchronization by augmenting tonic inhibition. Indeed, such a mechanism may explain in part the well-described exacerbation of generalized spike-waves in animals and humans by AEDs such as vigabatrin (30–32) or tiagabine (33–36), both of which increase GABA concentrations. Clinical reports suggest that this effect is seen in children as well as adults.

Recent studies have suggested that α4- or α6-containing GABA-A receptors often contain the δ subunit rather than the γ subunit and are thus insensitive to BZD, exhibit high affinity for GABA, and do not inactivate rapidly (29,37). Given this fact, one may need to reevaluate the implications of older data addressing GABA receptor subunit expression patterns during development (as well as during epileptogenesis), especially as these relate to strategies employed during AED development.

Finally, what can we say about the ontogeny of GABA systems that may explain the distinctive efficacy of vigabatrin (38–40), an inhibitor of GABA-transaminase (GABA-T), against infantile spasms? A study in human fetal brains suggests that all the key enzymes involved in GABA neurochemistry show peak expression around 25–26 weeks gestational age (41). However, the typical age of onset of spasms is postnatal, peaking between 3 and 7 months. Sankar and colleagues had demonstrated that, under conditions of stress imposed by status epilepticus, GABA synthesis is maintained maximally in the immature hippocampus and declines with development (42). However, there does not appear to be a major role for the hippocampus in the genesis of these seizures. It is increasingly likely that the effect of vigabatrin in infantile spasms, especially those associated with tuberous sclerosis, could be independent of its effect on GABA-T and brain GABA levels. Certainly, other GABA-ergic drugs (e.g., phenobarbital, benzodiazepines, and even tiagabine) are clearly not as efficacious as vigabatrin in the treatment of infantile spasms.

NOVEL MOLECULAR TARGETS AND CONCEPTS

Interaction of an AED with Currents Mediated by nAChR

In 1995, Steinlein and associates were the first to demonstrate that autosomal-dominant nocturnal frontal lobe epilepsy (ADNFLE) was due to mutations in one of the subunits comprising the nicotinic acetylcholine receptor (nAChR) (43; see Chapter 4 by Cooper in this volume). The major brain nAChR assembly possesses the stoichiometry of two α4 and three β2 subunits. Bertrand et al. (44) studied the biophysical properties of mutated (α4 and β2 mutations found in humans with ADNFLE, homozygous and heterozygous) nAChRs expressed in *Xenopus* oocytes. Their results suggest that a gain-of-function mutation may be at the heart of the network dysfunction that causes the epileptic seizures. In general, all mutants exhibited a greater sensitivity to ACh and altered inactivation of the ACh-evoked Ca^{2+} currents.

It is known that most patients with ADNFLE respond well to CBZ (45). Picard and coworkers (46) had shown that CBZ blocks the ACh-mediated currents in a noncompetitive manner, suggesting a channel blocking mode of action. A recent study from Bertrand et al. (44), in which various known mutations were studied pharmacologically in an in vitro expression system, revealed that some mutations (α4S248F, α4L776ins3, and β2V287M) give rise to receptors that are more sensitive to CBZ than others (α4S252L). Interestingly, the α4S252L mutation was first encountered in a Japanese family (47), and it appears that the children in this pedigree often do not respond to AEDs (48). Thus, it appears that the nAChR-associated channel may constitute a novel target for AEDs.

Potassium Channels

The last decade has witnessed remarkable advances in our understanding of the genetics of epilepsy and other paroxysmal neurological disorders. The term "channelopathy" is now well accepted in scientific circles, referring to a disease state believed to arise from mutations in ion channel genes. As an example, benign familial neonatal convulsions (BFNC), a rare form of inherited seizure disorder, was recently linked to mutations in two novel potassium channel genes, KCNQ2 and KCNQ3 (49,50). These genes encode subunits that contribute to the KCNQ2/3 K^+ channel heteromultimer that mediates neuronal M-type currents. These currents are important regulators of membrane excitability. Retigabine, a novel AED with broad efficacy in animal seizure models (51), enhances activation of KCNQ2/Q3 potassium channels (52–55).

BFNC, attributed to mutations in KCNQ2/3 genes, tends to remit before 6 months of age in most patients. One might wonder whether the ability of retigabine to augment M-type K^+ currents is in fact relevant to modifying seizures in the mature organism, and if so, to what degree. As mentioned earlier, retigabine's efficacy in animal models is broad (51). Further, Rundfelt and Netzer (56) have shown that retigabine augments GABA mediated Cl^- currents only at a 100-fold greater concentration (10 μM) compared to that shown to be effective in promoting K^+ currents (0.1 μM). Inhibitory effects observed on voltage-activated Na^+ and Ca^{2+} channels, as well as on kainate-induced currents, were only observed at the highest concentration tested (100 μM), and can be considered nonspecific. No significant interaction with NMDA-induced currents was observed. Thus, the effect of retigabine on M-type K^+ currents may be quite important to its broad anticonvulsant action. None of the available AEDs are known to interact with M-type currents, but this target now represents an intense focus of interest for future drug development (57).

Hyperpolarization-Activated Cation Channels

The well-described phenomenon of use-dependent blockade of voltage-gated Na^+ channels is insufficient to explain the broader spectrum of clinical efficacy shown by lamotrigine (LTG) when compared to PHT or CBZ. Continuing interest in the exploration of novel targets for AED action has led to an exciting observation that could pharmacologically distinguish LTG from PHT and CBZ. Poolos et al. (58)

recently demonstrated that LTG selectively reduced action potential firing from dendritic depolarization while minimally affecting firing at the soma, an effect that was not demonstrable with either PHT or CBZ. The anatomically specific action of LTG resulted from an increase in the hyperpolarization-induced cation current (I_h), a voltage-gated current present predominantly in dendrites.

The importance of this particular effect of LTG is that these channels are critical in the generation of pacemaker currents within thalamocortical circuits (59,60). Since the thalamocortical pacemaker forms the basis for the generation of generalized oscillatory activity (more specifically, generalized spike-waves in the pathological condition), this property of LTG provides a reasonable explanation for its antiabsence activity. It should be emphasized, however, that the ability of LTG to affect I_h was not by rational design. Rather, it was a byproduct of continued efforts to correlate more closely the mechanistic profile of AEDs with the distinctive spectrum of activities encountered in clinical practice.

What do we know about I_h and development? The hyperpolarization-induced cationic currents are mediated by channel proteins called HCN channels. The genes for HCN1, HCN2, HCN3, and HCN4 have been cloned (61). Homomeric channels containing HCN1, HCN2, or HCN4 are differentially expressed in the developing hippocampus such that HCN-mediated pacing activity is generated in hippocampal interneurons associated with the Ammon's horn prior to those in the hilus of the dentate gyrus (62). It is conceivable that any disturbance in these currents during development, such as that caused by a prolonged seizure, may affect hippocampal development. Indeed, such appears to be the case when P10 rat pups are subjected to hyperthermic seizures (63). In these animals, I_h was permanently enhanced and interacted with the potentiated inhibition (64) to convert the system to frequency-dependent hyperexcitability.

What Is the Site of Action for Levetiracetam?

Levetiracetam (LEV) is novel in its drug development heritage as well as in its mode of action. Its heritage is unique because it survived the anticonvulsant screening process in spite of its lack of activity in both the electroshock convulsive model and the threshold pentylenetetrazol model (65). From reports that have appeared subsequent to its clinical development and regulatory approval, understanding of its action at very distinctive and novel sites is emerging. Levetiracetam has been shown to block *synchronization* in brain slice experiments in which conventional AEDs such as valproic acid, benzodiazepines, and CBZ were inactive (66). Klitgaard et al. (67) have also confirmed this finding by in vivo recordings in the rat pilocarpine model of temporal lobe epilepsy. This is quite exciting because conventional AEDs impact mainly neuronal hyperexcitability, even though the two sine qua non conditions of the epileptic state are hypersynchrony and hyperexcitability. How does LEV accomplish this? Could it be antagonize currents mediated by gap junctions that are responsible for "local" synchrony? We do not know for certain, but more thoughts on this fascinating concept can be found in the chapter by Dr. Dudek that discusses nonsynaptic mechanisms of synchronization.

While hyperexcitability may underlie some of the genetic epilepsies now recognized as ion channelopathies, the acquired epilepsies seem to reveal anatomic and physiologic evidence of seizure-associated circuit rearrangement which may be, in part, the basis for their intractability. While space does not permit extensive discussion of the role of mossy fiber sprouting in the epileptogenic process in this chapter, it should be mentioned that mossy fiber sprouting is seen in experimental models of temporal lobe epilepsy as well as in human hippocampi resected during surgical treatment of mesial temporal lobe epilepsy.

Mossy fiber synapses release zinc, and zinc antagonizes GABA-mediated inhibition. Coulter (68) has shown that the GABA receptors in the granule cells of the epileptic hippocampus have undergone subunit changes that render them even more sensitive to the antagonism of GABA-ergic inhibition by zinc. It turns out that LEV can reverse the inhibitory effect of zinc on GABA-mediated currents (69). This selective effect of LEV on a brain that has already undergone circuit rearrangement is consistent with the intriguing preclinical observation that LEV was ineffective in acute seizure models, but was active in a chronic epileptic brain. Once again, the lesson learned from the study of LEV is that we have become aware of two other novel sites as potential targets for anticonvulsant action, but LEV was not specifically developed with an understanding of these as target sites!

It Is Déjà Vu All Over Again! Carbonic Anhydrase as a Target?

The use of acetazolamide as an adjunctive anticonvulsant, especially in specific situations such as catamenial epilepsy and absence epilepsy is a time-honored tradition. Clinicians are familiar with the technique of hyperventilation to induce alkalosis, which can precipitate a paroxysm of absence seizure activity in susceptible children. In most discussions reviewing the modes of action of agents such as TPM and zonisamide (ZNS), their ability to inhibit carbonic anhydrase has been relegated to minor importance, but is usually invoked to explain the annoying side effects. However, there may be more to this than just funny taste and tingling.

It has been shown that GABA-A receptors are sensitive to extracellular pH (70). In expression studies conducted with *Xenopus* oocytes, acidic extracellular pH (6.4) augmented the current evoked by $100\,\mu$M GABA, whereas basic pH (8.4) decreased it relative to the current evoked at a pH 7.4. Aram and Lodge (71) showed years ago that epileptiform activity could be induced in a slice preparation by alkalosis, and that even a change in pH of 0.2 units produced a substantial increase in discharges. Subsequently, Velíšek et al. (72) confirmed that acidosis suppressed epileptiform discharges evoked by low Mg^{2+} in a combined entorhinal cortex-hippocampus slice preparation. They attributed the effect to proton blockade of NMDA receptors. Consistent with that notion, mild acidosis was shown to be neuroprotective to cerebellar granule cells in primary culture (73). Thus, it appears that even a mild downward shift in extracellular pH could simultaneously augment GABA-ergically mediated Cl^- currents and suppress NMDA receptor-mediated excitatory currents.

Another interesting observation was made by Staley and colleagues (74). They demonstrated that when GABA-A receptors are intensely activated by barbiturates or benzodiazepines, the dendritic receptors excite, rather than inhibit. Owing to collapse of the concentration gradient, Cl^- accumulated intracellularly through dendritic receptors, and concomitantly, bicarbonate efflux was observed. This is a depolarizing effect as such, but the shift in extracellular pH accompanying this could lower the voltage-dependent Mg^{2+} block of the NMDA-mediated Ca^{2+} current. This sequence of events can be abolished by inhibiting intracellular carbonic anhydrase, which is required to form bicarbonate ion from CO_2. It remains to be seen whether the clinical success of TPM and ZNS will encourage further attempts to capitalize on carbonic anhydrase inhibition as a strategy to manipulate neuronal excitability.

Revisiting an Old Friend—The Voltage-Gated Sodium Channel

Genetic studies of the syndrome of Generalized Epilepsy with Febrile Seizures Plus (GEFS+) have led to the identification of several mutations subunits that comprise the voltage-gated sodium channel. Additionally, the Dravet syndrome, otherwise known as Severe Myoclonic Epilepsy of Infancy (SMEI), is considered within the spectrum of ion channelopathies involving the voltage-gated sodium channel. This subject is discussed in detail in Chapter 4 by Cooper in this volume.

In general, there is a paucity of information on the ontogeny of brain sodium channels. Further, it is interesting to note that the classic AEDs that modulate voltage-gated Na^+ channel are not particularly useful in treating febrile convulsions or myoclonic epilepsies. In fact, the latter may be exacerbated by available Na^+ channel antagonists (75). One would have to conclude that present state of knowledge does not permit targeting these channels for novel anticonvulsant action.

What Underlies the Unique Efficacy of Zonisamide in Progressive Myoclonic Epilepsies?

There have been numerous reports describing the unusual efficacy of ZNS in treating the progressive myoclonic epilepsies (76–78), all of which are considered neurodegenerative conditions arising from diverse etiologies. Why certain neurodegenerative syndromes produce myoclonus (and more specifically, myoclonic seizures) is unknown. Further, the manner in which certain AEDs interact with the pathogenic process to produce amelioration is incompletely understood.

In considering the known mechanisms of action of ZNS, two aspects of its pharmacology distinguish it from other AEDs. First, it appears to have an ability to function as an antioxidant and quench free radicals (79,80), which implies a neuroprotective action. Secondly, it has been shown to enhance serotonin levels at plasma concentrations associated with anticonvulsive activity (81). Given the prominent role of serotonergic systems in rodent models of myoclonus (82), it has been speculated that this unique action of ZNS might underlie its effects against myoclonic seizures. However, nonepileptic or subcortical myoclonus involving serotonergic modulation is considered somewhat distinct from myoclonic seizures that are associated with cortical epileptiform discharges. Therefore, one should remain cautious about invoking serotonergic modulation as the relevant mechanism of ZNS's efficacy against myoclonic seizures. It should be further noted that, in general, commercial enthusiasm for targeting serotonergic systems has been more focused on the lucrative migraine and psychiatric markets than on symptoms affecting rare neurodegenerative disorders.

IMPACT ON DRUG CHOICE

How does the previous information affect our decision making with regard to AED choice? At a clinical level, it is unclear whether choosing medications based on mechanisms alone affords any particular advantages. The basic problem is that every AED in fact possesses multiple mechanisms; what is more difficult is to determine which of the mechanisms are clinically relevant. Further, there are likely additional mechanisms for both old and newer AEDs that have yet to be defined.

Nevertheless, some attempt has been made to address this question clinically at the Western Infirmary in Glasgow, Scotland (83–85). Brodie and Yuen (83) found that, among a group of refractory patients, the addition of LTG to VPA (64% responders) produced a significantly better response ($P < .001$) than adding it to CBZ (41% responders) or PHT (38% responders). This effect was seen for partial (VPA, 57%; CBZ, 39%; PHT, 39%; $P < .02$) as well as tonic-clonic seizures (VPA, 70%; CBZ, 53%; PHT, 50%; NS). These data suggested to the authors the possibility of therapeutic synergy between LTG and VPA. Stephen et al. (84) reported a couple cases in which addition of a small dose of TPM to the patients' regimen of LTG resulted in dramatic improvement in seizure control, even though these patients had failed other combinations that included LTG. Indeed, we have encountered cases of youngsters with the Lennox-Gastaut syndrome who responded in such a manner. Stephen and colleagues (84) also provided animal data in which the combination of LTG and TPM prevented seizures provoked by pentylenetetrazol during the observation period, even though neither of the drugs demonstrated the ability to do so independently.

Inspired by such observations, Kwan and Brodie (85) compared the effect of treating patients with combinations of AEDs who were refractory to the first tolerated AED or an AED substitution. Of the patients treated with AED combinations ($n = 42$), 36% of those treated with the combination of a sodium channel blocker with a drug with multiple mechanisms of action became seizure free, compared to 7% treated with other combinations ($p = .05$). The authors are gratified by this study and the ongoing prospective studies under way in Glasgow, since we have argued unabashedly for some time that a mechanistic understanding of AED action, applied to clinical scenarios, can potentially improve patient outcomes. Conversely, such mechanistic knowledge can help avoid seizure exacerbation in certain clinical situations. As a concrete example, we now understand that certain GABA-ergic drugs, based on preclinical data in animal models and the GABA pharmacology, can have the potential for seizure deterioration or nonconvulsive status epilepticus in some patients.

There are, of course, other factors that modify the selection of an AED for specific circumstances. Age-dependent idiosyncratic toxicities have been described for some AEDs (see chapter in this volume by Glauser) and a consideration of the impact of induction or inhibition of drug-metabolizing enzymes may guide choices based as well on concomitant medications. The ontogenetic aspects of the drug-metabolizing systems presently influence pharmacokinetic parameters pertaining to dosing strategies more than the absolute choice of an AED.

Another interesting new finding pertains to the role of genes responsible for the expression of multiple drug resistance (MDR) proteins in epilepsy (for further details, see chapter in this volume by Kapur and Bertram). These proteins were initially described in the oncology literature, specifically from investigations aimed at determining the mechanisms of resistance to chemotherapeutic agents. Multiple drug resistance proteins (e.g., MDR1) may restrict the access of certain drugs (e.g., phenytoin) to the site of action in the brain of certain patients. Siddiqui et al. (86)

found that, when compared to drug-responsive patients, AED-refractory patients were more likely to exhibit a specific genetic polymorphism in the MDR1 gene. Others have shown overexpression of MDR1 protein in experimental seizures in animals (87,88), in the capillary endothelium of resected human epileptic tissue (89), and in several common causes of refractory epilepsy, including dysembryoplastic neuroepithelial tumors, focal cortical dysplasia, and hippocampal sclerosis (90).

Our present understanding is that MDRs play a role in "buffering" and possibly extruding certain drugs, and not others. We also suspect that increased expression may be a feature of chronic, and presumably drug-refractory epilepsy. We know very little about the developmental aspects of this system. In a simple experiment, we showed that developing rat pups subjected to SE did not show enhanced expression of MDR1 in the astrocytes and that these animals thus maintained their sensitivity to PHT well into a bout of SE (91), a finding at variance with that seen in mature rats (92). Our present knowledge of manipulating this system to enhance clinical efficacy is mostly incomplete. Nevertheless, this field of inquiry is raising questions about variables in drug selection that go beyond the activity of drugs on ion channels, native and mutated, to a plastic system that may exclude certain drugs with progressively increasing efficiency. Can this system be manipulated to help the patient with epilepsy and improve the safety profile of AEDs?

SUMMARY

In the past decade, numerous studies have identified basic structural and functional alterations in epileptic tissue from animals and humans (93). Among these, include changes in the expression of immediate early genes, alterations in cellular and network inhibition, cell- and region-specific cell damage/death, differential molecular composition of receptor channels, and aberrant synaptic reorganization. With further characterization of these changes, new targets for intervention in the processes of seizure genesis and/or epileptogenesis are likely to be identified. However, it has been difficult to link a specific molecular or cellular change in a causal manner to the condition that generates spontaneous recurrent seizures. The challenge will be to delineate which basic changes are required and sufficient for producing the epileptic state, and which are merely epiphenomena. In so doing, development of new AEDs may be directed not only in a more rational manner, but will also reflecting the unique changes that occur normally and pathologically in the developing brain.

Yet despite the explosion of information regarding molecular alterations associated with the epileptic condition, in both animal models and human epileptic tissue, this information has not translated yet to a better understanding of how current AED choices can be made on the basis of changes in the pharmacosensitivity and responsiveness of molecular targets, changes that likely reflect (at least in developing brain) an interplay of normal ontogeny superimposed with pathophysiological insults.

REFERENCES

1. Porter RJ, Rogawski MA. New antiepileptic drugs: from serendipity to rational discovery. Epilepsia 1992; 33(suppl 1):S1–S6.

2. Rho JM, Sankar R. The pharmacological basis of antiepileptic drug action. Epilepsia 1999; 40:1471–1483.

3. Brooks-Kayal AR, Shumate MD, Jin H, Rikhter TY, Coulter DA. Selective changes in single cell GABA$_A$ receptor subunit expression and function in temporal lobe epilepsy. Nat Med 1998; 10:1166–1172.

4. Coulter DA. Epilepsy-associated plasticity in gamma-aminobutyric acid receptor expression, function, and inhibitory synaptic properties. Int Rev Neurobiol 2001; 45:237–252.

5. Rho JM, Donevan SD, Rogawski MA. Mechanism of action of the anticonvulsant felbamate: opposing effects on N-methyl-D-aspartate and γ-aminobutyric acid$_A$ receptors. Ann Neurol 1994; 35:229–234.

6. Sanchez RM, Jensen FE. Maturational aspects of epilepsy mechanisms and consequences for the immature brain. Epilepsia 2001; 42:577–585.

7. Harty TP, Rogawski MA. Felbamate block of recombinant N-methyl-D-aspartate receptors: selectivity for the NR2B subunit. Epilepsy Res 2000; 39:47–55.

8. Ritter FJ et al. Efficacy of felbamate in childhood epileptic encephalopathy (Lennox-Gastaut syndrome). The Felbamate Study Group in Lennox-Gastaut Syndrome. N Engl J Med 1993; 328:29–33.

9. Koh S, Jensen FE. Topiramate blocks perinatal hypoxia-induced seizures in rat pups. Ann Neurol 2001; 50:366–372.

10. Cha BH, Silveira DC, Liu X, Hu Y, Holmes GL. Effect of topiramate following recurrent and prolonged seizures during early development. Epilepsy Res 2002; 51:217–232.

11. Ikonomidou C, Bittigau P, Ishimaru MJ, et al. Ethanol-induced neurodegeneration and fetal alcohol syndrome. Science 2000; 287:1056–1060.

12. Bittigau P, Sifringer M, Genz K, et al. Antiepileptic drugs and apoptotic neurodegeneration in the developing brain. Proc Natl Acad Sci USA 2002; 99:15089–15094.

13. McLean MJ, Bukhari AA, Wamil AW. Effects of topiramate on sodium-dependent action-potential firing by mouse spinal cord neurons in cell culture. Epilepsia 2000; 41(suppl 1):S21–S24.

14. Jensen FE, Blume H, Alvarado S, Firkusny I, Geary C. NBQX blocks acute and late epileptogenic effects of perinatal hypoxia. Epilepsia 1995; 36:966–972.

15. Ikonomidou C, Bosch F, Miksa M, Bittigau P, Vockler J, Dikranian K, Tenkova TI, Stefovska V, Turski L, Olney JW. Blockade of NMDA receptors and apoptotic neurodegeneration in the developing brain. Science 1999; 283:70–74.

16. Ikonomidou C, Stefovska V, Turski L. Neuronal death enhanced by N-methyl-D-aspartate antagonists. Proc Natl Acad Sci USA 2000; 97:12885–12890.

17. Cherubini E, Rovira C, Gaiarsa JL, Corradetti R, Ben Ari Y. GABA mediated excitation in immature rat CA3 hippocampal neurons. Int J Dev Neurosci 1990; 8:481–490.

18. Plotkin MD, Snyder EY, Hebert SC, Delpire E. Expression of the Na-K-2Cl cotransporter is developmentally regulated in postnatal rat brains: a possible mechanism underlying GABA's excitatory role in immature brain. J Neurobiol 1997; 33:781–795.

19. Clayton GH, Owens GC, Wolff JS, Smith RL. Ontogeny of cation-Cl-cotransporter expression in rat neocortex. Brain Res Dev Brain Res 1998; 109:281–292.

20. Lu J, Karadsheh M, Delpire E. Developmental regulation of the neuronal-specific isoform of K$^+$-Cl$^-$-cotransporter KCC2 in postnatal rat brains. J Neurobiol 1999; 39:558–568.

21. Rivera C, Voipio J, Payne JA, Ruusuvuori E, Lahtinen H, Lamsa K, Pirvola U, Saarma M, Kaila K. The K$^+$-Cl$^-$-cotransporter KCC2 renders GABA hyperpolarizing during neuronal maturation. Nature 1999; 397:251–255.

22. Simeone TA, Donevan SD, Rho JM. Molecular biology and ontogeny of GABA$_A$ and GABA$_B$ receptors in the mammalian central nervous system. J Child Neurol 2003; 18:39–48.

23. Hornung JP, Fritschy JM. Developmental profile of GABA-A receptors in the marmoset monkey: expression of distinct subtypes in pre- and postnatal brain. J Comp Neurol 1996; 367:413–430.

24. Kapur J, Macdonald RL. Postnatal development of hippocampal dentate granule cell γ-aminobutyric acid$_A$ receptor pharmacological properties. Mol Pharmacol 1999; 55:444–452.

25. White HS, Brown SD, Woodhead JH, Skeen GA, Wolf HH. Topiramate enhances GABA-mediated chloride flux and GABA-evoked chloride currents in murine brain neurons and increases seizure threshold. Epilepsy Res 1997; 28:167–179.

26. Gibbs JW 3rd, Sombati S, DeLorenzo RJ, Coulter DA. Cellular actions of topiramate: blockade of kainate-evoked inward currents in cultured hippocampal neurons. Epilepsia 2000; 41(suppl 1):S10–S16.

27. Skradski S, White HS. Topiramate blocks kainate-evoked cobalt influx into cultured neurons. Epilepsia 2000; 41(suppl 1):S45–S47.

28. Simeone TA, McClellan AML, Twyman RE, White HS. Direct activation of the recombinant $\alpha_4\beta_3\gamma_{2S}$ GABA$_A$ receptor by the novel anticonvulsant topiramate. Soc Neurosci Abstr 2000.

29. Nusser Z, Mody I. Selective modulation of tonic and phasic inhibition in dentate gyrus granule cells. J Neurophysiol 2002; 87:2624–2628.

30. Vergnes M, Marescaux C, Micheletti G, Depaulis A, Rumbach L, Warter JM. Enhancement of spike and wave discharges by GABAmimetic drugs in rats with spontaneous petit-mal-like epilepsy. Neurosci Lett 1984; 44:91–94.

31. Panayiotopoulos CP, Agathonikou A, Sharoqi IA, Parker AP. Vigabatrin aggravates absences and absence status. Neurology 1997; 49:1467.

32. Yang MT, Lee WT, Chu LW, Shen YZ. Anti-epileptic drug-induced de novo absence seizures. Brain Dev 2003; 25:51–56.

33. Coenen AM, Blezer EH, Van Luijtelaar EL. Effects of the GABA-uptake inhibitor tiagabine on electroencephalogram, spike-wave discharges and behaviour of rats. Epilepsy Res 1995; 21:89–94.

34. Schapel G, Chadwick D. Tiagabine and non-convulsive status epilepticus. Seizure 1996; 5:153–156.

35. Knake S, Hamer HM, Schomburg U, Oertel WH, Rosenow F. Tiagabine-induced absence status in idiopathic generalized epilepsy. Seizure 1999; 8:314–317.

36. Balslev T, Uldall P, Buchholt J. Provocation of non-convulsive status epilepticus by tiagabine in three adolescent patients. Eur J Paediatr Neurol 2000; 40:169–170.

37. Stell BM, Mody I. Receptors with different affinities mediate phasic and tonic GABA(A) conductances in hippocampal neurons. J Neurosci 2002; 22:RC223.

38. Chiron C, Dulac O, Beaumont D, Palacios L, Pajot N, Mumford J. Therapeutic trial of vigabatrin in refractory infantile spasms. J Child Neurol 1991; (suppl 2):S52–S59.

39. Aicardi J, Mumford JP, Dumas C, Wood S. Vigabatrin as initial therapy for infantile spasms: a European retrospective survey. Sabril IS Investigator and Peer Review Groups. Epilepsia 1996; 37:638–642.

40. Elterman RD, Shields WD, Mansfield KA, Nakagawa J. US Infantile Spasms Vigabatrin Study Group. Randomized trial of vigabatrin in patients with infantile spasms. Neurology 2001; 57:1416–1421.

41. Das SK, Ray PK. Ontogeny of GABA pathway in human fetal brains. Biochem Biophys Res Commun 1996; 228:544–548.

42. Sankar R, Shin DH, Wasterlain CG. GABA metabolism during status epilepticus in the developing rat brain. Dev Brain Res 1997; 98:60–64.

43. Steinlein OK, Mulley JC, Propping P, Wallace RH, Phillips HA, Sutherland GR, Scheffer IE, Berkovic SF. A missense mutation in the neuronal nicotinic acetylcholine

receptor alpha 4 subunit is associated with autosomal dominant nocturnal frontal lobe epilepsy. Nat Genet 1995; 11:201–203.

44. Bertrand D, Picard F, Le Hellard S, Weiland S, Favre I, Phillips H, Bertrand S, Berkovic SF, Malafosse A, Mulley J. How mutations in nAChRs can cause ADNFLE epilepsy. Epilepsia 2002; 43(suppl 5):112–122.

45. Scheffer IE, Bhatia KP, Lopes-Cendes I, Fish DR, Marsden CD, Andermann E, Andermann F, Desbiens R, Keene D, Cendes F. Autosomal dominant nocturnal frontal lobe epilepsy. A distinctive clinical disorder. Brain 1995; 118(Pt 1):61–73.

46. Picard F, Bertrand S, Steinlein OK, Bertrand D. Mutated nicotinic receptors responsible for autosomal dominant nocturnal frontal lobe epilepsy are more sensitive to carbamazepine. Epilepsia 1999; 40:1198–1209.

47. Hirose S, Iwata H, Akiyoshi H, Kobayashi K, Ito M, Wada K, Kaneko S, Mitsudome A. A novel mutation of CHRNA4 responsible for autosomal dominant nocturnal frontal lobe epilepsy. Neurology 1999; 53:1749–1753.

48. Ito M, Kobayashi K, Fujii T, Okuno T, Hirose S, Iwata H, Mitsudome A, Kaneko S. Electroclinical picture of autosomal dominant nocturnal frontal lobe epilepsy in a Japanese family. Epilepsia 2000; 41:52–58.

49. Biervert C, Schroeder BC, Kubisch C, Berkovic SF, Propping P, Jentsch TJ, Steinlein OK. A potassium channel mutation in neonatal human epilepsy. Science 1998; 279: 403–406.

50. Singh NA, Charlier C, Stauffer D, DuPont BR, Leach RJ, Melis R, Ronen GM, Bjerre I, Quattlebaum T, Murphy JV, McHarg ML, Gagnon D, Rosales TO, Peiffer A, Anderson VE, Leppert M. A novel potassium channel gene, KCNQ2, is mutated in an inherited epilepsy of newborns. Nat Genet 1998; 18:25–29.

51. Rostock A, Tober C, Rundfeldt C, Bartsch R, Engel J, Polymeropoulos EE, Kutscher B, Loscher W, Honack D, White HS, Wolf HH. D-23129: a new anticonvulsant with a broad spectrum activity in animal models of epileptic seizures. Epilepsy Res 1996; 23:211–223.

52. Rundfelt C. The new anticonvulsant retigabine (D-23129) acts as an opener of K+ channels in neuronal cells. Eur J Pharmacol 1997; 336:243–249.

53. Rundfelt C, Netzer R. The novel anticonvulsant retigabine activates M-currents in Chinese hamster ovary-cells tranfected with human KCNQ2/3 subunits. Neurosci Lett 2000; 282:73–76.

54. Main MJ, Cryan JE, Dupere JR, Cox B, Clare JJ, Burbidge SA. Modulation of KCNQ2/3 potassium channels by the novel anticonvulsant retigabine. Mol Pharmacol 2000; 58:253–262.

55. Wickenden AD, Yu W, Zou A, Jegla T, Wagoner PK. Retigabine, a novel anti-convulsant, enhances activation of KCNQ2/Q3 potassium channels. Mol Pharmacol 2000; 58:591–600.

56. Rundfeldt C, Netzer R. Investigations into the mechanism of action of the new anticonvulsant retigabine. Interaction with GABAergic and glutamatergic neurotrans-mission and with voltage gated ion channels. Arzneimittelforschung 2000; 50:1063–1070.

57. Rogawski MA. KCNQ2/KCNQ3 K+ channels and the molecular pathogenesis of epilepsy: implications for therapy. Trends Neurosci 2000; 23(9):393–398.

58. Poolos NP, Migliore M, Johnston D. Pharmacological upregulation of h-channels reduces the excitability of pyramidal neuron dendrites. Nat Neurosci 2002; 5:767–774.

59. Pape HC, McCormick DA. Noradrenaline and serotonin selectively modulate thalamic burst firing by enhancing a hyperpolarization-activated cation current. Nature 1989; 340:715–718.

60. Soltesz I, Lightowler S, Leresche N, Jassik-Gerschenfeld D, Pollard CE, Crunelli V. Two inward currents and the transformation of low-frequency oscillations of rat and cat thalamocortical cells. J Physiol (Lond) 1991; 441:175–197.

61. Monteggia LM, Eisch AJ, Tang MD, Kaczmarek LK, Nestler EJ. Cloning and localization of the hyperpolarization-activated cyclic nucleotide-gated channel family in rat brain. Mol Brain Res 2000; 81:129–139.

62. Bender RA, Brewster A, Santoro B, Ludwig A, Hofmann F, Biel M, Baram TZ. Differential and age-dependent expression of hyperpolarization-activated, cyclic nucleotide-gated cation channel isoforms 1–4 suggests evolving roles in the developing rat hippocampus. Neuroscience 2001; 106:689–698.

63. Chen K, Aradi I, Thon N, Eghbal-Ahmadi M, Baram TZ, Soltesz I. Persistently modified h-channels after complex febrile seizures convert the seizure-induced enhancement of inhibition to hyperexcitability. Nat Med 2001; 7:331–337.

64. Chen K, Baram TZ, Soltesz I. Febrile seizures in the developing brain result in persistent modification of neuronal excitability in limbic circuits. Nat Med 1999; 5:888–894.

65. Klitgaard H, Matagne A, Gobert J, Wulfert E. Evidence for a unique profile of levetiracetam in rodent models of seizures and epilepsy. Eur J Pharmacol 1998; 353: 191–206.

66. Margineanu D, Klitgaard H. Inhibition of neuronal hypersynchrony in vitro differentiates levetiracetam from classical antiepileptic drugs. Pharmacol Res 2000; 42:281–285.

67. Klitgaard H, Matagne A, Grimee R, Vanneste-Goemaere J, Margineanu DG. Electrophysiological, neurochemical and regional effects of levetiracetam in the rat pilocarpine model of temporal lobe epilepsy. Seizure 2003; 12:92–100.

68. Coulter DA. Mossy fiber zinc and temporal lobe epilepsy: pathological association with altered "epileptic" gamma-aminobutyric acid A receptors in dentate granule cells. Epilepsia 2000; 41(suppl 6):S96–S99.

69. Rigo JM, Hans G, Nguyen L, Rocher V, Belachew S, Malgrange B, Leprince P, Moonen G, Selak I, Matagne A, Klitgaard H. The anti-epileptic drug levetiracetam reverses the inhibition by negative allosteric modulators of neuronal GABA- and glycine-gated currents. Br J Pharmacol 2002; 136:659–672.

70. Robello M, Balduzzi R, Cupello A. Modulation by extracellular pH of GABAA receptors expressed in *Xenopus* oocytes injected with rat brain mRNA. Int J Neurosci 2000; 103:41–51.

71. Aram JA, Lodge D. Epileptiform activity induced by alkalosis in rat neocortical slices: block by antagonists of N-methyl-D-aspartate. Neurosci Lett 1987; 83:345–350.

72. Velísek L, Dreier JP, Stanton PK, Heinemann U, Moshé SL. Lowering of extracellular pH suppresses low-Mg^{2+}-induced seizures in combined entorhinal cortex-hippocampal slices. Neurosci Lett 2002; 326:61–63.

73. Leahy JC, Chen Q, Vallano ML. Chronic mild acidosis specifically reduces functional expression of N-methyl-D-aspartate receptors and increases long-term survival in primary cultures of cerebellar granule cells. Neuroscience 1994; 63:457–470.

74. Staley KJ, Soldo BL, Proctor WR. Ionic mechanisms of neuronal excitation by inhibitory GABA$_A$ receptors. Science 1995; 269:977–981.

75. Guerrini R, Belmonte A, Genton P. Antiepileptic drug-induced worsening of seizures in children. Epilepsia 1998; 39(suppl 3):S2–S10.

76. Henry TR, Leppik IE, Gumnit RJ, Jacobs M. Progressive myoclonus epilepsy treated with zonisamide. Neurology 1988; 38:928–931.

77. Kyllerman M, Ben-Menachem E. Zonisamide for progressive myoclonus epilepsy: long-term observations in seven patients. Epilepsy Res 1998; 29:109–114.

78. Yoshimura I, Kaneko S, Yoshimura N, Murakami T. Long-term observations of two siblings with Lafora disease treated with zonisamide. Epilepsy Res 2001; 46:283–287.

79. Mori A, Noda Y, Packer L. The anticonvulsant zonisamide scavenges free radicals. Epilepsy Res 1998; 30:153–158.

80. Tokumaru J, Ueda Y, Yokoyama H, Nakajima A, Doi T, Mitsuyama Y, Ohya-Nishiguchi H, Kamada H. In vivo evaluation of hippocampal anti-oxidant ability of zonisamide in rats. Neurochem Res 2000; 25:1107–1111.

81. Okada M, Hirano T, Kawata Y, Murakami T, Wada K, Mizuno K, Kondo T, Kaneko S. Biphasic effects of zonisamide on serotonergic system in rat hippocampus. Epilepsy Res 1999; 34:187–197.

82. Welsh JP, Placantonakis DG, Warsetsky SI, Marquez RG, Bernstein L, Aicher SA. The serotonin hypothesis of myoclonus from the perspective of neuronal rhythmicity. Adv Neurol 2002; 89:307–329.

83. Brodie MJ, Yuen AW. Lamotrigine substitution study: evidence for synergism with sodium valproate? 105 Study Group. Epilepsy Res 1997; 26:423–432.

84. Stephen LJ, Sills GJ, Brodie MJ. Lamotrigine and topiramate may be a useful combination. Lancet 1998; 351:958–959.

85. Kwan P, Brodie MJ. Epilepsy after the first drug fails: substitution or add-on? Seizure 2000; 9:464–468.

86. Siddiqui A, Kerb R, Weale ME, Brinkmann U, Smith A, Goldstein DB, Wood NW, Sisodiya SM. Association of multidrug resistance in epilepsy with a polymorphism in the drug-transporter gene ABCB1. N Engl J Med 2003; 348:1442–1448.

87. Löscher W, Potschka H. Role of multidrug transporters in pharmacoresistance to antiepileptic drugs. J Pharmacol Exp Ther 2002; 301:7–14.

88. Seegers U, Potschka H, Löscher W. Transient increase of P-glycoprotein expression in endothelium and parenchyma of limbic brain regions in the kainate model of temporal lobe epilepsy. Epilepsy Res 2002; 51:257–268.

89. Dombrowski SM, Desai SY, Marroni M, Cucullo L, Goodrich K, Bingaman W, Mayberg MR, Bengez L, Janigro D. Overexpression of multiple drug resistance genes in endothelial cells from patients with refractory epilepsy. Epilepsia 2001; 42:1501–1506.

90. Sisodiya SM, Lin WR, Harding BN, Squier MV, Thom M. Drug resistance in epilepsy: expression of drug resistance proteins in common causes of refractory epilepsy. Brain 2002; 125(Pt 1):22–31.

91. Sankar R, Mazarati L, Shin D, Suchomelova L, Wasterlain CG. Multidrug resistance protein-1 is acutely altered by status epilepticus in the developing rat brain. Epilepsia 2002; 43(suppl 7):257–258.

92. Mazarati AM, Shin DH, Mazarati LG, Sankar R, Wasterlain CG. Status epilepticus–induced changes in P-glycoprotein expression in the rat brain. Epilepsia 2002; 43(suppl 7):220.

93. Delgado-Escueta AV, Wilson WA, Olsen RW, Porter RJ. Jasper's Basic Mechanisms of the Epilepsies. 3rd ed. Philadelphia: Lippincott Williams & Wilkins, 1999.

6

Epilepsy and Disease Modification: Animal Models for Novel Drug Discovery

H. Steve White

University of Utah
Salt Lake City, Utah, U.S.A.

INTRODUCTION

Worldwide, approximately 1–3% of the general population suffers from epilepsy. For the most part, pharmacotherapy represents the mainstay of patient treatment. Vagus nerve stimulation represents a potential option for those patients who are not viable candidates for surgery or whose seizures cannot be controlled by existing anticonvulsant drugs. Advances in brain imaging and seizure mapping techniques have made surgery an option for patients in whom a resectable seizure focus can be identified. Unfortunately, despite the availability of these new therapeutic options, a significant fraction of the patients with epilepsy continue to live with uncontrolled seizures, often at the expense of significant drug-induced adverse effects. Clearly, there is a need for more efficacious therapies that will not infringe on a patient's quality of life.

As with any other class of drugs, the discovery and development of new AEDs rely heavily on the employment of animal models to demonstrate efficacy and safety prior to their introduction in human volunteers. Obviously, the more predictive an animal model for a particular seizure type or syndrome, the greater the likelihood that the investigational AED will demonstrate efficacy in human clinical trials. Herein lies one of the most often discussed issues in the current-day AED discovery process: what is the most appropriate animal model to employ when attempting to screen for efficacy against human epilepsy?

This chapter will review briefly the different approaches employed in the AED discovery process. Furthermore, an attempt will be made to address some of the issues surrounding the development of more appropriate models of pharmacoresistant epilepsy. Lastly, attention will be paid to the employment of strategies being discussed

Table 1. Proposed Characteristics for an Animal Model of Human Epilepsy

Pathology consistent with human epilepsy (e.g., cell loss, gliosis, neurogenesis, axonal and
    synaptic reorganization)
Species-appropriate latent period following initial insult
Chronic hyperexcitability
Expression of spontaneous seizures following latent period
Resistance to one or more AEDS

that may lead to the identification and development of the truly novel drug that prevents the development of epilepsy, i.e., the "antiepileptogenic" compound. An extensive discussion of these issues is beyond the scope of this chapter. Where possible, the reader will be referred to pertinent reviews for a more detailed discussion.

THE IDEAL MODEL SYSTEM

The "ideal" screening model should reflect a similar pathophysiology and phenomenology to human epilepsy. Based on our current understanding of the factors contributing to the development of temporal lobe epilepsy, there are a number of characteristics that can be suggested (Table 1). For example, the ideal animal model would be expected to display spontaneous seizures within some time frame following an initiating insult. The "latent" period between initiating insult and expression of a behavioral seizure would be expected to be days to weeks in duration (which would be analogous to months to years in humans). The latent period should reflect a period of "clinical quiescence" in which the animal does not display behavioral seizures. The latent period also defines the time frame in which functional and structural reorganization occurs as a consequence of a specific series of pathological events set in motion by the activation of a series of critical modulators. As such, the functional and structural changes that contribute to the expression of spontaneous seizures should also be consistent with that observed in human tissue. The ideal model of human temporal lobe epilepsy may also be characterized by additional neuroplastic changes that manifest as pharmacological resistance to existing anticonvulsant drugs or neurobehavioral or cognitive impairment.

From a drug discovery perspective, the ideal model would provide an opportunity to assess efficacy against a pharmaco-resistant seizure phenotype and permit the early evaluation of a drug's ability to modify the course of epilepsy following an epileptogenic insult. Because human epilepsy is a heterogeneous neurological disorder that encompasses many seizure phenotypes and syndromes , it is highly unlikely that any one animal model will ever predict the full therapeutic potential of an investigational AED. This necessitates the evaluation of an investigational AED in several syndrome-specific model systems.

IDENTIFICATION OF "ANTICONVULSANT" ACTIVITY

The current era of AED discovery was ushered in by Merritt and Putnam in 1937, when they demonstrated the feasibility of using the maximal electroshock seizure (MES) model to identify the anticonvulsant potential of phenytoin (1). Subsequently, a number of animal models have been employed in the search for more efficacious and tolerable AEDs. In the early 1970s, the National Institute of Neurological Disorders and Stroke (NINDS) embarked on a mission to encourage basic research aimed at a greater understanding of the factors that contribute to the initiation, propagation, and amelioration of seizures. As part of this effort, the Anticonvulsant Drug Development (ADD) Program was created to foster the development of new drugs for the treatment of epilepsy.

Since 1975, the ADD program has accessioned >25,000 investigational anticonvulsant drugs from the academic community and the pharmaceutical industry. This ongoing effort has led to the identification and development of nine new anticonvulsant drugs including felbamate (1993), gabapentin (1993), lamotrigine (1994), fosphenytoin (1996), topiramate (1996), tiagabine (1997), levetiracetam (1999), zonisamide (2000), and oxcarbazepine (2000). The introduction of this "second generation" of anticonvulsant drugs has had a clear impact on the lives of many hundreds of thousands of epilepsy patients. Many have benefited from improved seizure control and/or fewer drug-induced adverse events. In addition, many of the newer drugs have demonstrated a more favorable pharmacokinetic profile.

Unfortunately, two of the newer AEDs (felbamate and vigabatrin) have been associated with potential long-term safety concerns that have limited their clinical utility. Nonetheless, despite the introduction of several new AEDs, it is estimated that the percentage of patients with partial epilepsy that remain pharmacoresistant to the existing AEDs has not changed significantly since the early 1970s and remains relatively stable between 25% and 40% (2).

In addition to the advancements made at the therapeutic level, significant progress has also been made at basic science level as well. For example, results from basic research have led to greater insight into the biology of epilepsy at both the molecular and genetic levels. Why then, given our current level of understanding of the pathophysiology of epilepsy, the introduction of several new drugs, greater access and improvements in neurosurgery, and the introduction of the vagus nerve stimulator, does there still remain such a significant unmet clinical need?

Will it ever be possible to translate findings at the bench to an effective therapy for the treatment of therapy-resistant seizures or, better yet, devise a therapy that will prevent or modify the development of epilepsy in the susceptible population? Addressing this question will require appropriate model systems wherein proposed therapies can be systematically evaluated. Unfortunately, raising this as an issue leads to the suggestion that the model systems currently employed in the search for new therapies are inadequate.

Having said this, a multitude of clinical trials and vast clinical experience would support the validity of the current approach. For example, as mentioned above, nine new drugs have been identified and developed on the basis of preclinical findings using two easy-to-conduct animal seizure models, i.e., the maximal electroshock (MES) seizure and the subcutaneous pentylenetetrazol (scPTZ) seizure tests (Table 2). Clearly, these models have been effective in identifying and characterizing several new and novel therapies for the symptomatic treatment of epilepsy. Moreover, the registration of the newer anticonvulsant drugs by the FDA or other regulatory agencies requires demonstrated proof of efficacy in randomized double-blind placebo controlled "add-on" trials employing patients with "refractory" epilepsy. As such, it is hard to argue that these newer AEDs are not pharmacologically different from the first-generation AEDs.

Table 2. Correlation Between Anticonvulsant Efficacy and Clinical Utility of the Established and Second-Generation AEDs in Experimental Animal Models[a]

Experimental model	Clinical seizure type			
	Tonic and/or clonic generalized seizures	Myoclonic/generalized absence seizures	Generalized absence seizures	Partial seizures
MES (tonic extension)[b]	CBZ, PHT, VPA, PB [FBM, GBP, LTG, TPM, ZNS]			
scPTZ (clonic seizures)[b]		ESM, VPA, PB[c], BZD [FBM, GBP, TGB[c], VGB[c]]		
Spike-wave discharges[d]			ESM, VPA, BZD [LTG, TPM, LVT]	
Electrical kindling (focal seizures)				CBZ, PHT, VPA, PB, BZD [FBM, GBP, LTG, TPM, TGB, ZNS, LVT, VGB]
Phenytoin-resistant kindled rat[e]				[LVT, GBP, TPM, FBM, LTG]
6-Hz (44 mA)[f]				VPA [LVT]

[a]BZD, benzodiazepines; CBZ, carbamazepine; ESM, ethosuximide; FBM, felbamate; GBP, gabapentin; LTG, lamotrigine; LVT, levetiracetam; PB, phenobarbital; PHT, phenytoin; TGB, tiagabine; TPM, topiramate; VPA, valproic acid; ZNS, zonisamide; VGB, vigabatrin.

[b]Data summarized from White et al., 2002 (5).

[c]PB, TGB, and VGB block clonic seizures induced by scPTZ but are inactive against generalized absence seizures and may exacerbate spike-wave seizures.

[d]Data summarized from GBL, GAERS, and lh/lh spike-wave models (7–10).

[e]Data summarized from Loescher, 2002 (2).

[f]Data summarized from Barton et al., 2001 (11).

[ ] Second-generation AEDs.

However, one must keep in mind that efficacy is defined by the ability of a drug to reduce the seizure frequency in 50% or more of the patient population and not by a drug's ability to produce complete seizure freedom. Indeed, the seizure-free rate from most add-on clinical trials is <10%. Based on these findings, it becomes easier to appreciate why there still remains a significant therapy-resistant patient population. A reasonable question to ask is whether the new drugs have made a significant impact in the "newly diagnosed" patient population. It is perhaps too early to answer this question because very few patients are treated with one of the second-generation AEDs as a first line of therapy. Only when a sufficient number of newly diagnosed patients are successfully treated early in the course of their epilepsy with the second-generation AEDs will their full impact on the incidence of therapy resistance be realized.

In addition to the MES and scPTZ models, there are several other animal model systems that may ultimately lead to the identification and development of novel therapies for the treatment of "refractory" epilepsy and prevention of epileptogenesis (Table 2). Nonetheless, the MES and subcutaneous PTZ seizure models continue to represent the two most widely used animal seizure models employed in the search for new AEDs (3–5). As mentioned above, Merritt and Putnam successfully employed the MES test in a systematic screening program to identify phenytoin (1). This observation, when coupled with the subsequent success of phenytoin in the clinical management of generalized tonic-clonic seizures, provided the validation necessary to consider the MES test as a reasonable model of human generalized tonic-clonic seizures.

In 1944, Everett and Richards demonstrated that PTZ-induced seizures could be blocked by trimethadione and phenobarbital but not by phenytoin (11a). A year later, Lennox demonstrated that trimethadione was effective in decreasing or preventing petit mal (absence) attacks in 50 patients but was ineffective or worsened grand mal attacks in 10 patients (6). Trimethadione's success in the clinic and its ability to block threshold seizures induced by PTZ provided the necessary correlation to establish the PTZ test as a model of petit mal or generalized absence seizures. With these observations, the current era of AED screening using the MES and scPTZ tests was launched.

The MES and scPTZ tests are easily conducted with a minimal investment in equipment and technical expertise. They provide valuable data regarding the potential anticonvulsant activity of an investigational drug, and with one exception (i.e., levetiracetam) all of the currently available AEDs have been found to be active in one or both of these tests (Table 2). Furthermore, both tests are amenable to high-volume screening with widely available relatively inexpensive normal rodents.

Although amenable to high-volume screening, the MES and scPTZ tests fail to meet any of the remaining criteria described above (Table 1). For example, there are now several examples wherein the pharmacological profile of an AED can be affected by the disease state. Because the MES and scPTZ tests are conducted in "pathologically normal" rodents, there is no guarantee that they will be equally effective in "pathologically abnormal" rodents. The best example to illustrate this point is levetiracetam. As mentioned above, the MES and scPTZ tests failed to identify levetiracetam's anticonvulsant activity. Subsequent investigations demonstrated that levetiracetam was active in pathologically abnormal models of partial and primary generalized seizures (12–16). In this regard, levetiracetam appears to represent the first "truly" novel AED to be identified in recent years. The identification and subsequent development of levetiracetam as an efficacious AED for the treatment of partial seizures underscore the need for flexibility when screening for efficacy and the need to incorporate levetiracetam-sensitive models into the early evaluation process.

One distinct disadvantage of the MES and scPTZ tests is that they do not possess a pharmacological profile consistent with therapy-resistant human epilepsy. For example, the MES test is sensitive to all of the first-generation AEDs with demonstrated clinical efficacy in the treatment of generalized tonic-clonic seizures (e.g., phenytoin, carbamazepine, valproate, and phenobarbital). In contrast, the scPTZ test is sensitive to those first-line AEDs used in the management of generalized absence seizures (i.e., ethosuximide, valproate, and the benzodiazepines). As mentioned above, this is due in part to the fact that these two models were developed and validated initially using the older, established AEDs phenytoin, phenobarbital, and trimethadione (17,18). This particular validation process led to their selection on the basis that these two model systems displayed a pharmacological profile consistent with established medical practice at the time (see 17,18 for historical review and discussion).

However, the lack of any demonstrable efficacy by tiagabine, vigabatrin, and levetiracetam in the MES test argues against its utility as a predictive model of partial seizures. Consistent with this conclusion is the observation that NMDA antagonists are very effective against tonic extension seizures induced by MES; however, they were found to be without benefit in patients with partial seizures (19).

Historically, positive results obtained in the scPTZ seizure test were considered suggestive of potential clinical utility against generalized absence seizures. Based on this argument, phenobarbital, gabapentin, and tiagabine, which are all effective in the scPTZ test, should all be effective against spike-wave seizures; and lamotrigine, which is inactive in the scPTZ test, should be inactive against spike-wave seizures. However, clinical experience has demonstrated that this is an invalid prediction. For example, the barbiturates, gabapentin, and tiagabine all aggravate spike-wave seizure discharge, whereas lamotrigine has been found to be effective against absence seizures. Thus, the overall utility of the scPTZ test in predicting activity against human spike-wave seizures is limited. Thus, before any conclusion concerning potential clinical utility against spike-wave seizures is made, positive results in the scPTZ test should be corroborated by positive findings in other models of absence such as the γ-butyrolactone (7) seizure test, the genetic absence epileptic rat of Strasbourg (8), and the lethargic (*lh/lh*) mouse (9,10). Another important advantage of all three of these models is that they accurately predict the potentiation of spike-wave seizures by drugs that elevated GABA concentrations (e.g., vigabatrin and tiagabine), drugs that directly activate the GABA-B receptor, and the barbiturates.

One might ask, then, what if any benefit these two tests might provide when screening for novel AEDs. First, both tests provide some insight into the CNS bioavailability of a particular investigational AED. Furthermore, both models are nonselective with respect to mechanism of action. As such, they are very well suited for the early evaluation of anticonvulsant activity because neither model assumes that a particular drug's pharmacodynamic activity is dependent on its molecular mechanism of action. Lastly, both model systems display clear and definable seizure endpoints and require minimal technical expertise. This, coupled with lack of dependence on molecular mechanism, makes them ideally suited to screen large numbers of chemically diverse entities. However, levetiracetam taught the community that lack of efficacy in either of these tests does not translate into lack of human efficacy. As such, there is no longer any reason to limit further screening on the basis of results obtained in the MES and scPTZ. In fact, there is no a priori reason to assume that a novel AED will be active in the MES, scPTZ, or other acute seizure tests.

BEYOND THE MES AND PTZ TESTS

In recent years, the kindling model of partial epilepsy has been frequently employed in the AED development process (Table 2). Kindling refers to the process whereby there is a progressive increase in electrographic and behavioral seizure activity in response to repeated stimulation of a limbic brain region such as the amygdala or hippocampus with an initially subconvulsive current (20). Furthermore, the kindling process is associated with a progressive increase in seizure severity and duration, a decrease in the focal seizure threshold, and neuronal degeneration in limbic brain regions that resemble human mesotemporal lobe epilepsy (Table 3). Both electrographic and behavioral components of the kindled seizure begin locally at the site of stimulation, and quickly become secondarily generalized.

From a therapeutic perspective, the kindled rat model offers perhaps the best predictive value for efficacy against partial seizures. For example, it is the only model that adequately predicted the clinical utility of the first- and second-generation AEDs, including tiagabine and vigabatrin (Table 2). Furthermore, the kindled rat is the only model that accurately predicted the lack of clinical efficacy of NMDA antagonists (21). Given the predictive nature of the kindled rat, one might legitimately ask why this model or a similarly predictive chronic model is not utilized as a primary screen rather than a secondary screen for the early identification and evaluation of novel AEDs? The answer is primarily one of logistics. Any chronic animal model such as kindling is labor-intensive and requires adequate facilities and resources to surgically implant the stimulating/recording electrode, and to kindle and to house sufficient rats over a chronic period of time. Furthermore, unlike the acute seizure models, the time required to conduct a drug study with a chronic model far exceeds the time required to conduct a similar study with the MES or scPTZ tests, thereby severely limiting the number of AEDs that can be screened in a timely manner. However, if our goal is to provide novel therapeutic options that will meet the needs of the therapy-resistant patient population, we should no longer let these reasons be a barrier to testing of drugs in chronic epilepsy models.

WHAT IS THE FUTURE OF AED DISCOVERY AND DEVELOPMENT?

Therapy-Resistant Epilepsy

Since its inception in 1975, the ASP has screened over 25,000 investigational AEDs. In addition to the compounds that have been successfully developed, a number of additional compounds are in various stages of clinical development. Each of these drugs has brought about substantial benefit to the patient population in the form of increased seizure control, increased tolerability, and better safety and

Table 3. Chronic Animal Models of Epileptogenesis and Secondary Hyperexcitability

Model	Neuronal degeneration	Mossy fiber sprouting	Chronic hyperexcitability	Latent period	Spontaneous seizures	References
Kindling	present	present	yes	no[a]	no	31–33
Status epilepticus (i.e., kainic acid, pilocarpine, Li+-pilocarpine, PPS,[b] SAS[c])	marked	marked	yes	days-weeks	yes	32,34–38
Neonatal hypoxia	no	minimal	yes	no	no	35,39,40
Neonatal hyperthermia	no	no	yes	no	no	35,39,41
Traumatic brain injury Cortical undercut	yes	?	yes	yes	yes	42–45
FeCl$_2$	yes	?	yes	yes	yes	46,47
Fluid percussion	yes	yes	yes	no	no	48–50

[a]Spontaneous seizures do develop with prolonged kindling stimulation.
[b]Perforant path stimulation.
[c]Sustained amygdala stimulation.

pharmacokinetic profiles. Unfortunately for 25–40% of epilepsy patients, there remains a need to identify therapies that will more effectively treat their therapy resistant seizures. As such, there is a continued need to identify and incorporate more appropriate models of refractory epilepsy into the AED screening process. At the present time, there are several model systems that could be suggested including: the phenytoin-resistant kindled rat (22); the carbamazepine-resistant kindled rat (23); the 6-Hz psychomotor seizure model (11,24); and the in vitro low-magnesium entorhinal-hippocampal slice preparation (25).

As discussed above, levetiracetam is unique among all of the clinically available AEDs in that it is inactive in both the MES and scPTZ tests. This fact underscores why there is a continued need to identify and characterize new screening models to minimize the chance of missing other potentially novel AEDs. Interestingly, the phenytoin-resistant kindled rat displays a unique sensitivity to the anticonvulsant action of levetiracetam (Table 2). Furthermore, the pharmacological profile of the phenytoin-resistant kindled rat includes topiramate, gabapentin, felbamate, and lamotrigine but not phenytoin, valproate, or phenobarbital. This finding alone suggests that these newer drugs are at the very least mechanistically different from the latter group of older drugs.

While the high-frequency, short-duration stimulation employed in the MES test has become a standard for screening AEDs, it was only one of several electroshock paradigms initially developed in the 1940s and 1950s (26). An alternative stimulation paradigm was the low-frequency (6-Hz) long-duration (3 sec) corneal stimulation model that was stated to produce "psychic" or "psychomotor" seizures (Table 2). Instead of the tonic extension seizure characteristic of the MES test, the 6-Hz seizure was reported to involve a minimal, clonic phase followed by stereotyped automatisms reminiscent of human complex partial seizures (24,27,28).

At the time of its initial description, the authors were attempting to validate the 6-Hz model as a screening test for partial seizures; however, the pharmacological profile was not consistent with clinical practice (24). For example, phenytoin was found to be inactive in the 6-Hz seizure test. This observation led the authors to suggest that it was no more predictive of clinical utility than the other models available at the time (i.e., the MES and scPTZ tests). Subsequent investigations in our laboratory confirmed the relative insensitivity of the 6-Hz test to phenytoin, and extended this observation to include carbamazepine, lamotrigine, and topiramate (11). The relative resistance of some patients to phenytoin and other AEDs in today's clinical setting and the lack of sensitivity of the MES and scPTZ to levetiracetam prompted studies to reevaluate the 6-Hz seizure test as a potential screen for therapy resistant epilepsy (11). Subsequent investigations demonstrated that levetiracetam afforded protection against the 6-Hz seizure at a stimulus intensity where other AEDs display little to no efficacy (Table 2). This observation clearly demonstrates the potential utility of this model as a screen for novel AEDs that may be useful for the treatment of therapy-resistant partial seizures.

In addition to the phenytoin-resistant rat and the 6-Hz seizure model, the late-recurrent discharges associated with in vitro low-Mg^{2+} slice model also displays a unique pharmacological profile that includes resistance to phenytoin, carbamazepine, phenobarbital, and valproic acid. Interestingly, the late-recurrent discharges are uniquely sensitive to block by the investigational AED retigabine, which targets

KCNQ$_{2/3}$ channels. This is of particular interest because this particular channel has been associated with human benign familial neonatal convulsions (29,30).

Unfortunately, it will take the successful clinical development of a drug with demonstrated clinical efficacy in the management of refractory epilepsy before any one of these (or other) model systems will be clinically validated. Nonetheless, this should not preclude the community at large from continuing the search for a more effective therapy using these and any other viable models that are currently available. In fact, until there is a validated model, it becomes even more important to characterize and incorporate several of the available models into the drug discovery process while at the same time continuing to identify new models of refractory epilepsy.

Disease Modification: Moving Beyond the Symptomatic Treatment of Epilepsy

Today, there are several animal models of epileptogenesis that share many similarities with Mesial Temporal Lobe Epilepsy (MTLE) and which have been utilized to study the underlying molecular biology of the epileptogenic process (Table 3). These studies have led to the identification of a number of factors that either increase or decrease in response to the initiating insult. Numerous investigations are attempting to assess whether observed changes are causative or simply an epiphenomenon of the initiating event. Beyond their value for understanding the molecular biology of epilepsy, animal models are also extremely valuable for assessing the potential neuroprotective and "disease-modifying" potential of existing and future drugs.

At present, there are no known therapies that are capable of modifying the course of acquired epilepsy. Attempts to prevent the development of epilepsy following febrile seizures, traumatic brain injury, and craniotomy with the older, established drugs have been disappointing [see Temkin (51) for review]. At the same time, discoveries at the molecular level have provided greater insight into the pathophysiology of certain seizure disorders. As such, it may be possible in the not so distant future to identify a treatment strategy that will slow or halt the progressive nature of epilepsy and prevent the development of epilepsy in susceptible individuals. However, any successful human therapy will necessarily be identified and characterized in a model system that closely approximates human epileptogenesis. At the present time, several of the chronic animal models display spontaneous seizures secondary to a particular insult or genetic manipulation (for review and references, see 2,52). To be successful in identifying a novel, disease-modifying therapy, we must become intentional in our efforts to characterize and incorporate models of epileptogenesis into our screening protocols.

Specific models of epileptogenesis include kindling, status epilepticus, and traumatic brain injury (Table 3). All of these models display varying degrees of cell loss, synaptic reorganization, network hyperexcitability, and a latent period that is followed by the expression of spontaneous seizures. As such, they fulfill some important characteristics of a model of acquired partial epilepsy. In addition, there are two age-specific models of hyperexcitability worthy of mention—neonatal hyperthermic seizures, and neonatal hypoxia. These particular models have provided valuable insights into the functional and pathological consequences associated with an age-specific insult. Unfortunately, they remain somewhat limited because they are not associated with the development of chronic spontaneous seizures. However, this is not to imply that they are not useful models. On the contrary, they may actually be more relevant to the development of human epilepsy because not every individual exposed to a precipitating insult will develop chronic epilepsy.

Clearly, comparative data is urgently needed from these and other models of acquired epilepsy before any conclusions regarding their overall utility can be assessed. In this regard, it is important to note that each model system will bring certain strengths to epilepsy research and therapy development. At the present time, it is not clear whether any of the aforementioned models are pharmacoresistant to one or more of the available AEDs. As such, it is important that comprehensive pharmacological studies be conducted to assess their relative sensitivity to the existing AEDs.

A greater understanding of the pathophysiology of acquired epilepsy at the molecular and genetic level may lead to the development of a new therapeutic approach that reaches beyond the symptomatic treatment of epilepsy to modify the progression or, dare we suggest, prevent the development of epilepsy in the susceptible patient. The realization of such a possibility will necessitate a change in our current AED discovery approach. For the most part, the existing approach is effective for identifying drugs that are effective for treating seizures, but is not likely to be effective in identifying the "disease-modifying" therapeutic agents. Furthermore, the evidence to date would suggest that the MES and scPTZ tests, though useful, are not likely to identify drugs that will effectively manage the patient with refractory seizures. As such, new models should be considered that more closely approximate the pathophysiology and phenotypic features associated with acquired human epilepsy.

SUMMARY

The current utility of the existing AEDs is limited by their ineffectiveness against refractory seizures. For the most part, their preclinical efficacy was defined by the MES, scPTZ, and kindled rat models. The phenytoin- and carbamazepine-resistant rat models, the 6-Hz seizure model, and the in vitro entorhinal-hippocampal slice model display some degree of pharmacoresistance to several of the available AEDs. Whether activity in these resistant models will translate into improved treatment for the therapy-resistant patient population has yet to be defined by clinical studies. Nonetheless, their utility should not be dismissed, but rather endorsed as part of a comprehensive screen to thoroughly evaluate the anticonvulsant potential of an investigational AED.

Furthermore, significant progress in our understanding of the factors that contribute to human epileptogenesis has been made in recent years. These advances have in large part been made possible through the development and characterization of insult- and age-specific animal models of epileptogenesis and secondary neuronal hyperexcitability. As we gain additional insight into the molecular biology and genetics of the acquired and genetic epilepsies, the day may come wherein new therapies that target the epileptogenic process will be developed.

Therapeutics designed to modify the course of epilepsy or prevent the development of epilepsy in the susceptible patient will require testing in appropriate animal models. Numerous models of acute status epilepticus display many similarities with the human condition including pathology, a species-appropriate latent period, and the development of spontaneous seizures following the latent period. The kindling model and traumatic brain injury models also display some of these same characteristics. Lastly, two age-specific models (i.e., neonatal hyperthermia- and hypoxia-induced seizures) display similar pathological and phenotypic features to their human counterparts (i.e., febrile seizures and neonatal hypoxia-ischemia, respectively). There are numerous subtle and gross differences across the various syndrome-specific models that necessitates their continued evaluation to access their validity to the human condition. The true validation of a given model of epileptogenesis requires the development of an effective therapy that prevents or delays the development of epilepsy or second hyperexcitability in the human condition, and whose activity was predicted by preclinical testing.

REFERENCES

1. Putnam TJ, Merritt HH. Experimental determination of the anticonvulsant properties of some phenyl derivatives. Science 1937; 85:525–526.
2. Loscher W. Animal models of epilepsy for the development of antiepileptogenic and disease-modifying drugs. A comparison of the pharmacology of kindling and models with spontaneous recurrent seizures. Epilepsy Res 2002; 50:105–123.
3. White HS, Woodhead JH, Franklin MR, Swinyard EA, Wolf HH. General principles: experimental selection, quantification, and evaluation of antiepileptic drugs. In: Levy RH, Mattson RH, Meldrum BS, eds. Antiepileptic Drugs, 4th ed. New York: Raven Press, 1995:99–110.
4. White HS. Mechanisms of antiepileptic drugs. In: Porter R, Chadwick D, eds. Epilepsies II. Boston: Butterworth-Heinemann, 1997:1–30.
5. White HS, Woodhead JH, Wilcox KS, Stables JP, Kupferberg HJ, Wolf HH. Discovery and preclinical development of antiepileptic drugs. In: Levy RH, Mattson RH, Meldrum B, Perucca E, eds. Antiepileptic Drugs. Philadelphia: Lippincott, 2002:36–48.
6. Lennox WG. The petit mal epilepsies. Their treatment with Tridione. JAMA 1945; 129:1069–1074.
7. Snead OC. Pharmacological models of generalized absence seizures in rodents. J Neural Transm 1992; 35:7–19.
8. Marescaux C, Vergnes M. Genetic absence epilepsy in rats from Strasbourg (GAERS). Ital J Neurol Sci 1995; 16:113–118.
9. Hosford DA, Clark S, Cao Z, Wilson WAJ, Lin FH, Morrisett RA, Huin A. The role of GABAB receptor activation in absence seizures of lethargic (lh/lh) mice. Science 1992; 257:398–401.
10. Hosford DA, Wang Y. Utility of the lethargic (*lh/lh*) mouse model of absence seizures in predicting the effects of lamotrigine, vigabatrin, tiagabine, gabapentin, and topiramate against human absence seizures. Epilepsia 1997; 38:408–414.
11. Barton ME, Klein BD, Wolf HH, White HS. Pharmacological characterization of the 6-Hz psychomotor seizure model of partial epilepsy. Epilepsy Res 2001; 47:217–227.
11a. Everett GM, Richards RK. Comparative anticonvulsive action of 3,5,5-trimethyl-oxazolidine-2,4-dione (Tridione), Dilantin and phenobarbital. J. Pharmacol. Exp. Ther., 1997; 81:402–407.
12. Gower AJ, Noyer M, Verloes R, Gobert J, Wulfert E. ucb LO59, a novel anticonvulsant drug: pharmacological profile in animals. Eur J Pharmacol 1992; 222:193–203.

13. Loscher W, Honack D. Profile of ucb-L059, a novel anticonvulsant drug, in models of partial and generalized epilepsy in mice and rats. Eur J Pharmacol 1993; 232:147–158.

14. Gower AJ, Hirsch E, Boehrer A, Noyer M, Marescaux C. Effects of levetiracetam, a novel antiepileptic drug, on convulsant activity in two genetic rat models of epilepsy. Epilepsy Res 1995; 22:207–213.

15. Klitgaard H, Matagne A, Gobert J, Wulfert E. Evidence for a unique profile of levetiracetam in rodent models of seizures and epilepsy. Eur J Pharmacol 1998; 353:191–206.

16. Loscher W, Honack D, Rundfeldt C. Antiepileptogenic effects of the novel anticonvulsant levetiracetam (ucb L059) in the kindling model of temporal lobe epilepsy. J Pharmacol Exp Ther 1998; 284:474–479.

17. White HS, Johnson M, Wolf HH, Kupferberg HJ. The early identification of anticonvulsant activity: role of the maximal electroshock and subcutaneous pentylenetetrazol seizure models. Ital J Neurol Sci 1995; 16:73–77.

18. Kupferberg H. Animal models used in the screening of antiepileptic drugs. Epilepsia 2001; 42:7–12.

19. Meldrum BS. Neurotransmission in epilepsy. Epilepsia 1995; 36:S30–S35.

20. Goddard GV, McIntyre DC, Leech CK. A permanent change in brain function resulting from daily electrical stimulation. Exp Neurol 1969; 25:295–330.

21. Loscher W, Honack D. Responses to NMDA receptor antagonists altered by epileptogenesis. Trends Pharmacol Sci 1991; 12:52.

22. Loscher W, Reissmuller E, Ebert U. Anticonvulsant efficacy of gabapentin and levetiracetam in phenytoin-resistant kindled rats. Epilepsy Res 2000; 40:63–77.

23. Nissinen J, Halonen T, Koivisto E, Pitkanen A. A new model of chronic temporal lobe epilepsy induced by electrical stimulation of the amygdala in rat. Epilepsy Res 2000; 38:177–205.

24. Brown WC, Schiffman DO, Swinyard EA, Goodman LS. Comparative assay of antiepileptic drugs by "psychomotor" seizure test and minimal electroshock threshold test. J Pharmacol Exp Ther 1953; 107:273–283.

25. Armand V, Rundfeldt C, Heinemann U. Effects of retigabine (D-23129) on different patterns of epileptiform activity induced by low magnesium in rat entorhinal cortex hippocampal slices. Epilepsia 2000; 41:28–33.

26. Swinyard EA. Electrically induced convulsions. In: Purpura DB, Penry JK, Tower D, Woodbury DM, Walter R, eds. Experimental Models of Epilepsy. New York: Raven Press, 1972:443–458.

27. Toman JEP. Neuropharmacologic considerations in psychic seizures. Neurology 1951; 1:444–460.

28. Toman JEP, Everett GM, Richards RK. The search for new drugs against epilepsy. Tex Rep Biol Med 1952; 10:96–104.

29. Singh NA, Charlier C, Stauffer D, DuPont BR, Leach RJ, Melis R, Ronen GM, Bierre I, Quattlebaum T, Murphy JV, McHarg ML, Gagnon D, Rosales TO, Pciffer A, Anderson VE, Leppert M. A novel potasssium channel gene, KCNQ2, is mutated in an inherited epilepsy of newborns. Nat Genet 1998; 18:25–29.

30. Biervert C, Schroeder BC, Kubisch C, Berkovic SF, Propping P, Jentsch TJ, Steinlein OK. A potassium channel mutation in neonatal human epilepsy. Science 1998; 279:403–406.

31. Loscher W. Animal models of intractable epilepsy. Prog Neurobiol 1997; 53:239–258.

32. Dalby NO, Mody I. The process of epileptogenesis: a pathophysiological approach. Curr Opin Neurol 2001; 14:187–192.

33. McNamara JO. Analyses of the molecular basis of kindling development. Psychiatry Clin Neurosci 1995; 49:S175–S178.

34. Pitkanen A, Sutula TP. Is epilepsy a progressive disorder? Prospects for new therapeutic approaches in temporal-lobe epilepsy. Lancet 2002; 1:173–181.

35. Lado FA, Sankar R, Lowenstein D, Moshe SL. Age-dependent consequences of seizures: relationship to seizure frequency, brain damage, and circuitry reorganization. Ment Retard Dev Disabil Res Rev 2000; 6:242–252.

36. Sankar R, Shin D, Mazarati AM, Liu H, Katsumori H, Lezama R, Wasterlain CG. Epileptogenesis after status epilepticus reflects age- and model-dependent plasticity. Ann Neurol 2000; 48:580–589.

37. Andre V, Ferrandon A, Marescaux C, Nehlig A. Vigabatrin protects against hippocampal damage but is not antiepileptogenic in the lithium-pilocarpine model of temporal lobe epilepsy. Epilepsy Res 2001; 47:99–117.

38. Andre V, Ferrandon A, Marescaux C, Nehlig A. The lesional and epileptogenic consequences of lithium-pilocarpine-induced status epilepticus are affected by previous exposure to isolated seizures: effects of amygdala kindling and maximal electroshocks. Neuroscience 2000; 99:469–481.

39. Jensen FE, Baram TZ. Developmental seizures induced by common early-life insults: short- and long-term effects on seizure susceptibility. Ment Retard Dev Disabil Res Rev 2000; 6:253–257.

40. Jensen FE, Blume H, Alvarado S, Firkusny I, Geary C. NBQX blocks acute and late epileptogenic effects of perinatal hypoxia. Epilepsia 1995; 36:966–972.

41. Baram TZ, Gerth A, Schlutz L. Febrile seizures: an appropriate-aged model suitable for long-term studies. Dev Brain Res 1997; 98:265–270.

42. Echlin F, Battista J. Epileptiform seizures from chronic isolated cortex. Arch Neurol 1963; 9:154–170.

43. Sharpless S, Halpern L. The electrical excitability of chronically isolated cortex studied by means of chronically implanted electrodes. Electroencephalogr Clin Neurophysiol 1962; 14:244–255.

44. Prince DA, Jacobs K. Inhibitory function in two models of chronic epileptogenesis. Epilepsy Res 1998; 32:83–92.

45. Bush PC, Prince DA, Miller KD. Increased pyramidal excitability and NMDA conductance can explain postraumatic epileptogenesis without disinhibition: a model. J Neurophysiol 1999; 82:1748–1758.

46. Willmore LJ, Sypert GW, Munson JV, Hurd RW. Chronic focal epileptiform discharges induced by injection of iron into rat and cat cortex. Science 1978; 200:1501–1503.

47. Willmore LJ, Rubin JJ. Effects of antiperoxidants on $FeCl_2$-induced lipid-peroxidation and focal edema in rat-brain. Exp Neurol 1984; 83:62–70.

48. Lowenstein DH, Thomas MJ, Smith DH, McIntosh TK. Selective vulnerability of dentate hilar neurons following traumatic brain injury: a potential mechanistic link between head trauma and disorders of the hippocampus. J Neurosci 1992; 12:4846–4853.

49. Laurer HL, McIntosh TK. Experimental models of brain trauma. Curr Opin Neurol 1999; 12:715–721.

50. Golarai G, Greenwood AC, Feeney DM, Connor JA. Physiological and structural evidence for hippocampal involvement in persistent seizure susceptibility after traumatic brain injury. J Neurosci 2001; 21:8523–8537.

51. Temkin NR. Antiepileptogenesis and seizure prevention trials with antiepileptic drugs: meta-analysis of controlled trials. Epilepsia 2001; 42:515–524.

52. Loscher W. Current status and future directions in the pharmacotherapy of epilepsy. TIPS 2002; 23:113–118.

7

Nonsynaptic Mechanisms in Seizures and Epileptogenesis: Targets for Clinical Management?

F. Edward Dudek
Colorado State University
Fort Collins, Colorado, U.S.A.

WHICH "NONSYNAPTIC" MECHANISMS MAY PLAY A ROLE IN SEIZURES?

Most research on the generation and propagation of seizures and on the mechanisms of epileptogenesis has centered around the role of chemical synaptic transmission, specifically the glutamatergic and GABA-ergic systems. Research on the role of nonsynaptic mechanisms in epilepsy, particularly in the synchronization of electrical activity during seizures, has a long and controversial history. Over 15 years ago, electrical mechanisms of neuronal interaction were proposed to play an important role in synchronization during epileptiform activity (see 1,2 for reviews), and comparable analyses of the potential role of ionic mechanisms were also available (3,4). The widely used expression "nonsynaptic" has come to refer to those mechanisms that are independent of *active chemical synaptic transmission*. One mechanism included in this description would be electrotonic coupling through gap junctions, which many workers would consider to be *electrical synapses* (5–7). Another mechanism is electrical-field effects (i.e., ephaptic interactions), which are mediated by current flow in the extracellular space. These two mechanisms are distinctly different because the former involves a specialized membrane structure (i.e., gap junctions, which are intercellular channels composed of connexin proteins), whereas the latter is due to neuronal orientation and the size of the extracellular space (i.e., tightly packed neurons that are arranged in parallel are susceptible to the effects of activity-induced electrical fields). A third mechanism involves activity-dependent shifts in the intracellular and extracellular concentration of ions. The intense electrical activity of seizures is associated with transmembrane ionic currents, which cause a redistribution of ions such as potassium and calcium. Increases in the concentration of extracellular potassium and decreases in extracellular calcium, both of which would usually increase membrane excitability, would have a slow synchronizing effect on neurons in a network. The goal of this chapter is to summarize (1) the evidence for the presence of these mechanisms in the hippocampus, (2) their possible role in synchronization of electrical activity during seizures, and (3) how these mechanisms may be targets for clinical intervention. It should be noted that nonsynaptic interactions amongst neocortical neurons may not be as relevant owing to their lower packing density and relative lack of gap junctions.

Electrotonic Junctions

Considerable experimental support for the hypothesis that some vertebrate neurons, including those in several subcortical areas in mammals (e.g., mesenchephalic nucleus, lateral vestibular nucleus, inferior olive), are electrotonically coupled through gap junctions has been available for decades (see 1,2,6,7 for reviews). During the 1980s, several studies suggested that hippocampal pyramidal cells and dentate granule cells are also electrotonically coupled through gap junctions (8–12). Intracellular injections of low-molecular-weight tracers have suggested that intracellular acidification reduces tracer coupling (13), and alkanization increases tracer coupling (14). Although this concept remains controversial, several aspects of the experimental evidence have been replicated and extended with other techniques (see 15–17 for reviews). In particular, recent experiments with patch pipettes in hippocampal slices have shown that antidromic stimulation evokes "spikelets" in CA1 pyramidal cells, and gap junction blockers reduce the amplitude of these events without directly altering evoked action potentials (Fig. 1) (19). Furthermore, tracer injections under direct visual observation confirmed the presence of tracer coupling. The site of apparent junctional coupling appeared to be axo-axonal, which is consistent with computer modeling studies (20–22). Early observations of freeze-fracture replicas of hippocampal pyramidal cells (11) and dentate granule cells (10) suggested that gap junctions were located on the somata and dendrites of these neurons, but after reanalysis of the published data based on more specific criteria for cellular identification, the gap junctions appear to have been on oligodendrocytes (23).

More recent freeze-fracture data have confirmed the presence of gap junctions in the hippocampus, but neuronal identity (i.e., principal neurons vs. interneurons) has been unclear (15). Thin-section ultrastructual studies, however, have clearly shown gap junctions between hippocampal interneurons (24,25). Therefore, several lines of evidence have suggested that some hippocampal pyramidal cells, granule cells, and associated interneurons are electrotonically coupled through gap junctions, but more rigorous ultrastructural data with immunogold labeling of specific connexins and identified neurons are needed. Furthermore, the relative number and size of gap junctions for different cell types is essentially unknown. The available evidence, however, strongly suggests that if gap junctions are present on principal neurons in the hippocampus, they are low in number (or have a small number of connexins), so that any one pyramidal or granule cell is normally coupled to only one or a few other neurons (see 1,2,22 for reviews). Several lines of evidence suggest that nonsynaptic synchronization of epileptiform events (26) and electrotonic coupling

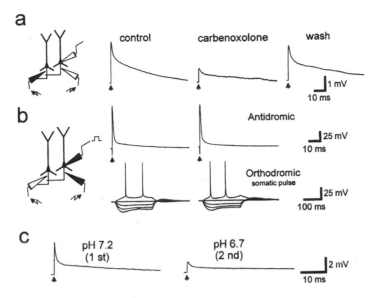

Figure 1. Bath application of carbenoxolone blocked partial spikes in response to antidromic stimulation of CA1 pyramidal cells. (A) Application of the gap junction blocker carbenoxolone (100 μM) reversibly reduced the amplitude of the spikelets evoked through extracellular stimulation at a distant site (filled electrode). (B) Carbenoxolone did not affect the antidromically evoked action potential (i.e., direct stimulation of the axon, filled electrode) or the somatically evoked action potentials (i.e., through the recording electrode). (C) Similar data were obtained from a neuron first recorded in whole-cell configuration with the standard pipette solution (pH = 7.2), and then subsequently with another pipette with pH 6.7. The partial spikes were greatly reduced when the pipette contained a solution with a lower pH. Subsequent recordings with two other patch pipettes as a control showed no significant alteration in the amplitude or waveform of the spikelets. (From Ref. 19.)

through gap junctions are more prominent in the immature hippocampus and cortex (27), but the issue of developmental differences will not be considered in this chapter.

Electrical-Field Effects

Electrical-field or ephaptic interactions depend on the orientation and density of neurons within a population. For over half a century, electrophysiologists have known that the hippocampus generates large field potentials during synchronous activity because of the tight packing and parallel orientation of the hippocampal pyramidal cells and dentate granule cells. The extracellular space in the hippocampus is comparatively small (28), and this leads to high extracellular resistance, which effectively shunts current across the membrane of some neurons (2,29,30). This spatial arrangement of neurons augments the amplitude of the extracellular field potentials and their associated currents. The technique of transmembrane recording (i.e., intracellular minus focal extracellular) revealed that hippocampal population spikes generate an intracellular depolarization that can be recorded in the inactive neurons (reviewed in 2; see 29–31). These field-effect depolarizations are roughly half of the amplitude of the population spike (i.e., a 10-mV population spike generates a

5-mV depolarization). These electrical-field effects may act in concert with electrotonic coupling through gap junctions to synchronize the action potentials of hippocampal pyramidal cells (31–33).

Ionic Mechanisms

Intense neuronal activity, as occurs during electrographic seizures, is known to cause increases in the concentration of extracellular potassium and decreases in the concentration of extracellular calcium (see 3,4 for reviews). Numerous studies with ion-selective electrodes have corroborated earlier findings that major shifts in the concentration of extracellular potassium and calcium occur during seizures. Furthermore, experiments with hippocampal slices show that changes in the concentration of these ions alter the susceptibility to seizure activity (see below). These ionic mechanisms would generally be expected to have a powerful but slower effect than the electrical interactions described above.

ARE NONSYNAPTIC MECHANISMS IMPORTANT IN SEIZURES?

Numerous experimental studies with a variety of preparations and techniques have provided overwhelming evidence that (1) GABA receptor-mediated mechanisms effectively raise seizure threshold, (2) pharmacological agents that block GABA-A receptors generally induce epileptiform activity, and (3) chronic alterations in the GABA-ergic systems have been proposed to underlie or contribute to epileptogenesis. Excitatory glutamate receptor-mediated synaptic mechanisms also contribute importantly to seizure generation, and synaptic reorganization of these pathways has been hypothesized to be an important mechanism in epileptogenesis. Nonetheless, experiments from numerous laboratories have clearly shown that robust seizurelike activity can occur in hippocampal slices after active chemical synaptic transmission has been blocked pre- and postsynaptically with ionic and pharmacological treatments, respectively (see below and 15–18 for reviews).

Low-Calcium Seizure Models

Initial Experiments in the CA1 Area

In the early 1980s, three research groups showed nearly simultaneously that solutions containing little or no extracellular calcium, which effectively block active chemical synaptic transmission, induce "hyperexcitability," and promote seizurelike activity. Taylor and Dudek (31) showed that low-calcium solutions containing manganese, which demonstrably blocked EPSPs in CA1 pyramidal cells from Schaffer collateral stimulation, led to a progressive increase in excitability that was manifest as long antidromically evoked afterdischarges and prolonged spontaneous bursts (Fig. 2). Simultaneous intracellular and extracellular recordings showed that intracellular action potentials were synchronous with extracellular population spikes, and that partial spikes (i.e., fast prepotentials or spikelets) also occurred synchronously with small population spikes. Furthermore, differential transmembrane recording revealed that extracellular population spikes generated field-effect depolarizations (29–31). This work showed that (1) synchronous spontaneous bursts could occur in low-calcium solutions without active chemical transmission, (2) partial spikes (suggestive

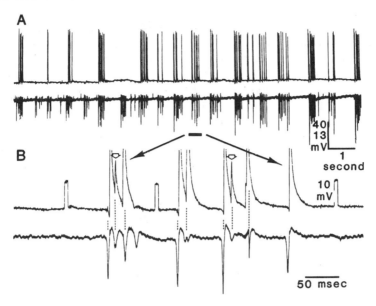

Figure 2. Simultaneous intracellular and extracellular recording of spontaneous bursts of synchronous action potentials from the CA1 area of a hippocampal slice preparation that was bathed in a low-calcium solution containing manganese. This solution was shown to block active chemical transmission. (A) Spontaneous bursts of action potentials recorded intracellularly (upper trace) occurred synchronously with the bursts of population spikes recorded extracellularly (lower trace). (B) Expansion of the time scale (see bar in A) showed that the action potentials and population spikes occurred synchronously (see the vertical dashed lines). Fast depolarizations that were subthreshold (open arrowheads) and resembled fast prepotentials (or spikelets) were also recorded synchronously with the population spikes. (From Ref. 31.)

of electrotonic coupling) were synchronous with population spikes, and (3) synchronization involved electrical-field effects (i.e., ephaptic interactions). Jefferys and Haas (34) showed nearly simultaneously that spontaneous bursts of population spikes could occur in low-calcium solutions that blocked chemical transmission (35). Konnerth, et al. (36,37) clearly showed with ion-selective electrodes that these prolonged nonsynaptic bursts were associated with an increase in the concentration of extracellular potassium, and that the propagation of these events coincided with shifts in the concentration of extracellular ions. Spontaneous release of transmitter (i.e., miniature postsynaptic potentials) occurs in low-calcium solutions. To confirm that spontaneous miniature postsynaptic potentials were not required for low-calcium bursting, experiments were conducted in a medium containing GABA-A, NMDA, and AMPA receptor antagonists such as bicuculline, AP-5, and DNQX (which alone were shown to block fast evoked chemical postsynaptic potentials in hippocampal slices) (38). The observation that epileptiform activity still occurred in the presence of the GABA-A, NMDA, and AMPA receptor antagonists indicated that spontaneous spike-independent release of "fast" amino acid transmitters (i.e., miniature postsynaptic potentials) is not required for nonsynaptic bursting. These results have been replicated and extended by several other laboratories (see 15–18 for reviews).

Other Hippocampal Regions

One important concern regarding the experiments described above on the CA1 area of hippocampal slices is whether neocortical regions, or even other hippocampal areas, show nonsynaptic mechanisms of synchronization during epileptiform activity. Normally, CA1 pyramidal cells are more tightly packed than other pyramidal cells in hippocampus and neocortex, and their resting potential is relatively close to threshold; therefore, CA1 pyramidal cells would seem particularly susceptible to low-calcium solutions, which essentially lower spike threshold in addition to blocking spike-mediated release of neurotransmitters. Dentate granule cells are also tightly packed, but generally have a more negative resting potential (39); they were also shown to be susceptible to low-calcium solutions (Fig. 3A), particularly when extracellular potassium was elevated to higher levels (40,41). Based on histological observations, CA3 pyramidal cells would be expected to be less susceptible to electrical-field and ionic interactions because of their lower packing density, but CA3 pyramidal cells also show low-calcium bursting (Fig. 3A) (41). Studies using both field-potential and multiple-unit recordings have revealed that these "field bursts" are preceded by an increase in spontaneous action-potential activity, and that this phenomenon can also occur in the medial entorhinal cortex, a cortical region that is not as laminated or densely packed as the hippocampus (42).

These experiments also showed that spontaneous multiple-unit activity occurred when CA1 pyramidal cells generated slow negative shifts in the field potential without superimposed population spikes, which are likely the result of ionic

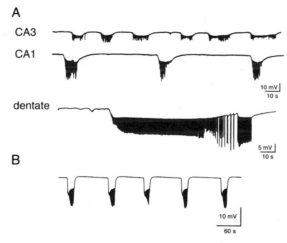

Figure 3. Spontaneous bursts of population spikes recorded throughout the hippocampus after active chemical transmission was blocked. (A) Bursts of population spikes occurred in the CA3 area in the presence of low-calcium and high-potassium medium. Under these conditions, the CA1 area and the dentate gyrus also showed spontaneous bursts of synchronous action potentials. (B) Prolonged bursts of population spikes recorded in a normal extracellular concentration of calcium (i.e., 1.3 mM) and high extracellular potassium (i.e., 12 mM). Chemical synaptic transmission involving GABA-A, NMDA, and AMPA receptors was blocked with 30 µM bicuculline, 50 µM AP-5, and 50 µM DNQX. (From Refs. 41,43.)

interactions. Medial entorhinal cortex, with its decreased lamination and packing density, showed slow negative shifts in the extracellular field potential with coincident multiple-unit activity, but without population spikes. These experiments indicate that all of the major fields of the hippocampus, and even some of the parahippocampal regions like the entorhinal cortex, are susceptible to low-calcium bursting. Therefore, nonsynaptic mechanisms appear to involve (1) ionic mechanisms that affect both membrane potential and action potential threshold, and mediate "slow" synchronization that generates the negative field-potential shifts, and (2) faster electrical mechanisms that generate spontaneous population spikes.

Nonsynaptic Seizure Activity in Normal Concentrations of Extracellular Calcium

One potential criticism of the work described above is that the extracellular ionic concentrations are abnormal, and thus may not reflect what normally happens in epileptic brain. As reviewed above, however, a variety of studies have shown that seizure activity causes an increase in extracellular potassium and a decrease in the concentration of extracellular calcium (3,4). Therefore, these levels of extracellular ions at least partially mimic the changes that would be expected to occur during a seizure. Furthermore, other studies have used relatively normal calcium concentrations to evaluate the potential role of nonsynaptic mechanisms in the generation and synchronization of seizurelike activity in a more normal ionic environment. Synchronous bursts could be generated in the presence of GABA-A, NMDA, and AMPA receptor antagonists when calcium was maintained at more physiological concentrations, if potassium was also raised to higher levels (Fig. 3B) (41,43). Thus, prolonged bursts can occur in normal calcium concentrations if excitability is raised, even when chemical synaptic transmission is blocked pharmacologically (see 44,45 for additional information on this issue). These studies suggest that ionic and electrical mechanisms, such as electrotonic coupling through gap junctions and/or electrical field effects, contribute importantly to seizure generation under a wide range of ionic conditions that include relatively normal concentrations of extracellular calcium (46). Thus, these nonsynaptic mechanisms, particularly when operative together, are powerful and can synchronize hyperexcitable cortical neurons independent of chemical transmission.

EXPERIMENTAL APPROACHES TO BLOCK NONSYNAPTIC MECHANISMS OF SEIZURE GENERATION AND SYNCHRONIZATION

The concept that these nonsynaptic interactions between neurons could play an important role in seizure activity suggests that these mechanisms could be new targets for clinical intervention. At present, the pharmacological mechanisms of antiepileptic drugs (AEDs) are thought to involve primarily either voltage-gated ion channels or ligand-activated channels. Drugs that would target neuronal gap junctions or modulate the size of the extracellular space (and thus influence electrical-field effects and activity-induced ion shifts) would potentially represent novel ways to control seizures.

Electrotonic Junctions

The experimental approaches to evaluate whether gap junctions mediate electrotonic coupling has largely included the use of gap junction blockers in brain slice experiments. Recent studies aimed at providing evidence that CA1 pyramidal cells are electrically coupled by axonal gap junctions showed that antidromic stimulation evoked "spikelets" or partial action potentials. Bath application of $100\,\mu M$ carbenoxolone, a relatively specific gap junction blocker (19), reduced the amplitude of these events (Fig. 1). Three independent studies using different seizure models in hippocampal slices have provided evidence that gap junction blockers, including carbenoxolone, halothane, and octanol, depress or even block epileptiform activity (47–49). A critical issue when using these pharmacological agents is to determine whether the gap junction blocker alters membrane excitability, which would also influence seizure susceptibility. These studies have provided different types of evidence to suggest that excitability was unaltered and did not account for the blocking effect of these agents on epileptiform activity.

Although these studies support the hypothesis that gap junctions between neurons, particularly hippocampal pyramidal cells, play a role in the synchronization of electrical activity during epileptiform events, additional experiments are warranted to ensure that slight decreases in excitability do not contribute to depression of seizure activity. For example, recordings that show a loss of *synchrony during electrical activity* after application of the gap junction blocker would be stronger evidence that the gap junction blockers specifically blocked junctional transmission and did not elevate spike threshold. Future studies ultimately need to test the specificity of particular pharmacological agents on *neuronal* gap junctions, because an added complication for the above experiments is the extensive gap junctional coupling known to occur between glial cells, particularly astrocytes.

An important conceptual difficulty with gap junction blockers as potential AEDs, in addition to the problem with glial cells, is that gap junctions connect many other types of cells in a variety of tissues. Compared to these other tissues, neurons display a relative *lack* of gap junctions, even in neuronal structures where electrotonic coupling is thought to be present. Thus, treatments that block gap junctions would be expected to have widespread physiological effects, including functional disruption of critical structures such as the heart. A large body of data, however, has begun to identify which connexins are in gap junctions from different tissues, and neuronal gap junctions appear to have specific connexins (50).

Electrical and Ionic Mechanisms Involving Extracellular Space

Pharmacological mechanisms directed at electrical-field effects or changes in the concentration of extracellular ions may be more difficult to implement for selective control of seizures than agents directed at gap junctions. Classic studies have shown that seizurelike activity causes neuronal swelling that is manifest as a decrease in the size of the extracellular space (51; see 3 for review). Using potassium-induced electrographic seizures in the CA1 area of hippocampal slices, Traynelis and Dingledine (52) showed that hyperosmotic solutions suppressed electrographic seizure activity, and this was associated with a decrease in extracellular resistance that arose from a reduction in extracellular space. Nonsynaptic mechanisms were considered likely to be responsible for these effects of hyperosmotic solutions. Experiments with low-calcium

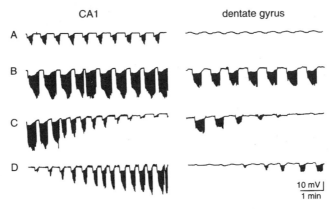

Figure 4. Nonsynaptic seizurelike activity in CA1 and the dentate gyrus was sensitive to changes in the osmolality of the extracellular medium. (A) Spontaneous burst discharges were present in CA1, but not the dentate gyrus in low-calcium solution. (B) The CA1 bursts increased in amplitude and duration and spontaneous bursts began to occur in the dentate gyrus after the osmolality of the extracellular medium was reduced from 308 mOsm to 254 mOsm. (C) Bursts were blocked in both the CA1 area and the dentate gyrus when mannitol (20 mM) was added to the extracellular fluid to increase the osmolality. (D) Bursts began to occur again when the extracellular fluid was diluted. (From Ref. 40.)

solutions and pharmacological treatments that blocked synaptic transmission both pre- and postsynaptically showed that hyperosmolar solutions with membrane impermeant solutes could block nonsynaptic seizurelike activity (Fig. 4), whereas hyperosmolar solutions with membrane permeant solutes did not (38,40). Those slices that did not generate low-calcium bursts were treated with hypoosmolar solutions, which would be expected to cause cell swelling; these hypoosmolar solutions induced synchronous burst discharges (Fig. 4). Therefore, hyperosmolar solutions, such as mannitol, appear to depress seizures by causing cell shrinkage and an increase in extracellular space, which would be expected to reduce electrical-field effects and dampen the effects of activity-induced changes in ion concentrations. Dilute media, or hypoosmolar solutions that would cause cell swelling, promote seizure activity. These results support the hypothesis that nonsynaptic mechanisms involving the extracellular space, in particular electrical-field effects and shifts in the extracellular concentration of potassium, contribute to synchronization of epileptiform activity (53). Similar to studies with gap junction blockers, additional experiments are needed to demonstrate that the effects of these changes in osmolality are specifically on cell volume and the size of the extracellular space.

Other approaches have been used to test this hypothesis. Hochman et al. (54) showed that furosemide, a loop diuretic that would be expected to reduce activity-dependent increases in cell volume, depressed several different types of seizure activity in vivo and in vitro. The effect of furosemide was observed in low-calcium solutions, further suggesting that nonsynaptic mechanisms involving extracellular space could hypothetically be used to manage clinical seizures. Furosemide, similar to the gap junction blockers, however, may have other mechanisms of action. Transient electrical fields can block or disrupt epileptiform activity (55–57), and this effect could be due to a disruption of electrical-field effects. Nonsynaptic epileptiform activity can cross a knife-cut lesion that would eliminate gap-junctional communication and reduce electrical-field effects, which supports the hypothesis of an important role for ionic interactions in the synchronization and propagation of slow epileptiform activity (58). These experiments suggest that nonsynaptic mechanisms are potential clinical targets for future AEDs.

ARE NONSYNAPTIC MECHANISMS ALTERED DURING EPILEPTOGENESIS?

Most hypotheses concerning the cellular mechanisms of chronic epileptogenesis, at least in regard to temporal lobe epilepsy, have focused on synaptic mechanisms, and few studies have tested hypotheses concerning nonsynaptic mechanisms of *chronic epileptogenesis* (vs. seizure generation and synchronization). This is important because one must separate the concepts of blocking seizures through a mechanism that is *not* part of the epileptogenic mechanism versus one that is. If epileptogenesis were hypothetically to depend—at least in part—on alterations in nonsynaptic mechanisms, and one could find a selective therapeutic intervention strategy, one might have a way to depress epileptic seizures with minimal side effects.

Electrotonic Coupling and Gap Junctions

Whereas numerous studies have addressed the issue of whether gap junctions between neurons are present and contribute to synchronization of epileptiform events, relatively few experiments have been directed at the hypothesis that epileptogenesis is associated with an increase in neuronal gap junctions. Colling et al. (59) reported increased dye coupling between rat hippocampal CA1 pyramidal cells in the tetanus-toxin model of epilepsy. These data suggest that the increased seizure susceptibility associated with this model may be due in part to increased gap junctional coupling between CA1 pyramidal cells. Additional experiments, however, are needed to address this issue in other models of temporal lobe epilepsy and in other cortical areas.

Gap junctions among glial cells could also be altered in epileptogenesis. Gap junctions between astrocytes are thought to participate in spatial buffering of extracellular potassium and other ions. A decrease in gap-junctional communication might be expected to impede this process. Lee et al. (60) isolated astrocytes from human surgical tissue, and reported an increase in gap-junctional coupling among astrocytes, based on the propagation of intracellular calcium oscillations and fluorescence recovery after photobleach. A subsequent analysis of functional coupling in gliomas using fluorescence recovery after photobleach showed reduced coupling among cultured astrocytes obtained from human surgical tissue (i.e., gliomas and mesial temporal sclerosis) (61). Using a freeze-lesion model of cortical dysplasia, Bordey et al. (62) found *reduced* dye coupling among proliferative astrocytes at the site of injury and *enhanced* coupling among astrocytes in a hyperexcitable zone near the cortical injury. These studies suggest altered junctional coupling among the glia around a focal injury or in an area of mesial temporal sclerosis. Additional experiments are needed to test these hypotheses, and it is unclear whether these changes are compensatory or they contribute to chronic seizures.

Numerous studies over the last decade have suggested an increase in the expression of different connexins, particularly connexins 43 and 32, in human tissue from surgical treatment for temporal lobe epilepsy or in animal models of this disorder. Many of these studies have suggested that this may reflect an increase in neuronal coupling, but recent evidence from Rash et al. (50), using freeze-fracture immunogold labeling of specific connexins on gap junctions of identified cells in the central and peripheral nervous system, indicates (at least in normal brain) that connexin 43 is specific for astrocytes and connexin 32 for oligodendrocytes. The data concerning these two connexins in various animal models and in tissue from human surgery is unclear on whether the gliosis in epileptic lesions is associated with normal, reduced, or enhanced expression of connexin proteins and gap junctions in glia (63–70).

Ionic and Electrical-Field Mechanisms

Several hypothetical mechanisms could be responsible for an enhanced contribution of ionic or electrical-field effects in epileptogenesis (71). For example, a decrease in extracellular space, as might be expected to occur with gliosis and seizure-induced cell swelling, could increase seizure susceptibility similar to the application of dilute media. However, neuronal loss, as is known to occur in mesial temporal sclerosis, would reduce neuronal density and the amplitude of the field potentials, which would thus reduce electrical-field effects. An increase in astrocytes associated with mesial temporal sclerosis might better buffer changes in the concentration of extracellular ions associated with seizure activity, although this hypothesis has not been tested directly. Therefore, little or no direct evidence is available concerning the hypothesis that changes in ionic mechanisms or electrical-field effects are responsible for or contribute to chronic epileptogenesis. This lack of evidence should not be interpreted as evidence *against* such mechanisms contributing to chronic epileptogenesis, but only the need for additional research.

CONCLUSION

This chapter has reviewed the different types of nonsynaptic mechanisms that may contribute to seizure generation and synchronization. Electrotonic coupling through gap junctions and/or electrical field effects via currents in the extracellular space appear to synchronize action potentials and be responsible for the fast oscillations (i.e., "fast ripples") seen at seizure onset in animal models of temporal lobe epilepsy and in patients with this disorder (21,22,72,73). Seizurelike activity after active chemical transmission is blocked in hippocampal slices represents a possible experimental model for testing AEDs that would hypothetically target nonsynaptic mechanisms. Several laboratories have conducted experiments aimed at blocking this type of seizure activity with either gap junction blockers or treatments that increase the size of the extracellular space, and the potential to use this approach with several different types of in vitro seizure models may be useful for identifying the cellular mechanism of action of new AEDs. Future research in this area could identify AEDs that act specifically on nonsynaptic mechanisms and hypothetically do not impact negatively on normal brain function. Relatively few data suggest that the chronic mechanism of epileptogenesis involves nonsynaptic mechanisms, but further experiments are required to test this hypothesis.

REFERENCES

1. Dudek FE, Andrew RD, MacVicar BA, Snow RW, Taylor CP. Recent evidence for and possible significance of gap junctions and electrotonic synapses in the mammalian brain. In: Jasper HH, Van Gelder NM, eds. Basic Mechanisms of Neuronal Hyperexcitability. New York: Alan R. Liss, 1983:31–73.

2. Dudek FE, Snow RW, Taylor CP. Role of electrical interactions in synchronization of epileptiform bursts. Adv Neurol 1986; 44:593–617.

3. Lux HD, Heinemann U, Dietzel I. Ionic changes and alterations in the size of the extracellular space during epileptic activity. Adv Neurol 1986; 44:619–639.

4. Heinemann U, Konnerth A, Pumain R, Wadman WJ. Extracellular calcium and potassium concentration changes in chronic epileptic brain tissue. Adv Neurol 1986; 44:641–661.

5. Bennett MVL. A comparison of electrically and chemically mediated transmission. In: Pappas GD, Purpura DP, eds. Structure and Function of Synapses. New York: Raven Press, 1972:221–256.

6. Bennett MVL. Electrical transmission: a functional analysis and comparison with chemical transmission. In: Kandel ER, ed. Handbook of Physiology. Section I: The Nervous System, Vol. I, Cellular Biology of Neurons, Part I. Bethesda: American Physiological Society, 1977:357–416.

7. Bennett M. Gap junctions as electrical synapses. J Neurocytol 1997; 26:349–366.

8. MacVicar BA, Dudek FE. Dye-coupling betwen CA3 pyramidal cells in slices of rat hippocampus. Brain Res 1980; 196:494–497.

9. MacVicar BA, Dudek FE. Electrotonic coupling between pyramidal cells: a direct demonstration in rat hippocampal slices. Science 1981; 213:782–785.

10. MacVicar BA, Dudek FE. Electrotonic coupling between granule cells of rat dentate gyrus: physiological and anatomical evidence. J Neurophysiol 1982; 47:579–592.

11. Schmalbruch H, Jahnsen H. Gap junctions on CA3 pyramidal cells of guinea pig hippocampus shown by freeze-fracture. Brain Res 1981; 217:175–178.

12. Taylor CP, Dudek FE. A physiological test for electrotonic coupling between CA1 pyramidal cells in rat hippocampal slices. Brain Res 1982a; 235:351–357.

13. MacVicar BA, Jahnsen H. Uncoupling of CA3 pyramidal neurons by propionate. Brain Res 1985; 330:141–145.

14. Church J, Baimbridge KG. Exposure to high-pH medium increases the incidence and extent of dye coupling between rat hippocampal CA1 pyramidal neurons in vitro. J Neurosci 1991; 11:3289–3295.

15. Dudek FE, Yasumura T, Rash JE. '"Nonsynaptic" mechanisms in seizures and epileptogenesis. Cell Biol Int 1998; 22:793–805.

16. Jefferys JG. Nonsynaptic modulation of neuronal activity in the brain: electric currents and extracellular ions. Physiol Rev 1995; 75:689–723.

17. Carlen PL, Perez-Velazquez JL, Valiante TA, Jahroml SS, Bardakjian BL. Electric coupling in epileptogenesis. In: Spray DC and Dermietzel R, eds. Gap Junctions in the Nervous System. Austin, TX: R.G. Landes Company, 1996:289–299.

18. Carlen PL, Skinner F, Zhang L, Naus C, Kushnir M, Perez Velazquez JL. The role of gap junctions in seizures. Brain Res Rev 2000; 32:235–241.

19. Schmitz D, Schuchmann S, Fisahn A, Draguhn A, Buhl EH, Petrasch-Parwez E, Dermietzel R, Heinemann U, Traub RD. Axo-axonal coupling: a novel mechanism for ultrafast neuronal communication. Neuron 2001; 31:831–840.

20. Traub RD, Schmitz D, Jefferys JG, Draguhn A. High-frequency population oscillations are predicted to occur in hippocampal pyramidal neuronal networks interconnected by axoaxonal gap junctions. Neuroscience 1999; 92:407–426.

21. Traub RM, Miles AW, Buhl EH, LeBeau FEN, Bibbig A, Boyd S, Cross H, Baldeweg T. A possible role for gap junctions in generation of very fast EEG

oscillations preceding the onset of, and perhaps initiating, seizures. Epilepsia 2001; 42:153–170.

22. Traub RD, Draguhn A, Whittington MA, Baldeweg T, Bibbig A, Buhl EH, Schmitz D. Axonal gap junctions between principal neurons: a novel source of network oscillations, and perhaps epileptogenesis. Rev Neurosci 2002; 13:1–30.

23. Rash JE, Duffy HS, Dudek FE, Bilhartz BL, Whalen LR, Yasumura T. Grid-mapped freeze-fracture analysis of gap junctions in gray and white matter of adult rat central nervous system, with evidence for a "panglial syncytium" that is not coupled to neurons. J Comp Neurol 1997; 388:265–292.

24. Kosaka T. Neuronal gap junctions in the polymorph layer of the rat dentate gyrus. Brain Res 1983; 277:347–351.

25. Kosaka T, Hama K. Gap junctions between non-pyramidal cell dendrites in the rat hippocampus (CA1 and CA3 regions): a combined Golgi-electron microscopy study. J Comp Neurol 1985; 231:150–161.

26. Roper SN, Obenaus A, Dudek FE. Increased propensity for nonsynaptic epileptiform activity in immature rat hippocampus and dentate gyrus. J Neurophysiol 1993; 70:857–862.

27. Rorig B, Sutor B. Regulation of gap junction coupling in the developing neocortex. Mol Neurobiol 1996; 12:225–249.

28. McBain CJ, Traynelis SF, Dingledine R. Regional variation of extracellular space in the hippocampus. Science 1990; 249:674–677.

29. Taylor CP, Dudek FE. Excitation of hippocampal pyramidal cells by an electrical field effect. J Neurophysiol 1984; 52:126–142.

30. Taylor CP, Dudek FE. Synchronization without active chemical synapses during hippocampal afterdischarges. J Neurophysiol 1984; 52:143–155.

31. Taylor CP, Dudek FE. Synchronous neural afterdischarges in rat hippocampal slices without active chemical synapses. Science 1982; 218:810–812.

32. Traub RD, Dudek FE, Taylor CP, Knowles WD. Simulation of hippocampal afterdischarges synchronized by electrical interactions. Neuroscience 1985; 14:1033–1038.

33. Traub RD, Dudek FE, Snow RW, Knowles WD. Computer simulations indicate that electrical field effects contribute to the shape of the epileptiform field potential. Neuroscience 1985; 15:947–958.

34. Jefferys JG, Haas HL. Synchronized bursting of CA1 hippocampal pyramidal cells in the absence of synaptic transmission. Nature 1982; 300:448–450.

35. Haas HL, Jefferys JG. Low calcium field burst discharges of CA1 pyramidal neurones in rat hippocampal slices. J Physiol 1984; 354:185–201.

36. Konnerth A, Heinemann U, Yaari Y. Slow transmission of neural activity in hippocampal area CA1 in absence of active chemical synapses. Nature 1984; 307:69–71.

37. Konnerth A, Heinemann U, Yaari Y. Nonsynaptic epileptogenesis in the mammalian hippocampus in vitro. I. Development of seizurelike activity in low extracellular calcium. J Neurophysiol 1986; 56:409–423.

38. Dudek FE, Obenaus A, Tasker JG. Osmolality-induced changes in extracellular volume alter epileptiform bursts independent of chemical synapses in the rat: importance of non-synaptic mechanisms in hippocampal epileptogenesis. Neurosci Lett 1990; 120:267–270.

39. Fricke RA, Prince DA. Electrophysiology of dentate gyrus granule cells. J Neurophysiol 1984; 51:195–209.

40. Roper SN, Obenaus A, Dudek FE. Lowered osmolality causes nonsynaptic epileptiform bursts in rat dentate gyrus: a comparison with area CA1. Ann Neurol 1992; 31:81–85.

41. Schweitzer JS, Patrylo PR, Dudek FE. Prolonged field bursts in the dentate gyrus: dependence on low calcium, high potassium, and nonsynaptic mechanisms. J Neurophysiol 1992; 68:2016–2025.

42. Patrylo PR, Kuhn AJ, Schweitzer JS, Dudek FE. Multiple-unit recordings during slow field-potential shifts in low-$[Ca^{2+}]_0$ solutions in rat hippocampal and cortical slices. Neuroscience 1996; 74:107–118.

43. Patrylo PR, Schweitzer JS, Dudek FE. Potassium-dependent prolonged field bursts in the dentate gyrus: effects of extracellular calcium and amino acid receptor antagonists. Neuroscience 1994; 61:13–19.

44. Xiong ZQ, Stringer JL. Prolonged bursts occur in normal calcium in hippocampal slices after raising excitability and blocking synaptic transmission. J Neurophysiol 2001; 86:2625–2628.

45. Bikson M, Baraban SC, Durand DM. Conditions sufficient for nonsynaptic epileptogenesis in the CA1 region of hippocampal slices. J Neurophysiol 2002; 87:62–71.

46. Jensen MS, Yaari Y. Role of intrinsic burst firing, potassium accumulation, and electrical coupling in the elevated potassium model of hippocampal epilepsy. J Neurophysiol 1997; 77:1224–1233.

47. Kohling R, Gladwell SJ, Bracci E, Vreugdenhil M, Jefferys JG. Prolonged epileptiform bursting induced by 0-Mg^{2+} in rat hippocampal slices depends on gap junctional coupling. Neuroscience 2001; 105:579–587.

48. Ross FM, Gwyn P, Spanswick D, Davies SN. Carbenoxolone depresses spontaneous epileptiform activity in the CA1 region of rat hippocampal slices. Neuroscience 2000; 100:789–796.

49. Margineanu DG, Klitgaard H. Can gap-junction blockade preferentially inhibit neuronal hypersynchrony vs. excitability? Neuropharmacology 2001; 41:377–383.

50. Rash JE, Yasumura T, Dudek FE, Nagy JI. Cell-specific expression of connexins and evidence of restricted gap junctional coupling between glial cells and between neurons. J Neurosci 2001; 21:1983–2000.

51. Dietzel I, Heinemann U, Hofmeier G, Lux HD. Transient changes in the size of the extracellular space in the sensorimotor cortex of cats in relation to stimulus-induced changes in potassium concentration. Exp Brain Res 1980; 40:432–439.

52. Traynelis SF, Dingledine R. Role of extracellular space in hyperosmotic suppression of potassium-induced electrographic seizures. J Neurophysiol 1989; 61:927–938.

53. Andrew RD, Fagan M, Ballyk BA, Rosen AS. Seizure susceptibility and the osmotic state. Brain Res 1989; 498:175–180.

54. Hochman DW, Baraban SC, Owens JW, Schwartzkroin PA. Dissociation of synchronization and excitability in furosemide blockade of epileptiform activity. Science 1995; 270:99–102.

55. Bikson M, Kian J, Hahn PJ, Stacey WC, Sciortino C, Durand DM. Suppression of epileptiform activity by high frequency sinusoidal fields in rat hippocampal slices. J Physiol 2001; 531:181–191.

56. Richardson TL, O'Reilly CN. Epileptiform activity in the dentate gyrus during low-calcium perfusion and exposure to transient electric fields. J Neurophysiol 1995; 74:388–399.

57. Weinstein S. The anticonvulsant effect of electrical fields. Curr Neurol Neurosci Rep 2001; 1:155–161.

58. Lian J, Bikson M, Shuai J, Durand DM. Propagation of non-synaptic epileptiform activity across a lesion in rat hippocampal slices. J Physiol 2001; 537:191–199.

59. Colling SB, Man WD, Draguhn A, Jefferys JG. Dendritic shrinkage and dye-coupling between rat hippocampal CA1 pyramidal cells in the tetanus toxin model of epilepsy. Brain Res 1996; 741:38–43.

60. Lee SH, Magge S, Spencer DD, Sontheimer H, Cornell-Bell AH. Human epileptic astrocytes exhibit increased gap junction coupling. Glia 1995; 15:195–202.

61. Soroceanu L, Manning TJ Jr, Sontheimer H. Reduced expression of connexin-43 and functional gap junction coupling in human gliomas. Glia 2001; 33:107–117.

62. Bordey A, Lyons SA, Hablitz JJ, Sontheimer H. Electrophysiological characteristics of reactive astrocytes in experimental cortical dysplasia. J Neurophysiol 2001; 85: 1719–1731.

63. Aronica E, Gorter JA, Jansen GH, Leenstra S, Yankaya B, Troost D. Expression of connexin 43 and connexin 32 gap-junction proteins in epilepsy-associated brain tumors and in the perilesional epileptic cortex. Acta Neuropathol (Berl) 2001; 101: 449–459.

64. Elisevich K, Rempel SA, Smith BJ, Edvardsen K. Hippocampal connexin 43 expression in human complex partial seizure disorder. Exp Neurol 1997; 145:154–164.

65. Elisevich K, Rempel SA, Smith B, Hirst K. Temporal profile of connexin 43 mRNA expression in a tetanus toxin-induced seizure disorder. Mol Chem Neuropathol 1998; 35:23–37.

66. Fonseca CG, Green CR, Nicholson LF. Upregulation in astrocytic connexin 43 gap junction levels may exacerbate generalized seizures in mesial temporal lobe epilepsy. Brain Res 2002; 929:105–116.

67. Khurgel M, Ivy GO. Astrocytes in kindling: relevance to epileptogenesis. Epilepsy Res 1996; 26:163–175.

68. Li J, Shen H, Naus CC, Zhang L, Carlen PL. Upregulation of gap junction connexin 32 with epileptiform activity in the isolated mouse hippocampus. Neuroscience 2001; 105:589–598.

69. Naus CC, Bechberger JF, Paul DL. Gap junction gene expression in human seizure disorder. Exp Neurol 1991; 111:198–203.

70. Sohl G, Guldenagel M, Beck H, Teubner B, Traub O, Gutierrez R, Heinemann U, Willecke K. Expression of connexin genes in hippocampus of kainate-treated and kindled rats under conditions of experimental epilepsy. Brain Res Mol Brain Res 2000; 83:44–51.

71. Schwartzkroin PA, Baraban SC, Hochman DW. Osmolarity, ionic flux, and changes in brain excitability. Epilepsy Res 1998; 32:275–285.

72. Draguhn A, Traub RD, Schmitz D, Jefferys JG. Electrical coupling underlies high-frequency oscillations in the hippocampus in vitro. Nature 1998; 394:189–192.

73. Bragin A, Mody I, Wilson CL, Engel J Jr. Local generation of fast ripples in epileptic brain. J Neurosci 2002; 22:2012–2021.

8

A Mechanistic Approach to Antiepileptic Drug Interactions

Gail D. Anderson
University of Washington
Seattle, Washington, U.S.A.

INTRODUCTION

Antiepileptic drugs (AEDs) are associated with a wide range of drug interactions. Although monotherapy with AEDs is preferred, patients with multiple seizure types or intractable epilepsy generally require various combinations of AEDs AEDs also are used to treat other, nonepileptic conditions, including affective disorders, migraine, and pain. Long-term treatment is common, and concurrent treatment is often prescribed by multiple caregivers during AED therapy. Thus, the risk for the development of AED-associated drug interactions is increased. Drug interactions can occur by pharmacokinetic and/or pharmacodynamic mechanisms. Pharmacodynamic interactions occur when the pharmacology of one agent alters the pharmacology or effect of the other drugs without altering plasma concentrations of the drugs. For example, the additive sedative properties of drinking alcohol and taking a sedating antihistamine, diphenyhydramine (Benadryl), or combining phenobarbital with a benzodiazepine. The most commonly occurring AED interactions are pharmacokinetic in nature, where one drug alters the plasma concentrations of another. Pharmacokinetic interactions include hepatic enzyme induction and inhibition, and displacement of protein binding.

MECHANISMS OF DRUG INTERACTIONS

Hepatic Enzyme Induction

Hepatic enzyme induction is generally the result of an increase in the amount of enzyme protein (1,2). In most cases, enzyme induction results in an increase in the rate of metabolism of the affected drug, a decrease in the serum concentration of a parent drug, and possibly a loss of clinical efficacy. If the affected drug has an active metabolite, induction can result in increased metabolite concentrations and potentially an increase in the drug's therapeutic effect and toxicity. Enzyme induction causes major effects on a limited number of extensively metabolized drugs (i.e., >75% metabolized) with a low therapeutic index. For the drugs listed in Table 1, addition or removal of an inducer could result in loss of efficacy or toxicity if plasma concentrations are not adjusted (3). Dosage adjustments of ~50–100%, with careful clinical monitoring, may be required.

Table 1. Drugs in Which Addition or Discontinuation of a Hepatic Enzyme Inducer Could Cause Clinically Significant Effects

Drug category	Specific drugs	
Antiepileptic drugs	Carbamazepine	Tiagabine
	Ethosuximide	Topiramate
	Felbamate	Valproate
	Lamotrigine	Zonisamide
	Phenytoin	
Anti-infectious agents	Itraconazole	Mebendazole
	Ketoconazole	
Antipsychotic agents	Clozapine	Risperidone
	Haloperidol	Quetiapine
Antiviral agents	Amprenavir	Ritonavir
	Delavirdine	Saquinavir
	Indinavir	Zidovudine
	Nelfinavir	
Benzodiazepines	Alprazolam	Lorazepam
	Clonazepam	Midazolam
	Diazepam	Triazolam
Calcium channel blockers	Amlodipine	Nifedipine
	Belpridil	Nimodipine
	Diltiazem	Nisodipine
	Felodipine	Nitrendipine
	Isradipine	Verapamil
	Nicardipine	
Cardioactive drugs	Digoxin	Propranolol
	Disopyramide	Quinidine
	Procainamide	
Corticosteroids	Cortisone	Methylprednisolone
	Betamethasone	Prednisolone
	Dexamaethasone	Prednisone
	Hydrocortisone	Triamcinolone
Immunosuppresants	Cyclosporine	Tacrolimus
	Sirolimus	
Oral anticoagulants	Dicumarol	Warfarin
Oral contraceptives	Conjugated estrogens	Levonorgestrel
	Ethinyl estradiol	Norethindrone
Miscellaneous	Methadone	Vincristine
	Theophylline	

Source: Ref. 3

The time required for induction depends on both the time to reach steady state of the inducing agent and the rate of synthesis of new enzymes. The amount of enzyme induction is proportional to the dose of the inducing agent. This has been shown for phenytoin (4), phenobarbital (4), and carbamazepine (5). In contrast to the dose relationship, induction is not strictly additive when patients are receiving multiple inducers (4,6). In a group of patients receiving both carbamazepine and phenytoin, the elimination half-life of antipyrine was determined (as a marker used to assess oxidative metabolism) before and after discontinuation of either carbamazepine or phenytoin (6). In patients in whom carbamazepine was discontinued, the antipyrine half-life did not change. However, when phenytoin was discontinued instead of carbamazepine, the antipyrine half-life increased. Assuming no change in the volume of distribution, this suggests that phenytoin has stronger inducing properties than carbamazepine and that induction is not additive.

Because induction is a gradual process, allowing time for gradual increases in the dose of the affected drug is required. The time course of deinduction is dependent on the rate of degradation of the enzyme and the time required eliminating the inducing drug. For the AEDs, the rate-limiting step in deinduction is generally dependent on the elimination of the inducing drug. When the inducer is removed, plasma concentrations of the affected drug will increase. Serious adverse events can occur if the dose of the affected drug is not reduced.

Three different situations exist in which hepatic enzyme induction plays a role in therapeutic decision making: (1) addition of a medication when an inducer is present; (2) addition of an inducer to existing therapy; and (3) removal of an inducer from chronic therapy. As an example, consider the interaction between warfarin and carbamazepine, an inducer of warfarin metabolism. If a patient is on chronic therapy with carbamazepine and warfarin is subsequently added, the patient will require larger doses of warfarin to achieve a clinical response. If a patient is stabilized on chronic warfarin therapy and carbamazepine is added, warfarin doses will need to be increased. Finally, if a patient is stabilized on concomitant warfarin and carbamazepine, and carbamazepine is then removed, the warfarin dosage will need to be reduced to prevent toxicity. The magnitude and timing of these interactions are critical to allow clinicians to adjust doses in such a way to maintain therapeutic effect and avoid toxicity.

Hepatic Enzyme Inhibition

Hepatic enzyme inhibition usually occurs because of competition at the enzyme active site and results in a decrease in the rate of metabolism of the affected drug (7). Clinically, this is associated with an increased plasma concentration of the affected drug and potentially an increased pharmacologic response. The onset of the interaction is frequently rapid, and the extent of the interaction is highly variable. The initial effects of hepatic enzyme inhibition usually occur within 24 h of addition of the inhibitor, but the time to maximal inhibition will depend on the time needed to achieve steady state of both the affected drug and the inhibiting drug.

Most commonly used AEDs are eliminated via hepatic metabolism. Metabolic reactions are catalyzed by the cytochrome P450 (CYP) and UDP glucuronosyl-transferase (UGT) enzymes. CYPs are a family of multiple enzymes with the individual isozymes being composed of three major families (CYP1, CYP2, and CYP3).

Seven primary isozymes are involved in the hepatic metabolism of most drugs: CYP1A2, CYP2A6, CYP2C8/9, CYP2C19, CYP2D6, CYP2E1, and CYP3A4 (8,9). The most abundant isozyme, CYP3A4, which accounts for ~30% of the total hepatic CYP (8), has the broadest substrate specificity and is involved in the metabolism of >50% of all drugs (9).

The UGTs are a family of enzymes that catalyze the transfer of a glucuronic acid moiety from a donor cosubstrate UDPGA to an aglycone (10). The UGT1 family members are capable of glucuronidating a wide range of drugs, xenobiotics, and endobiotics (11). The UGT2 family of isoforms has long been considered to be more involved in the glucuronidation of endobiotics including steroids and bile acids. UGT2 isoenzymes seem to favor these types of compound as substrates but can glucuronidate other chemical types as well.

Recent knowledge of the specific CYP isozymes involved in the metabolism of the AEDs allows prediction of potential inhibition interactions (Table 2). However, research involving drug interactions of specific isozymes of UGT has lagged behind. The extent of inhibition is more difficult to predict than the type of interaction. A large number of patient and drug factors will influence the extent of the inhibition. The extent of inhibition is dependent on the dose of the inhibitor as the majority of inhibition interactions are competitive. Intersubject variability in the expression of the CYP isozymes will influence the fraction of the dose associated with each metabolic pathway that is inhibited. The expression of the isozymes is dependent on both genetic and environmental influences including concurrent disease states (9,12).

Displacement of Protein Binding

Drug interactions related to protein binding result from the displacement of one drug with less affinity for the protein by another drug with greater affinity. Clinically significant interactions occur only with highly protein-bound drugs (i.e., >90%). For highly protein-bound drugs that are primarily eliminated by low extraction hepatic metabolism, protein-binding displacement causes a decrease in total plasma concentrations of the displaced drug and no change in the unbound drug. Transient increases in unbound drug can be associated with acute toxicity. For most AEDs, total plasma concentrations are used for clinical monitoring. Interpretation of total concentrations in the context of protein binding interactions will result in dosing adjustments that will possibly lead to AED toxicity. In the case of AEDs, phenytoin and valproate are the only drugs involved in clinically important protein-binding interactions. Tiagabine is also highly protein bound. As tiagabine plasma concentrations are not routinely monitored, misinterpretation of total plasma concentrations is not a clinically significant issue.

ANTIEPILEPTIC DRUG INTERACTIONS

Carbamazepine

Effect of Carbamazepine on Other Drugs

Carbamazepine induces the metabolism of drugs metabolized by the CYP1A2 (13), CYP2C (14), and CYP3A (15) families and UGT (16). In addition to inducing the

Table 2. Inhibitors of Uridine Diphosphate Glucuronosyltranferases (UGT) and Cytochrome P450 (CYP) Isozymes Involved in AED Metabolism

Isozyme	AED substrate	Inhibitors[a]	References
CYP 1A2	Carbamazepine	Fluvoxamine	22
CYP 2C8	Carbamazepine		22
CYP 2C9	Carbamazepine	Sulfaphenazole	22,108,121,193
	Phenobarbital	Fluconazole	
	Phenytoin	Amiodarone	
	Valproate	Miconazole	
		Propoxyphene	
		Valproate	
		Cimetidine	
CYP 2C19	Phenobarbital	Felbamate	47,108,121,134,193,221
	Phenytoin	Fluoxetine	
	Valproate	Fluvoxamine	
		Isoniazid	
		Ticlopidine	
CYP 3A4	Carbamazepine	Erythromycin	22,44,160,221
	Ethosuximide[b]	Cimetidine	
	Tiagabine[a]	Clarithromycin	
		Diltiazem	
		Fluconazole	
		Grapefruit juice	
		Indinavir	
		Isoniazid	
		Itraconazole	
		Ketoconazole	
		Miconazole	
		Propoxyphene	
		Ritonavir	
		Troleandomycin	
		Verapamil	
UGTs	Lamotrigine	Valproate	68,189
	Lorazepam		
	Valproate		

[a]The drugs listed below have been shown to be inhibitors of the various CYP isozymes. Not all interactions have been demonstrated for all drugs. Caution should be used with concurrent therapy of known inhibitors.
[b]Data in rat microsomes only.

metabolism of other drugs, carbamazepine induces its own metabolism (17). The plasma clearance of carbamazepine more than doubles during the initial weeks of therapy. Autoinduction of carbamazepine occurs via induction of CYP3A4-catalyzed metabolism to carbamazepine epoxide (CBZ epoxide). The time course of auto-induction provides evidence regarding the expected time course of carbamazepine induction of other CYP-metabolized drugs. In pharmacokinetic modeling studies, carbamazepine demonstrated an induction half-life of 4 days (17,18). The majority of the induction occurs within 1 week of initiation of carbamazepine and should be completed within ~3 weeks. The time course of the deinduction is approximately the same (19). Reductions in plasma concentrations of other AEDs and non-AEDs will occur when carbamazepine is added to existing therapy (Table 1).

With the increased use of carbamazepine in affective and peripheral pain syndromes, interactions with the tricyclic antidepressants (TCAs) are important to consider. Carbamazepine induces the metabolism of TCAs, resulting in decreased plasma concentrations of the parent drugs and increased metabolite concentrations. Because many TCAs have active metabolites, it is not clear whether dosage adjustments are necessary (20). Carbamazepine is moderately protein bound (75%). Protein-binding interactions can occur, but are usually not clinically significant.

Effect of Other Drugs on Carbamazepine

Carbamazepine is extensively metabolized, with <1% excreted unchanged in the urine. CBZ epoxide is the predominant metabolite, accounting for ~25% of the dose in monotherapy and 50% in polytherapy with other inducing AEDs (21). In human liver microsomal preparations, carbamazepine is a substrate for CYP3A4 (major) with minor metabolism by CYP1A2 and CYP2C8 (22). CBZ epoxide is pharmacologically active and contributes to the therapeutic effects of carbamazepine as well as to its neurotoxicity. When considering effects of other drugs on carbamazepine, one also must consider the effects on the active metabolite, which is rarely clinically measured. For example, fluoxetine inhibits the metabolism of carbamazepine but does not inhibit CYP3A4 formation of CBZ epoxide within the concentration range attained with routine therapeutic doses (23). By inhibiting carbamazepine metabolism through unknown alternative pathways, fluoxetine added to carbamazepine causes increased plasma concentrations of both carbamazepine and CBZ epoxide (23,24). Clinically, the patients may show significant signs of carbamazepine toxicity with what might appear to be small increases in carbamazepine plasma concentrations. The inhibition of carbamazepine metabolism by both fluoxetine, (a CYP2C19 and CYP2D6 inhibitor) and phenytoin (a CYP2C9 and CYP2C19 substrate) suggests that carbamazepine may be a substrate for CYP2C19. However, a CYP2C19 pathway has not been identified.

Increases in serum concentrations of CBZ epoxide are seen with either an increase or no change in carbamazepine concentrations when valproate is added to carbamazepine therapy. Valproate inhibits epoxide hydrolase, the enzyme that catalyzes the metabolism of CBZ epoxide, and addition of valproate may result in carbamazepine related toxicity (25,26).

The macrolide antibiotics also are potent inhibitors of CYP3A4; case reports of interactions with carbamazepine have been reported for erythromycin (27,28), clarithromycin (29), and troleandomycin (30), resulting in increased carbamazepine and decreased CBZ epoxide plasma concentrations. Despite extensive literature establishing that the elevations in carbamazepine plasma concentrations and the serious clinical toxicity that can result, this combination is still commonly prescribed (31).

The calcium channel blockers verapamil and diltiazem have been reported to decrease the metabolism of carbamazepine and result in carbamazepine toxicity (32,33). There have been several case reports of addition of propoxyphene (34), danazol (35), and nicotinamide (36) resulting in carbamazepine toxicity because of elevations in carbamazepine plasma concentrations. All five drugs have been shown to be CYP3A4 inhibitors in vitro demonstrating the ability of in vitro data (22) to predict the occurrence of in vivo interactions.

Herbal/Carbamazepine Interactions

The effect of St. John's wort, an inducer of CYP3A metabolism (37,38), on carbamazepine pharmacokinetics demonstrated no significant interaction (39). The induction of carbamazepine plus St. John's wort is not additive, as St. John's wort was not able to increase the induction already produced by carbamazepine. A study in rabbits evaluated the potential pharmacokinetic interaction of carbamazepine and Mentat, an herbal medication used in psychiatric conditions in India. Mentat significantly increased the plasma concentrations of carbamazepine, suggesting a possible inhibitor effect (40).

Ethosuximide

Effect of Ethosuximide on Other Drugs

Therapeutic doses of ethosuximide do not cause induction of enzymes in humans, and ethosuximide has not been associated with inhibition of other drugs (41,42). A recent report, however, suggests that ethosuximide administration may reduce valproate concentrations by approximately one-third through an unknown mechanism (43). The negligible protein binding of ethosuximide eliminates the potential for protein-binding interactions. Overall, ethosuximide has a low capacity to alter the pharmacokinetics of other drugs.

Effect of Other Drugs on Ethosuximide

Ethosuximide is eliminated primarily by hepatic metabolism (42). In rats, ethosuximide is a major substrate for CYP3A4 with minor metabolism by CYP2B, CYP2C, and CYP2E (44). Human data are unavailable at this time, and it is not possible to accurately extrapolate animal data to humans. Only 20% of a given dose is excreted unchanged. Valproate (45) and isoniazid (46) have been reported to inhibit the metabolism of ethosuximide and cause small increases in ethosuximide plasma concentration; however, a dosage adjustment of ethosuximide usually is not required. In general, interactions with ethosuximide are few.

Felbamate

Effect of Felbamate on Other Drugs

Felbamate is both an inhibitor of drugs metabolized by CYP2C19 (47) and β-oxidation (48) and an inducer of drugs metabolized by CYP3A4 (47). An in vitro study in human liver microsomes demonstrated that of the CYPs evaluated; only CYP2C19-metabolized drugs are inhibited (47). This is consistent with clinical experience with felbamate. Felbamate reduces the concentrations of carbamazepine but increases CBZ epoxide concentrations, which may require a decrease in carbamazepine dose when felbamate is added (49). Felbamate also significantly decreases the concentrations of gestodene, a low-dose contraceptive (50). Phenytoin (51,52), phenobarbital (53), and valproate doses may need to be reduced when felbamate therapy is initiated owing to inhibition by felbamate of CYP2C19 (phenytoin, phenobarbital) and β-oxidation (valproate). The moderate protein binding of felbamate (30%) makes protein-binding interactions unlikely.

Effect of Other Drugs on Felbamate

Felbamate is eliminated via renal excretion of unchanged drug (50%), glucuronidation (20%), and is a substrate for CYP3A4 (20%) and CYP2E1 (47). Plasma concentrations of felbamate are decreased by carbamazepine (49), phenytoin (52), and phenobarbital (53) Erythromycin (a CYP3A4 inhibitor) did not result in a significant increase in felbamate plasma concentrations (54). Owing to the small percent of felbamate metabolized by CYP3A4, this is not unexpected. A retrospective evaluation of felbamate plasma concentrations found that dose-normalized concentrations of felbamate with concurrent therapy with gabapentin were 37% higher than in patients receiving monotherapy (55). A pharmacokinetic study of felbamate and gabapentin has not been done in order to confirm this retrospective observation.

Gabapentin

Effect of Gabapentin on Other Drugs

Gabapentin is not an inducer of CYP (56) or UGT-dependent metabolism, and does not significantly affect the elimination of the commonly used AEDs (57) or oral contraceptives (58). Gabapentin may decrease the plasma clearance of felbamate (see above); however, the mechanism is unclear (55). Administration of gabapentin with lithium, another drug that is exclusively eliminated by renal excretion, does not alter the pharmacokinetics of lithium (59). The lack of protein binding ($<$5%) of gabapentin makes protein-binding interactions unlikely.

Effect of Other Drugs on Gabapentin

Gabapentin is eliminated almost completely unchanged by the kidneys. There are no clinically significant interactions reported regarding gabapentin elimination. Administration of aluminum hydroxide and magnesium hydroxide (Maalox TC) simultaneously and within 2 h of a single dose of gabapentin reduced gabapentin bioavailability by ~10–20% (60). Therefore, separating the administration of antacids and gabapentin by more than 2 h is recommended.

Food/Gabapentin Interactions

Gabapentin is transported across membranes in the intestinal membrane and the blood–brain barrier via the L-amino acid transporter system. This results in saturable intestinal absorption of gabapentin. Evaluation of the interaction with food, especially high-protein meals, becomes a clinically relevant question. Two studies have evaluated the effects of a high protein meal on gabapentin pharmacokinetics. In a study of 12 patients with epilepsy, a high-protein meal did not significantly alter gabapentin serum or saliva concentrations or urinary excretion (61). In contrast, a study in 10 healthy subjects did find a 36% increase in C_{max} and decreased T_{max} with a nonstatistically significant 11% increase in AUC (62). The overall effect on AUC is small enough and should not result in a clinically significant effect on steady state gabapentin plasma concentrations. Administration of gabapentin mixed with food of varied protein composition did not significantly alter gabapentin absorption.

Lamotrigine

Effect of Lamotrigine on Other Drugs

Lamotrigine is an inducer of UGT. It induces its own metabolism (63) and causes a small decrease (~25%) in valproate plasma concentrations when added to therapy (64). An increase in CBZ epoxide plasma concentrations was reported in case reports (65), but was not confirmed in larger clinical studies (66). Carbamazepine toxicity presents with only small changes in carbamazepine and CBZ epoxide concentrations, suggesting that the interaction with lamotrigine may be pharmacodynamic rather than pharmacokinetic (67). The moderate protein binding (55%) of lamotrigine makes protein-binding interactions unlikely.

Effect of Other Drugs on Lamotrigine

Lamotrigine is extensively metabolized to two N-glucuronide metabolites through a reaction catalyzed by UGT1A4 (68) with only minor renal elimination (69). Lamotrigine plasma concentrations are reduced by carbamazepine, phenytoin, and phenobarbital (70,71). In a retrospective analysis, dose-corrected plasma concentrations of lamotrigine in patients receiving methsuximide and oxcarbazepine were significantly lower than in patients receiving lamotrigine monotherapy (72). The inducing properties of oxcarbazepine were less (29%) than carbamazepine (54%). Therefore, replacement of carbamazepine with oxcarbazepine should result in an increase in lamotrigine plasma concentrations and a reduction in lamotrigine dose is necessary (72). Methsuximide is not a known inducer of UGTs; however, a similar decrease in lamotrigine plasma concentrations was found in a pharmacokinetic study in 16 patients. Subchronic dosing of acetaminophen, a drug that is ~55% eliminated by glucuronide conjugation, resulted in unexplained increase in lamotrigine clearance. The clinical significance and mechanism of this interaction is unknown (73).

Valproate significantly increases lamotrigine plasma concentrations, presumably by competitively inhibiting lamotrigine glucuronidation. The magnitude of the inhibition is not dependent on the valproate dose or concentration (74). The maximum inhibition of lamotrigine plasma clearance at the lowest measured valproate plasma concentration is consistent with the approximately 20-fold higher molar concentrations of valproate used compared to lamotrigine. In addition, the lamotrigine-valproate combination has been notoriously associated with hypersensitivity reactions (75). The incidence of rash in children is significantly higher than that in adults. In some cases, the rash has been potentially life-threatening. Patients should be carefully counseled to report any rash or other symptom of hypersensitivity (e.g., fever, lymphadenopathy) to their clinician. Because lamotrigine-valproate combination therapy has been reported to have significant efficacy in refractory patients with atypical absence and complex partial seizures (76), the combination should not be contraindicated in adult patients. By decreasing the initial starting dose and the rate of dose escalation of lamotrigine, the incidence of the rash is significantly decreased (75).

A case report of two patients receiving sertraline and lamotrigine cotherapy reported that sertraline significantly increased plasma concentrations of lamotrigine (77).

Levetiracetam

Effect of Levetiracetam on Other Drugs

Levetiracetam is not an inducer of CYP- or UGT dependent metabolism and does not appear to alter the plasma concentrations of the other AEDs measured in most clinical studies—including carbamazepine, clobazam, phenobarbital, phenytoin, primidone, and valproate (78–81). Even though phenytoin concentrations increased 27–52% in four of six patients after levetiracetam was added in an efficacy/safety clinical trial (78), a clinical pharmacokinetic study in six male patients found there was no effect of levetiracetam on phenytoin serum concentrations or pharmacokinetics (82). Levetiracetam does not affect the pharmacokinetics of warfarin, oral contraceptives (83), or digoxin (84).

Effect of Other Drugs on Levetiracetam

Levetiracetam is eliminated predominately by renal excretion of unchanged drug (~2/3) and by hydrolysis of the acetamide group, a reaction catalyzed by amidases, which are present in a number of tissues. As levetiracetam is not significantly metabolized by either CYP or UGTs, induction by other inducing AEDs does not occur. In vitro evaluation of potential drug interactions with levetiracetam on 11 different drug-metabolizing enzyme activities demonstrated that levetiracetam is unlikely to inhibit the metabolism of other drugs by CYPS, UGTs, or epoxide hydrolase (85). Digoxin does not alter the pharmacokinetics of levetiracetam (84).

Oxcarbazepine

Effect of Oxcarbazepine on Other Drugs

Unlike carbamazepine, oxcarbazepine is not a broad-spectrum inducer of CYP enzymes; however, it does induce the metabolism of drugs that are catalyzed by CYP3A4 and UGT. The extent of induction is less than that reported with carbamazepine. Oral contraceptives need to be used cautiously in patients receiving any AED that causes induction of CYP3A4. Two weeks of oxcarbazepine cotherapy with an oral contraceptive resulted in a significant decrease in the plasma concentrations of ethinylestradiol and levonorgestrel (86,87). Consistent with CYP3A4 induction, a case report found that oxcarbazepine decreased cyclosporine plasma concentrations (88). Felodipine plasma concentrations were significantly reduced by coadministration of oxcarbazepine (89). In a retrospective analysis of samples obtained during therapeutic drug monitoring, oxcarbazepine appeared to reduce the plasma concentrations of lamotrigine by 29%; however, the decrease was significantly less than found with carbamazepine cotherapy (54%) (72). Both phenobarbital and phenytoin plasma concentrations may increase when oxcarbazepine is added in a dose-dependent manner. This is consistent with inhibition of CYP2C19 (see package insert). Oxcarbazepine does not alter the pharmacokinetics of warfarin (90).

Effect of Other Drugs on Oxcarbazepine and 10-Monohydroxy Metabolites (MHD)

Oxcarbazepine is a pro-drug which is rapidly converted to a monohydroxy derivative (MHD) upon oral administration, a reaction catalyzed by cytosolic arylketone reductase. MHD is predominantly excreted unchanged in the urine or conjugated by UGT and then excreted, with only minor oxidation metabolism to dihydroxy derivative (DHD). The conversion of oxcarbazepine to MHD appears to be via a noninducible pathway (91). Phenobarbital and phenytoin decrease the plasma concentration of MHD, presumably owing to induction of UGT, or by increasing the minor CYP metabolism to DHD (91,92). Valproate slightly decreases the elimination of MHD, most likely owing to inhibition of UGT-catalyzed metabolism (93). Verapamil coadministration resulted in a small decrease in MHD (94). Neither cimetidine (95), erythromycin (96), nor propoxyphene (97) affected the pharmacokinetics of oxcarbazepine.

Phenobarbital

Effect of Phenobarbital on Other Drugs

Phenobarbital induces the metabolism of drugs metabolized by CYP1A (98), CYP2A6 (99), CYP2B (100), CYP2C (101), and CYP3A (102) families, and UGT (16,103). The time course of induction and deinduction is primarily dependent on the long elimination half-life of phenobarbital. Induction usually begins in ~1 week, with maximal induction occurring 2–3 weeks after phenobarbital therapy is initiated (104). The time course of the deinduction will follow a similar course, as phenobarbital plasma concentrations decline over 2–3 weeks following removal of drug (105). Decreases in the plasma concentrations of other AEDs and non-AEDs will occur when phenobarbital is added to therapy (Table 1).

Effect of Other Drugs on Phenobarbital

Phenobarbital is eliminated by both renal excretion of unchanged drug and hepatic metabolism (106). The primary metabolites of phenobarbital are parahydroxyphenobarbital (PbOH) and phenobarbital N-glucoside (107). CYP2C9 plays a major role in the formation of PbOH, with minor metabolism by CYP2C19 and CYP2E1 (108). The diversity of the elimination pathways of phenobarbital and the low protein binding (50%) minimize the effects of other drugs on phenobarbital. For example, inhibitors of CYP2C9 should alter the formation of PbOH. However, because the fraction of the dose of phenobarbital metabolized by CYP2C9 to PbOH is low (20%), CYP2C9 inhibitors do not cause clinically significant increases in phenobarbital plasma concentrations. Valproate causes the only clinically significant increase in phenobarbital plasma concentrations because of its broad spectrum of inhibition. Valproate inhibits both major metabolic pathways of phenobarbital, the formation of PbOH and phenobarbital N-glucoside (109).

Phenytoin

Effect of Phenytoin on Other Drugs

Phenytoin increases the metabolism of drugs that are metabolized by the CYP2C (110) and CYP3A (102,111) families and UGT enzymes (15,16,112). Maximal induction or deinduction occurs ~1–2 weeks after initiation of phenytoin therapy, corresponding to the approximate time to steady-state concentrations (113). Theoretically, deinduction requires a similar period of time. Decreases in the

Table 3. Induction and Inhibition Effect of AEDs on Hepatic Enzymes

AED	Effect	Enzyme involved	Reference
Carbamazepine	Inducer	CYP1A2, CYP2C, CYP3A, UGT	13–16
Ethosuximide	No effect		41,42
Felbamate	Inducer	CYP3A4	47,48
	Inhibitor	CYP2C19, β-oxidation	
Gabapentin	No effect		56
Lamotrigine	Inducer	UGT	63,64
Levetiracetam	No effect		78–81
Oxcarbazepine	Inducer	CYP3A4, UGT	72,86–89
	Inhibitor	CYP2C19	
Phenobarbital/ primidone	Inducer	CYP1A, CYP2A6, CYP2B, CYP2C, CYP3A, UGT	16,98–103
Phenytoin	Inducer	CYP2C, CYP3A, UGT	15,16,102,110–112
Tiagabine	No effect		157–160
Topiramate	Inducer	β-Oxidation	169,170,172,173
	Inhibitor	CYP2C19	
Valproate	Inhibitor	CYP2C9, UGT, epoxide hydrolase	63,177,178,180
Vigabatrin	No effect		199
Zonisamide	No effect		203

plasma concentrations of other AEDs and non-AEDs can occur when phenytoin is added to therapy (see Table 1).

Oral contraceptives should be used cautiously in patients receiving any AED that causes induction of CYP3A4 (Table 3). Phenytoin decreases the area under the concentration (AUC) time curve of ethinylestradiol and levonorgestrel (114). A number of unplanned pregnancies have occurred in women taking phenytoin or other inducing AEDs (115,116). Breakthrough bleeding and spotting may be a sign of inadequate contraception, and an alternative form of birth control may be advisable.

Although phenytoin is considered an inducer of hepatic metabolism, competition by phenytoin at the site of metabolism can occur with other drugs metabolized by the same CYP (see Table 2). Both phenytoin and phenobarbital are metabolized by CYP2C9. Phenobarbital plasma concentrations reportedly decrease when phenytoin is discontinued in some patients (117,118). Therefore, combined use of phenytoin and phenobarbital may decrease the concentrations of both drugs, or in some patients, phenobarbital concentrations and/or phenytoin concentrations may increase.

Initiation of phenytoin in a patient receiving warfarin requires special consideration. There have been case reports of a hypoprothrombinemic response after phenytoin was given to patients receiving chronic warfarin therapy (119,120). Two proposed mechanisms could account for this response. First, when phenytoin therapy is started in a patient stabilized on warfarin therapy, phenytoin may displace warfarin from albumin-binding sites and cause a transient increase in warfarin effect (119,120). Second, phenytoin initially may competitively inhibit the metabolism of warfarin because both phenytoin and S-warfarin are CYP2C9 substrates (121).

After the initial increased effect of S-warfarin, plasma concentrations may decline within 1–2 weeks after phenytoin is added because of CYP219 induction. Therefore, an initial decrease and then increase in warfarin dose may be needed in order to maintain the desired anticoagulation effect.

Effect of Other Drugs on Phenytoin

Phenytoin is eliminated predominantly by CYP2C9- and CYP2C19-dependent hepatic metabolism (121). Clinically significant increases in phenytoin plasma concentrations have been demonstrated for the following inhibitors of CYP2C9 and CYP2C19 enzymes (see Table 2). CYP2C9 inhibitors are amiodarone (122), fluconazole (123), miconazole (124), propoxyphene (125), sulfaphenazole (126), and valproate (127). CYP2C19 inhibitors are felbamate (52), omeprazole (128), cimetidine (129,130), fluoxetine, fluvoxamine (131), isonizaid (132,133), and ticlopidine (134,135).

When carbamazepine and phenytoin are given concurrently, the serum concentrations of both drugs may decrease. Similar to phenytoin–phenobarbital interactions, phenytoin concentrations may increase in some patients when carbamazepine is added; the mechanism underlying this effect is unclear (136).

The effect of valproate on phenytoin is a combination of a protein-binding displacement and enzyme inhibition (127). If valproate only displaced phenytoin from albumin, total phenytoin concentrations would decrease and unbound phenytoin concentrations would not change. If valproate only caused inhibition of phenytoin metabolism, both total and unbound phenytoin concentrations would increase. The interactions result in a disruption of the relationship between unbound and total phenytoin concentrations. Total phenytoin concentrations can increase, decrease, or not change when valproate is added. The unbound phenytoin concentrations, however, will increase. Ideally, unbound phenytoin concentrations should be monitored in a patient receiving both valproate and phenytoin. If unbound phenytoin concentrations are not available, Haidukewych et al. (137) propose the following method of predicting unbound phenytoin concentrations from a measured total phenytoin and valproate plasma concentration, which is a reliable predictor of unbound phenytoin concentrations (138):

$$\text{PHT unbound} = (0.095 + 0.001 * [\text{VPA}] * [\text{PHT total}])$$

Herbal/Phenytoin Drug Interactions

There is one case report of two patients receiving phenytoin who both lost seizure control after Shankapulshipi, an Ayurvedic preparation used for treatment of epilepsy, was added (139). In a follow-up study in rats, coadministration resulted in a 50% decrease in plasma phenytoin concentration (139). Another study in rats evaluated the effect of a traditional Chinese medicine, Paeoniae Radix, used in the treatment of epilepsy in Asian countries on phenytoin pharmacokinetics. Paeoniae Radix cotherapy resulted in no significant difference in phenytoin pharmacokinetics (140). In yet another study involving rabbits, the potential pharmacokinetic interaction of phenytoin and Mentat, an herbal medication used in psychiatric conditions in India, was evaluated. Mentat significantly increased the plasma concentrations of phenytoin, suggesting a possible inhibitor effect (40). The Chinese herb *Angelica dahurica* significantly inhibited the metabolism of tolbutamide (a CYP2C9 substrate) after intravenous administration in rats (141). In vitro studies of human CYP enzymes have demonstrated that St. John's wort (142) and Ginkgo Biloba (personal communication) inhibit CYP2C9. Therefore, these studies suggest there is a significant potential interaction between herbal preparations and phenytoin; however, clinical data are still lacking.

Primidone

Effect of Primidone on Other Drugs

Primidone therapy results in the formation of phenobarbital, one of its active metabolites (143). Therefore, the interactions described above for phenobarbital also relate to administration of primidone (144).

Effect of Other Drugs on Primidone

Fifty percent of primidone is eliminated unchanged via urinary excretion. The remainder is metabolized by CYP to two active metabolites, phenobarbital and phenylethylmalonamide (PEMA) (143). The specific CYPs involved have not been identified. A decreased ratio of primidone to phenobarbital occurs with concurrent administration of CYP inducers such as phenytoin (145) and carbamazepine (146). Valproate inhibits the formation and elimination of phenobarbital, resulting in variable effects on the primidone–phenobarbital ratio (36,147). Isoniazid (148) inhibits the formation of phenobarbital, causing an increased primidone-to-phenobarbital ratio. As both primidone and phenobarbital are active, the clinical significance of the interactions is unclear.

Stiripentol

Effect of Stiripentol on Other Drugs

Stiripentol is a potent inhibitor of the majority of the CYPs involved in drug metabolism. In vitro studies have demonstrated inhibition of CYP1A2, CYP2C9, CYP2C19, CYP2D6, and CYP3A4 (149). Clinically, stiripentol has been shown to significantly reduce the clearance of many AEDs, including carbamazepine (150), phenytoin (151), and phenobarbital (151). There is a small, but not clinically significant, increase in valproate plasma concentrations, as stiripentol does not affect the major pathways of valproate elimination (glucuronidation and β-oxidation) (152). Since stiripentol inhibits all the major CYPs involved in drug metabolism, caution should be used when stiripentol is coadministered with any drug eliminated predominantly by CYP-catalyzed metabolism.

Effect of Other Drugs on Stiripentol

Stiripentol is eliminated extensively by hepatic metabolism and displays Michaelis-Menten nonlinear pharmacokinetics within the range of plasma concentrations found clinically (153). Thirteen metabolites have been identified including UGT-catalyzed conjugation with glucuronic acid (22–33%), oxidative cleavage of the methylenedeioxy ring system, O-demethylation, and hydroxylation (154). Plasma concentrations of stiripentol are significantly decreased in patients receiving concurrent and inducing AEDs (carbamazepine, phenytoin, and phenobarbital) (153,155,156). Stiripentol is also highly protein bound (>99%); however, there are no studies addressing displacement of protein binding.

Tiagabine

Effect of Tiagabine on Other Drugs

Tiagabine appears to be neither an inducer nor an inhibitor. Tiagabine did not affect the plasma concentrations and/or pharmacokinetics of carbamazepine, valproate, and phenytoin (157); triazolam (158); theophylline (159); warfarin (160); digoxin (161); cimetidine (160); oral contraceptives (160); or ethanol (160). Tiagabine coadministration resulted in a slight, but clinically insignificant, reduction in valproate plasma concentrations (~10%); however, the mechanism of this reduction is unknown (162).

Effect of Other Drugs on Tiagabine

Tiagabine is extensively metabolized, with <2% excreted unchanged in the urine (163). After administration of and oral dosing of ^{14}C-tiagabine to four subjects, the 5-oxo-tiagabine isomers (~22% of the dose) and two unidentified metabolites (40%) were recovered (164). CYP3A4 has been identified as the primary isozyme responsible for metabolism of tiagabine to 5-oxo-tigabine (160). In patients with epilepsy treated with enzyme-inducing AEDs (carbamazepine, phenobarbital, phenytoin, primidone), tiagabine clearance is significantly increased (157,165). In vitro, inhibitors of CYP3A4 (erythromycin, ketoconazole) significantly decreased the metabolism of tiagabine (160). However, in a study in normal subjects, erythromycin did not significantly alter the clearance of tiagabine (166). These observations suggest that there is only a small fraction of the dose metabolized by CYP3A4, consistent with the ^{14}C-tiagabine study. Temazepam, a CYP3A4 substrate, did not alter the pharmacokinetics of tiagabine (158). Tiagabine is extensively protein bound (96%) to albumin and α_1-acid glycoprotein (167). Valproate, naproxen, and salicylates decreased tiagabine binding in vitro from 96.3% to 94.8%, but the clinical relevance of this is unknown (168).

Topiramate

Effect of Topiramate on Other Drugs

Topiramate does not significantly affect the plasma concentrations of carbamazepine or phenobarbital (169), but does cause a modest decrease in valproate plasma concentrations by inducing the β-oxidation of valproate (170). Reduced ethinyl estradiol plasma concentrations also occur with concurrent topiramate, suggesting the need for higher doses of oral contraceptives (171). The mechanism of the reduced ethinyl estradiol plasma concentrations is unknown. As topiramate does not induce CBZ epoxide formation, induction of CYP3A4 is presumably not the mechanism. In one study, an increase (≈25%) in phenytoin plasma concentrations occurred in six of 12 patients when topiramate was added (172). The inhibition spectrum of topiramate was evaluated in human liver microsomes (173). Topiramate significantly inhibited the model substrate of CYP2C19 with no effect on any of the other CYPs evaluated. The in vitro study was consistent with the inhibitory effect of topiramate on phenytoin, and lack of inhibitory effect on the other AEDs. The intersubject variability in the phenytoin–topiramate interaction reflects the intersubject variability in the fraction of phenytoin metabolized by CYP2C9 versus CYP2C19 (121). A slight increase in digoxin oral clearance (13%) was also found in a small single-dose trial (174). The low protein binding (15%) of topiramate makes protein-binding interactions unlikely.

Effect of Other Drugs on Topiramate

In a single dose study of ^{14}C-topiramate, topiramate was predominantly eliminated unchanged in the urine (70%) (175). However, concurrent use of enzyme-inducing drugs (e.g., carbamazepine, phenytoin, and phenobarbital) has been reported to decrease topiramate plasma concentrations by ~40–50% (176). This suggests that, at least in patients on multiple doses of topiramate and receiving enzyme-inducing drugs, hepatic metabolism of topiramate accounts for a larger percentage of topiramate elimination than originally suggested by the single-dose study.

Valproate

Effect of Valproate on Other Drugs

Valproate is a broad-spectrum inhibitor of hepatic metabolism, including inhibition of CYP2C9 (177), UGT (178,179), and epoxide hydrolase (180). Valproate increases the plasma concentrations of phenobarbital and phenytoin, presumably via inhibition of CYP2C9 (phenytoin, phenobarbital) and N-glucosidation (phenobarbital) (109,127). Valproate does not inhibit cyclosporine (181) or oral contraceptives (182), suggesting a lack of inhibition of CYP3A metabolized drugs. Valproate significantly inhibits the glucuronide conjugation of lamotrigine (179), lorazepam (178), and zidovudine (183), resulting in significant increases in plasma concentrations of the affected drugs. A case report of elevated clomipramine and desmethylclomipramine plasma concentrations after addition of valproate suggests that valproate can inhibit the parallel glucuronidation pathway of clomipramine elimination (184).

Compared to a group of patients receiving clozapine monotherapy, patients receiving clozapine with valproate had higher clozapine plasma concentrations and lower plasma concentrations of desmethylclozapine, an active metabolite. The interaction should not be clinically significant (185). Both CYP3A4 and CYP1A2 are predominantly responsible for catalyzing the formation of desmethylclozapine from clozapine (186). The lack of effect of valproate in vitro and in vivo on other CYP3A4 substrates suggests that valproate can inhibit the CYP1A2 in vivo. In vitro, valproate was found to be a weak inhibitor of CYP1A2 (177).

Valproate is highly protein bound to albumin (>90%). Because of the high molar concentrations of valproate obtained clinically, valproate displaces other AEDs (phenytoin, carbamazepine, and diazepam) from albumin binding sites. [See the phenytoin section for discussion on phenytoin–valproate interaction (127).] Valproate decreases the renal clearance of diflunisal and diflunisal glucuronide, decreasing the plasma concentrations of diflunisal (187). Valproate displaces naproxen from plasma protein-binding sites and possibly decreases the glucuronidation and desmethylation of naproxen (188). Because of the wide therapeutic range of naproxen, this is probably not a clinically significant interaction.

Effect of Other Drugs on Valproate

Valproate undergoes predominately hepatic metabolism, with <5% of the dose excreted unchanged in the urine (189). Major metabolism occurs by UGT-catalyzed glucuronide conjugation and β-oxidation, with minor CYP-dependent metabolism (189). Three UGT isoforms have been reported to be capable of glucuronidating VPA: UGT1A6 (190), UGT1A9 (191), and UGT2B7 (192). Valproate is a substrate for CYP2C9 and CYP2C19 (193), but not CYP3A4 (194), consistent with the lack of competitive inhibition of valproate on CYP3A4 drugs found in vitro (177). Valproate plasma concentrations are decreased in the presence of CYP2 and UGT-inducing drugs (carbamazepine, phenobarbital, and phenytoin) (127). Felbamate significantly inhibits valproate metabolism (195) by inhibiting the β-oxidation pathway (48). In a case report of two patients, guanfacine significantly increased the plasma concentrations of valproate (196). Guanfacine is predominantly eliminated by glucuronide conjugate, suggesting a competition at the UGT enzyme(s) (197). Diflunisal (187) and naproxen (188), coadministered with valproate, results in significant displacement of protein-bound valproate. Unbound valproate plasma concentrations are not affected and therefore, the interaction should not clinically significant.

Herbal/Valproate Drug Interactions

A study in healthy subjects evaluating the effect of a traditional Chinese medicine, Paeoniae Radix (used in the treatment of epilepsy in Asian countries), found that there was no effect on the pharmacokinetics of valproate (198).

Vigabatrin

Effect of Vigabatrin on Other Drugs

Vigabatrin is available in almost all countries except the United States. Vigabatrin is neither an inducer (199) nor an inhibitor of drug metabolism, and is not associated with any significant drug interactions with one exception (200). A clinically significant decrease of 25–40% in phenytoin plasma concentrations occurs in approximately one-third of the patients receiving both drugs. A study with administration of both intravenous and oral phenytoin with and without vigabatrin concluded that the oral availability was unaffected (201). In this study, the percent of the administered dose recovered in the urine as the primary metabolite of phenytoin, parahydroxyphenytoin (HPPH), was unchanged in spite of a decrease of 25–48% in phenytoin plasma concentrations. The fraction of dose metabolized to a specific metabolite is proportional to the ratio of the formation clearance of the metabolite and the plasma clearance of the parent compound. Therefore, an increase in plasma clearance with no change in the fraction of the metabolite recovered as HPPH suggests an induction of either CYP2C9 or CYP2C19.

Effect of Other Drugs on Vigabatrin

Vigabatrin is eliminated almost completely unchanged by the kidneys (202). There are no reported interactions significantly affecting the plasma concentrations of vigabatrin. The lack of protein binding of vigabatrin makes protein-binding interactions unlikely.

Zonisamide

Effect of Zonisamide on Other Drugs

Zonisamide does not significantly affect the plasma concentrations of carbamazepine, phenytoin, phenobarbital, primidone, or valproate (203). One study did find that zonisamide increased plasma concentrations of carbamazepine (204). However, in many of the patients, phenytoin and/or phenobarbital were withdrawn concurrently with addition of zonisamide. Plasma protein binding of phenytoin and valproate (205) or carbamazepine (204) was not affected by zonisamide coadministration.

Effect of Other Drugs on Zonisamide

Zonisamide is eliminated by a combination of renal excretion of unchanged drug (~35%), metabolism via N-acetylation (~15%), and ~50% undergoes reduction to 2-sulfamoyolacetylphenol (SMAP) (206). Studies using expressed human CYPs demonstrated that CYP3A4, CYP3A5, and CYP2C19 are all capable of catalyzing zonisamide reduction. The intrinsic clearance of CYP2C19 and CYP3A5 were low compared to CYP3A4, indicating that the relative contribution of CYP2C19 and CYP3A5 may be low in vivo (207). In vitro studies showed that drugs that can inhibit CYP3A4 metabolism may decrease zonisamide plasma clearance. Based on the in vitro inhibition constants, Nakasa et al. predicted that ketoconazole, cyclosporine, and miconazole could decrease zonisamide plasma clearance by 31%, 23%, and 17%, respectively (207). Clinical studies of CYP3A4 interactions have not been reported. Therefore, zonisamide should be used cautiously with CYP3A4 inhibitors until further clinical data are available. Zonisamide plasma clearance is increased in the presence of enzyme-inducing AEDs (carbamazepine, phenytoin, and phenobarbital) (204,208,209). Zonisamide is only moderately protein-bound (40–50%) and is unaffected by the presence of carbamazepine, phenytoin, or phenobarbital (210,211).

ANTIEPILEPTIC DRUG INTERACTIONS OF DRUGS IN DEVELOPMENT

By the time a new AED is released to market, basic information regarding the elimination of the drug, as well as a potential drug interaction spectrum, is usually established. However, detailed clinical studies may or may not be found in the literature at the same time.

Pregabalin

Effect of Pregabalin on Other Drugs

Steady-state plasma concentrations of carbamazepine, lamotrigine, phenobarbital, phenytoin, topiramate, and valproate were not altered when pregabalin was evaluated as add-on therapy in clinical efficacy/safety studies (212). Therefore, pregabalin is neither an inducer nor an inhibitor of metabolic enzymes.

Effect of Other Drugs on Pregabalin

Pregabalin is eliminated by renal excretion of unchanged drug with little or no metabolism, and is not bound to plasma proteins. Clinically significant drug interactions are not expected (213).

Remacemide

Effect of Remacemide on Other Drugs

In vitro studies employing human liver microsomes have revealed that remacemide inhibits CYP3A4 and CYP2C19 isozymes. Consistent with the in vitro inhibition spectrum in human microsomes, remacemide cotherapy resulted in a modest increase in phenobarbital (214), phenytoin (215), and carbamazepine plasma concentrations (216). Remacemide does not affect the pharmacokinetics of valproate (217).

Effect of Other Drugs on Remacemide

Remacemide is metabolized by CYP-dependent oxidation and UGT-dependent glucuronidation. Remacemide undergoes significant first-pass metabolism to a desglycinated metabolite, a reaction catalyzed by aminopeptidases, which occur in many tissues. The desglycinated metabolite is active and is also extensively metabolized by oxidation and conjugation reactions with little excreted unchanged in the urine of either parent or active metabolite (218). Carbamazepine (216), phenytoin (215), and phenobarbital (214) significantly decrease the plasma concentrations of both remacemide and its metabolite. Valproate does not significantly affect remacemide pharmacokinetics (217).

Retigabine

Effect of Retigabine on Other Drugs

Retigabine did not alter the pharmacokinetics of lamotrigine in healthy subjects, suggesting that retigabine is not a broad-spectrum inducer of UGT-catalyzed metabolism (213). The CYP inhibition and induction spectrum of retigabine has not been reported.

Effect of Other Drugs on Retigabine

Retigabine is eliminated predominately by metabolism via N-glucuronidation and acetylation, with no involvement of CYP-dependent oxidation pathways (219). Drug interaction studies have not been reported. Based on knowledge of the induction and inhibition spectrum of the other AEDs, valproate may increase retigabine plasma concentrations by inhibition of UGT-catalyzed metabolism, while AED inducers of UGT (carbamazepine, phenytoin, and phenobarbital) may decrease the plasma concentrations of retigabine.

Rufinamide

Effect of Rufinamide on Other Drugs

In vitro studies in human liver microsomes have demonstrated that rufinamide does not inhibit model substrates of CYP1A2, CYP2A6, CYP2C9, CYP2C19, CYP2D6, CYP2E1, CYP3A4/5, or CYP4A9/11 (220). In efficacy/safety studies, rufinamide did not affect the trough plasma concentrations of any of the coadministered AEDs, including carbamazepine, clobazam, clonazepam, phenobarbital, phenytoin, primidone, oxcarbazepine, and valproate (213).

Effect of Other Drugs on Rufinamide

Rufinamide is extensively metabolized, with <2% of the dose excreted in the urine or feces as unchanged drug. The primary metabolic pathway is a hydrolysis of the carboxylamide group to an inactive metabolite, which is subsequently excreted in the urine (213). In a population pharmacokinetic analysis, cotherapy with CYP enzyme-inducing AEDs, rufinamide oral clearance was increased by ~25%. Valproate reduced the oral clearance of rufinamide by 22% (213).

CONCLUSIONS

Drug interactions in patients receiving AEDs are a common complication of therapy. AED induction of the metabolism of drugs with narrow therapeutic ranges will lead to patients receiving suboptimal doses of concurrent therapy if standard doses are not adjusted. By understanding the time course of induction and deinduction, serious adverse events, as well as loss of efficacy, can be avoided. Owing to the rapid onset and unpredictable extent of inhibitory drug interactions, they are the leading cause of clinically significant drug interactions. Interactions involving inhibition of the AEDs often result in toxicity. Increased knowledge regarding the specific isozymes of CYPs and UGTs involved in the metabolism of the AEDs enables the qualitative prediction of interactions for both the new AEDs, as well as interactions of new non-AEDs. The recent correlation between the findings of the in vitro studies and the clinical interaction studies have demonstrated the value of in vitro studies in predicting and directing clinical interaction studies.

REFERENCES

1. Conney AH. Pharmacological implications of microsomal enzyme induction. Pharmacol Rev 1967; 19:317–366.
2. Dogra S, Whitelaw ML, May BK. Transcriptional activation of cytochrome P450 genes by different classes of chemical inducers. Clin Exp Pharmacol Physiol 1998; 25:1–9.
3. Hansten PD, Horn JR. The Top 100 Drug Interactions: a Guide to Patient Management. Edmonds, WA: H&H Publications, 2001.
4. Perucca E, Hedges A, Makki KA, Ruprah M, Wilson JF, Richens A. A comparative study of the relative enzyme inducing properties of anticonvulsant drugs in epileptic patients. Br J Clin Pharmacol 1984; 18:401–410.
5. Tomson T, Svensson JO, Hilton-Brown P. Relationship of intra-individual dose to plasma concentration of carbamazepine: indication of dose-dependent induction of metabolism. Ther Drug Monitor 1989; 11:537–539.
6. Patsalos PN, Duncan JS, Shorvon SD. Effect of the removal of individual antiepileptic drugs on antipyrine kinetics, in patients taking polytherapy. Br J Clin Pharmacol 1988; 26:253–259.
7. Testa B, Jenner P. Inhibitors of cytochrome P450s and their mechanism of action. Drug Metab Rev 1981; 21:1–117.
8. Shimada T, Yamazaki H, Mimura M, Inui T, Guengerich FP. Interindividual variation in human liver cytochrome P450 enzymes involved in the oxidation of drugs, carcinogens, and toxic chemicals: studies with the microsomes of 30 Japanese and 30 Caucasians. J Pharmacol Exp Ther 1994; 270:414–423.
9. Wrighton SA, Stevens JC. The human hepatic cytochrome P450 involved in drug metabolism. Crit Rev Toxicol 1992; 22:1–21.

10. Clarke DJ, Burchell B. The uridine diphosphate glucuronosyltransferase multigene family; function and regulation. Handb Exp Pharmacol 1994; 112:3–43.

11. Burchell B, Brierley CH, Rance D. Specificity of human UDP-glucuronosyltransferases and xenobiotic glucuronidation. Life Sci 1995; 57:1819–1831.

12. Bertz RJ, Granneman GR. Use of in vitro and in vivo data to estimate the likelihood of metabolic pharmacokinetic interactions. Clin Pharmacokinet 1997; 32:210–258.

13. Parker AC, Pritchard P, Preston T, Choonara I. Induction of CYP1A2 activity by carbamazepine in children using the caffeine breath test. Br J Clin Pharmacol 1998; 45:176–178.

14. Cropp JS, Bussey HI. A review of enzyme induction of warfarin metabolism with recommendations for patient management. Pharmacotherapy 1997; 17:917–928.

15. Tomlinson B, Young RP, Ng MC, Anderson PJ, Kay R, Critchley JA. Selective liver enzyme induction by carbamazepine and phenytoin in Chinese epileptics. Eur J Clin Pharmacol 1996; 50:411–415.

16. Miners JO, MacKenzie PI. Drug glucuronidation in humans. Pharmacol Ther 1991; 51:347–369.

17. Gérardin AP, Abadie FV, Campestrini JA, Theobald W. Pharmacokinetics of carbamazepine in normal humans after single and repeated doses. J Pharmacoket Biopharm 1976; 5:521–535.

18. Levy RH, Lai AA. A pharmacokinetic model for drug interaction by enzyme induction and its application to carbamazepine-clonazepam. In: Johannessen SI, Morselli PL, Pippenger CE, Richens A, Schmidt D, Meinardi H, eds. Antiepileptic Therapy. Advances in Drug Monitoring. New York: Raven Press, 1980:315–323.

19. Schäffler L, Bourgeois BFD, Luders HO. Rapid reversibility of autoinduction of carbamazepine metabolism after temporary discontinuation. Epilepsia 1994; 35: 195–198.

20. Baldessarini RJ, Teicher MH, Cassidy JW, Stein MH. Anticonvulsant cotreatment may increase toxic metabolites of antidepressants and other psychotropic drugs. J Clin Psychopharmacol 1988; 8:381–382.

21. Faigle JW, Feldmann KF. Carbamazepine: chemistry and biotransformation. In: Levy RH, Mattson RH, Meldrum BS, eds. Antiepileptic Drugs. New York: Raven Press, 1995:499–514.

22. Kerr BM, Thummel KE, Wurden CJ, Klein SM, Kroetz DL, Gonzales FL, Levy RH. Human liver carbamazepine: role of CYP3A4 and CYP2A8 in 10,11 epoxide formation. Biochem Pharmacol 1994; 47:1769–1779.

23. Gidal BE, Anderson GD, Seaton TL, Miyoshi RH, Wilensky AJ. Evaluation of the effect of fluoxetine on the formation of carbamazepine epoxide. Ther Drug Monitor 1993; 15:405–409.

24. Grimsley SR, Jann MW, Carter JG, D'Mello AP, D'Souza MJ. Increased carbamazepine plasma concentrations after fluoxetine administration. Clin Pharmacol Ther 1991; 50:10–15.

25. Rambeck B, Salke-Treumann A, May T, Boenigk HE. Valproic acid induced carbamazepine 10,11-epoxide toxicity in children and adolescents. Eur Neurol 1990; 30:79–83.

26. McKee PJW, Blacklaw J, Butler E, Gillham RA, Brodie MJ. Variability and clinical relevance of the interaction between sodium valproate and carbamazepine in epileptic patients. Epilepsy Res 1992; 11:193–198.

27. Hedrick R, Williams F, Morin R, Lamb WA, Cate JC. Carbamazepine-erythromycin interaction leading to carbamazepine toxicity in epileptic children. Ther Drug Monit 1983; 5:405–407.

28. Wroblewski BA, Singer WD, Whyte J. Carbamazepine-erythromycin interaction: case studies and clinical significance. JAMA 1986; 255:1165–1167.

29. Albani F, Riva R, Baruzzi A. Clarithromycin-carbamazepine interaction: a case report. Epilepsia 1993; 34:161–162.

30. Dravet C, Mesdijian E, Cenraud B, Roger J. Interaction between carbamazepine and triacetyloeandomycin. Lancet 1977; 1:810–811.

31. Stafstrom CE, Nohria V, Loganbill H, Nahouraii R, Boustany RM, DeLong GR. Erythromycin-induced carbamazepine toxicity: a continuing problem. Arch Pediatr Adolesc Med 1995; 149:99–101.

32. Bahls FH, Ozuna J, Ritchie DE. Interactions between calcium channel blockers and the anticonvulsants carbamazepine and phenytoin. Neurology 1991; 41:740–742.

33. Hunt BA, Self TH, Lalonde RL, Bottorff MB. Calcium channel blockers as inhibitors of drug metabolism. Chest 1989; 96:393–399.

34. Dam M, Christiansen J. Interaction of propoxyphene with carbamazepine. Lancet 1977; 2:509.

35. Kramer G, Theisohn M, Von Unruh GE, Eichelbaum M. Carbamazepine-danazol interaction: its mechanism examined by stable isotope technique. Ther Drug Monitor 1986; 8:387–392.

36. Bourgeois BF, Dodson WE, Ferrendelli JA. Interactions between primidone, carbamazepine, and nicotinamide. Neurology 1982; 32:1122–1126.

37. Roby CA, Anderson GD, Kantor ED, Dryer DA, Burstein AH. St. John's wort: effect on CYP3A4 activity. Clin Pharmacol Ther 2000; 67:451–457.

38. Durr D, Stieger B, Kullak-Ublick GA, Rentsch KM, Steinert HC, Meier PJ, Fattinger K. St John's wort induces intestinal P-glycoprotein/MDR1 and intestinal and hepatic CYP3A4. Clin Pharmacol Ther 2000; 68:598–604.

39. Burstein AH, Horton RL, Dunn T, Alfaro RM, Piscitelli SC, Theodore W. Lack of effect of St John's wort on carbamazepine pharmacokinetics in healthy volunteers. Clin Pharmacol Ther 2000; 68:605–612.

40. Tripathi M, Sundaram R, Rafiq M, Venkataranganna MV, Gopumadhavan S, Mitra SK. Pharmacokinetic interactions of Mentat with carbamazepine and phenytoin. Eur J Drug Metab Pharmacokinet 2000; 25:223–226.

41. Gilbert JC, Scott AK, Galloway DB, Petrie JC. Ethosuximide: liver enzyme induction and D-glucaric acid excretion. Br J Clin Pharmacol 1974; 1:249–252.

42. Bialer M, Xiaodong S, Perucca E. Ethosuximide: absorption, distribution and excretion. In: Levy RH, Mattson RH, Meldrun BS, eds. Antiepileptic Drugs. New York: Raven Press, 1995:659–665.

43. Salke-Kellermann RA, May T, Boenigk HE. Influence of ethosuximide on valproic acid concentrations. Epilepsy Res 1997; 26:345–359.

44. Bachmann K, Chu CA, Greear VP. In vivo evidence that ethosuximide is a substrate for cytochrome P450IIIA. Pharmacology 1992; 45:121–128.

45. Bauer LA, Harris C, Wilensky AJ, Raisys VA, Levy RH. Ethosuximide kinetics: possible interaction with valproic acid. Clin Pharmacol Ther 1982; 31:741–745.

46. Van Wieringer A, Vrijlandt CM. Ethosuximide intoxication cause by interaction with isoniazid. Neurology 1983; 33:1227–1228.

47. Glue P, Banfield CR, Perhach JL, Mather GG, Racha JK, Levy RH. Pharmacokinetic interactions with felbamate: in vitro–in vivo correlation. Clin Pharmacokinet 1997; 33:214–224.

48. Hooper WD, Franklin ME, Glue P, Banfield CR, Radwanski E, McLaughlin DB, McIntyre ME, Dickinson RG, Eadie MJ. Effect of felbamate on valproic acid disposition in healthy volunteers: inhibition of β-oxidation. Epilepsia 1996; 37:91–97.

49. Albani F, Theodore WH, Washington P, Devinsky O, Bromfield E, Porter RJ, Nice FJ. Effect of felbamate on plasma levels of carbamazepine and its metabolites. Epilepsia 1981; 32:130–132.

50. Saano V, Glue P, Banfield CR, Reidenberg P, Colucci RD, Meehan JW, Haring P, Radwanski E, Nomeir A, Lin CC, Jense PK, Affrime MB. Effects of felbamate on the pharmacokinetics of a low-dose combination oral contraceptive. Clin Pharmacol Ther 1995; 58:523–531.

51. Fuerst RH, Graves NM, Leppik IE, Brundage RC, Holmes GB, Remmel RP. Felbamate increases phenytoin but decreases carbamazepine concentrations. Epilepsia 1988; 29:488–491.

52. Sachedeo R, Wagner ML, Sachdeo S, Shumaker RC, Lyness WH, Rosenberg A, Ward D, Perhach JL. Coadministration of phenytoin and felbamate: evidence of additional phenytoin dose-reduction requirements and tolerability with increasing doses of felbamate. Epilepsia 1999; 40:1122–1128.

53. Reidenberg P, Glue P, Banfield CR, Colucci RD, Meehan JW, Radwanski E, Mojavarian P, Lin CC, Nezamis J, Guillaume M, Affrime MB. Effects of felbamate on the pharmacokinetics of phenobarbital. Clin Pharmacol Ther 1995; 58:279–287.

54. Sachdeo RC, Narang-Sachdeo S, Montgomery PA, Shumaker RC, Perhach JL, Lyness WH, Rosenberg A. Evaluation of the potential interaction between felbamate and erythromycin in patients with epilepsy. J Clin Pharmacol 1998; 38:184–190.

55. Hussein G, Troupin AS, Montourls G. Gabapentin interaction with felbamate. Neurology 1996; 47:1106.

56. Allen E, Tsanaclis LM, Wroe SJ, Reece PA, Sedman AJ. Gabapentin does not affect antipyrine clearance. J Clin Pharmacol 1999; 39:934–935.

57. Radulovic LL, Wilder BJ, Leppik IE, Bockbrader HN, Chang T, Posvar EL, Sedman AJ, Uthman BM, Erdman GR. Lack of interaction of gabapentin with carbamazepine or valproate. Epilepsia 1994; 35:155–161.

58. Eldon MA, Underwood BA, Randinitis EJ, Sedman AJ. Gabapentin does not interact with a contraceptive regimen of norethindrone acetate and ethinyl estradiol. Neurology 1998; 50:1146–1148.

59. Frye MA, Kimbrell TA, Dunn RT, Piscitelli S, Grothe D, Vanderham E, Cora-Locatelli G, Post RM, Ketter TA. Gabapentin does not alter single-dose lithium pharmacokinetics. J Clin Psychopharmacol 1998; 18:461–464.

60. Busch JA, Radulovic LL, Bockbrader HN, Underwood BA, Sedman AJ, Chang TsS. Effect of Maalox TC on single-dose pharmacokinetics of gabapentin capsules in healthy subjects (abstract). Pharm Res 1992; 9(suppl 2):S315.

61. Benetello P, Furlanut M, Fortunato M, Baraldo M, Pea F, Tognon A, Testa G. Oral gabapentin disposition in patients with epilepsy after a high-protein meal. Epilepsia 1997; 38:1140–1142.

62. Gidal BE, Maly MM, Budde J, Lensmeyer GL, Pitterle ME, Jones JC. Effect of a high-protein meal on gabapentin pharmacokinetics. Epilepsy Res 1996; 23:71–76.

63. Yau MK, Adams MA, Wargin WA, Lai AA. A single dose and steady state pharmacokinetic study of lamotrigine in healthy male volunteers. Third International Cleveland Clinic–Bethel Epilepsy Symposium on Antiepileptic Drug Pharmacology, Cleveland, OH, June 1992.

64. Anderson GD, Yau MK, Gidal BE, Harris SJ, Levy RH, Lai AA, Drehn AT. Bidirectional interaction of valproate and lamotrigine in healthy subjects. Clin Pharmacol Ther 1996; 60:145–156.

65. Warner T, Patsalos PN, Prevett M, Elyas AA, Duncan JS. Lamotrigine-induced carbamazepine toxicity: an interaction with carbamazepine-10,11-epoxide. Epilepsy Res 1992; 11:147–150.

66. Pisani F, Xiao B, Fazio A, Spina E, Perucca E, Tomson T. Single dose pharmacokinetics of carbamazepine-10,11-epoxide in patients on lamotrigine monotherapy. Epilepsy Res 1994; 19:245–248.

67. Besag FM, Berry DJ, Pool F, Newbery JE, Subel B. Carbamazepine toxicity with lamotrigine: pharmacokinetic or pharmacodynamic interaction? Epilepsia 1998; 39:183–187.

68. Green MD, Bishop WP, Tephley TR. Expressed human UGT1.4 protein catalyzes the formation of quaternary ammonium-linked glucuronides. Drug Metab Dispos 1995; 23:299–302.

69. Dickins M, Sawyer DA, Moreley TJ, Parsons DN. Lamotrigine: chemistry and biotransformation. In: Levy RH, Mattson RH, Meldrun BS, eds. Antiepileptic Drugs. New York: Raven Press, 1995:871–875.

70. Eriksson AS, Hoppu K, Nergardh A, Boreus L. Pharmacokinetic interactions between lamotrigine and other antiepileptic drugs in children with intractable epilepsy. Epilepsia 1996; 37:769–773.

71. May TW, Rambeck B, Jurgens U. Serum concentrations of lamotrigine in epileptic patients: the influence of dose and comedication. Ther Drug Monit 1996; 18:523–531.

72. May TW, Rambeck B, Jurgens U. Influence of oxcarbazepine and methsuximide on lamotrigine concentrations in epileptic patients with and without valproic acid comedication: results of a retrospective study. Ther Drug Monit 1999; 21:175–181.

73. Depot M, Powell JR, Messenheimer JA, Gloutier G, Dalton MJ. Kinetic effects of multiple oral doses of acetaminophen on a single oral dose of lamotrigine. Clin Pharmacol Ther 1990; 48:346–355.

74. Gidal BE, Anderson GD, Rutecki PR, Shaw R, Lanning A. Lack of an effect of valproate concentration on lamotrigine pharmacokinetics in developmentally disabled patients with epilepsy. Epilepsy Res 2000; 42:23–31.

75. Guberman AH, Besag FMC, Brodie MJ, Dooley JM, Duchowny MS, Pellock JM, Richens A, Stern RS, Trevathan E. Lamotrigine-associated rash: risk/benefit considerations in adults and children. Epilepsia 1999; 40:985–991.

76. Brodie MJ, Yuen AWC, Group S. Lamotrigine substitution study: evidence for synergism with sodium valproate. Epilepsy Res 1997; 26:423–432.

77. Kaufman KR, Gerner R. Lamotrigine toxicity secondary to sertraline. Seizure 1998; 7:163–165.

78. Sharief MK, Singh P, Sander JWAS, Patsalos PN, Shorvon SD. Efficacy and tolerability study of ucb L059 in patients with refractory epilepsy. J Epilepsy 1996; 9:106–112.

79. Betts T, Waegemans T, Crawford P. A multicenter double-blind, randomized, parallel group study to evaluate the tolerability and efficacy of two oral doses of levetiracetam, 2000 mg daily and 4000 mg daily, without titration in patients with refractory epilepsy. Seizure 2000; 9:80–87.

80. Cereghino JJ, Biton V, Abou-Khalil B, Dreifuss F, Gauer LJ, Leppik I. Levetiracetam for partial seizures: results of a double-blind, randomized clinical trial. Neurology 2000; 55:236–242.

81. Perucca E, Gidal BE, Ledent E, Baltes E, Botta P. Levetiracetam does not interact with other antiepileptic drugs (abstract). Epilepsia 2000; 41(suppl 7):254.

82. Browne TR, Szabo GK, Leppik IE, Josephs E, Paz J, Baltes E, Jensen CM. Absence of pharmacokinetic drug interaction of levetiracetam with phenytoin in patients with epilepsy determined by new technique. J Clin Pharmacol 2000; 40:590–595.

83. Patsalos PN. Pharmacokinetic profile of levetiracetam: toward ideal characteristics. Pharmacol Ther 2000; 85:77–85.

84. Levy RH, Ragueneau-Majlessi I, Baltes E. Repeated administration of the novel antiepileptic agent levetiracetam does not alter digoxin pharmacokinetics and pharmacodynamics in healthy volunteers. Epilepsy Res 2001; 46:93–99.

85. Nicolas J-M, Collart P, EGerin B, Mather G, Trager W, Levy RH, Roba J. In vitro evaluation of potential drug interactions with levetiracetam, a new antiepileptic agent. Drug Metab Dispos 1999; 27:250–254.

86. Klosterskov Jensen P, Saano V, Haring P, Svenstrup B, Menge GP. Possible interaction between oxcarbazepine and an oral contraceptive. Epilepsia 1992; 33:1149–1152.

87. Fattore C, Cipolla G, Gatti G, Limido GL, Sturm Y, Perucca E, Bernasconi C. Induction of ethinylestradiol and levonorgestrel metabolism by oxcarbazepine in healthy women. Epilepsia 1999; 40:783–787.

88. Rosche J, Froscher W, Abendroth D, Liebel J. Possible oxcarbazepine interaction with cyclosporine serum levels: a single case study. Clin Neuropharmacol 2001; 24:113–116.

89. Zaccara G, Gangemi PF, Bendoni L, Menge GP, Schwabe S, Monza GC. Influence of single and repeated doses of oxcarbazepine on the pharmacokinetic profile of felodipine. Ther Drug Monit 1993; 15:39–42.

90. Kramer G, Tettenborn B, Klosterskov Jensen P, Menge GP, Stoll KD. Oxcarbazepine does not affect the anticoagulant activity of warfarin. Epilepsia 1992; 33:1145–1148.

91. Kumps A, Wurth C. Oxcarbazepine disposition: preliminary observations in patients. Biopharm Drug Dispos 1990; 11:365–370.

92. Van Parys JAP, Meijer JWA, Segers JP. Dose-concentration proportionality in epileptic patients stabilized on oxcarbazepine: effects of comedication (abstract). Epilepsia 1991; 32(suppl 1):70.

93. Tartara A, Galimberti CA, Manni R, Morini R, Limido G, Gatti G, Bartoli A, Strada G, Perucca E. The pharmacokinetics of oxcarbazepine and its active metabolite 10-hydroxy-carbazepine in healthy subjects and in epileptic patients treated with phenobatbital or valproic acid. Br J Clin Pharmacol 1993; 36:366–368.

94. Kramer G, Tettenborn B, Flesch G. Oxcarbazepine-verapamil drug interaction in healthy volunteers (abstract). Epilepsia 1991; 32(suppl 1):70.

95. Keranen T, Jolkkonen J, Klosterskov-Jensen P, Menge GP. Oxcarbazepine does not interact with cimetidine in healthy volunteers. Acta Neurol Scand 1992; 85:239–242.

96. Keranen T, Jolkkonen J, Jensen PK, Menge GP, Andersson P. Absence of interaction between oxcarbazepine and erythromycin. Acta Neurol Scand 1992; 86:120–123.

97. Mogensen PH, Jorgensen L, Boas J, Dam M, Vesterager A, Flesch G, Jensen PK. Effects of dextropropoxyphene on the steady-state kinetics of oxcarbazepine and its metabolites. Acta Neurol Scand 1992; 85:14–17.

98. Miners JO, McKinnon RA. CYP1A. In: Levy RH, Thummel KE, Trager WF, Hansten PD, Eichelbaum M, eds. Metabolic Drug Interactions. Philadelphia. Lippincott Williams & Wilkins, 2000:61–73.

99. Maurice M, Emiliani S, Dalet-Beluche I, Derancourt J, Lange R. Isolation and characterization of a cytochrome P450 of the IIA subfamily from human liver microsomes. Eur J Biochem 1991; 200:511–517.

100. Chang TK, Yu L, Maurel P, Waxman DJ. Enhanced cyclophosphamide and ifosfamide activation in primary human hepatocyte cultures: response to cytochrome P-450 inducers and autoinduction by oxazaphosphorines. Cancer Res 1997; 57:1946–1954.

101. Miners JO, Birkett DJ. Cytochrome P4502C9: an enzyme of major importance in human drug metabolism. Br J Clin Pharmacol 1998; 45:525–538.

102. Pichard L, Fabre I, Fabre G, Domergue J, Saint Aubert B, Mourad G, Maure IP. Cyclosporin A drug interactions. Screening for inducers and inhibitors of cytochrome P-450 (cyclosporin A oxidase) in primary cultures of human hepatocytes and in liver microsomes. Drug Metab Dispos 1990; 18:595–606.

103. Bock KW, Bock-Hennig BS. Differential induction of human liver UDP-glucuronosyl-transferase activities by phenobarbital-type inducers. Biochem Pharmacol 1987; 36:4137–4143.

104. Ohnhaus EE, Breckenridge A, Park B. Urinary excretion of 6β-hydroxycortyisol and time course measurement of enzyme induction in man. Eur J Clin Pharmacol 1989; 36:39–46.

105. Dossing M, Pilsgaard H, Rasmussen B, Poulsen HE. Time course of phenobarbital and cimetidine mediated changes in hepatic drug metabolism. Eur J Clin Pharmacol 1983; 25:215–222.

106. Anderson GD, Levy RH. Phenobarbital: chemistry and biotransformation. In: Levy RH, Mattson RH, Meldrum BS, eds. Antiepileptic Drugs. New York: Raven Press, 1995:371–377.

107. Tang BK, Yilmaz B, Kalow W. Determination of phenobarbital, p-hydroxyphenobarbital and phenobarbital-N-glucoside in urine by gas chromatography chemical ionization mass spectrometry. Biomed Mass Spectrom 1983; 11:462–465.

108. Hargraves JA, Howald WN, Racha JK, Levy RH. Identification of enzymes responsible for the metabolism of phenobarbital (abstract). Int Soc Stud Xenobiotics Proc 1996; 10:259.

109. Bernus I, Dickinson G, Hooper WD, Eadie MJ. Inhibition of phenobarbitone N-glucosidation by valproate. Br J Clin Pharmacol 1994; 38:411–416.

110. Chetty M, Miller R, Seymour M. Phenytoin auto-induction. Ther Drug Monit 1998; 20:60–62.

111. Schuetz EG, Schuetz JD, Strom SC, Thompson MT, Fisher RA, Molowa DT, Li D, Guzelian PS. Regulation of human liver cytochromes P-450 in family 3A in primary and continuous culture of human hepatocytes. Hepatology 1993; 18:1254–1262.

112. Scott AK, Khir AS, Steele WH, Hawksworth GM, Petrie JC. Oxazepam pharmacokinetics in patients with epilepsy treated long-term with phenytoin alone or in combination with phenobarbitone. Br J Clin Pharmacol 1983; 16:441–444.

113. Fleishaker JC, Pearson LK, Peters GR. Phenytoin causes a rapid increase in 6 beta-hydroxycortisol urinary excretion in humans—a putative measure of CYP3A induction. J Pharm Sci 1995; 84:292–294.

114. Crawford P, Chadwick DJ, Martin C, Tjia J, Back D, Orme M. The interaction of phenytoin and carbamazepine with combined oral contraceptive steroids. Br J Clin Pharmacol 1990; 30:892–896.

115. Kenyon IE. Unplanned pregnancy in an epileptic. BMJ 1972; 1:686–687.

116. Janz D, Schmidt D. Antiepileptic drugs and failure of oral contraceptives (letter). Lancet 1974; 1:1113.

117. Morselli PL, Rizzo M, Garattini S. Interaction between phenobarbital and diphenylhydantoin in animals and in epileptic patients. Ann NY Acad Sci 1971; 179:88–107.

118. Lambie DG, Johnson RH, Nanda RN, Shakir RAL. Therapeutic and pharmacokinetic effects of increasing phenytoin in chronic epileptics on multiple drug therapy. Lancet 1976; 2:386–389.

119. Panegyres PK, Rischbieth RH. Fatal phenytoin warfarin interaction. Postgrad Med J 1991; 67:98.

120. Nappi JM. Warfarin and phenytoin interaction. Ann Intern Med 1979; 90:852.

121. Bajpai M, Roskos LK, Shen DD, Levy RH. Roles of cytochrome P4502C9 and cytochrome P4502C19 in the stereoselective metabolism of phenytoin to its major metabolites. Drug Metab Disp 1996; 24:1401–1403.

122. Nolan PE, Erstad BL, Hoyer GL, Bliss M, Gear K, Marcus FI. Steady-state interaction between amiodarone and phenytoin in normal subjects. Am J Cardiol 1990; 65:1252–1257.

123. Blum, AR, Wilton JH, Hilligoss DM, Gardner MJ, Henry EB, Harrison NJ, Schentag JJ. Effect of fluconazole on the disposition of phenytoin. Clin Pharmacol Ther 1991; 49:420–425.

124. Rolan PE, Somogyi AA, Drew MJ, Cobain WG, South D, Bochner F. Phenytoin intoxication during treatment with parenteral miconazole. Br Med J Clin Res Ed 1983; 287:1760.

125. Hansen BS, Dam M, Brandt J, Hvidberg EF, Angelo HR, Christensen JM, Lous P, Skovsted L. Influence of dextropropoxyphene on steady state serum levels and protein binding of three anti-epileptic drugs in man. Acta Neurol Scand 1980; 61:357–367.

126. Hansen JM, Kampmann JP, Siersbaek-Nielsen K, Lumholtz IB, Arroe M, Abildgaard U. The effect of different sulfonamides on phenytoin metabolism in man. Acta Med Scand Suppl 1979; 624:106–110.

127. Levy RH, Koch KM. Drug interactions with valproic acid. Drugs 1982; 24:543–546.

128. Andersson T, Lagerstrom P-O, Unge P. A study of the interaction between omeprazole and phenytoin in epileptic patients. Ther Drug Monit 1990; 12:329–333.

129. Bartle WR, Walker SE, Shapero T. Dose-dependent effects of cimetidine on phenytoin kinetics. Clin Pharmacol Ther 1983; 33:649–655.

130. Levine M, Jones MW, Sheppard I. Differential effect of cimetidine on serum concentrations of carbamazepine and phenytoin. Neurology 1985; 35:562–565.

131. Mamiya K, Kojima K, Yukawa E, Higuchi S, Ieiri I, Ninomiya H, Tashiro N. Phenytoin intoxication induced by fluvoxamine. Ther Drug Monit 2001; 23:75–77.

132. Kutt H, Brennan R, Dehejia H, Verebely K. Diphenylhydantoin intoxication. A complication of isoniazid therapy. Am Rev Respir Dis 1970; 101:377–384.

133. Miller RR, Porter J, Greenblatt DJ. Clinical importance of the interaction of phenytoin and isoniazid: a report from the Boston Collaborative Drug Surveillance Program. Chest 1979; 75:356–358.

134. Privitera M, Welty TE. Acute phenytoin toxicity followed by seizure breakthrough from a ticlopidine-phenytoin interaction. Arch Neurol 1996; 53:1191–1192.

135. Donahue S, Flockhart DA, Abernethy DR. Ticlopidine inhibits phenytoin clearance. Clin Pharmacol Ther 1999; 66:563–568.

136. Browne TR, Szabo GK, Evans JE, Evans BA, Greenblatt DJ, Mikati MA. Carbamazepine increases phenytoin serum concentrations and reduces phenytoin clearance. Neurology 1988; 38:1146–1150.

137. Haidukewych D, Rodin EA, Zielinski JJ. Derivation and evaluation of an equation for prediction of free phenytoin concentrations in patients co-medicated with valproic acid. Ther Drug Monit 1989; 11:134–139.

138. Kerrick JM, Wolff DL, Graves NM. Predicting unbound phenytoin concentrations in patients receiving valproic acid: a comparison of two prediction methods. Ann Pharmacother 1995; 29:470–474.

139. Dandekar UP, Chandra RS, Dalvi SS, Joshi MV, Gokhale PC, Sharma AV, Kshirsager NA. Analysis of a clinically important interaction between phenytoin and Shankhapushpi, an Ayurvedic preparation. J Ethnopharm 1992; 35:285–288.

140. Chen LC, Chou MH, Lin MF, Yang LL. Effects of Paeoniae Radix, a traditional Chinese medicine, on the pharmacokinetics of phenytoin. J Clin Pharm Ther 2001; 26:271–278.

141. Ishihara K, Kushida H, Yuzurihara M, Wakui Y, Yanagisawa T, Kamei H, Ohmori S, Kitada M. Interaction of drugs and chinese herbs: pharmacokinetic changes of tolbutamide and diazepam caused by extract of *Angelica dahurica*. J Pharm Pharmacol 2000; 52:1023–1029.

142. Obach RS. Inhibition of human cytochrome P450 enzymes by constituents of St. John's wort, an herbal preparation used in depression. J Pharmacol Exp Ther 2000; 294:88–95.

143. Bourgeois BFD. Primidone: chemistry and biotransformation. In: Levy RH, Mattson RH, Meldrum BS, eds. Antiepileptic Drugs. New York: Raven Press, 1995:449–457.

144. Fincham RW, Schottelius DD. Primidone: interactions with other drugs. In: Levy RH, Mattson RH, Meldrum BS, eds. Antiepileptic Drugs. New York: Raven Press, 1995:467–475.

145. Sato J, Sekizawa Y, Yoshida A, Owada E, Sakuta N, Yoshihara M, Goto T, Kobayashi Y, Ito K. Single-dose kinetics of primidone in human subjects: effect of phenytoin on formation and elimination of active metabolites of primidone, phenobarbital and phenylethylmalonamide. J Pharmacobio-Dyn 1992; 15:467–472.

146. Callaghan N, Feely M, Duggan F, M OC, Seldrup J. The effect of anticonvulsant drugs which induce liver microsomal enzymes on derived and ingested phenobarbitone levels. Acta Neurol Scand 1977; 56:1–6.

147. Bruni J. Valproic acid and plasma levels of primidone and derived phenobarbital. Can J Neurol Sci 1981; 8:91–92.

148. Sutton G, Kupferberg HJ. Isoniazid as an inhibitor of primidone metabolism. Neurology 1975; 25:1179–1181.

149. Tran A, Rey E, Pons G, Rousseau M, d'Athis P, Olive G, Mather GG, Bishop FE, Wurden CJ, Labroo R, Trager WF, Kunze KL, Thummel KE, Vincent JC, Gillardin J-M, Lepage F, Levy RH. Influence of stiripentol on cytochrome P450– mediated metabolic pathways in humans: in vitro and in vivo comparison and calculation of in vivo inhibition constants. Clin Pharmacol Ther 1997; 62:490–504.

150. Kerr BM, Martinez-Lage JM, Viteri C, Tor J, Eddy AC, Levy RH. Carbamazepine dose requirements during stiripentol therapy: influence of cytochrome P-450 inhibition by stiripentol. Epilepsia 1991; 32:267–274.

151. Levy RH, Loiseau P, Guyot M, Blehaut HM, Tor J, Moreland TA. Stiripentol kinetics in epilepsy: nonlinearity and interactions. Clin Pharmacol Ther 1984; 36:661–669.

152. Levy RH, Rettenmeier AW, Anderson GD, Wilensky AJ, Friel PN, Baille TA, Acheampong A, Torr J, Guyot M, Loiseau P. Effects of polytherapy with phenytoin, carbamazepine, and stiripentol on formation of 4-ene-valproate, a hepatotoxic metabolite of valproic acid. Clin Pharmacol Ther 1990; 48:225–235.

153. Levy RH, Loiseau P, Guyot M, Blehaut HM, Tor J, Moreland TA. Michaelis-Menten kinetics of stiripentol in normal humans. Epilepsia 1984; 25:486–491.

154. Moreland TA, Astoin J, Lepage F, Tombret F, Levy RH, Baillie TA. The metabolic fate of stiripentol in man. Drug Metab Dispos 1986; 14:654–662.

155. Rascol O, Squalli A, Montastruc JL, Garat A, Houin G, Lachau S, Tor J, Blehaut H, Rascol A. A pilot study of stiripentol, a new anticonvulsant drug, in complex partial seizures uncontrolled by carbamazepine. Clin Neuropharmacol 1989; 12:119–123.

156. Farwell JR, Anderson GD, Kerr BM, Tor JA, Levy RH. Stiripentol in atypical absence seizures in children: an open trial. Epilepsia 1993; 34:305–311.

157. So EL, Wolff D, Graves NM, Leppik IE, Cascino GD, Pixton GC, Gustavson LE. Pharmacokinetics of tiagabine as add-on therapy in patients taking enzyme-inducing antiepilepsy drugs. Epilepsy Res 1995; 22:221–226.

158. Richens A, Marshall RW, Dirach J, Jansen JA, Snel S, P PC. Absence of interaction between tiagabine, a new antiepileptic drug, and the benzodiazepine triazolam. Drug Metabol Drug Interact 1998; 14:159–177.

159. Mengel HB, Jansen JA, Sommerville KW, Jonkman JHG, Wesnes K, Cohen A, Carlson GF, Marshall R, Snel S, Dirach J, Kastberg H. Tiagabine: evaluation of the risk of interaction with theophylline, warfarin, digoxin, cimetidine, oral contraceptives, triazolam or ethanol (abstract). Epilepsia 1995; 36(suppl 3):S160.

160. Bopp BA, Nequist GD, Rodrigues AD. Role of the cytochrome P450 3A subfamily in the metabolism of [14C]tiagabine by human hepatic microsomes (abstract). Epilepsia 1995; 36(suppl 3):S158–S159.

161. Snel S, Jansen JA, Pedersen PC, Jonkman JH, van Heiningen PN. Tiagabine, a novel antiepileptic agent: lack of pharmacokinetic interaction with digoxin. Eur J Clin Pharmacol 1998; 54:355–357.

162. Gustavson LE, Sommerville KW, Boellner SW, Witt GF, Guenther HJ, Granneman GR. Lack of a clinically significant pharmacokinetic drug interaction between tiagabine and valproate. Am J Ther 1998; 5:73–79.

163. Gustavson LE, Mengel HB. Pharmacokinetics of tiagabine, a gamma-aminobutyric acid-uptake inhibitor, in healthy subjects after single and multiple doses. Epilepsia 1995; 36:605–611.

164. Bopp BA, Gustavson L, Johnson MK, Hightower BA, Mulford D, Chasseud LF, Wood SG, Freedman PS, Hounslow NJ. Disposition and metabolism of orally administered ^{14}C-tiagabine in humans (abstract). Epilepsia 1992; 33(suppl 3):83.

165. Samara EE, Gustavson LE, El-Shourbagy T, Locke C, Granneman GR, Sommerville KW. Population analysis of the pharmacokinetics of tiagabine in patients with epilepsy. Epilepsia 1998; 39:868–873.

166. Thomsen MS, Groes L, Agerso H, Kruse T. Lack of pharmacokinetic interaction between tiagabine and erythromycin. J Clin Pharmacol 1998; 38:1051–1056.

167. Lau AH, Gustavson LE, Sperelakis R, Lam NP, El-Shourbagy T, Qian JX, Layden T. Pharmacokinetics and safety of tiagabine in subjects with various degrees of hepatic function. Epilepsia 1997; 38:445–451.

168. Brodie BJ. Tiagabine pharmacology in profile. Epilepsia 1995; 36(suppl 6):S7–S9.

169. Bourgeois BF. Drug interaction profile of topiramate. Epilepsia 1996; 37(suppl 2):S14–S17.

170. Rosenfeld WE, Liao S, Kramer LD, Anderson G, Palmer M, Levy RH, Nayak RK. Comparison of the steady-state pharmacokinetics of topiramate and valproate in patients with epilepsy during monotherapy and concomitant therapy. Epilepsia 1997; 38:324–333.

171. Rosenfeld WE, Doose DR, Walker SA, Nayak RK. Effect of topiramate on the pharmacokinetics of an oral contraceptive containing norethindrone and ethinyl estradiol in patients with epilepsy. Epilepsia 1997; 38:317–323.

172. Gisclon LC, Curtin CR, Kramer LD. The steady-state pharmacokinetics of phenytoin (Dilantin) and topiramate (Topamax) in male and female epielptic patients on monotherapy and during combination therapy. Epilepsia 1994; 35(suppl 8):S4.

173. Levy RH, Bishop F, Streeter AJ, Trager WF, Kunze KL, Thummel KT, Mather GG. Explanation and prediction of drug interactions with topiramate using CYP450 inhibition spectrum. Epilepsia 1995; 36(suppl 4):47.

174. Liao S, Palmer M. Digoxin and topiramate drug interaction study in male volunteers. Pharm Res 1993; 11(suppl):S405.

175. Wu WN, Heebner JB, Streeter AJ, Moyer MD, Takacs AR, Doose DR, Ferraiolo BL. Evaluation of the absorption, excretion, pharmacokinetics and metabolism of the anticonvulsant topiramate in healthy men. Pharm Res 1994; 11(suppl):S336.

176. Sachdeo RC, Sachdeo SK, Walker SA, Kramer LD, Nyak RK, Doose DR. Steady-state pharmacokinetics of topiramate and carbamazepine in patients with epilepsy during monotherapy and concomitant therapy. Epilepsia 1996; 37:774 780.

177. Hurst SI, Labroo R, Carlson SP, Mather GG, Levy RH. In vitro inhibition profile of valproic acid for cytochrome P450. International Society for the Study of Xenobiotics, Hilton Head, SC, October 26 30, 1997, Vol 12.

178. Anderson GD, Gidal BE, Kantor ED, Wilensky AJ. Lorazepam-valproate interaction: studies in normal subjects and isolated perfused rat liver. Epilepsia 1994; 35:221–225.

179. Yuen AW, Land G, Weatherley BC, Peck AW. Sodium valproate acutely inhibits lamotrigine metabolism. Br J Clin Phrmacol 1992; 33:511–513.

180. Kerr BM, Rettie AE, Eddy AC, Loiseau P, Guyot M, Wilensky AJ, Levy RH. Inhibition of human liver microsomal epoxide hydrolase by valproate and valrpomide: in vitro/in vivo correlation. Clin Pharmacol Ther 1989; 46:82–93.

181. Fischman MA, Hull D, Bartus SA, Schweizer RT. Valproate for epilepsy in renal transplant recipients receiving cyclosporine. Transplantation 1989; 48:542.

182. Crawford P, Chadwick D, Cleland P, Tjia J, Cowie A, Back DJ, Orme ML. The lack of effect of sodium valproate on the pharmacokinetics of oral contraceptive steroids. Contraception 1986; 33:23–29.

183. Lertora JJ, Rege AB, Greenspan DL, Akula S. Pharmacokinetic interaction between zidovudine and valproic acid in patients infected with immunodeficiency virus. Clin Pharmacol Ther 1994; 56:272–278.

184. Fehr C, Grunder G, Hiemke C, Dahmen N. Increase in serum clomipramine concentrations caused by valproate. J Clin Psychopharmacol 2000; 20:493–494.

185. Facciola G, Avenoso A, Scordo MG, Madia AG, Ventimiglia A, Perucca E, Spina E. Small effects of valproic acid on the plasma concentrations of clozapine and its major metabolites in patients with schizophrenic or affective disorders. Ther Drug Monit 1999; 21:341–345.

186. Eiermann B, Engel G, Johansson I, Zanger UM, Bertilsson L. The involvement of CYP1A2 and CYP3A4 in the metabolism of clozapine. Br J Clin Pharmacol 1997; 44:439–446.

187. Addison RS, Parker-Scott SL, Eadie MJ, Hooper WD, Dickinson RG. Steady-state dispositions of valproate and diflunisal alone and coadministered to healthy volunteers. Eur J Clin Pharmacol 2000; 56:715–721.

188. Addison RS, Parker-Scott SL, Hooper WD, Eadie MJ, Dickinson RG. Effect of naproxen co-administration on valproate disposition. Biopharm Drug Dispos 2000; 21:235–242.

189. Baille TA, Sheffels PR. Valproic acid: chemistry and biotransformation. In: Levy RH, Mattson RH, Meldrun BS, eds. Antiepileptic Drugs. New York: Raven Press, 1995:589–604.

190. Soars MG, Smith DJ, Riley RJ, Burchell B. Cloning and characterization of a canine UDP-glucuronosyltransferase. Arch Biochem Biophys 2001; 391:218–224.

191. Ebner T, Burchell B. Substrate specificities of two stably expressed human liver UDP-glucuronosyltransferases of the UGT1 gene family. Drug Metab Dispos 1993; 21:50–55.

192. Jin C, Miners JO, Lillywhite KJ, Mickenzie PI. Complementary deoxyribonucleic acid cloning and expression of human liver uridine diphosphate-glucuronosyltrans-ferase glucuronidating carboxylic acid-containing drugs. J Pharm Exp Ther 1993; 264:475–579.

193. Sadeque AJM, Korzekwa KR, Gonzalez FJ, Rettie AE. Identification of human liver cytochrome P450 isozymes responsible for the formation of 4-ene-valproic acid (abstract). ISSX Proc 1984; 8:87.

194. Sadeque AJM, Korzekwa KR, Gonzalez F, Rettie AE. Metabolism of valproic acid by human liver microsomes (abstract). ISSX Proc 1994; 6:273.

195. Wagner ML, Graves NM, Leppik IE, Remmel RP, Schumaker RC, Ward DL, Perhach JL. The effect of felbamate on valproic disposition. Clin Pharmacol Ther 1994; 56:494–502.

196. Ambrosini PJ, Sheikh RM. Increased plasma valproate concentrations when coadministered with guanfacine. J Child Adolesc Psychopharmacol 1998; 8:143–147.

197. Kiechel JR. Pharmacokinetics and metabolism of guanfacine in man: a review. Br J Clin Pharmacol 1980; 10(suppl 1):25S–32S.

198. Chen LC, Chou MH, Lin MF, Yang LL. Lack of pharmacokinetic interaction between valproic acid and a traditional Chinese medicine, Paeoniae Radix, in healthy volunteers. J Clin Pharm Ther 2000; 25:452–459.

199. Bartoli A, Gatti G, Cipolli G, Barzaghi N, Veliz G, Fattore C, Mumford J, Perucca E. A double-blind, placeo-controlled study on the effect of vigabatrin on in vivo parameters of hepatic microsomal enzyme induction and on the kinetics of steroid oral contraceptives in healthy female volunteers. Epilepsia 1997; 38:702–707.

200. Rey G, Pons G, Olive G. Vigabatrin. Clin Pharmacokinet 1992; 23:267–278.

201. Gatti G, Bartoli A, Marchiselli R, Michellucci R, Tassinari C, Pisani F, Zaccara G, Timmings P, Richens A, Perucca E. Vigabatrin-induced decrease in serum phenytoin concentration does not involve a change in phenytoin bioavailability. Br J Clin Pharmacol 1993; 36:603–606.

202. Haegele KD, Huebert ND, Ebel M, Tell GP, Schechter PJ. Pharmacokinetics of vigabatrin: implications of creatinine clearance. Clin Pharmacol Ther 1988; 44:558–565.

203. Schmidt D, Jacob R, Loiseau P, Deisenhammer E, Klinger D, Despland A, Egli M, Bauer G, Stenzel E, Blankenhorn V. Zonisamide for add-on treatment of refractory partial epilepsy: a European double-blind trial. Epilepsy 1993; 15:67–73.

204. Sackellares JC, Donofrio PD, Wagner JG, Abou-Khalil B, Berent S, Aasved-Hoyt K. Pilot study of zonisamide (1,2-benzisoxazole-3-methanesulfonamide) in patients with refractory partial seizures. Epilepsia 1985; 26:206–211.

205. Tasaki K, Minami T, Ieiri I, Ohtsubo K, Hirakawa Y, Ueda K, Higuchi S. Drug interactions of zonisamide with phenytoin and sodium valproate: serum concentrations and protein binding. Brain Dev 1995; 17:182–185.

206. Ito T, Yamaguchi T, Miyazaki H, Sekine Y, Shimizu M, Ishida S, Yagi K, Kakegawa N, Seino M, Wada T. Pharmacokinetic studies of AD-810, a new antiepileptic compound. Phase I trials. Arzneimittelforschung 1982; 32:1581–1586.

207. Nakasa H, Nakamura H, Ono S, Tsutsui M, Kiuchi M, Ohmori S, Kitada M. Prediction of drug-drug interactions of zonisamide metabolism in humans from in vitro data. Eur J Clin Pharmacol 1998; 54:177–183.

208. Ojemann LM, Shastri RA, Wilensky AJ, Friel PN, Levy RH, McLean JR, Buchanan RA. Comparative pharmacokinetics of zonisamide (CI-912) in epileptic patients on carbamazepine or phenytoin monotherapy. Ther Drug Monit 1986; 8:293–296.

209. Shinoda M, Akita M, Hasegawa M, Hasegawa T, Nabeshima T. The necessity of adjusting the dosage of zonisamide when coadministered with other anti-epileptic drugs. Biol Pharm Bull 1996; 19:1090–1092.

210. Matsumoto K, Miyazaki H, Fujii T, Kagemoto A, Maeda T, Hashimoto M. Absorption, distribution and excretion of 3-(sulfamoyl[^{14}C]methyl)-1,2-benziosoxazole (AD-810) in rats, dogs and monkeys and of AD-810 in men. Arzneimittelforschung 1983; 33:961–968.

211. Kimura M, Tanaka N, Kimura Y, Miyake K, Kitaura T, Fukuchi H. Pharmacokinetic interaction of zonisamide in rats. Effect of other antiepileptics on zonisamide. J Pharmacobiodyn 1992; 15:631–639.

212. Bockbrader HN, Burger PJ, Kugler AR, Knapp LE, Garofalo EA, Lalonde RL. Population pharmacokinetic (PK) analysis of commonly prescribed antiepileptic drugs (AEDs) coadminstered with pregabalin (PGB) in adult patients with refractory partial seizures. Epilepsia 2001; 42(suppl 7):84.

213. Bialer M, Johannessen SI, Kupferberg HJ, Levy RH, Loiscau P, Perucca E. Progress report on new antiepileptic drugs: a summary of the Fifth Eilat Conference (EILAT V). Epilepsy Res 2001; 43:11–58.

214. Hooper WD, Eadie MJ, Blakey GE, Lockton JA, Manun'Ebo M. Evaluation of a pharmacokinetic interaction between remacemide hydrochloride and phenobarbitone in healthy males. Br J Clin Pharmacol 2001; 51:249–255

215. Leach JP, Girvan J, Jamieson V, Jones T, Richens A, Brodie MJ. Mutual interaction between remacemide hydrochloride and phenytoin. Epilepsy Res 1997; 26:381–388.

216. Leach JP, Blacklaw J, Jamieson V, Jones T, Richens A, Brodie MJ. Mutual interaction between remacemide hydrochloride and carbamazepine: two drugs with active metabolites. Epilepsia 1996; 37:1100–1106.

217. Leach JP, Girvan J, Jamieson V, Jones T, Richens A, Brodie MJ. Lack of pharmacokinetic interaction between remacemide hydrochloride and sodium valproate in epileptic patients. Seizure 1997; 6:179–184.

218. Clark B, Hutchison JB, Jamieson V, Jones T, Palmer GC, Scheyer RD. Remacemide Hydrochloride. In: Levy RH, Mattson RH, Meldrum BS, eds. Antiepileptic Drugs. New York: Raven Press, 1995:1035–1044.

219. Hempel R, Schupke H, McNeilly PJ, Heinecke K, Kronbach C, Grunwald C, Zimmermann G, Griesinger C, Engel J, Kronbach T. Metabolism of retigabine (D-23129), a novel anticonvulsant. Drug Metab Dispos 1999; 27:613–622.

220. Kapeghian JC, Madan A, Parkinson A, Tripp SL, Probst A. Evaluation of rufinamide, a novel anticonvulsant for potential drug interactions in vitro. Epilepsia 1996; 37(suppl 5):26.

221. Desta Z, Soukhova NV, Flockhard DA. Inhibition of cytochrome P450 (CYP450) isoforms by isonizaid: potent inhibition of CYP2C19 and CYP3A. Antimicrob Agents Chemother 2001; 45:382–392.

9
Toxicology of Idiosyncratic Organ Toxicities of AEDs

Tracy A. Glauser
Cincinnati Children's Hospital Medical Center
Cincinnati, Ohio, U.S.A.

INTRODUCTION

Although the signs and symptoms of antiepileptic drug (AED)-induced idiosyncratic organ toxicities (also called idiosyncratic drug reactions, or IDRs) are well documented, clinical and genetic susceptibility factors are poorly understood. By understanding the mechanisms underlying the interaction between specific AEDs and an individual patient's clinical and genetic characteristics, treatment approaches can be developed to reduce the risk of developing these severe life-threatening reactions. The goal of this chapter is to narrow this knowledge gap and to help improve clinical care. The chapter is divided into four interrelated sections. The first section will describe the general characteristics of idiosyncratic drug reactions, while the second section will address the mechanisms through which they occur. In the third section, the clinical characteristics, patient-related clinical risk factors and—if known—potential mechanisms of life-threatening IDRs associated with specific AEDs (e.g., phenobarbital, phenytoin, carbamazepine, oxcarbazepine, valproic acid, felbamate, lamotrigine, ethosuximide, and zonisamide) will be discussed. Gabapentin, levetiracetam, tiagabine, and topiramate will not be discussed since they have not been associated with life-threatening IDRs. Lastly, the future role of pharmacogenetics in the identification of patients at high risk for IDRs will be briefly addressed.

GENERAL CHARACTERISTICS OF IDIOSYNCRATIC DRUG REACTIONS

Overview of Adverse Drug Reactions

In addition to their desired effect on decreasing neuronal hyperexcitability, antiepileptic drugs (AEDs) can cause unwanted adverse effects. Adverse drug reactions can be organized using a classification scheme with four categories: types A, B, C, and D (1). Type A adverse drug reactions are directly related to the primary and secondary pharmacologic effect of the drug. They are usually predictable, dose dependent, host independent, and resolve with dose reduction (1,2). An example is sedation with benzodiazepine use.

Type B adverse drug reactions cannot be predicted based upon the known pharmacologic effect of the drug. These idiosyncratic drug reactions (IDRs) do not demonstrate a simple dose-response relationship, are host dependent, organ specific, and can be serious and life-threatening. Preclinical animal toxicology testing may not detect these reactions and these reactions cannot be reproduced in animal models (1,2). An example is the development of aplastic anemia with felbamate use.

Type C adverse drug reactions represent effects of long-term therapy and are related to the cumulative dose (1,2). An example is the development of coarsening facial features with chronic phenytoin use. Type D adverse side effects denote delayed effects of a drug (such as teratogenicity and carcinogenicity) and are dose independent but host dependent (1,2). An example is the development of spina bifida in a newborn of a woman with epilepsy taking valproic acid.

Overview of Idiosyncratic Organ Toxicities

Idiosyncratic reactions to medications are considered unpredictable, dose-independent reactions that occur in <0.1% of the general population but account for ~10% of all adverse drug reactions (3,4). For any one particular medication, the typical incidence of an IDR ranges from one in 100 exposures to one in 100,000 exposures (5). The skin is the most commonly affected site followed by the formed elements of the blood and the liver, and to a lesser extent the nervous system and kidneys (1,4). These reactions can be organ specific or present with generalized nonspecific symptoms, such as lymphadenopathy, arthralgias, eosinophilia, and fever (1,3).

Traditional antiepileptic medications, such as phenobarbital, phenytoin, carbamazepine, valproic acid, and ethosuximide, have been associated (to varying degrees) with a wide variety of IDRs, including agranulocytosis, aplastic anemia, Stevens-Johnson syndrome, allergic dermatitis and rash, hepatic failure, serum sickness reaction, and pancreatitis (Table 1) (6–18). Overall, the profile of IDRs noted in patients taking the newer AEDs (felbamate, gabapentin, lamotrigine, levetiracetam, topiramate, tiagabine, oxcarbazepine, and zonisamide) is less striking than that seen in association with the older AEDs (Table 2). There are two notable

Table 1.

Reaction	CBZ	ETX	PB	PHT	VPA
Agranulocytosis	×	×	×	×	×
Stevens-Johnson syndrome	×	×	×	×	×
Aplastic anemia	×	×		×	×
Hepatic failure	×		×	×	×
Allergic dermatitis/rash	×	×	×	×	×
Serum sickness reaction	×	×	×	×	×
Pancreatitis	×			×	×

CBZ, carbamazepine; ETX, ethosuximide; PB, Phenobarbital; PHT, phenytoin; VPA, valproate.
Source: Ref. 14.

Table 2.

Reaction	FBM	GBP	LTG	TPM	TGB	ZNS	LEV	OXC
Agranulocytosis	×							
Stevens-Johnson			×			×		
Aplastic anemia	×							
Hepatic failure	×							
Dermatitis/rash	×	×	×	×	×	×	×	×
Serum sickness								
Pancreatitis								

FBM, felbamate; GBP, gabapentin; LTG, lamotrigine; TPM, topiramate; TGB, tiagabine; OXC, oxcarbazepine; ZNS, zonisamide; LEV, levetiracetam.
Source: Ref. 48.

exceptions: Felbamate is associated with hematologic and hepatic reactions while lamotrigine is (19,20) linked to severe cutaneous reactions (6,9,10,17,18,21). All AEDs in Table 2 are approved in the United States and have been used in over 100,000 patients.

In general, cutaneous reactions, such as allergic dermatitis and rash, are usually mild and resolve upon withdrawal of the drug. The more severe cutaneous reactions, including Stevens-Johnson syndrome (SJS) and toxic epidermal necrolysis, require more aggressive inpatient therapy and are potentially life threatening. Anticonvulsants rank among the top three drugs (along with antibacterials and nonsteroidal anti-inflammatories) in their incidence of severe cutaneous reactions (1).

MECHANISMS OF IDIOSYNCRATIC DRUG REACTIONS

Idiosyncratic drug reactions develop through multiple, often interrelated, pathways (Fig. 1). Following absorption and distribution throughout the body, AEDs undergo metabolism. This metabolism is conventionally divided into two phases, phase I and phase II reactions (2). Phase I reactions can be oxidative (catalyzed by a number of enzymes including cytochrome P450 enzymes, prostaglandin synthetases, and tissue peroxidases), reductive, or hydrolytic reactions (2,22). Phase I reactions are considered bioactivating reactions.

Phase II reactions conjugate a drug either directly or after the drug has undergone phase I reactions with moieties (such as sulfate, glucuronic acid, and glutathione) to increase its water solubility and subsequent excretion (2). Enzymes such as epoxide hydrolase, glutathione-S-transferase and N-acetyltransferase are often involved in these phase II reactions (22). Phase II reactions are considered a form of detoxification (2).

These phase I and phase II metabolic reactions can result in the formation of metabolites which can be nonreactive, water-soluble and excreted without further effects on body tissues, or the metabolites can be reactive and potentially harmful. When a reactive metabolite is formed, there are four possible consequences (2):

1. Further detoxification of the reactive metabolite to a nonreactive metabolite
2. Direct toxicity to cells, tissues, and organs by the reactive metabolite

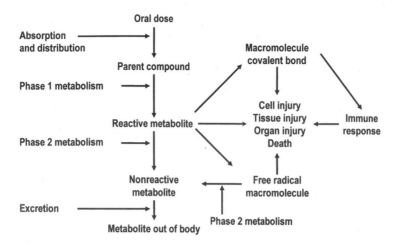

Figure 1.   Mechanisms of development of idiosyncratic drug reactions.

3.   Covalent binding to a macromolecule with subsequent development of an immunologic response
4.   Formation of a free radical with subsequent cellular membrane disruption

The most common consequence is the further detoxification of the reactive metabolite to a nonreactive metabolite, which is then excreted, and no clinical symptoms are noted. The remaining three scenarios can result in significant clinical symptomatology. If detoxificiation of the reactive metabolite is inadequate, the metabolite can directly affect cells, tissues, or organs, usually in the organ where it was formed. The liver is at greatest risk for direct organ toxicity from a reactive metabolite owing to its anatomical location and central role in detoxification (1). The formed elements of the blood are also at high risk for direct reactive metabolite toxicity due to the bioactivating ability of the NADPH oxidase/myeloperoxidase system found in monocytes and neutrophils (4,7,23,24).

Another pathway for toxicity involves the reactive metabolite covalently binding to a macromolecule and the subsequent development of an immunologic response (25). Anticonvulsant molecules (and their reactive metabolites) are not immunogenic by themselves since they are low molecular weight compounds (MW < 1000) (4). However, if the reactive metabolite covalently binds to a macromolecular carrier, the new molecule can be immunogenic, i.e., a hapten, and can produce an immunologic response mediated either through specific antibodies or a T-cell response (4,9). An individual's immune responsiveness appears to be largely under genetic control. IDRs that occur through drug-induced immune responses are typically called drug hypersensitivity reactions (9).

These two mechanisms for development of idiosyncratic drug reactions (deficient detoxification of a reactive metabolite and the immunologic response to formation of a hapten) have been extensively described in the past for many drugs. The role of an imbalance between free radical production and destruction in the development of an idiosyncratic drug reaction has been significantly less well described.

Free radicals, first discovered by Gomberg in 1900, are naturally occurring highly reactive molecules or ions with an unpaired electron (26–28). When a drug is metabolized, its reactive metabolites are often electrophilic, resulting in the formation of highly reactive free radical polyunsaturated fatty acid macromolecules on nearby cell membranes (26). In the presence of oxygen, a free radical chain reaction can occur on these cell membranes which, if unchecked, can result in alteration and eventual destruction of membrane integrity. If this destruction occurs on a large enough scale, organ toxicity and death can result. The major antioxidant defenses are provided by five intracellular enzymes, three associated trace elements, and the cellular antioxidant reduced glutathione (GSH). These five crucial enzymes are glutathione peroxidase (GSH-Px), glutathione reductase (GSSR), glutathione-S-transferase (GST), catalase (CAT), and superoxide dismutase (SOD) (26,29). Trace elements selenium, copper, and zinc are essential for the proper functioning of these enzymes (26,30).

Figure 2 illustrates the cascade of propagation and detoxification of oxygen-based free radicals (26). Once a biological process has generated a superoxide ion radical O_2^- (e.g., by metabolism of an anticonvulsant medication), the superoxide ion radical (O_2^-) can react with SOD to form hydrogen peroxide (H_2O_2). Either GSH-Px or CAT can neutralize this hydrogen peroxide. If the hydrogen peroxide is not neutralized, it can then react with another superoxide ion radical (O_2^-) to form a hydroxyl radical (OH^-). If the hydroxyl radical attacks a polyunsaturated fatty acid (PUFA) cell membrane, a chain reaction can begin which generates another lipid membrane radical and a lipid hydroperoxide. The lipid hydroperoxide can be detoxified by GSH-Px or GST into a nondestructive PUFA alcohol (26). If the lipid hydroperoxide is not detoxified it can cause further alteration of membrane integrity that, if on a large enough scale, can lead to organ failure and possibly death.

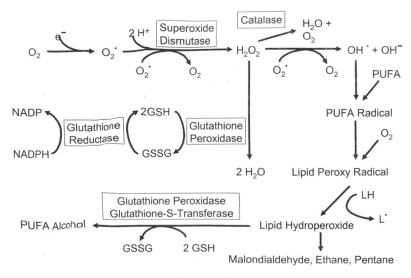

Figure 2. Cascade of free radical propagation and detoxification. O_2^-, superoxide ion radical; H_2O_2, hydrogen peroxide; OH^-, hydroxyl radical; PUFA, polyunsaturated fatty acid; LH, lipid hydroperoxide.

Erythrocyte GSH-Px and SOD are the most important enzymes involved in the pathophysiology of free radical-mediated neurologic diseases (31). GSH-Px is actually a superfamily of at least four selenium-containing peroxidases which are differentially expressed in various tissues (32). There is a close connection between the GSH-Px superfamily and the cellular antioxidant reduced GSH. GSH is not only a cofactor for GSH-Px, but GSH can also exert its own antioxidant effect, through enzymatic or direct action, by blocking destruction and alteration of lipids, proteins, and nucleic acids (33,34). GSH exerts a protective effect against injury from oxygen-derived free radicals, heavy metals, radiation, and toxic substances (33,34). Factors which elevate levels of GSH increase the body's resistance to an oxidative challenge. Conversely, some toxicants may only cause cellular injury if there is depletion of available GSH (34–36).

Selenium may influence the body's ability to handle oxidative stress in various ways. Selenium is the cofactor for GSH-Px governing its turnover at the level of translation. When a patient is selenium deficient, GSH-Px synthesis is profoundly suppressed; when selenium is replenished, GSH-Px enzyme activity rebounds (26,32,37). In experimental systems, selenium deficiency may enhance oxidative injury (32). Lastly, selenium may also influence the regulation of other antioxidant proteins such as selenoprotein P and GST (32).

Three facts support investigating the role of free radical-mediated injury in patients on AEDs who have suffered an IDR:

1. Free radical production is increased in patients taking AEDs either by direct effect or indirectly (i.e., generated during AED metabolism). Valproic acid, for example, can promote oxidative stress through disruption of mitochondria (which releases endogenous superoxide) or generation of electrophiles from unstable Co A- and glucuronide esters of VPA (26,32).

2. Free radical enzyme scavenging activity (FRESA) is genetically determined and varies with age, race, gender, and ethnic background (26,38–46). This raises the possibility that some patients may have barely adequate baseline detoxification abilities that become inadequate during times of increased free radical burden and result in the patient suffering a free radical-mediated injury (26,47).

3. Case reports have found deficient FRESA in both patients on AEDs who have suffered an IDR and their immediate family members (26).

The balance between the free radical propagation and detoxification cascades has been quantitated in two ratios, termed the calculated oxidative protection (COP) 1 and 2 ratios (48):

COP1: $k_3(\text{GSH-Px})/k_2(\text{SOD}) = (O_2^-)/2(H_2O_2)$

COP2: $k_9(\text{GSH-Px})^2/k_2(\text{SOD}) = k_5(O_2^-)^2/2k_3$ (lipid hydroperoxide)

The left-hand side of the COP1 and COP2 ratio equations is calculated using the patient's measured GSH-Px and SOD activity. For convenience, the calculated ratio is multiplied by 1000 (units are adjusted accordingly). Using this convention, COP1 ratios usually range between 1 and 6 while COP2 ratios range from 10 to 350. The right hand side of the COP1 and COP2 ratio equations represent a ratio of superoxide ion radical to later produced reactive species at two different steps in the antioxidant protection pathway. Theoretically, the higher the ratio, the more protected the individual as fewer superoxide radicals have escaped neutralization. The application of these ratios for specific AEDs is described below in the valproic acid and felbamate sections.

GENERAL CHARACTERISTICS OF IDIOSYNCRATIC DRUG REACTIONS

Aromatic Anticonvulsants (Phenobarbital, Phenytoin, Carbamazepine)

Specific IDRs

Aromatic anticonvulsants (phenytoin, carbamazepine, phenobarbital) are the most commonly used AEDs, but unfortunately are associated with a wide variety of IDRs (11,22). Nonlife threatening rash is the most common aromatic AED IDR affecting 8.5–16.6% of patients (49–52). The rash can appear as fine punctate erythema, large erythematous macules, or erythroderma. Some patients progress to develop erythema multiforme, exfoliative dermatitis, SJS, or toxic epidermal necrolysis (53–56). Stevens-Johnson syndrome and toxic epidermal necrolysis are considered to be related severe mucocutaneous disorders with mortality rates of <5% and 30%, respectively (57).

The anticonvulsant hypersensitivity syndrome (AHS), another major aromatic AED IDR, is a multisystem process often composed of the triad of fever, rash, and internal organ involvement (58). Organ involvement can be symptomatic or asymptomatic and involve the liver, spleen, blood (e.g., eosinophilia, blood dyscrasias, lymphocytosis), kidney (e.g., interstitial nephritis, renal failure), heart (myocarditis), muscles (polymyositis), or brain (e.g., encephalitis, aseptic meningitis) (58–60). The frequency of AHS for patients receiving aromatic AEDs is between 1:1000 to 1:10,000 persons (15,61). Symptoms usually occur within the first 2–3 months of therapy (62). Following removal of the aromatic AED, recovery over a few weeks usually occurs, but death occurs in as many as 10% of affected patients (63).

Aromatic AED IDRs can occur in other organ systems such as the hematopoetic system, the gastrointestinal system, connective tissue, and the nervous system. Agranulocytosis, pure red cell aplasia, and aplastic anaemia have been reported (54,64–68). Gastrointestinal IDRs include hepatitis, jaundice, liver failure, and pancreatitis (12,69,70). Symptoms of aromatic AED hepatoxicity often start following "a rather short duration of exposure" (12). Aromatic AED-induced lupus erythematosus, connective tissue disorders, fibromyalgia, and the shoulder-hand syndrome have been reported (54,71–75). Neurologic IDRs include dyskinesias, tics, Tourette's syndrome, ophthalmoplegia, asterixis, nonepileptic myoclonus, and reflex sympathetic dystrophy (76–83).

Patient-Related Clinical Risk Factors

A history of a cutaneous IDR to one aromatic AED is a risk factor for the development of a cutaneous IDR when exposed to another aromatic AED. The in vivo and in vitro cross-reactivity among phenytoin, phenobarbital, and carbamazepine is as high as 70–80% (60,84).

Proposed IDR Mechanisms

Aromatic AED idiosyncratic reactions are proposed to result from the formation of a reactive metabolite, such as an arene oxide intermediate, in a patient with inadequate detoxification capability (9,85). Usually arene oxide intermediates are either converted to nonreactive *trans*-dihydrodiols by microsomal epoxide hydrolase, spontaneously decompose to nontoxic phenols, or form a glutathione conjugate by glutathione-S-transferase (9). One proposed mechanism for the development of an aromatic AED IDR is that deficient arene oxide detoxification by microsomal epoxide hydrolase leads to excessive arene oxide that can cause direct cytotoxicity or stimulate an immunological response through hapten formation (1,9,86).

The role that deficient epoxide hydrolase activity plays in this IDR pathogenesis was elegantly demonstrated in a series of in vitro experiments by Spielberg (Fig. 3) (85,86). In the Spielberg model, lymphocytes are mixed with murine liver microsomes, $NADP^+$, G6P, G6PD, K^+, Mg^{2+}, and the AED to be tested (86). Depending on the experiment's hypothesis, lymphocytes can be from normal healthy controls or subjects who have experienced an IDR. In vitro, the AED undergoes bioactivation, and a potentially toxic metabolite is formed. If the lymphocyte detoxification defenses are intact, the lymphocytes survive; if the defenses are inadequate, the lymphocytes die. Lymphocytes normally contain adequate epoxide hydrolase and glutathione-S-transferase to detoxify arene oxides. The cytotoxicity of the proposed reactive metabolites is expressed as the percentage of dead lymphocytes following mixture of lymphocytes, AED, and murine liver microsomes (86).

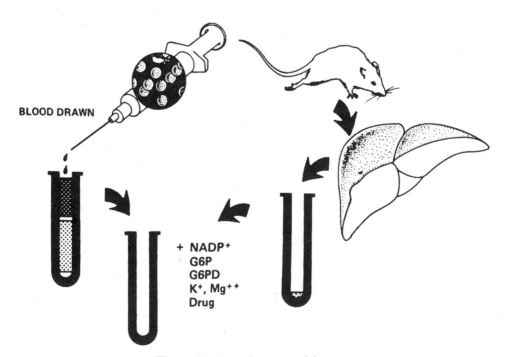

BLOOD DRAWN

+ $NADP^+$
G6P
G6PD
K^+, Mg^{++}
Drug

Figure 3. Lymphocyte toxicity test.

Spielberg initially studied phenobarbital, phenytoin, mephenytoin, and phenacemide using lymphocytes from normal controls (85,86). In humans, the first two AEDs have a low incidence of IDRs while the latter two have a much greater risk. None of these AEDs was directly toxic to the normal control lymphocytes. However, when each AED was separately incubated in the model, lymphocyte toxicity occurred in a dose-response manner that paralleled the toxicity of each AED in humans. When an inhibitor of epoxide hydrolase (trichloropropene oxide) was added and the experiments were repeated, the lymphocyte toxicity of each drug was enhanced. Subsequent addition of purified epoxide hydrolase abolished this enhanced lymphocyte toxicity (85,86).

Spielberg then repeated the experiments using lymphocytes from three patients who recovered from phenytoin hepatotoxicity compared to lymphocytes from 20 control subjects (including patients on long-term phenytoin without an IDR). A series of trials was performed with varying PHT concentrations (8–32 μg/mL). Cells from patients with a history of PHT hepatotoxicity had a dose dependent increase in lymphocyte death whereas the control group exhibited no toxicity. When an inhibitor of epoxide hydrolase (trichloropropene oxide) was added to the control group's mixture and the experiments were repeated, the control group's lymphocytes demonstrated dose-response curves similar to those seen for the lymphocytes from the three affected patients (86).

This series of experiments led to the conclusion that inherited deficiencies in epoxide hydrolase significantly increase a patient's susceptibility to an aromatic AED IDR from arene oxides (3,85,86). Although elegant, these experiments are difficult to perform, time-consuming, and not readily available to the clinician.

Lamotrigine (LTG)

Specific IDRs

Idiosyncratic reactions to lamotrigine predominantly involve the skin. The most common skin manifestation is a nonspecific rash affecting 10–12% of LTG patients (10,21,57). The rash, initially described as being maculopapular or erythematous, usually appears within the first 2–8 weeks of LTG therapy, and may be associated with additional clinical symptoms such as fever, myalgia, malaise, lymphadeno-pathy, and eosinophilia (57,87). Following LTG withdrawal, the rash rapidly resolves. Sometimes the rash may even resolve without changing LTG dosage (87).

This dermatologic IDR can present in some patients as AHS, erythema multiforme, Stevens-Johnson syndrome, or even toxic epidermal necrolysis (21,57,87). The risk of a potentially life-threatening rash (based on clinical trials and postmarketing reports) in adults is 0.3% and ~1% in children 16 years old and younger (87).

Patient-Related Clinical Risk Factors

Risk factors for LTG-associated severe dermatologic reactions include younger age (children more than adults), comedication with valproic acid, a rapid rate of LTG dose escalation, and a high LTG starting dose (Table 3) (21,57,87). Clinically, the risk of LTG-associated rash is greatest when VPA and LTG are used concurrently followed in frequency by LTG and enzyme inducing AEDs. LTG monotherapy is the clinical situation least likely to be associated with rash (88).

Table 3. Clinical Profile for Patients at High Risk for Idiosyncratic Reactions to Valproic Acid, Lamotrigine, and Felbamate

Valproic acid (Hepatotoxicity)	Felbamate (Aplastic anemia)	Lamotrigine (Stevens-Johnson or toxic epidermal necrolysis)
Children under age 2 years	Caucasian	Children > adults
Multiple concomitant AEDs	Adults > children	Concurrent valproic acid use
Underlying metabolic disease	Females > males	High starting dose
Developmental delay	Previous cytopenia	Rapid titration
	History of an AED allergy or toxicity	On lamotrigine <1 year
	History of an immune disorder	
	On felbamate <1 year	

In the current LTG package insert in the United States, it is recommended that LTG "should be discontinued at the first sign of rash, unless the rash is clearly not drug-related" (89). In all cases, careful attention should be given to initial LTG starting dose, LTG titration rate, and comedications. The prompt evaluation of any rash is prudent.

Proposed IDR Mechanisms

One study of the clinical characteristics of 26 patients (nine published and 17 unpublished) experiencing LTG-associated AHS concluded that the features were comparable to the AHS induced by aromatic AEDs (90). Animal studies suggest part of LTG's metabolism is through a reactive arene oxide intermediate metabolite (similar to the aromatic AEDs); the arene oxide intermediate is detoxified by GSH (91). One patient with LTG-associated hypersensitivity syndrome had a positive lymphocyte toxicity test similar to that noted with the aromatic AEDs (92).

Analysis of the LTG metabolic pathways can help explain the clinical risk factors underlying LTG-associated rash (e.g., concomitant VPA use, a rapid rate of LTG dose escalation). LTG is predominantly metabolized by uridine diphosphate glucuronsyltransferase (UDPGT1A4) to a LTG N-glucuronide and to a lesser extent by hepatic microsomal P450 enzymes to a reactive arene oxide intermediate metabolite (91). VPA inhibits UDPGT1A4 activity. When LTG is administered concomitantly with VPA, a greater fraction of the LTG dose will be metabolized to the arene oxide reactive intermediate, increasing the risk for rash. Enzyme-inducing AEDs will induce both UDPGT1A4 and the P450 enzymes that metabolize LTG. The induction will be greater for the P450 enzymes, causing a greater fraction of LTG to be metabolized to the reactive metabolite compared to the noninduced (i.e., monotherapy) situation (88).

LTG induces its own metabolism (autoinduction) through induction of UDPGT1A4 (88). Additionally, LTG induces VPA glucoronidation. A low LTG starting dose and a slow LTG dosage escalation would allow time for UDPGT enzyme induction to occur and lead to a slow rather than rapid rate of increase for both LTG and its reactive metabolite. A high LTG starting dose and rapid LTG dosage escalation would lead to disproportionately elevated LTG and reactive metabolite concentration compared to the low–starting dose, slow-titration scenario.

In these clinical situations, the mechanism of LTG IDRs is probably some combination of the direct effects of a reactive metabolite and an immune-mediated reaction (57,88).

Oxcarbazepine

Specific IDRs

Oxcarbazepine (OXC) is a 10-keto analog of carbamazepine. Although it is structurally an aromatic anticonvulsant, there is not an association between OXC and severe idiosyncratic reactions such as hepatic failure, pancreatitis, aplastic anemia, SJS, or toxic epidermal necrolysis (93,94). In monotherapy comparative trials, allergic skin reactions are less frequent with OXC than with phenytoin (95) or carbamazepine (96), but more frequent than with valproic acid (97).

Patient-Related Clinical Risk Factors

In one report of 51 patients experiencing allergic skin reactions to carbamazepine, 27% experienced allergic cross-reactivity when switched to OXC (98). A similar study showed that 16% (9/55) of patients who were switched from carbamazepine to OXC because of skin reactions or "evidently allergic" reactions experienced a recurrence on OXC treatment (99). In a large Danish retrospective survey of 947 patients, 6% of patients treated with OXC developed a rash, but half of these patients had a previous allergic reaction to carbamazepine (100).

Proposed IDR Mechanisms

Although oxcarbazepine is an aromatic AED, it undergoes rapid and almost complete reductive metabolism of its keto group to form the pharmacologically active 10-monohydroxy derivative instead of oxidation to form an arene oxide intermediate. The lack of an arene oxide intermediate is the most likely explanation for the difference in IDR profiles between oxcarbazepine and other aromatic anticonvulsants.

Valproic Acid

Specific IDRs

Idiosyncratic reactions to valproic acid most frequently involve the liver (8,11,101,102), pancreas (103), and formed elements of the blood (aplastic anemia, leucopenia) (104). In contrast to the aromatic AEDs, the incidence of rash with valproic acid therapy is <1% (15,105).

Among these, the most comprehensively studied IDR is hepatotoxicity (8,11,101,102). The most common presenting symptoms in patients with fatal VPA associated hepatotoxicity are gastrointestinal (nausea, vomiting, anorexia) and central nervous system related (lethargy, drowsiness, coma, and even seizure exacerbation) (11,105,106). These signs and symptoms usually appear within 3–6 months after VPA is initiated (11,12,107–109). If clinical symptoms occur after VPA therapy is begun, immediate metabolic assessment is recommended. Carnitine supplementation is reasonable to consider owing to the risk of VPA-induced carnitine deficiency (106).

Patient-Related Clinical Risk Factors

Through retrospective analyses of different cohorts of affected patients a profile of "at-risk" patient characteristics can be constructed (Table 3). Risk factors for valproic associated hepatotoxicity include young age (<2 years old), concurrent use of multiple anticonvulsants (especially P450 enzyme inducers), severe organic brain disease with mental retardation, and underlying congenital metabolic disorders (2,8,101,102,105,106). The risk of death from VPA associated hepatotoxicity in high-risk patients has been reported to be as great as one in 500 (8,101,102).

Some experienced clinicians recommend pursuing further laboratory screening (focusing on the identification of a potential underlying congenital metabolic disorder) prior to initiating VPA therapy in a child with risk factors such as mental retardation or one receiving polypharmacy. These tests may include serum lactate, serum pyruvate, serum carnitine, urinary organic acids, and serum amino acids, along with baseline routine hematology, chemistry screens, prothrombin time and partial thromboplastin time, arterial blood gases, and ammonia (106). Unfortunately, laboratory monitoring of liver function during VPA therapy does not anticipate "fulminant and irreversible hepatic failure" (106). VPA-associated hepatotoxicity is different from the more commonly encountered dose-related reversible VPA induced abnormalities in liver enzymes without clinical symptoms (105). Overall, clinical monitoring is more important than laboratory monitoring in anticipation of VPA-associated hepatotoxicity (11,12,106).

In contrast to VPA-associated hepatotoxicity, the at-risk characteristics for patients to develop VPA-associated pancreatitis were younger patients (age <20 years), polytherapy, history of a chronic encephalopathy, and recent onset of VPA use (within the first 3 months in almost half of the cases, within a year of onset in 69% of cases) (103,105).

Proposed IDR Mechanisms

Valproic acid (VPA) hepatotoxicity is proposed to result from the formation of a reactive metabolite, such as the 4-en-VPA or possibly the 2,4-dien-VPA metabolites, in a patient with inadequate detoxification capability (88,110,111). There are two major metabolic pathways for VPA: glucuronidation (mediated by uridine diphosphatylglucuronyl transferase) that produces a VPA-glucuronide metabolite, and beta oxidation (mediated by a series of mitochondrial-based reactions), which leads to the formation of multiple metabolites including the 2-en-VPA, the 3-OH-VPA, and the 3-oxo-VPA metabolites (111). Other minor pathways exist, including carnitine ester formation, conjugation with glycine, conjugation with coenzyme A, and oxygenation pathways. One of the oxygenation pathways is hydroxylation that is mediated by a variety of CYP450 enzymes (CYP2A6, CYP2B6, CYP2C9, CYP2C19, CYP2E1). This pathway produces multiple metabolites including the 3-OH-VPA, 4-OH-VPA, 5-OH-VPA and most importantly the proposed hepatotoxic 4-en-VPA metabolite with a potential free radical intermediate (112,113).

It is proposed that if a patient has inadequate ability to metabolize VPA through beta-oxidation (e.g., due to an underlying mitochondrial defect) coupled with induction of their P450 enzyme system (due to concomitant enzyme inducing AEDs), the balance of VPA metabolism can shift to increased production of the hepatotoxic 4-en-VPA metabolite and free radical intermediates. If the patient has deficient detoxification capability, then the risk of VPA hepatotoxicity increases. Patients with the clinical risk factors for VPA hepatoxicity described in the previous section would be at risk to have an altered balance between the multiple metabolic pathways and overproduce the hepatotoxic metabolite without adequate ability to detoxify it.

The hypothesis that patients on VPA suffering IDRs have deficiencies in FRESA and associated trace element concentrations compared to matched controls has been examined by Graf and colleagues (32,114). This study focused on 15 children taking valproic acid who suffered a "severe adverse event" (32). Although this study termed these events as severe adverse events, these events fulfilled the criteria for idiosyncratic drug reactions: unpredictable, not dose-dependent, severe and life-threatening, and not predictable based on the pharmacologic effect of valproic acid. Some of the IDRs seen included acute, severe behavioral changes with persistent vomiting shortly after beginning treatment, pancreatitis, and unexplained death. Erythrocyte glutathione peroxidase, glutathione reductase, glutathione-S-transferase, catalase, and superoxide dismutase activities and plasma concentrations of selenium, copper, and zinc were measured in the 15 affected patients on VPA and compared to enzyme activities and trace element concentrations in 35 age-matched patients with good clinical tolerance of VPA, and 50 healthy, age-matched subjects (32).

Erythrocyte GSH-Px activity, plasma selenium concentrations, and plasma zinc concentrations were significantly lower in the 15 patients in the IDR group than in the 35 age-matched patients with good clinical tolerance of VPA, and 50 healthy, age-matched subjects (GSH-Px, $P < .001$; Se, $P < .001$; Zn, $P < .05$). Erythrocyte GSSG-R activity was significantly higher in the IDR group compared to both control groups ($P < .005$). There was no difference in erythrocyte catalase, SOD, GST activity, or plasma copper concentrations among the three study groups (32). These results imply that low erythrocyte GSH-Px activity and low concentrations of plasma selenium may enhance a person's susceptibility to VPA-associated IDRs.

The clinical applicability of the COP1 and COP2 ratios were also examined in the Graf study (32). The COP1 ratio was significantly lower in the affected group (1.7 ± 0.5) compared to the other two groups (healthy control group, 2.6 ± 0.6; children on VPA without clinical problems, 2.5 ± 0.7, $P = .001$). Similarly, the COP2 ratio was significantly lower in the affected group (31 ± 10) compared to the other two groups (healthy control group, 75 ± 37; children on VPA without clinical problems, 74 ± 35, $P = 0.001$). These results suggest that the COP1 and COP2 ratios may be useful in identifying patients at high risk for IDRs to VPA (48).

Felbamate

Specific IDRs

Idiosyncratic reactions to felbamate (FBM) can involve the formed elements of the blood, liver, or skin. The most common severe FBM associated IDR is aplastic anemia, seen to date in 34 patients receiving FBM (115). Detailed studies of the first 31 reported cases estimate that the incidence of FBM associated aplastic anemia is ~127 cases per million treated with felbamate (about one in 4000–8000 FBM treated patients) versus 2–2.5 per million persons in the general population (21,115,116).

Another report estimates the risk of aplastic anemia in patients receiving FBM to be 1:3000 with a death rate of one in 10,000 FBM treated patients (21,117). To provide a proper perspective, this estimated risk is roughly up to 20 times greater than that for carbamazepine-associated aplastic anemia (115).

The second most common severe FBM associated IDR is hepatotoxicity. Reported in 18 patients receiving FBM, its estimated incidence is 64–164 per million (approximately one in 18,500–25,000 FBM treated patients) (115). This suggests that the frequency of FBM-associated hepatotoxicity and VPA-associated hepatotoxicity are roughly the same (115).

Patient-Related Clinical Risk Factors

Patients with FBM-associated aplastic anemia ranged in age between 13 and 75 years (mean 42.5 years). All were postpubertal. Most (94%) were Caucasian and two-thirds were female. Neither the daily FBM dose (mean 3,129 mg) nor the FBM treatment duration prior to anemia onset (173 days, range 23–339 days) was related to onset of the aplastic anemia (115). Three historical/clinical factors occurred disproportionately and frequently in the FBM-associated aplastic anemia group: a history of an allergy or significant toxicity to a prior antiepileptic drug in 52% of affected patients, a history of cytopenia in 42% of affected patients, and clinical or serologic evidence of an immune disorder such as lupus erythematosus in 33% of affected patients (115). In retrospect, a patient's relative risk was quadrupled for aplastic anemia if two of the above three factors were present. Only three patients had all three factors (115).

This retrospective analysis of the FBM-associated aplastic anemia cohorts permits constructions of a profile of "at risk" patient characteristics (Table 3). Risk factors for FBM-associated aplastic anemia are Caucasian, adult, female, a history of an immune disorder, a history of prior AED toxicity or allergy, prior cytopenia and treatment, with FBM for <1 year (115,118).

Among the patients who experienced hepatotoxicity, half were older than 17 years, a majority were female, and most were on concomitant medications. The mean time to presentation was 217 days with a range of 25–939 days (115). Upon detailed review by a hepatologist, only seven patients (39%) experienced hepatotoxicity deemed "likely due" to felbamate (115). This subset of patients were primarily adult females with a mean age of 36 years receiving FBM for an average of ~4 months at onset of hepatotoxicity. The remaining patients either had hepatotoxicity identified as being "unlikely due" to felbamate (50%) or insufficient data to make a determination (11%) of causality. This second subgroup consisted mostly of children (mean age 16.6 years) receiving FBM for ~10 months with concomitant factors such as status epilepticus (N = 5), increased seizures, acute hepatitis A, acetaminophen toxicity, and "shock liver." Although these data suggest adult females recently placed on FBM may be characteristic of an "at-risk" patient, the small numbers in the "likely due" category suggest caution in using this data to construct an "at-risk" profile for FBM-associated hepatotoxicity (115).

There is no evidence that laboratory monitoring of blood counts and liver function during FBM therapy anticipates these severe IDRs (115). A suggested management strategy is to employ careful clinical monitoring and routine laboratory testing and discontinue the drug if no substantial clinical benefit is observed after 3–6 months of therapy.

Proposed IDR Mechanisms

There have been multiple hypotheses proposed and tested for the cause(s) of felbamate IDRs. One hypothesis is that FBM IDRs are initiated by the formation of a toxic metabolite by a bioactivation pathway unrecognized prior to felbamate's release. Initially, four metabolites of FBM had been identified and none appeared to be toxic (119): 2-(4-hydroxyphenyl)-1,3-propanediol dicarbamate (pOH-FBM), 2-hydroxy-2-phenyl-1,3-propanediol dicarbamate (2OH-FBM), 2-phenyl-1,3-propanediol monocarbamate (MCF), and 3-carbamoyl-2-phenylpropionic acid (CPPA). Subsequently, mercapturic acid metabolites of FBM were identified in rat and human urine (120). This discovery led Thompson to propose a metabolic scheme that expanded on the previously recognized metabolites (120). In the previously established pathways, MCF was metabolized to CPPA which was then excreted in the urine. In the newly proposed pathways, a reactive aldehyde called atropaldehyde (2-phenylpropenal, or simply ATPAL) would be formed from the monocarbamate metabolite MCF through first oxidation and then spontaneous or catalyzed β-elimination. ATPAL is a potent electrophile and cytotoxic agent that could lead to an IDR either through direct toxicity or protein conjugation provoking an immunologic response. However, in the presence of adequate stores of glutathione (an intracellular antioxidant that detoxifies electrophilic compounds), ATPAL could be converted into mercapturic acid derivatives that would be excreted in the urine (119,121).

Direct evidence of the proposed metabolic scheme was provided when the proposed metabolites of the monocarbamate metabolite MCF were demonstrated using human liver S9 fractions and microsomes (119). This study also demonstrated that the ATPAL reactive metabolite could form an adduct with protein molecules (119).

Since glutathione conjugates (detoxifies) the reactive metabolite ATPAL and forms easily excretable mercapturic acid derivatives, a urine test was devised to measure both CPPA (the major nontoxic metabolite formed from metabolism of MCF) and the mercapturic acid derivatives of ATPAL (121). The proposed biomarker is the ratio of CPPA to the mercapturic acid derivatives of ATPAL. The hypothesis is that this ratio can increase if the patient is forming less mercapturic acid derivatives of ATPAL due to decreased detoxification of ATPAL by glutathione (121). This situation may imply the patient has excessive ATPAL which could result in an IDR (121). Although logically derived, further validation of this biomarker should occur before it becomes a standard measure of susceptibility to FBM-associated IDRs (121).

One study examined whether patients on FBM suffering IDRs have deficiencies in FRESA and associated trace element concentrations compared to matched controls (114). This study investigated whether seven patients with a history of FBM-associated aplastic anemia had deficiencies in erythrocyte FRESA and associated plasma trace element concentrations compared to two control groups (normal healthy adults, and patients on felbamate without evidence of an IDR) (114). Each control group contained seven patients who were matched for age, race, sex, and geography for the seven affected patients. The activities of glutathione peroxidase, glutathione reductase, glutathione-S-transferase, catalase, and super-oxide dismutase in erythrocytes and plasma concentrations of three associated trace elements (selenium, copper, and zinc) were measured for each patient in the three groups and compared. Two-way analysis of variance accounting for matched patients was performed (114).

Patients with a history of felbamate-associated aplastic anemia had significantly lower erythrocyte glutathione peroxidase activity ($P < 0.005$), erythrocyte superoxide dismutase activity ($P < 0.001$), and erythrocyte glutathione reductase activity ($P < 0.05$) compared to the two control groups. There were no group differences found in erythrocyte glutathione-S-transferase activity, catalase activity, or plasma selenium concentrations, copper concentrations, or zinc concentrations. This study concluded that patients with a history of felbamate-associated aplastic anemia have multiple significant abnormalities in FRESA compared to matched controls (114).

The clinical applicability of the COP1 and COP2 ratios was examined in this study. The COP1 ratios of the three groups were not statistically different ($P = 0.0874$) while the COP2 ratios were at the threshold of statistical significance ($P = 0.0500$). There are two potential explanations for the lack of a clear statistical difference in COP1 and COP2 ratio in the affected group in the FBM study. First, the FBM study had few patients (total 21); a larger sample size probably would have given a more definitive statistical difference between the groups. Secondly, since both COP1 and COP2 ratios involve only GSH-Px and SOD activities, the clinical usefulness of the ratio is affected if the specific AED IDR occurs in patients with significant alterations in both GSH-Px and SOD activities. In these patients, depending on the relative reductions in GSH-Px and SOD activities, the COP1 and COP2 ratio may appear higher than, equal to, or lower than control values. In patients with FBM IDRs, both GSH-Px and SOD activities were significantly reduced. The ratios' clinical utility for patients taking FBM is not yet completely clear. Interpretation of the COP1 and COP2 ratios should always include an analysis of the absolute activities of the GSH-Px and SOD activities upon which they are calculated (48).

Pellock reported preliminary results of HLA typing of patients on felbamate (122). One allele, not specified in the report, was overrepresented in the group of patients on FBM without serious side effects (122). In contrast, a rare allele was found in three patients with FBM-associated aplastic anemia (122). Whether these alleles represent "protection" or "at-risk" markers require additional study.

Ethosuximide

Specific IDRs

Ethosuximide have been associated (to varying degrees) with a wide variety of idiosyncratic reactions (14,18,123,124), including allergic dermatitis, rash, erythema multiforme, Stevens-Johnson syndrome (125), systemic lupus erythematosus (126–128), a lupuslike syndrome (123,129–131), blood dyscrasias (aplastic anemia, agranulocytosis) (132–141), dyskinesia (142,143), akathisia (142), autoimmune thyroiditis (144), and diminished renal allograft survival (145). The mild cutaneous reactions, allergic dermatitis and rash, are the most common ETX-associated idiosyncratic reactions. These reactions frequently resolve with withdrawal of ETX but some patients may require steroid therapy. Patients developing Stevens-Johnson syndrome, a potentially life-threatening condition, require more aggressive management in the hospital.

The symptoms of the lupuslike syndrome are described as "fever, malar rash, arthritis, lymphadenopathy, and, on occasion, pleural effusions, myocarditis, and pericarditis" (123). Following ethosuximide discontinuation, patients with a lupuslike syndrome usually fully recover, but recovery may be prolonged (123).

The manifestations of ethosuximide associated blood dyscrasias range from thrombocytopenia to pancytopenia and aplastic anemia (132–140). Between 1958 and 1994, only eight cases of ETX associated aplastic anemia were reported, with onset 6 weeks to 8 months after ethosuximide initiation (139). Six patients were on polypharmacy, five taking either phenytoin or ethotoin in combination with ethosuximide (139). Despite therapy, five of the eight patients died (132–140).

Patient-Related Clinical Risk Factors

There are no identified patient-related clinical risk factors for the development of idiosyncratic reactions to ethosuximide.

Proposed IDR Mechanisms

The mechanism of some of the ethosuximide-associated IDRs (e.g., lupus, thyroiditis) is proposed to be immunologic (144). The details of the immunological cascade involved have not been elucidated. There is no evidence to date that a reactive metabolite is formed although metabolism is the main method of ethosuximide elimination in humans. Ethosuximide undergoes extensive hepatic oxidative biotransformation (80–90%) to pharmacologically inactive metabolites. Its oxidation is catalyzed mainly by enzymes of the CYP3A subfamily (146). There is no evidence to date that ethosuximide IDRs are primarily a result of free radical–mediated injury.

Zonisamide

Specific IDRs

Idiosyncratic reactions to zonisamide predominantly involve the skin. The most common skin manifestation is a rash. In Japanese clinical trials, a serious rash or a rash that resulted in discontinuation from the trial was seen in 2% of study patients; the rash began within 2 weeks of initiating therapy in 90% of these patients. A rash leading to discontinuation from U.S. and European randomized controlled clinical trials occurred in 2.2% of study patients. In the U.S. and European clinical trials, 85% of patients who developed a rash noted it began within 16 weeks of initiating zonisamide therapy. The rash is dose independent (147).

During the first 11 years of marketing in Japan, the rate of zonisamide-related Stevens Johnson syndrome or toxic epidermal necrolysis was 46 per million patient-years of exposure. One case of "mild" Stevens-Johnson syndrome was reported during a clinical trial in the United States early in zonisamide's clinical development (148). Although no patients died from zonisamide-related Stevens Johnson syndrome or toxic epidermal necrolysis during the Japanese, U.S., or European controlled clinical trial program, in postmarketing Japanese report, seven deaths were reported from zonisamide-related Stevens-Johnson syndrome or toxic epidermal necrolysis. All seven patients were also receiving other AEDs (147).

Patient-Related Clinical Risk Factors

A proposed clinical risk factor for the development of severe dermatological reactions to zonisamide is the prior history of a dermatologic reaction to a sulfonamide antibiotic. However, a recent abstract reported eight patients with "good evidence" of a history of a rash to sulfonamide antibiotics who were started on zonisamide but did not develop a rash or other manifestations of an allergic reaction (149).

Unlike lamotrigine, there does not appear to be a relationship between the development of dermatologic reactions and either the initial zonisamide starting dose, rate of zonisamide titration, or concomitant AEDs.

Proposed IDR Mechanisms

Sulfonamide medications ("sulfa" drugs) have an SO_2NH_2 in its structure. Sulfonamide antibiotics, such as sulfamethoxazole, not only have the SO_2NH_2 in their structure but also an aromatic amine group (NH_2 plus a benzene ring) at the N4 position (150). It is thought that the aromatic amine, not the SO_2NH_2 portion, is the immunogenic component leading to the development of rashes and more severe dermatologic reactions (e.g., Stevens-Johnson syndrome or toxic epidermal necrolysis) (150).

Multiple medications, including zonisamide, contain a sulfa core (SO_2NH_2) but are not aromatic amines. In patients with a history of dermatologic reactions to sulfonamides whose strucuture contains an aromatic amine, there should not be cross-reactivity with nonaromatic amine sulfonamides such as zonisamide (150).

There is no evidence that a stable active metabolite is formed during zonisamide's metabolism. Zonisamide is primarily metabolized by two major pathways: (1) acetylation (by N-acetyl transferase) to form N-acetyl zonisamide, and (2) reduction (mediated by CYP3A4) to form 2-sulfamoylacetylphenol (SMAP) (151–153). There is variation in the relative contributions of each metabolic pathway between Japanese and non-Japanese groups. In Japanese patients, 29% of a recovered dose is represented by the parent compound, 52% as N-acetyl zonisamide, and 19% as the inactive glucuronide, SMAP (154). In U.S. studies, the proportion of parent compound recovered was 35%; N-acetyl zonisamide represented 15%, and SMAP represented 50% of the recovered dose (153). Given the relatively high proportion of slow acetylators in the U.S. population (compared with the Japanese population) (155–157), it is likely that hepatic biotransformation by CYP3A4 is the main metabolic pathway for zonisamide in the U.S. population. There is no evidence to date that zomisamide IDRs are primarily a result of free radical–mediated injury.

PHARMACOGENETICS

Overview

First coined by Friedrich Vogel in 1959, pharmacogenetics is the study of the genetic basis of therapeutics (158). Controversy exists regarding the exact difference between pharmacogenetics and the more recent term, pharmacogenomics (158–160), as the terms are often used interchangeably (161). Both pharmacogenetics and pharmacogenomics are subsumed under the broader concept of ecogenetics, which is the study of the effects of genetic variation on individual responses to any environmental substance (162). The goal of pharmacogenetics in epilepsy therapy is to apply the advances in the understanding of human genetics (specifically genetic polymorphism information about drug-metabolizing enzymes, drug transporters and receptors) to improve AED efficacy and tolerability.

As detailed in the section on Mechanisms of Idiosyncratic Drug Reactions, IDRs develop through multiple, often interrelated, pathways. Following absorption and distribution throughout the body, antiepileptic drugs undergo metabolism. Phase I and phase II metabolic reactions can result in the formation of metabolites which can be nonreactive, water soluble, and excreted without further effects on body tissues or the metabolites can be reactive and potentially harmful. The drug-metabolizing enzymes involved with phase I or phase II embolic reactions can have polymorphic variations in DNA sequences that can affect enzyme activity.

By definition, a polymorphism exists if there are two or more phenotypes in a defined population. Traditionally, these phenotypes must affect at least 1% of the population for the polymorphism to be recognized. Polymorphisms represent variations in DNA sequences that can take various forms, including single-nucleotide polymorphisms (SNPs), deletions or insertions of at least one (and often hundreds or thousands) of DNA bases, or deletions or insertions of repetitive DNA (159).

More than 70 pharmacogenetic differences have been described (161,163). Polymorphisms in drug-metabolizing enzyme (DME) genes are responsible for most of these identified differences, while polymorphisms in the DME receptor and drug transporter genes account for most of the rest (161,163). A molecular basis has not been identified to explain some of the observed pharmacogenetic differences (159).

P450 Genetic Variability

Genetic variability in phase I metabolizing enzymes can result in the under-production or overproduction of a toxic metabolite. The best-studied example of this is the hepatic microsomal cytochrome P450 group of enzymes. These P450 enzymes play a key role in the phase I metabolism of multiple AEDs including the aromatic anticonvulsants (phenytoin, phenobarbital, carbamazepine).

The cytochrome P450 class of enzymes metabolizes compounds by catalyzing the insertion of an oxygen atom from O_2 into an aromatic or aliphatic molecule to form a hydroxyl group. Cytochrome P450 enzymes are heme-thiolate proteins that occur in all living organisms (164,165). In mammals, cytochrome P450s are membrane bound and concentrated in the liver.

The superfamily of genes coding for P450 proteins is called CYP. Employing sequence similarities, a standardized nomenclature categorizes the P450 proteins into families and subfamilies (164,166). P450 proteins are in the same family if they exhibit >40% similarity in protein sequence. Proteins within the same family that exhibit >55% sequence homology are in the same subfamily (166). Families are given a unique Arabic number, subfamilies noted by a letter following the family's number, and individual genes in the subfamily are denoted by a second Arabic number after the subfamily letter, e.g., CYP2C9 (164,166–168). The most informative and current source for data about CYP450 allelic variants can be found at the following website: http://www.imm.ki.se/cypalleles.

The importance of CYP450 genetic variation in AED metabolism can be illustrated by CYP2C9. This enzyme is the major phase I enzyme involved with phenytoin and phenobarbital metabolism, and to a lesser extent valproic acid and diazepam metabolism (169). There are six allelic variants reported (including the normal or wild type) (http://www.imm.ki.se/cypalleles). Three of the six allelic variants (CYP2C9*2, CYP2C9*3, and CYP2C9*5) have been associated with decreased enzyme activity either in vivo or in vitro. In individuals with these variants, the subsequent altered enzyme activity could lead to less production of the arene oxide and subsequently a lower risk of developing a dermatologic IDRs.

Epoxide Hydrolase Genetic Variability

Human microsomal epoxide hydrolase (*hmEH*) catalyzes the conversion of epoxides to less toxic *trans*-dihydrodiols that can subsequently be conjugated with glucuronic acid or glutathione and excreted. This detoxification is critical during the metabolism of AEDs such as carbamazepine (that forms an 10,11 carbamazepine epoxide) or phenytoin or phenobarbital (that both form arene oxide intermediates). The enzyme is found in many tissues, including the liver, intestine, brain, kidney, lung, adrenal, and mononuclear leukocytes (170–172). An IDR can result if there is an overproduction of a reactive metabolite and epoxide hydrolase activity is insufficient.

Two single nucleotide polymorphisms (SNPs) have been described in the coding region of the *hmEH* gene (173). One SNP is in exon 3 at amino acid position 113 and changes tyrosine to histidine (His-113). The other SNP is in exon 4 at amino acid position 139 and changes histidine residue to arginine (Arg-139) (173). Despite initial data suggesting that these SNPs may alter enzyme function (173), further research using human liver microsomal preparations now indicate that these SNPs "may have only modest impact on the enzyme's specific activity in vivo" (174). Additional genetic studies have found that no single genetic defect altering the structure or function of the microsomal epoxide hydrolase gene predisposes patients for aromatic AEDs IDRs (9,175,176).

Extreme Discordant Phenotype Methodology

The use of the "extreme discordant phenotype" methodology provides a practical approach for assessing the contribution of specific genetic polymorphisms to a specific clinical response in a large clinical population of patients. This approach has been employed in one form or another for many years, but its most current form has recently been described in detail (159).

The extreme discordant phenotype methodology has five steps. First, a quantifiable phenotype needs to be selected. For example, in an AED pharmaco-genetic toxicity study, the variable assessed may be presence or absence of a particular idiosyncratic drug reaction (e.g., aplastic anemia). The second step in this approach is to identify "outliers." Children with an IDR to an AED after a short priod of exposure ("most sensitive") and children without any evidence of the same IDR after an extended AED exposure period ("most resistant") would be examples (Fig. 4). These subgroups represent the extreme condition, and most people fall in the midrange. This happens because most drug responses are not a single gene trait but rather polygenic, also called a multiplex phenotype. Idiosyncratic drug reactions

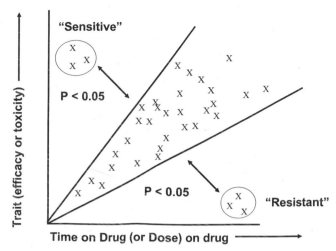

Figure 4. Extreme discordant phenotype diagram.

are probably influenced by dozens if not hundreds of genes that can result in a very complicated genotypes and corresponding phenotypes.

After identifying the outliers, candidate gene(s) must be selected and sequenced in each of the outliers. The candidate gene could be genes that code for drug-metabolizing enzymes, nuclear or postsynaptic receptors, or drug transporters. Correlations between genotypic differences in candidate DNA sequence and phenotypic profile are then performed. Completing the loop is to prove a functional correlation between the differences found in genotype and the clinically recognized differences in phenotype (159).

REFERENCES

1. Park BK, Pirmohamed M, Kitteringham NR. Idiosyncratic drug reactions: a mechanistic evaluation of risk factors. Br J Clin Pharmacol 1992; 34(5):377–395.
2. Pirmohamed M, Kitteringham NR, Park BK. The role of active metabolites in drug toxicity. Drug Saf 1994; 11(2):114–144.
3. Gibaldi M. Adverse drug effect—reactive metabolites and idiosyncratic drug reactions. Part I. T Ann Pharmacother 1992; 26:416–421.
4. Uetrecht JP. The role of leukocyte-generated reactive metabolites in the pathogenesis of idiosyncratic drug reactions. Drug Metab Rev 1992; 24(3):299–366.
5. Uetrecht J. New concepts in immunology relevant to idiosyncratic drug reactions: the "danger hypothesis" and innate immune system. Chem Res Toxicol 1999; 12(5):387–395.
6. Hamer H, Morris H. Hypersensitivity syndrome to antiepileptic drugs: a review including new anticonvulsants. Cleve Clin J Med 1999; 66(4):239–245.
7. Uetrecht JP. Idiosyncratic drug reactions: possible role of reactive metabolites generated by leukocytes. Pharm Res 1989; 6(4):265–273.
8. Bryant AE 3rd, Dreifuss FE. Valproic acid hepatic fatalities. III. U.S. experience since 1986. Neurology 1996; 46(2):465–469.
9. Leeder JS. Mechanisms of idiosyncratic hypersensitivity reactions to antiepileptic drugs. Epilepsia 1998; 39(suppl 7):S8–S16.

10. Schlienger RG, Shapiro LE, Shear NH. Lamotrigine-induced severe cutaneous adverse reactions. Epilepsia 1998; 39(suppl 7):S22–S26.

11. Dreifuss FE, Langer DH. Hepatic considerations in the use of antiepileptic drugs. Epilepsia 1987; 28(suppl 2):S23–S29.

12. Gram L, Bentsen K. Hepatic toxicity of antiepileptic drugs: a review. Acta Neurol Scand Suppl 1983; 97:81–90.

13. Pellock J. Carbamazepine side effects in children and adults. Epilepsia 1987; 28(suppl 3):S64–S70.

14. Pellock JM. Standard approach to antiepileptic drug treatment in the United States. Epilepsia 1994; 35(suppl 4):S11–S18.

15. Tennis P. Risk of serious cutaneous disorders after initiation of use of phenytoin, carbamazepine, or sodium valproate: a record linkage study. Neurology 1997; 49(2):542–546.

16. Booker H. Idiosyncratic reactions to the antiepileptic drugs. Epilepsia 1975; 16(1):171–181.

17. Rzany B, Correia O, Kelly JP, Naldi L, Auquier A, Stern R. Risk of Stevens-Johnson syndrome and toxic epidermal necrolysis during first weeks of antiepileptic therapy: a case-control study. Study Group of the International Case Control Study on Severe Cutaneous Adverse Reactions. Lancet 1999; 353(9171):2190–2194.

18. Wallace SJ. A comparative review of the adverse effects of anticonvulsants in children with epilepsy. Drug Saf 1996; 15(6):378–393.

19. Pharmacogenetics. Humangenetik 1970; 9(3):197–280.

20. Pharmacogenetics. Report of a WHO scientific group. Hoppe Seylers Z Physiol Chem 1973; 354(1):8–9.

21. Pellock JM. New antiepileptic drugs in pediatric epilepsy syndromes. Pediatrics 1999; 104(5 Part 1):1106–1116.

22. Shapiro L, Shear N. Mechanisms of drug reactions: the metabolic track. Semin Cutan Med Surg 1996; 15(4):217–227.

23. Uetrecht J. Myeloperoxidase as a generator of drug free radicals. Biochem Soc Symp 1995; 61:163–170.

24. Furst S, Sukhai P, McClelland R, Uetrecht J. Covalent binding of carbamazepine oxidative metabolites to neutrophils. Drug Metab Dispos 1995; 23(5):590–594.

25. Uetrecht J. Current trends in drug-induced autoimmunity. Toxicology 1997; 119(1):37–43.

26. Pippenger CE, Meng X, Rothner AD, Cruse RP, Erenberg G, Solano R. Free radical scavenging enzyme activity profiles in risk assessment of idiosyncratic drug reactions. In: Levy RH, Penry JK, eds. Idiosyncratic Reactions to Valproate: Clinical Risk Pattterns and Mechanisms of Toxicity. 1st ed. New York: Raven Press, 1991:75–87.

27. Warner BB, Wispe JR. Free radical-mediated diseases in pediatrics [review]. Semin Perinatol 1992; 16(1):47–57.

28. Roberfroid M, Buc Caldron P. Definitions, properties, and reactions of radicals. In: Roberfroid M, Buc Calderon P, eds. Free Radicals and Oxidation Phenomena in Biological Systems. 1st ed. New York-Basel-Hong Kong: Marcel Dekker; 1995:13–31.

29. Halliwell B, Gutteridge J. Free Radicals in Biology and Medicine. 3rd ed. Oxford: Oxford University Press, 1999.

30. Neve J. Biological Functions of Selenium. In: Neve J, Favier A, eds. Selenium in Medicine and Biology. 1st ed. Berlin-New York: de Gruyter, 1989:97–111.

31. Kurekci AE, Alpay F, Tanindi S, Gokcay E, Ozcan O, Akin R, et al. Plasma trace element, plasma glutathione peroxidase, and superoxide dismutase levels in epileptic children receiving antiepileptic drug therapy. Epilepsia 1995; 36(6):600–604.

32. Graf WD, Oleinik OE, Glauser TA, Maertens P, Eder DN, Pippenger CE. Altered antioxidant enzyme activities in children with a serious adverse experience related to valproic acid therapy. Neuropediatrics 1998; 29(4):195–201.

33. Spielberg S. Pharmacogenetics and blood dyscrasias. Eur J Haematol Suppl 1996; 60:93–97.
34. Meister A. Glutathione metabolism and its selective modification. J Biol Chem 1988; 263(33):17205–17208.
35. Mitchell JR, Jollow DJ, Potter WZ, Gillette JR, Brodie BB. Acetaminophen-induced hepatic necrosis. IV. Protective role of glutathione. J Pharmacol Exp Ther 1973; 187(1):211–217.
36. Nelson SD. Metabolic activation and drug toxicity. J Med Chem 1982; 25(7):753–765.
37. Pippenger C, Browne R, Armstrong D. Regulatory antioxidant enzymes. Methods Mol Biol 1998; 108:299–313.
38. Guemouri L, Artur Y, Herbeth B, Jeandel C, Cuny G, Siest G. Biological variability of superoxide dismutase, glutathione peroxidase, and catalase in blood. Clin Chem 1991; 37(11):1932–1937.
39. Jozwiak Z, Jasnowska B. Changes in oxygen-metabolizing enzymes and lipid peroxidation in human erythrocytes as a function of age of donor. Mech Ageing Dev 1985; 32:77–83.
40. Ceballos-Picot I, Trivier JM, Nicole A, Sinet PM, Thevenin M. Age-correlated modifications of copper-zinc superoxide dismutase and glutathione-related enzyme activities in human erythrocytes. Clin Chem 1992; 38(1):66–70.
41. Wasowicz W, Kantorski J, Perek D, Popadiuk S. Concentration of zinc and zinc-copper superoxide dismutase activity in red blood cells in normals and children with cancer. J Clin Chem Clin Biochem 1989; 27:413–418.
42. Ripalda MJ, Rudolph N, Wong SL. Developmental patterns of antioxidant defense mechanisms in human erythrocytes. Pediatr Res 1989; 26(4):366–369.
43. Perrin R, Briancon S, Jeandel C, Artur Y, Minn A, Penin F. Blood activity of Cu/Zn superoxide dismutase, glutathione peroxidase and catalase in Alzheimer's disease: a case-control study. Gerontology 1990; 36:306–313.
44. Neve J, Vertongen F, Peretz A, Carpentier YA. Valeurs usuelles du selenium et de la glutathione peroxidase dans une population belge. Ann Biol Clin 1989; 47:138–143.
45. Beutler E, Matsumoto F. Ethnic variation in red cell glutathione peroxidase activity. Blood 1975; 46(1):103–110.
46. Glauser TA, Titanic-Schefft M, Pippenger CE. Racial differences in free radical scavenging enzyme activity in children. J Child Neurol 1999; 14(6):382–387.
47. Pippenger CE, Meng X, Van Lente F. Alternative approaches to the prediction of antiepileptic, Idiosyncratic, or drug-drug interactions. In: Pitlick WH, ed. Antiepileptic Drug Interactions. 1st ed. New York: Demos Publications, 1989:293–307.
48. Glauser TA. Idiosyncratic reactions: new methods of identifying high-risk patients. Epilepsia 2000; 41(suppl 8):S16–S29.
49. Chadwick D, Shaw M, Foy P, Rawlins M, Turnbull D. Serum anticonvulsant concentrations and the risk of drug induced skin eruptions. J Neurol Neurosurg Psychiatry 1984; 47:642–644.
50. Leppik I, Lapora J, Loewenson R. Seasonal incidence of phenytoin allergy unrelated to plasma levels. Arch Neurol 1985; 42:120–122.
51. Leppik IE. Phenytoin. In: Resor SR, Kutt H, eds. The Medical Treatment of Epilepsy. New York: Marcel Dekker, 1992:279–291.
52. Kramlinger KG, Phillips KA, Post RM. Rash complicating carbamazepine treatment. J Clin Psychopharmacol 1994; 14(6):408–413.
53. Salomon D, Saurat JH. Erythema multiforme major in a 2-month-old child with human immunodeficiency virus (HIV) infection. Br J Dermatol 1990; 123(6):797–800.
54. Bruni J. Phenytoin: toxicity. In: Levy R, Mattson R, Meldrum B, eds. Antiepileptic Drugs. New York: Raven Press, 1995:345–350.

55. Friedmann PS, Strickland I, Pirmohamed M, Park BK. Investigation of mechanisms in toxic epidermal necrolysis induced by carbamazepine. Arch Dermatol 1994; 130(5):598–604.

56. Roujeau JC, Kelly JP, Naldi L, Rzany B, Stern RS, Anderson T. Medication use and the risk of Stevens-Johnson syndrome or toxic epidermal necrolysis. N Engl J Med 1995; 333(24):1600–1607.

57. Pellock JM. Overview of lamotrigine and the new antiepileptic drugs: the challenge. J Child Neurol 1997; 12(suppl 1):S48–S52.

58. Arroyo S, De la Morena A. Life-threatening adverse events of antiepileptic drugs. Epilepsy Res 2001; 47(1–2):155–174.

59. De Vriese AS, Philippe J, Van Renterghem DM, De Cuyper CA, Hindryckx PH, Matthys EG. Carbamazepine hypersensitivity syndrome: report of 4 cases and review of the literature. Medicine (Baltimore) 1995; 74(3):144–151.

60. Schlienger RG, Shear NH. Antiepileptic drug hypersensitivity syndrome. Epilepsia 1998; 39(suppl 7):S3–S7.

61. Vittorio C, Muglia J. Anticonvulsant hypersensitivity syndrome. Arch Intern Med 1995; 155(21):2285–2290.

62. Haruda F. Phenytoin hypersensitivity: 38 cases. Neurology 1979; 29(11):1480–1485.

63. Roujeau JC, Stern RS. Severe adverse cutaneous reactions to drugs. N Engl J Med 1994; 331(19):1272–1285.

64. Olcay L, Pekcan S, Yalnizoglu D, Buyukpamukcu M, Yalaz K. Fatal agranulocytosis developed in the course of carbamazepine therapy. A case report and review of the literature. Turk J Pediatr 1995; 37(1):73–77.

65. Spickett GP, Gompels MM, Saunders PW. Hypogammaglobulinaemia with absent B lymphocytes and agranulocytosis after carbamazepine treatment. J Neurol Neurosurg Psychiatry 1996; 60(4):459.

66. Kaufman DW, Kelly JP, Jurgelon JM, Anderson T, Issaragrisil S, Wiholm BE. Drugs in the aetiology of agranulocytosis and aplastic anaemia. Eur J Haematol suppl 1996; 60:23–30.

67. Franceschi M, Ciboddo G, Truci G, Borri A, Canal N. Fatal aplastic anemia in a patient treated with carbamazepine. Epilepsia 1988; 29(5):582–583.

68. Buitendag DJ. Pure red-cell aplasia associated with carbamazepine. A case report. S Afr Med J 1990; 78(4):214–215.

69. Jeavons P. Hepatotoxicity of antiepileptic drugs. In: Oxley JJD, Meinardi H, eds. Chronic Toxicity of Antiepileptic Drugs. New York: Raven, 1983:1–45.

70. Roberts EA, Spielberg SP, Goldbach M, Phillips MJ. Phenobarbital hepatotoxicity in an 8-month-old infant. J Hepatol 1990; 10(2):235–239.

71. Schmidt S, Welcker M, Greil W, Schattenkirchner M. Carbamazepine-induced systemic lupus erythematosus. Br J Psychiatry 1992; 161:560–561.

72. Drory VE, Yust I, Korczyn AD. Carbamazepine-induced systemic lupus erythematosus. Clin Neuropharmacol 1989; 12(2):115–118.

73. Goldman SI, Krings MS. Phenobarbital-induced fibromyalgia as the cause of bilateral shoulder pain. J Am Osteopath Assoc 1995; 95(8):487–490.

74. Mattson RH, Cramer JA, McCutchen CB. Barbiturate-related connective tissue disorders. Arch Intern Med 1989; 149(4):911–914.

75. Taylor LP, Posner JB. Phenobarbital rheumatism in patients with brain tumor. Ann Neurol 1989; 25(1):92–94.

76. Sechi GP, Piras MR, Rosati G, Zuddas M, Ortu R, Tanca S. Phenobarbital-induced buccolingual dyskinesia in oral apraxia. Eur Neurol 1988; 28(3):139–141.

77. Schwartzman MJ, Leppik IE. Carbamazepine-induced dyskinesia and ophthalmoplegia. Cleve Clin J Med 1990; 57(4):367–372.

78. Neglia JP, Glaze DG, Zion TE. Tics and vocalizations in children treated with carbamazepine. Pediatrics 1984; 73(6):841–844.

79. Robertson PL, Garofalo EA, Silverstein FS, Komarynski MA. Carbamazepine-induced tics. Epilepsia 1993; 34(5):965–968.

80. Sandyk R. Phenobarbitol-induced Tourette-like symptoms. Pediatr Neurol 1986(2):54–55.

81. Ng K, Silbert PL, Edis RH. Complete external ophthalmoplegia and asterixis with carbamazepine toxicity. Aust N Z J Med 1991; 21(6):886–887.

82. Aguglia U, Zappia M, Quattrone A. Carbamazepine-induced nonepileptic myoclonus in a child with benign epilepsy. Epilepsia 1987; 28(5):515–518.

83. Falasca GF, Toly TM, Reginato AJ, Schraeder PL, O'Connor CR. Reflex sympathetic dystrophy associated with antiepileptic drugs. Epilepsia 1994; 35(2):394–399.

84. Shear NH, Spielberg SP. Anticonvulsant hypersensitivity syndrome. In vitro assessment of risk. J Clin Invest 1988; 82(6):1826–1832.

85. Spielberg SP. In vitro analysis of idiosyncratic drug reactions. Clin Biochem 1986; 19(2):142–144.

86. Spielberg SP. In vitro assessment of pharmacogenetic susceptibility to toxic drug metabolites in humans. Fed Proc 1984; 43(8):2308–2313.

87. Matsuo F. Lamotrigine. Epilepsia 1999; 40(suppl 5):S30–S36.

88. Anderson GD. Children versus adults: pharmacokinetic and adverse-effect differences. Epilepsia 2002; 43(suppl 3):53–59.

89. GlaxoWellcome. Prescribing Information on Lamictal (lamotrigine), 1997.

90. Schlienger RG, Knowles SR, Shear NH. Lamotrigine-associated anticonvulsant hypersensitivity syndrome. Neurology 1998; 51(4):1172–1175.

91. Maggs JL, Naisbitt DJ, Tettey JN, Pirmohamed M, Park BK. Metabolism of lamotrigine to a reactive arene oxide intermediate. Chem Res Toxicol 2000; 13(11):1075–1081.

92. Schaub N, Bircher AJ. Severe hypersensitivity syndrome to lamotrigine confirmed by lymphocyte stimulation in vitro. Allergy 2000; 55(2):191–193.

93. Glauser TA. Oxcarbazepine in the treatment of epilepsy. Pharmacotherapy 2001; 21(8):904–919.

94. Gram L. Oxcarbazepine. In: Engel J, Pedley T, eds. Epilepsy: A Comprehensive Textbook. Philadelphia: Lippincott-Raven, 1997:1541–1546.

95. Bill PA, Vigonius U, Pohlmann H, Guerreiro CA, Kochen S, Saffer D. A double-blind controlled clinical trial of oxcarbazepine versus phenytoin in adults with previously untreated epilepsy. Epilepsy Res 1997; 27(3):195–204.

96. Dam M, Ekberg R, Loyning Y, Waltimo O, Jakobsen K. A double-blind study comparing oxcarbazepine and carbamazepine in patients with newly diagnosed, previously untreated epilepsy. J Neurol Neurosurg Psychiatry 1989; 52(4):472–476.

97. Christe W, Kramer G, Vigonius U, Pohlmann H, Steinhoff BJ, Brodie MJ. A double-blind controlled clinical trial: oxcarbazepine versus sodium valproate in adults with newly diagnosed epilepsy. Epilepsy Res 1997; 26(3):451–460.

98. Gram L, Klosterskov-Jensen P. Oxcarbazepine. In: Resor S, Kutt H, eds. Medical Treatment of Epilepsy. New York: Marcel-Dekker, 1992:307–312.

99. Van Parys JA, Meinardi H. Survey of 260 epileptic patients treated with oxcarbazepine (Trileptal) on a named-patient basis. Epilepsy Res 1994; 19(1):79–85.

100. Friis ML, Kristensen O, Boas J, Dalby M, Deth SH, Gram L. Therapeutic experiences with 947 epileptic out-patients in oxcarbazepine treatment. Clin Pharmacokinet 1993; 24(6):441–452.

101. Dreifuss FE, Santilli N, Langer DH, Sweeney KP, Moline KA, Menander KB. Valproic acid hepatic fatalities: a retrospective review. Neurology 1987; 37(3):379–385.

102. Dreifuss FE, Langer DH, Moline KA, Maxwell JE. Valproic acid hepatic fatalities. II. US experience since 1984. Neurology 1989; 39(2 Pt 1):201–207.

103. Asconape JJ, Penry JK, Dreifuss FE, Riela A, Mirza W. Valproate-associated pancreatitis. Epilepsia 1993; 34(1):177–183.

104. Schmidt D. Adverse effects of valproate. Epilepsia 1984; 25(suppl 1):S44–S49.

105. Davis R, Peters DH, McTavish D. Valproic acid. A reappraisal of its pharmacological properties and clinical efficacy in epilepsy. Drugs 1994; 47(2):332–372.

106. Willmore LJ, Triggs WJ, Pellock JM. Valproate toxicity: risk-screening strategies. J Child Neurol 1991; 6(1):3–6.

107. Jeavons P. Non-dose-related side effects of valproate. Epilepsia 1984; 25(suppl 1): S50–S55.

108. Zimmerman H. Valproate-induced hepatic injury: analyses of 23 fatal cases. Hepatology 1982; 2(5):591–597.

109. Wyllie E, Wyllie R. Routine laboratory monitoring for serious adverse effects of antiepileptic medications: the controversy [review]. Epilepsia 1991; 32(suppl 5):S74–S79.

110. Kesterson JW, Granneman GR, Machinist JM. The hepatotoxicity of valproic acid and its metabolites in rats. I. Toxicologic, biochemical and histopathologic studies. Hepatology 1984; 4(6):1143–1152.

111. Baillie T, Sheffels P. Valproic acid: chemistry and biotransformation. In: Levy R, Mattson R, Meldrum B, eds. Antiepileptic Drugs. New York: Raven Press, 1995: 589–604.

112. Rettie AE, Rettenmeier AW, Howald WN, Baillie TA. Cytochrome P-450–catalyzed formation of delta 4-VPA, a toxic metabolite of valproic acid. Science 1987; 235(4791):890–893.

113. Sadeque AJ, Fisher MB, Korzekwa KR, Gonzalez FJ, Rettie AE. Human CYP2C9 and CYP2A6 mediate formation of the hepatotoxin 4-ene-valproic acid. J Pharmacol Exp Ther 1997; 283(2):698–703.

114. Glauser T, Titanic M, Armstrong D, Pippenger C. Abnormalities in free radical scavenging enzyme activity in patients with felbamate-associated aplastic anemia. Epilepsia 1998; 39(suppl 2):40.

115. Pellock JM. Felbamate. Epilepsia 1999; 40(suppl 5):S57–S62.

116. Patton W, Duffull S. Idiosyncratic drug-induced haematological abnormalities. Incidence, pathogenesis, management and avoidance. Drug Saf 1994; 11(6):445–462.

117. Bourgeois BF. Felbamate. Semin Pediatr Neurol 1997; 4(1):3–8.

118. Pellock JM, Brodie MJ. Felbamate: 1997 update. Epilepsia 1997; 38(12):1261–1264.

119. Kapetanovic IM, Torchin CD, Thompson CD, Miller TA, McNeilly PJ, Macdonald TL. Potentially reactive cyclic carbamate metabolite of the antiepileptic drug felbamate produced by human liver tissue in vitro. Drug Metab Dispos 1998; 26(11):1089–1095.

120. Thompson CD, Gulden PH, Macdonald TL. Identification of modified atropaldehyde mercapturic acids in rat and human urine after felbamate administration. Chem Res Toxicol 1997; 10(4):457–462.

121. Thompson CD, Barthen MT, Hopper DW, Miller TA, Quigg M, Hudspeth C. Quantification in patient urine samples of felbamate and three metabolites: acid carbamate and two mercapturic acids. Epilepsia 1999; 40(6):769–776.

122. Pellock J. Progress in felbamate research: toxic metabolite test and HLA typing. Epilepsia 1999; 40(suppl 2):251.

123. Dreifuss F. Ethosuximide: toxicity. In: Levy R, Mattson R, Meldrum B, eds. Antiepileptic Drugs. New York: Raven Press, 1995:675–679.

124. Dreifuss F. Ethosuximide: toxicity. In: Levy R, Mattson R, Meldrum B, Penry J, Dreifuss F, eds. Antiepileptic Drugs. New York: Raven Press, 1989:699–705.

125. Taaffe A, O'Brien C. A case of Stevens-Johnson syndrome associated with the anticonvulsants sulthiame and ethosuximide. Br Dent J 1975; 138(5):172–174.

126. Dabbous IA, Idriss HM. Occurrence of systemic lupus erythematosus in association with ethosuccimide therapy. Case report. J Pediatr 1970; 76(4):617–620.

127. Alter BP. Systemic lupus erythematosus and ethosuccimide. J Pediatr 1970; 77(6): 1093–1095.

128. Ansell BM. Drug-induced systemic lupus erythematosus in a nine-year-old boy. Lupus 1993; 2(3):193–194.

129. Singsen B, Fishman L, Hanson V. Antinuclear antibodies and lupus-like syndromes in children receiving anticonvulsants. Pediatrics 1976; 57:529–534.

130. Teoh PC, Chan HL. Lupus-scleroderma syndrome induced by ethosuximide. Arch Dis Child 1975; 50(8):658–661.

131. Takeda S, Koizumi F, Takazakura E. Ethosuximide-induced lupus-like syndrome with renal involvement. Intern Med 1996; 35(7):587–591.

132. Buchanan R. Ethosuximide: toxicity. In: Woodbury D, Penry J, Schmidt R, eds. Antiepileptic Drugs. New York: Raven Press, 1972:449–454.

133. Cohn R. A neuropathological study of a case of petit mal epilepsy. Electroencephalogr Clin Neurophysiol 1968; 24:282.

134. Kiorboe E, Paludan J, Trolle E, Overvad E. Zarontin (ethosuximide) in the treatment of petit mal and related disorders. Epilepsia 1964; 5:83–89.

135. Kousoulieris E. Granulopenia and thrombocytopenia after ethosuximide. Lancet 1967; 2:310–311.

136. Spittler J. Agranulocytosis due to ethosuximide with a fatal outcome. Klin Paediatr 1974; 186:364–366.

137. Weinstein A, Allen R. Ethosuximide treatment of petit mal seizures. A study of 87 pediatric patients. Am J Dis Child 1966; 111:63–67.

138. Browne TR, Dreifuss FE, Dyken PR, Goode DJ, Penry JK, Porter RJ. Ethosuximide in the treatment of absence (petit mal) seizures. Neurology (Minneapolis) 1975; 25(6):515–524.

139. Massey GV, Dunn NL, Heckel JL, Myer EC, Russell EC. Aplastic anemia following therapy for absence seizures with ethosuximide [review]. Pediatr Neurol 1994; 11(1):59–61.

140. Mann L, Habenicht H. Fatal bone marrow aplasia associated with administration of ethosuximide (Zarontin) for petit mal epilepsy. Bull Los Angeles Neurol Soc 1962; 27:173–176.

141. Seip M. Aplastic anemia during ethosuximide medication. Treatment with bolus-methylprednisolone. Acta Paediatr Scand 1983; 72(6):927–929.

142. Ehyai A, Kilroy A, Fenicheal G. Dyskinesia and akathisia induced by ethosuximide. Am J Dis Child 1978; 132:527–528.

143. Kirschberg G. Dyskinesia—an unusual reaction to ethosuximide. Arch Neurol 1975; 32:137–138.

144. Nishiyama J, Matsukura M, Fugimoto S, Matsuda I. Reports of 2 cases of autoimmune thyroiditis while receiving anticonvulsant therapy. Eur J Pediatr 1983; 140:116–117.

145. Wassner S, Pennisi A, Malekzadeh M, Fine R. The adverse effect of anticonvulsant therapy on renal allograft survival. A preliminary report. J Pediatr 1976; 88:134–137.

146. Sabers A, Dam M. Ethosuximide and methsuximide. In: Shorvon S, Dreifuss F, Fish D, Thomas D, eds. The Treatment of Epilepsy. London: Blackwell Science, 1996:414–420.

147. Elan Pharmaceuticals. Zonegran (package insert). San Diego, CA: Author, 2000, 2002.

148. Wilensky AJ, Friel PN, Ojemann LM, Dodrill CB, McCormick KB, Levy RH. Zonisamide in epilepsy: a pilot study. Epilepsia 1985; 26(3):212–220.

149. Ritter R, Gustafson M, Karney V, Penovich P, Moriarty G, Frost M. Do allergic reactions to sulfonamide antibiotics predict allergy to zonisamide? Epilepsia 2002; 43(suppl 7):209.

150. Knowles S, Shapiro L, Shear NH. Should celecoxib be contraindicated in patients who are allergic to sulfonamides? Revisiting the meaning of 'sulfa' allergy. Drug Saf 2001; 24(4):239–247.

151. Nakasa H, Komiya M, Ohmori S, Kitada M, Rikihisa T, Kanakubo Y. Formation of reductive metabolite, 2-sulfamoylacetylphenol, from zonisamide in rat liver microsomes. Res Commun Chem Pathol Pharmacol 1992; 77(1):31–41.

152. Nakasa H, Komiya M, Ohmori S, Rikihisa T, Kiuchi M, Kitada M. Characterization of human liver microsomal cytochrome P450 involved in the reductive metabolism of zonisamide. Mol Pharmacol 1993; 44(1):216–221.

153. Glauser TA, Pellock JM. Zonisamide in pediatric epilepsy: review of the Japanese experience. J Child Neurol 2002; 17(2):87–96.

154. Mimaki T. Clinical pharmacology and therapeutic drug monitoring of zonisamide. Ther Drug Monit 1998; 20(6):593–597.

155. Lou YC. Differences in drug metabolism polymorphism between Orientals and Caucasians. Drug Metab Rev 1990; 22(5):451–475.

156. Lee EJ. Genetic polymorphisms in drug metabolism—its relevance to Asian populations. Ann Acad Med Singapore 1991; 20(1):56–60.

157. Wood AJ. Ethnic differences in drug disposition and response. Ther Drug Monit 1998; 20(5):525–526.

158. Norton RM. Clinical pharmacogenomics: applications in pharmaceutical R&D. Drug Discov Today 2001; 6(4):180–185.

159. Nebert DW. Extreme discordant phenotype methodology: an intuitive approach to clinical pharmacogenetics. Eur J Pharmacol 2000; 410(2–3):107–120.

160. Jacobs MP, Fischbach GD, Davis MR, Dichter MA, Dingledine R, Lowenstein DH. Future directions for epilepsy research. Neurology 2001; 57(9):1536–1542.

161. Nebert DW. Pharmacogenetics and pharmacogenomics: why is this relevant to the clinical geneticist? Clin Genet 1999; 56(4):247–258.

162. Nebert DWJ-N, Lucia F. Pharmacogenetics and pharmacogenomics. In: Emery and Remoin's Principles and Practice of Medical Genetics. 4th ed, 2001.

163. Vesell ES. Advances in pharmacogenetics and pharmacogenomics [In Process Citation]. J Clin Pharmacol 2000; 40(9):930–938.

164. Omiecinski CJ, Remmel RP, Hosagrahara VP. Concise review of the cytochrome P450s and their roles in toxicology. Toxicol Sci 1999; 48(2):151–156.

165. Evans D. Cytochrome P450—general features. In: Evans D, ed. Genetic Factors in Drug Therapy: Clinical and Molecular Pharmacogenetics. Cambridge: Cambridge University Press, 1993:9–18.

166. Nelson DR, Koymans L, Kamataki T, Stegeman JJ, Feyereisen R, Waxman DJ. P450 superfamily: update on new sequences, gene mapping, accession numbers and nomenclature. Pharmacogenetics 1996; 6(1):1–42.

167. Nebert DW, Nelson DR, Coon MJ, Estabrook RW, Feyereisen R, Fujii-Kuriyama Y. The P450 superfamily: update on new sequences, gene mapping, and recommended nomenclature. DNA Cell Biol 1991; 10(1):1–14.

168. Van der Weide J, Steijns LS. Cytochrome P450 enzyme system: genetic polymorphisms and impact on clinical pharmacology. Ann Clin Biochem 1999; 36(Pt 6):722–729.

169. Cloyd JC, Remmel RP. Antiepileptic drug pharmacokinetics and interactions: impact on treatment of epilepsy. Pharmacotherapy 2000; 20(8 Pt 2):139S–151S.

170. Farin FM, Omiecinski CJ. Regiospecific expression of cytochrome P-450s and microsomal epoxide hydrolase in human brain tissue. J Toxicol Environ Health 1993; 40(2–3):317–335.

171. De Waziers I, Cugnenc PH, Yang CS, Leroux JP, Beaune PH. Cytochrome P450 isoenzymes, epoxide hydrolase and glutathione transferases in rat and human hepatic and extrahepatic tissues. J Pharmacol Exp Ther 1990; 253(1):387–394.

172. Seidegard J, Ekstrom G. The role of human glutathione transferases and epoxide hydrolases in the metabolism of xenobiotics. Environ Health Perspect 1997; 105(suppl 4):791–799.

173. Hassett C, Aicher L, Sidhu JS, Omiecinski CJ. Human microsomal epoxide hydrolase: genetic polymorphism and functional expression in vitro of amino acid variants. Hum Mol Genet 1994; 3(3):421–428.

174. Omiecinski CJ, Hassett C, Hosagrahara V. Epoxide hydrolase—polymorphism and role in toxicology. Toxicol Lett 2000; 112–113:365–370.

175. Gaedigk A, Spielberg SP, Grant DM. Characterization of the microsomal epoxide hydrolase gene in patients with anticonvulsant adverse drug reactions. Pharmacogenetics 1994; 4(3):142–153.

176. Green VJ, Pirmohamed M, Kitteringham NR, Gaedigk A, Grant DM, Boxer M. Genetic analysis of microsomal epoxide hydrolase in patients with carbamazepine hypersensitivity. Biochem Pharmacol 1995; 50(9):1353–1359.

10

Advances in Structural and Functional Neuroimaging: How Are These Guiding Epilepsy Surgery?

Robert C. Knowlton
University of Alabama at Birmingham
Birmingham, Alabama, U.S.A.

BACKGROUND AND HISTORY

Epilepsy surgery has been revolutionized by modern neuroimaging. Prior to the advent of CT and early MR imaging, the task of localizing seizures was, for the most part, a *needle-in-the-haystack* search based on electrophysiologic localization methods with recording electrodes typically requiring placement in or directly on the brain. Even with tomographic imaging that became widely available in the late 1970s and early 1980s, the majority of pathologic lesions serving as epileptogenic substrates or pathology remained undetected (cryptogenic).

The main goal of epilepsy-related neuroimaging advances has been to identify a greater percentage of surgical candidates who would otherwise have "normal" or nonlocalizing brain imaging studies. The impact of these advances has been to allow more patients to avoid expensive, invasive intracranial EEG (IC EEG) investigation and, based on better accuracy, to improve selection of candidates (decreased inclusion of candidates with a likely low yield for successful surgery, and increased inclusion of those that may have been otherwise incorrectly excluded). Such advances in imaging will have either a direct or indirect effect on improved seizure-free outcome and decreased neurological morbidity. Figure 1 illustrates the concepts of the impact advanced imaging methods can have on the evaluation and treatment of candidates for epilepsy surgery.

The first major modern neuroimaging advance to widely reduce IC-EEG was the development of FDG-PET (1). This novel modality for relatively high-resolution tomographic imaging of brain metabolism began to influence presurgical epilepsy evaluation by demonstrating focal *functional* defects of glucose uptake in regions

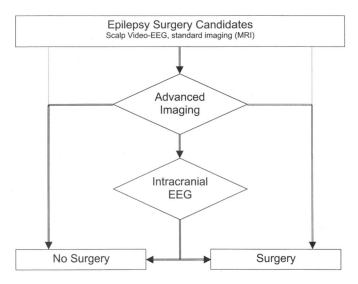

Figure 1. *Position of advanced imaging impact on epilepsy surgery.* Advances in neuroimaging methods have the opportunity to affect all outcomes of surgical decision making. If new imaging information informs clinicians that the patient would not be a good candidate for surgery, it may allow the patient to avoid any further evaluation and possibly even a failed surgery. Even if new localization information from imaging does not allow the patient to avoid intracranial EEG electrodes, it can direct optimal electrode placement, an effect that can avoid the result of false localization—either with respect to nonlocalized recordings whey they otherwise would have been localized (leading to in appropriate denial of surgery) or incorrect localization (leading to a failed surgical outcome). Additional information about the location or extent of epileptogenic substrate that would not be available without advanced imaging techniques affects all aspects of pre surgical decision making and ultimately optimal outcomes.

associated with epileptogenic tissue that did not appear abnormal on conventional *structural* imaging, including early MRI (2). This has been true for mesial temporal lobe epilepsy (MTLE), the most common form of intractable epilepsy, which in many cases is not associated with an obvious structural lesion. FDG-PET began to be applied in earnest to epilepsy surgery in the early 1980s, prior to the introduction of MRI, which became widely available in the late 1980s (3–9). In 1989 the UCLA group showed that focal ictal EEG patterns along with concordant relative focal temporal lobe hypometabolism reliably localized MTLE cases, and also that IC EEG recordings (at that time performed in nearly all evaluations—often referred to as "phase II" evaluations) provided no additional information (10). Thus, UCLA and other centers with FDG-PET advanced the concept of "skip candidates," a presurgical evaluation strategy that allowed patients to proceed directly to surgery skipping IC EEG or phase II evaluations.

Not long after the discovery of the value of FDG-PET in MTLE was the demonstration that it also revealed cryptogenic epileptogenic substrates in neonates and children with catastrophic partial epilepsies including infantile spasms (11). The role of FDG-PET was remarkable in these cases because it provoked the discussion and ultimate decision to offer radical resections (e.g., hemispherectomy or large multilobar resections), which afforded a seizure-free outcome and improved development in many patients who were otherwise doomed to severe mental retardation due to uncontrolled seizures during a critical window of brain development. From this experience arose the novel concept that as long as the epileptogenic pathology and relentless seizures affecting the entire brain remained, potential normal development of nonpathological brain was precluded. Indeed, in spite of major initial deficits from the radical resections (e.g., hemiparesis), the children made remarkable gains in brain development. Prior to FDG-PET revealing a focal or lateralized epileptogenic zone, these patients were not considered surgical candidates because EEG suggested global dysfunction of brain and generalized epilepsy.

In the late 1980s, MRI advanced to the point that subtle abnormalities of brain structure could be detected. Most importantly, this included MRI findings indicative of hippocampal sclerosis (12,13), the most common pathology of MTLE. Detection of relative hippocampal atrophy or prolonged T2 signal concordant with ictal scalp EEG had an analogous impact to that of PET with respect to skipping IC EEG (14). Because of the wide availability of MRI, however, the magnitude of the impact has been far greater than that of FDG-PET. Additionally, both hippocampal volumes (HV), and T2 relaxation times (T2 mapping) were used in imaging laboratories to objectively detect very subtle or questionable abnormalities, further optimizing sensitivity of MRI for this clinically critical brain structure in epilepsy (15–17). Shortly thereafter, correlations were demonstrated between HV and T2 mapping measures and clinical parameters, including surgical histopathology (hippocampal neuronal cell counts), prediction of seizure-free outcome, and memory dysfunction (18–23). Arguably, introduction of high-quality MRI capable of detecting evidence for hippocampal sclerosis and other previously cryptogenic epileptogenic lesions has had the greatest impact of any investigative tool used in the surgical treatment of epilepsy.

MRI advances in the past 10 years have continued to improve candidate selection and localization accuracy. The next most significant contribution of MRI was detection and delineation of malformations of cortical development (MCD) (24–26). This capability has provided for an entirely new in vivo imaging paradigm for classification of human brain development abnormalities, in addition to advanced detection of what was before not defined from an imaging standpoint (27). What remains as a challenge is to determine what part of the brain, although potentially extensive in distribution, is responsible for seizure onset, or to what extent abnormal cortical tissue remains undetected. For this challenge and others, the need for further improvement in structural imaging remains.

Functional imaging modalities have also evolved vastly over the past 10 years. The methodologies include those that are MR based, and others based on determinations of blood flow during seizures with ictal SPECT, biochemical mapping with PET neurotransmitter receptor ligands, etc. Many of these methods, previously considered to be developmental and resesarch-only, are rapidly being applied in clinical application for epilepsy localization. It is precisely the advances in these in vivo functional imaging methods that enable us to tackle the challenges that remain with advanced structural imaging: specifically, determining the significance of many ambiguous or subtle and questionable structural abnormalities; and for the detection of functional abnormalities, associated either indirectly or directly with epileptogenic substrates that remain invisible (cryptogenic), even on state-of-the-art high-resolution MRI.

This chapter will attempt to provide the reader with knowledge of more recent MR structural and functional imaging advances as they apply to the surgical evaluation of epilepsy. This will include developments to improve resolution or overall quality of images, either with improved acquisition or postprocessing techniques to gain information about subtle abnormalities that would otherwise be *missed.*

STRUCTURAL IMAGING

Improved Image Quality

MRI advances, whether applied to epilepsy or other disease states, begin first with enhancement of imaging quality. The main approaches to this are directed toward increasing the signal-to-noise ratio (SNR) and spatial resolution. Three different approaches that accomplish this task include the use of surface coils, image averaging, and high-field strength imaging. Each method has its merits and limitations when brought to clinical applications.

Phase-array surface coils can increase the SNR at the surface of cortical mantle as much as sixfold versus conventional quadrature head coils (28,29). The increase in signal allows for better contrast, or an increase in resolution can be readily achieved without compromise of the signal. In truth, the increase in spatial resolution is only significant for 2D imaging, for with an increase in 3D resolution, the drop-off in signal is proportional to the cube of the decrease in voxel size, an amount that cannot be overcome by even a 6-fold increase in signal. Furthermore, with surface coils SNR decreases with distance from coil; e.g., at a depth of the hippocampus the SNR increase is only 1.67-fold (30). Although this variation of signal strength as a function of distance away from the coils is one of the limitations of surface coils, the signal can be normalized by algorithms that correct for the variation such that signal intensity is uniform throughout the image (31). Other limitations associated with surface coils include limited brain coverage, potential motion problems, and an overall increase in scanning time. Still, the improvement in contrast and fine detail discrimination can be valuable in the assessment of very subtle abnormalities of cortical dysgenesis and hippocampal microstructural disturbances. In reality, the greatest limitation of surface coils is that they are not routinely available.

Image averaging is a novel method to improve SNR that can be performed without any special hardware (32). Improvement in image quality from increased SNR, mainly better gray-white matter contrast, is present throughout the brain (with no trade-off other than for deep vs. superficial tissue). The method requires the acquisition of several scans that are then coregistered and averaged. Gain in SNR is equal to the square root of the number of scans acquired. The same increase could be obtained in scans of the sum of "n" number of scans if patients could hold their head motionless for more than several minutes (usually even the most motivated subjects cannot keep their head perfectly still >10 min).

The optimal ways to take advantage of image averaging remain unclear. In the clinical setting, time in the scanner is of utmost importance. A preliminary report on the application of image averaging in patients with partial epilepsy and subtle or ambiguous lesions on conventional MRI showed a benefit in defining the suspected

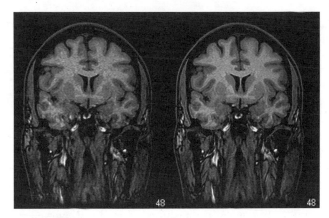

Figure 2. *Image averaging to improve signal to noise.* A subtle area of abnormal cortical migration is present in the right temporal stem, and is poorly visualized on the native single acquisition MRI scan on the left. The lesion is more clearly defined in the averaged image on the right (SPGR sequence × 4).

lesions of interest—greatly improved contrast allowed better delineation of very subtle abnormalities at the gray-white matter junction, yielding greater confidence in the interpretation (33). Figure 2 shows the improvement in image quality, mainly due to better contrast, in a patient with a small area of cortical migration disturbance that is not confidently visualized on the unaveraged native image. Realistically, only a few additional scans of several minutes duration can be allowed. A practical number of scans is four (only three additional) to yield a twofold increase in SNR. The greatest drawback for averaging is not the extra time required for the exam, but rather, that the image processing is not automated. Ultimately, to be practical for routine clinical use, the registration and averaging has to be done automatically immediately after acquisition of scans.

Another approach to improve MR image quality is to take advantage of higher field magnets (3–7 T). This approach provides the most effective method for increasing SNR with the least limitations. High-field imaging does not require special coils with limited brain coverage, nor does it require any postprocessing or extended time in the magnet. In the range of 1.5–7 T, increase in SNR is approximately linear. As with the other methods, by decreasing voxel size, the improvement in SNR can be traded for increased spatial resolution. Additionally, the dynamic range in T1 contrast can be increased using new pulse sequences that exploit the SNR advantage relative to standard field strength images. The main issue that remains with high-field MRI is that of limited availability of such scanners in the clinical environment. This is changing rapidly, however, and it should be expected that within the next five years, 3-T or greater scanners will likely be in routine use at most major medical centers.

Enhanced Visualization

Once optimal MRI acquisition is completed, postprocessing techniques can be exploited to extract more information from the anatomical data that may not be apparent on standard planar tomographic visualization. Multiplanar reconstruction, curvilinear reformating, surface reconstruction, and voxel-based morphometry (VBM) are either developed or emerging techniques that have been shown to benefit MRI interpretation, especially in imaging for epilepsy, which often requires detection of very subtle abnormalities.

Subtle focal lesions, particularly focal malformations of cortical development that involve thickening of the cortex and blurring of gray-white matter interfaces, can sometimes be best detected with multiplanar reformatting of 3D high-resolution MRI (34). However, the complex gyral anatomy causes oblique slicing of much of the cortical gray matter ribbon. Interactive on-line arbitrary reslicing by neuroimagers helps to handle this problem somewhat; however, it is extremely time-consuming to attempt correction of all oblique slicing of the entire brain cortex. Reslicing in an increasingly deep concentric fashion with serial curved slices using the recently developed method curvilinear multiplanar reformating (CMPR) solves the problem (35). This type of slicing results in an approximately perpendicular orientation of the slices in relation to inward-folding gyri. As a result, artificial cortical thickening and partial volume averaging are minimized or even eliminated in many regions.

Also, the method preserves topographical landmarks that are apparent from 3D reconstructions. In a report applying this technique to five patients in whom conventional 2D and 3D MRI analysis, including multiplanar reformating, was initially considered normal, five patients were found to have focal cortical dysplasia with CMPR (35). In four of these patients, histological diagnosis confirmed the finding. Figure 3 provides an example of CMPR in a patient with a questionable MCD in the right lateral frontal lobe region. With CMPR, a potential abnormal area of focal cortical thickening and blurring of the gray-white matter interface becomes unequivocal. CMPR offers a novel advance in image postprocessing to reduce the number of patients considered to have normal neuroanatomical imaging from even recent state-of-the-art MRI acquisitions.

Three-dimensional surface reconstruction of high-resolution MRI data sets allows a unique perspective for analysis of MCDs that cannot be appreciated by visual analysis of 2D tomographic slicing. Although variability and complex gyral patterns exist from person to person, abnormal patterns can still be easily detected, especially when the abnormalities are unilateral. Symmetrical images that preserve tomographic landmarks allow valid comparison between homologous gyri. Also, 3D surface visualization correlates best to what is actually seen in the operating room. Reflection of deeper abnormalities to the surface can also be performed such that surgeons can plan an accurate and exact strategy even beyond that provided by a better visual approach (36). The most logical use of 3D surface reconstructions is integrating the reconstructed volume into frameless stereotaxy systems.

Voxel-based morphometry (VBM) (37) in its simplest form is a voxel-by-voxel-based comparison of local concentration of gray matter between a patient (or within a patient group) and a normal control group using, for example, statistical parametric mapping (SPM) (38). VBM represents a morphometric feature analysis beyond that of simple volume measurements, such as hippocampal volumetry. It can detect structural abnormalities that are overlooked with visual inspection. Sisodiya and colleagues have shown that VBM can detect much more subtle structural disturbances beyond visually identified focal lesions of cortical dysplasia (39). Two

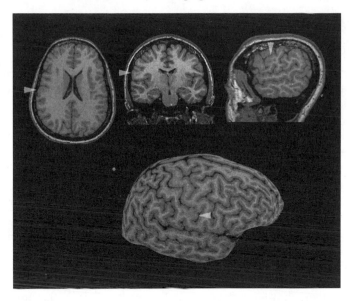

Figure 3. *Curvilinear multiplanar reformating (CMPR).* Cryptogenic cortical dysplasia: upper images are standard orthogonal multiplanar reformatted transverse, coronal, and sagittal slices. The lesion (white arrowheads) on these images cannot be unequivocally interpreted to show focal cortical gray mantle thickening or blurring of the gray-white matter junction because most of the gyri are not orthogonally sliced. The lower CMPR image definitively reveals the lesion, which histopathologic examination confirmed the diagnosis of Taylor type II cortical dysplasia. (Courtesy of Alexandre Bastos, Department of Neurology and Neurosurgery and Brain Imaging Center, Montreal Neurological Hospital and Institute, McGill University, Montreal, Quebec, Canada.)

important questions should be asked: (1) What is the true nature of the volumetric disturbance detected by VBM in these cases? (2) What impact does the presence or absence of such abnormalities have on the success of surgical resection of only the visible lesion? At least in patients with hippocampal sclerosis, the answer to the latter appears to be that patients with cryptic extrahippocampal structural disturbances detected by VBM are much less likely to be seizure-free than those who do not have such abnormalities outside of the typical resection volume (40).

VBM does not bias particular structures and includes assessment of the whole brain. Taking further advantage of nonlinear registration techniques, VBM can be used to identify differences in relative position of structures (deformation-based morphometry), or differences in local shape of brain structures (tensor-based morphometry) (37). These methods, however, are not computationally practical at this time for examining small local differences from one subject compared to a group, such as a group of normals. In the future, it can be envisioned that within a multivariate framework, VBM based feature analysis could include disturbances of local indices of gyrification and image gradients. In particular, the corrections computed for registration between a patient to an appropriate normal control group can be used to discern differences in gyral anatomy that are beyond the range of normal variation in regions of interest or the entire brain (37).

FUNCTIONAL IMAGING

Diffusion-Weighted Imaging

Diffusion-weighted imaging (DWI) is an alteration of standard MR sequences that results in image signals based on sensitivity to small displacement of water molecules. DWI is difficult to classify as either functional or structural-based imaging, for it really encompasses aspects of both. The main concept behind DWI is that imaging based on the measurement of water diffusion may offer the opportunity to explore cellular integrity and pathology (41). DWI measures both diffusivity (magnitude) and anisotropy (direction) of diffusional motion associated with small displacements of water molecules. As an advance with respect to presurgical epilepsy evaluations, it is expected that DWI should offer an opportunity to detect ultrastructural or cellular disturbances that may not be detected with conventional MRI sequences. As with other functional imaging techniques, the hope is that diffusion-weighted imaging methods may detect cryptic pathology in patients with normal MRI or delineate better the extent of pathology that is greater than that visibly seen on standard MRI.

The two parameters of DWI that are used for measurement of diffusion in anisotropy are the apparent diffusion coefficient (ADC) and the anisotropy index (AI). Changes in the ADC and AI are expected to be seen in ultrastructural changes of pathology that include neuronal swelling, shrinkage, or enlargement of extracellular space, or loss of cellular organization (41). Decreases in the ADC have been seen in patients with partial status epilepticus (42). Interictal disturbances of diffusivity have been shown with DWI in patients with mesial temporal lobe epilepsy with or without evidence for hippocampal sclerosis on MRI (43,44). More recent studies with diffusion tensor imaging (DTI), a derivative of DWI that allows better estimates of the magnitude of anisotropy in oblique as well as orthogonal directions, has shown abnormalities of diffusion indices in patients with MCDs and patients with pathologically proven true cryptogenic partial epilepsy (45,46). This new application of DWI methods points to the potential for increased sensitivity and specificity for detection of occult epileptogenic tissue that may more accurately identify the true epileptogenic zone, the extent of cortex that, when fully resected, results in seizure-free outcomes. Further work is needed to improve resolution in signal to noise, particularly at the region of gray-white matter interfaces.

PET

Positron emission tomography (PET) is the most established functional imaging modality in the evaluation of patients with epilepsy. Its largest clinical application involves 2-[^{18}F]fluoro-2-deoxy-D-glucose (FDG) PET. Imaging the tomographic distribution of glucose uptake in the brain with FDG PET has been equated with imaging cerebral metabolism. Ictal scans can be useful; however, the long duration for steady-state uptake of glucose (on the order of many minutes compared to partial seizures, which are typically less than a couple of minutes) often leads to scans that contain a difficult-to-interpret mixture of interictal, ictal, and postictal states. Presurgical epilepsy scans are typically performed in the interictal state with the goal of detecting relatively focal areas of decreased metabolism (i.e., *hypometabolism*) that is presumed to reflect focal functional disturbances of cerebral activity associated with the epileptogenic substrate. What is still enigmatic about FDG PET is that the cause of hypometabolism in and near epileptogenic regions of brain remains unclear. What is known is that it is not simply related to the presence of a structural lesion or frequency of epileptiform discharges as recorded by EEG.

From a purely imaging standpoint, FDG-PET provides a remarkable depiction of in vivo glucose metabolism. It offers relatively high resolution because positron-emitting isotopes emit two photons after annihilation between a positron and an electron. The distance of travel between a positron and electron annihilation is very small (on the order of 1 mm or less). This fact, along with the relatively good intrinsic signal-to-noise of FDG, and with state-of-the-art cameras and collimators, now allows images that can be obtained with full width at half maximum in-plane resolution as small as 2–3 mm (47).

It is in the evaluation of medically refractory epilepsy surgery candidates with clinically suspected temporal lobe epilepsy that FDG PET has been proven most valuable. Because the availability of PET arose before high-resolution structural imaging, it was for years the only modality that could show an abnormality of brain imaging in surgical epilepsy candidates. Sensitivity for detecting relative temporal lobe hypometabolism with FDG PET in MTLE ranges between 80% and 90% (48–53). Much of the variability in sensitivity reflects heterogeneity of the epilepsy more than the differences in quality or specifications of the PET camera (54). Specificity for delineating the exact location and extent of the epileptogenic zone is considered significantly less than sensitivity. This is due in part to the fact that more diffuse or regional relative hypometabolism is seen in the temporal lobe, even with additional involvement of extratemporal, basal ganglia, and thalamic regions (55). Still, the classic pattern for relative hypometabolism in mesial temporal lobe epilepsy (without lesions other than mesial temporal sclerosis) is that which involves mesial temporal, temporal polar, and anterior lateral temporal neocortical regions (55,56).

When structural lesions are present, presence of hypometabolism is effectively 100%, although it is commonly distributed over a larger area than the lesion itself (7,49). The question arises whether the distribution of hypometabolism beyond the lesion reflects a functional disturbance related directly to the epileptogenic zone. If not, then no clinical utility of FDG PET would exist for patients with focal epileptogenic lesions, including hippocampal sclerosis. The latter is the most common epileptogenic pathology in epilepsy surgery candidates, and it can be very reliably detected with MRI (19). Initially it was believed that the more extensive anterior temporal hypometabolism seen in patients with hippocampal sclerosis was a secondary functional disturbance, a finding that led to the conclusion that FDG PET was nonspecific with respect to localization of the epileptogenic zone and therefore should not guide epilepsy surgery without other supportive evidence for localization. In temporal lobe epilepsy, this long-held belief, however, has been brought into question by investigators who have pointed out that the region of seizure onset, as defined by intracranial EEG recordings in patients with classic evidence of hippocampal sclerosis, frequently involves the temporal polar region as much as the hippocampus (57). Thus, an important question arises as to whether the extent of temporal lobe hypometabolism should influence the surgical decision to pursue a standard anterior temporal lobectomy or a selective amygdalohippocampectomy.

The clinical value of FDG PET in neocortical epilepsy is less clear. Only series of uncontrolled, mostly retrospective studies have been reported (58,59), and only a few have been performed in the era of advanced MRI techniques (56–61).

Most importantly, FDG PET data from cases with nonlesional neocortical epilepsy are limited to a few patients scattered among the heterogeneous patients examined in series referenced above. In general, the sensitivity of detecting relative focal hypometabolism in nonlesional neocortical epilepsy appears to be significantly less than that of TLE. Part of FDG PET's limitation in the neocortex reflects poorer resolution of earlier generation cameras, and the difficulty in interpreting subtle focal abnormalities without coregistration to MRI.

The true sensitivity and specificity of relative focal hypometabolism in non-lesional extratemporal lobe epilepsy are less clear. Based on previous reports, the sensitivity is estimated to be generally ~50% (56,58–61). Still, it should be emphasized that focal defects in metabolism can be found in patients with medically intractable partial epilepsy that have cryptogenic lesions. Specifically, some focal cortical dysplasias that still cannot be detected with MRI can be detected with FDG PET. The question that remains is that of specificity. A recent study correlating neocortical focal hypometabolism with intracranial subdural grid EEG recordings found that not only is the distribution of hypometabolism often greater in extent, but also that it is more likely to be greatest on the margin of the region of seizure onset (62).

These persistent issues associated with FDG PET have spurred investigations into the use of flumazenil PET (FMZ PET) to see if GABA-A receptor binding disturbances are more focal and specific than glucose hypometabolism. Imaging GABA-A receptor binding was a logical choice for advanced functional imaging of epilepsy with PET due to the well-established relationship of disturbed GABA-ergic function in epileptogenic tissue. Indeed, early studies of temporal lobe epilepsy (small series with highly selected patients with unilateral hippocampal sclerosis) revealed that disturbances of GABA-A receptor binding were highly sensitive and more localized to epileptogenic mesial temporal-only tissue, contrasting the more diffuse anterior temporal hypometabolism seen with FDG PET (63–66).

More recently, the clinical utility of FMZ PET was investigated in a large series of patients with all types of partial epilepsy. Surprisingly, this study concluded that FMZ PET (53) was no more clinically useful than FDG PET, and that it could even be falsely lateralizing in temporal lobe epilepsy (67). However, a role for FMZ PET was noted for patients with bilateral hippocampal abnormalities on MRI. Also, the region of overlap of hypometabolism and decreased GABA-ergic function was highly specific for the epileptogenic zone as defined by intracranial ictal EEG.

In contrast, the imaging group at Wayne State University reported a greater specificity of FMZ PET over FDG PET in children with mostly extratemporal lobe epilepsy. In examining lesional epilepsy, they found that the distribution of abnormal FMZ PET in the perilesional region correlated with electrocortico-graphically defined epileptogenic tissue, the distribution of which is commonly eccentric in position with respect to the lesion (68). The conclusion for this finding was that FMZ PET offered the possibility of accurately identifying perilesional epileptogenic cortex, which should be removed in addition to the lesion for optimal surgical outcome.

In another study comparing PET abnormalities to intracranial EEG, it was concluded that FMZ PET, although not sufficient to preclude intracranial EEG recording, should be an effective tool for guiding placement of intracranial electrodes (69). Figure 4 provides an example of more localized abnormal GABA-A receptor binding as compared to widespread hypometabolism in a patient with cryptogenic

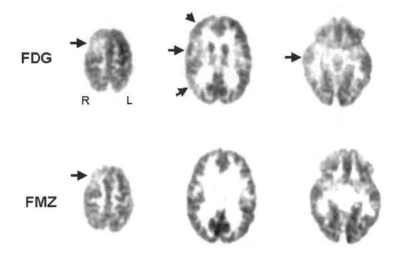

Figure 4. *FDG versus FMZ PET.* Top-row FDG PET images show widespread right frontal-parietal-temporal relative hypometabolism in this patient with frontal lobe onset-only seizures. The bottom row FMZ PET images show decreased benzodiazepine receptor binding that is confined to the right frontal lobe where this patient's seizures were confirmed to arise as defined by intracranial ictal EEG. (Courtesy of Csaba Juhasz, PET Center, Children's Hospital of Michigan, Department of Pediatrics, Wayne State University School of Medicine, Detroit, MI.)

frontal lobe epilepsy. Finally, in a more direct study addressing outcome, it was proposed that the main reason for surgical failure is residual epileptogenic tissue (70). FMZ PET's potential delineation of epileptogenic regions in lesional as well as nonlesional cases, even in patients with normal MRI, should positively affect surgical outcome. Indeed, it was found that a better outcome occurred when a greater extent of FMZ PET disturbance was included in the resection (70). In contrast, the extent of preop or nonresected cortex that was abnormal on FDG PET was not related to surgical outcome.

SPECT

Single photon emission computed tomography (SPECT) is the only modality practically suited for imaging brain activity changes specifically attributable to the ictus. In the clinical setting, all other functional imaging modalities remain confined to detecting metabolic or blood flow derangements as they may be present in the interictal state. This is because epileptic seizures are typically rare and occur in a random fashion. Two technetium [99m]-based isotopes have made ictal blood flow imaging possible. Technetium [99m]-hexanethylpropylene amine oxime (^{99m}Tc-HMPAO) has been the radiopharmaceutical used in the vast majority of ictal or peri-ictal SPECT studies in epilepsy. A more recently available and more convenient radiotracer is technetium [99m]-ethyl cysteinate diethylester (^{99m}Tc-ECD) that appears to be effectively as good as HMPAO, but does not require reconstitution just prior to injection (71). Both possess intravascular binding properties such

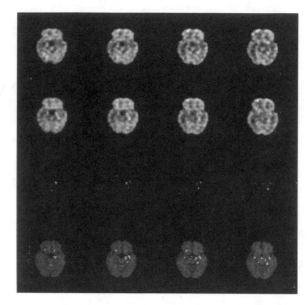

Figure 5. *Subtraction ictal SPECT and coregistration to MRI.* Third row shows the pixel data remaining after precise SPECT-SPECT coregistration, pixel intensity normalization, and subtraction of interictal (top row) from ictal (second row) of cerebral blood flow images. Bottom row images with coregistered MRI reveal the anatomic localization of increased blood flow associated with a complex partial seizure in this patient with left mesial temporal lobe epilepsy. Localization is remarkably confined to the left amygdalohippocampal region, where the seizure was confirmed to arise and remain with little spread with recording by scalp-sphenoidal EEG electrodes.

that most of the labeled isotope becomes trapped in the distribution of brain flow within the first pass following intravenous injection. This unique feature of these isotopes allows what can be conceptually considered a *snapshot* of cerebral blood flow at a given moment of interest, in this case at the earliest time possible that an injection can be performed following the signs or symptoms of a seizure. As such, ictal SPECT has been shown to provide reliable novel localizing information in the presurgical epilepsy evaluation in all types of partial epilepsies (72–79).

A recent advance that has dramatically improved ictal SPECT is image-digital subtraction of an interictal from an ictal scan (80–82). Subtraction ictal SPECT and coregistration to MRI (SISCOM) overcomes the main limitations of interpreting ictal scans. Subtraction allows detection of changes in blood flow that may not be reflective of an absolute increase but a relative one from an interictal state of relatively low blood flow. Second, with coregistration to MRI, the difficulty of recognizing anatomical landmarks for precise localization that was not possible with relatively low resolution SPECT is overcome. Figure 5 demonstrates the concept of perceived normal blood flow in an ictal scan that truly is a relative increase from that which is below normal from the scan in the interictal state. The figure further shows the precise localization of this relative increase in blood flow to that which is remarkably confined to the hippocampus, the small specific region of brain that was exclusively involved as the region of seizure activity.

Limitations of ictal SPECT center mainly around the logistics of successfully infusing the isotope as early as possible after the onset of a seizure. The very patients who are likely to benefit from ictal SPECT are those with seizures that arise outside of the temporal lobe, the type of seizures that typically spread very rapidly and frequently leading to ambiguous ictal blood flow changes. In fact, the changes may be misleading if an area of brain remote from the seizure onset zone takes over as the main generator of seizure activity. Another consequence of the difficult logistics associated with ictal SPECT is the high cost of resources necessary to have healthcare staff sitting at the patient's bedside waiting for the onset of a seizure. Some centers have devised and implemented automated or semiautomated injection systems with the help of basic engineering groups. Still, this remains an area in need of developments to bring down cost, improve accuracy, and ultimately bring this true advance in presurgical evaluation to more patients. Another area of research is to improve methods of objective analysis rather than subjective visual interpretation. One strategy is to use statistical comparison of a given patient's scan against a group of normal controls that has been coregistered in to a common space (83). If such quantitative analysis methods are successful then the second interictal scan required for SISCOM might be avoided.

MRS

Magnetic resonance spectroscopy (MRS) is the use of nuclear magnetic resonance to perform serial in vivo metabolite and macromolecule measurements. Protein- and phosphorus-based metabolites have been the main chemicals of interest in the study of epilepsy with MRS. Studies use either a single-voxel technique, simultaneous acquisition of an array of voxels, or regions using chemical shift imaging. When the latter is used, the technique is labeled "magnetic resonance spectroscopic imaging" (MRSI).

Proton spectroscopy is primarily based on the detection of N-acetyl compounds (primarily N-acetyl aspartate; NAA), creatine, choline, lactate, and glutamate. NA compounds are of particular interest because NAA is found specifically in neurons or their processes in the fully developed central nervous system (84). The cellular biochemical function of NAA is unknown, although there is a suggestion that it is involved in cell volume regulation and electrolyte homeostasis (85–87). Measurement of lactate and glutamate provide information about cellular energy status and localized information about excitatory amino acid concentration, respectively. These are valuable tools that have yet to be fully exploited in studies directed toward further understanding of mechanisms underlying focal cellular biochemical disturbances associated with epileptogenic tissue. They have played no role yet in localization of epileptic foci for surgical treatment.

Phosphorus-based MRS techniques detect phosphocreatine (PCr), ATP, inorganic phosphate (P_i), pH (from the chemical shift of P_i), free magnesium Mg^{2+} (from the chemical shift of ATP), phosphomonoesters (PME), and phosphodiesters (PDE). PCr, ATP, P_i, and pH provide information concerning bioenergetics. PDE and PME provide information concerning lipid metabolism.

Proton MRS and MRSI studies of temporal lobe epilepsy have demonstrated a remarkable sensitivity for the detection of relative depletion of NAA, both ipsilateral and contralateral to the side of predominant seizure onsets (52,88–96).

The sensitivity for detecting an ipsilateral depletion of NAA is relatively high, 85–100%. Most interesting is the high detection of contralateral abnormalities with sensitivity of 30–50%. Relative decreases in NAA are measured in either absolute concentration or as a ratio of NAA to Cr, Cho, or the sum of Cr and Cho. This high sensitivity for detecting abnormalities of NAA is seen with both single-voxel and spectroscopic imaging techniques. NAA abnormalities are also seen whether or not hippocampal atrophy or other evidence for mesial temporal sclerosis (a disease that is predominantly defined by hippocampal neuronal cell loss) exists (52,95,97,98). As an imaging tool, it is hoped that the predominantly lateralized NAA abnormalities can help provide information regarding the site of epilepsy and surgical decision making. The latter includes the possibility that the degree of disturbance may predict seizure-free outcome as well as postoperative neurological memory function (99–101).

Proton MRS and MRSI studies are generally performed interictally for the obvious reason that it is difficult to allow a patient have a seizure while inside the magnet. A preliminary report of a couple of patients with partial seizures of temporal lobe origin that occurred in the magnet showed an increase in lactate, but no NAA changes (102). Further, a report of postictal MRSI in patients with temporal lobe epilepsy showed no changes (103). Also to be emphasized, and in contradiction to what was initially believed about the concentration of NAA reflecting neuronal cell density, is the unequivocal evidence that decreases in NAA concentrations are reversible (104). This has been demonstrated in the evaluation of patients who have and have not become seizure free after anterior temporal lobectomy (105,106). It was shown that in patients who became seizure free after surgical treatment that their abnormally decreased NAA concentrations in the residual ipsilateral and contralateral temporal lobe (prior to surgery) increased or approached the normal range. Thus emerges the important concept that MRS imaging of NAA may be utilized more than just as a sensitive tool for in vivo detection of microscopic neuronal cell loss—rather, that it reflects functional neuronal disturbance. As such, it may provide much more predictive information of cognitive dysfunction and even recovery following temporal lobe surgery (101).

Relatively little work has been published with spectroscopic imaging of extratemporal partial epilepsy (107,108). One recent report looked at proton MRSI in the evaluation of patients with malformations of cortical development (109,110). These studies examined small numbers of patients with focal cortical dysplasia, polymicrogyria, and subcortical heterotopia with proton MRSI protocols. Interestingly, only the cortical dysplasias showed abnormal decreases in NAA compounds. Also revealed in both studies was the finding of abnormally low NAA measures into neighboring cortex beyond the visible lesions on MRI, an important finding that holds promise for proton MRSI to provide clinically valuable information about the true extent of the epileptogenic zone in patients with cortical dysplasia. The surgical outcome of patients with cortical dysplasias is not very high, and the most common reason for failure is inadequacy of resection as proven by a higher success rate with second surgeries in these cases. In spite of all the potential for proton MRSI based on NA measures, for it to be exploited as a more routine presurgical epilepsy imaging tool, development of fast acquisition whole-slice, multislice or whole-brain techniques will be required.

In contrast to proton MRS, the regions of interest studied by ^{31}P-MRSI are rather large owing to the small magnitude of signal for phosphorus-based compounds compared to those which are proton-based. Thus, most studies have generally confined interpretation of findings to lobar disturbances of ^{31}P metabolites. Common findings from the two main groups publishing on this work in partial epilepsy include the following: an elevation of inorganic phosphate, and a decrease in the phosphocreatine to inorganic phosphate ratio (111,112). Controversy remains as to whether changes in pH exist in the epileptogenic lobar region (113,114). With a high-field magnet (4.1 T), the decrease in phosphocreatine to inorganic phosphate ratio was consistently demonstrated in temporal lobe regions ipsilateral to the seizure onset (115). This abnormality was specific to temporal lobe regions with no relative disturbances in extratemporal regions. One study involved patients with frontal lobe epilepsy (116). Although only a small number of patients were studied, in seven of eight cases a decrease in phosphomonoesters was seen. In contrast to temporal lobe epilepsy, there was no significant change in inorganic phosphate. It should be emphasized that ^{31}P-MRSI is an evolving technology that is far from being ready for clinical application toward localization or lateralization of either temporal or extratemporal lobe epilepsy.

Overall, MRS and MRSI represent an active area of research for their role in both clinical application and in basic investigations aimed at understanding the in vivo pathophysiology of human epilepsy. Specifically, along with improvements in acquisition for better resolution, future advances in MRS for epilepsy imaging will be directed toward greater understanding of the nature and significance of NAA disturbances and their correlation with measures of changes in cellular bioenergetics (with both PET and MRS).

Functional MRI

By taking advantage of blood oxygen level dependency (BOLD), functional (f) MRI can image neuronal activation (117). Increased relative neuronal activity is linked with a localized relative increase in cerebral blood flow (CBF) (118). The increase in CBF is greater in magnitude relative to the increase in oxygen consumption. Therefore, the ratio of increased oxyhemoglobin to deoxyhemoglobin causes a change in paramagnetic effect on T2 relaxation time. This is due to the fact that deoxyhemoglobin is paramagnetic while oxyhemoglobin is not. The magnitude of signal change is small, on the order of 1–5%, with imaging at 1.5 Tesla.

The fMRI applications in epilepsy include mapping of interictal (or even ictal) epileptiform disturbances of cerebral activity recorded with EEG and localization of important cortical function (especially memory and language). PET using ^{15}O is also capable of imaging blood flow changes associated with stimulus-induced cortical activation, in some ways even better than fMRI. However, its requirement for repeated radioactive exposure and rare availability due to expense of an on-site cyclotron relegate its use mostly to research study of brain function.

Functional MRI imaging of epileptiform disturbances of cerebral activity is a novel application still in development (119,120). The first hurdle was the need to develop techniques that would allow safe and artifact-free EEG recording in the MRI environment (120,121). The second hurdle was the issue of how the low signal changes associated with epileptiform discharges could be detected. It was clear that large numbers of discharge-triggered acquisitions would be needed to gain adequate signal-to-noise ratio. This latter problem has been aided by the increasing availability of three Tesla magnets. In an initial study of application to localization of EEG spikes in patients with partial epilepsy, 12 of 24 patients had successful fMRI localization that was concordant that of EEG-defined seizure onset and associated structural lesions. In 10 patients who did not show significant fMRI activation, spike amplitudes were observed to be much smaller than to those with positive fMRI results. The potential for this technology as a noninvasive tool in the presurgical epilepsy evaluation is great because of the higher spatial resolution compared to EEG. Yet, it is important to remember that spikes may not represent localization of seizure onsets. A case report confirms the ability of EEG-triggered fMRI to successfully localize the region of cortical activity involved during a seizure (122), however, capturing seizures in MRI units is not logistically applicable for most patients.

Somatotopic mapping of sensory and motor function was demonstrated early in investigations of fMRI (123–128). For epileptogenic lesions neighboring the primary motor or sensory cortex, advance knowledge of critical motor and sensory function has obvious implications for optimal surgery—maximal extent of resection with minimal neurological morbidity (129). Conventionally, identifying primary motor and sensory cortex is based on identification of the central sulcus on anatomic structural imaging (130,131). However, this can be difficult in pathological conditions—e.g., tumors and strokes—which may distort normal landmarks. Additionally, in other types of lesions (dysplasia, developmental tumors, trauma, and ischemia), function may be shifted from that expected on normal anatomy. Over the past several years, numerous groups have shown successful somatotopic mapping in the setting of various pathologies with fMRI, and in many centers it is being used routinely for clinical mapping of function (132–137). Most paradigms use simple movement, which robustly activates M-I, S-I, and S-II.

Mapping of languages is of particular interest in epilepsy surgery owing to its elective nature and the fact that it occurs commonly in the dominant hemisphere. Language involves very complex special sensory systems that require distributed networks of neuronal populations, including regions in the nondominant hemisphere. Paradigms to activate language cortex must deal with this complex distribution of neuronal activation. The best results have been with word generation or fluency tasks (listening, reading, repeating, and object-naming tasks). Fluency tasks involve mainly word retrieval in response to a verbal cue. Semantic verbal fluency paradigms have demonstrated frontal activation asymmetry that correlates well with the intracarotid amobarbital injection test for determination of language dominance lateralization (the Wada exam) (138–143). Of note, temporal lobe areas of activation did not correlate with the Wada exam. Other approaches that have been successful involve word-pairing comprehension and semantic categorization tasks. One of the difficult issues in designing paradigms for activation of language involves the development of nonlinguistic tasks to act as controls such that primary auditory, attention, working memory, and motor aspects of language can be removed.

Although fMRI can provide relatively detailed maps of intrahemispheric activation, this degree of localization is not a reality yet for assisting surgical planning. Regions not activated by one task may be activated by another.

Just because a region is not activated does not mean it lacks important function. Conversely, because a region is activated does not mean it is critical for function. Thus, at this point, application of fMRI for language mapping in epilepsy should be confined to an attempt at lateralizing dominance that may ultimately replace the Wada. Even with respect to this application, it is emphasized that only a few atypical or cross-dominant subjects have been studied.

Memory functional lateralization and localization has obvious application for epilepsy surgery because the most common procedure is that of temporal lobe resections, including much of the hippocampus. The initial goals are to determine function of memory structures in pathological versus nonpathological temporal lobes such that the risk of amnestic complications can be avoided and that asymmetry of memory function may allow epilepsy lateralization. Early studies show promise for fMRI detection of lateralized asymmetries in memory activation (144,145). Also, as with the Wada, functional assessment of memory may provide information with respect to lateralization of temporal lobe epilepsy, as well as predictive power for seizure-free outcome (146). However, with regard to more specific localization, as with language, memory function is activated as a distributed network, and therefore, some regions may be critical for function while others may not. Most importantly, some paradigms may not activate all regions that are critical. Regardless, fMRI among all MR-based imaging advances is the area of greatest research for clinical application in neuroimaging and, without doubt, will increasingly impact the noninvasive presurgical evaluation of epilepsy more than any other imaging tool in the near future.

REFERENCES

1. Engel JJ, Kuhl DE, Phelps ME, Mazziotta JC. Interictal cerebral glucose metabolism in partial epilepsy and its relation to EEG changes. Ann Neurol 1982; 12:510–517.
2. Engel JJ, Kuhl DE, Phelps ME, Crandall PII. Comparative localization of epileptic foci in partial epilepsy by PCT and EEG. Ann Neurol 1982; 12:529–537.
3. Engel JJ. The use of positron emission tomographic scanning in epilepsy. Ann Neurol 1984; 15 Suppl:S180–S191.
4. Mazziotta JC, Engel JJ. The use and impact of positron computed tomography scanning in epilepsy. Epilepsia 1984; 25 Suppl 2:S86–S104.
5. Shimizu H, Ishijima B, Iio M. Diagnosis of temporal lobe epilepsy by positron emission tomography. No To Shinkei 1985; 37:507–512.
6. Sperling MR, Wilson G, Engel JJ, Babb TL, Phelps M, Bradley W. Magnetic resonance imaging in intractable partial epilepsy: correlative studies. Ann Neurol 1986; 20:57–62.
7. Theodore WH, Holmes MD, Dorwart RH, Porter RJ, Di CG, Sato S, Rose D. Complex partial seizures: cerebral structure and cerebral function. Epilepsia 1986; 27:576–582.
8. Abou KB, Siegel GJ, Sackellares JC, Gilman S, Hichwa R, Marshall R. Positron emission tomography studies of cerebral glucose metabolism in chronic partial epilepsy. Ann Neurol 1987; 22:480–486.
9. Stefan H, Pawlik G, Bocher SH, Biersack HJ, Burr W, Penin H, Heiss WD. Functional and morphological abnormalities in temporal lobe epilepsy: a comparison of interictal and ictal EEG, CT, MRI, SPECT and PET. J Neurol 1987; 234:377–384.
10. Engel JJ, Henry TR, Risinger MW, Mazziotta JC, Sutherling WW, Levesque MF, Phelps ME. Presurgical evaluation for partial epilepsy: relative contributions of chronic

depth-electrode recordings versus FDG-PET and scalp-sphenoidal ictal EEG. Neurology 1990; 40:1670–1677.

11. Chugani HT, Shewmon DA, Peacock WJ, Shields WD, Mazziotta JC, Phelps ME. Surgical treatment of intractable neonatal-onset seizures: the role of positron emission tomography. Neurology 1988; 38:1178–1188.

12. Jackson GD, Berkovic SF, Tress BM, Kalnins RM, Fabinyi GC, Bladin PF. Hippocampal sclerosis can be reliably detected by magnetic resonance imaging. Neurology 1990; 40:1869–1875.

13. Berkovic SF, Andermann F, Olivier A, Ethier R, Melanson D, Robitaille Y, Kuzniecky R, Peters T, Feindel W. Hippocampal sclerosis in temporal lobe epilepsy demonstrated by magnetic resonance imaging. Ann Neurol 1991; 29:175–182.

14. Sperling MR. Neuroimaging in epilepsy: contribution of MRI, PET and SPECT. Semin Neurol 1990; 10:349–356.

15. Jack JR, Sharbrough FW, Twomey CK, Cascino GD, Hirschorn KA, Marsh RW, Zinsmeister AR, Scheithauer B. Temporal lobe seizures: lateralization with MR volume measurements of the hippocampal formation. Radiology 1990; 175:423–429.

16. Watson C, Andermann F, Gloor P, Jones GM, Peters T, Evans A, Olivier A, Melanson D, Leroux G. Anatomic basis of amygdaloid and hippocampal volume measurement by magnetic resonance imaging. Neurology 1992; 42:1743–1750.

17. Jackson GD, Connelly A, Duncan JS, Grunewald RA, Gadian DG. Detection of hippocampal pathology in intractable partial epilepsy: increased sensitivity with quantitative magnetic resonance T2 relaxometry. Neurology 1993; 43:1793–1799.

18. Cascino GD, Jack CR, Parisi JE, Sharbrough FW, Hirschhorn KA, Meyer FB, Marsh WR, O'Orien PC. Magnetic resonance imaging-based volume studies in temporal lobe epilepsy: pathological correlations. Ann Neurol 1991; 30:31–36.

19. Jackson GD, Berkovic SF, Duncan JS, Connelly A. Optimizing the diagnosis of hippocampal sclerosis using MR imaging. Am J Neuroradiol 1993; 14:753–762.

20. Kuzniecky R, Burgard S, Faught E, Morawetz R, Bartolucci A. Predictive value of magne-tic resonance imaging in temporal lobe epilepsy surgery. Arch Neurol 1993; 50:65–69.

21. Trenerry MR, Jack CJ, Ivnik RJ, Sharbrough FW, Cascino GD, Hirschorn KA, Marsh WR, Kelly PJ, Meyer FB. MRI hippocampal volumes and memory function before and after temporal lobectomy. Neurology 1993; 43:1800–1805.

22. Loring DW, Murro AM, Meador KJ, Lee GP, Gratton CA, Nichols ME, Gallagher BB, King DW, Smith JR. Wada memory testing and hippocampal volume measurements in the evaluation for temporal lobectomy. Neurology 1993; 43:1789–1793.

23. Martin RC, Sawrie SM, Knowlton RC, Bilir E, Gilliam FG, Faught E, Morawetz RB, Kuzniecky R. Bilateral hippocampal atrophy: consequences to verbal memory following temporal lobectomy. Neurology 2001; 57:597–604.

24. Barkovich AJ, Maroldo TV. Magnetic resonance imaging of normal and abnormal brain development. Top Magn Reson Imag 1993; 5:96–122.

25. Barkovich AJ, Kuzniecky RI. Neuroimaging of focal malformations of cortical development. J Clin Neurophysiol 1996; 13:481–494.

26. Kuzniecky RI, Barkovich AJ. Pathogenesis and pathology of focal malformations of cortical development and epilepsy. J Clin Neurophysiol 1996; 13:468–480.

27. Barkovich AJ. Malformations of neocortical development: magnetic resonance imaging correlates. Curr Opin Neurol 1996; 9:118–121.

28. Grant PE, Barkovich AJ, Wald LL, Dillon WP, Laxer KD, Vigneron DB. High-resolution surface-coil MR of cortical lesions in medically refractory epilepsy: a prospective study. Am J Neuroradiol 1997; 18:291–301.

29. Maravilla K. Advances in MR imaging and MR spectroscopy evaluation of patients with temporal lobe epilepsy. Chonnam J Med Sci 1997; 10:162–170.

30. Hayes CE, Tsuruda JS, Mathis CM. Temporal lobes: surface MR coil phased-array imaging. Radiology 1993; 189:918–920.

31. Wald LL, Carvajal L, Moyher SE, Nelson SJ, Grant PE, Barkovich AJ, Vigneron DB. Phased array detectors and an automated intensity-correction algorithm for high-resolution MR imaging of the human brain. Magn Reson Med 1995; 34:433–439.

32. Holmes CJ, Hoge R, Collins L, Woods R, Toga AW, Evans AC. Enhancement of MR images using registration for signal averaging. J Comput Assist Tomogr 1998; 22:324–333.

33. Knowlton R, Kjos B. Enhanced visualization of anatomy and epileptogenic lesions using MR image registration and signal averaging. Epilepsia 1999; 40(suppl 7):182.

34. Barkovich AJ, Rowley HA, Andermann F. MR in partial epilepsy: value of high-resolution volumetric techniques. Am J Neuroradiol 1995; 16:339–343.

35. Bastos AC, Comeau RM, Andermann F, Melanson D, Cendes F, Dubeau F, Fontaine S, Tampieri D, Olivier A. Diagnosis of subtle focal dysplastic lesions: curvilinear reformatting from three-dimensional magnetic resonance imaging. Ann Neurol 1999; 46:88–94.

36. Chabrerie A, Ozlen F, Nakajima S, Leventon ME, Atsumi H, Grimson E, Keeve E, Helmers S, Riviello J, Jr., Holmes G, Duffy F, Jolesz F, Kikinis R, Black PM. Three-dimensional reconstruction and surgical navigation in pediatric epilepsy surgery. Pediatr Neurosurg 1997; 27:304–310.

37. Ashburner J, Friston KJ. Voxel-based morphometry—the methods. Neuroimage 2000; 11:805–821.

38. Acton PD, Friston KJ. Statistical parametric mapping in functional neuroimaging: beyond PET and fMRI activation studies. Eur J Nucl Med 1998; 25:663–667.

39. Sisodiya SM, Free SL, Stevens JM, Fish DR, Shorvon SD. Widespread cerebral structural changes in patients with cortical dysgenesis and epilepsy. Brain 1995; 118:1039–1050.

40. Sisodiya SM, Moran N, Free SL, Kitchen ND, Stevens JM, Harkness WF, Fish DR, Shorvon SD. Correlation of widespread preoperative magnetic resonance imaging changes with unsuccessful surgery for hippocampal sclerosis. Ann Neurol 1997; 41:490–496.

41. Hajnal JV, Doran M, Hall AS, Collins AG, Oatridge A, Pennock JM, Young IR, Bydder GM. MR imaging of anisotropically restricted diffusion of water in the nervous system: technical, anatomic, and pathologic considerations. J Comput Assist Tomogr 1991; 15:1–18.

42. Wieshmann UC, Symms MR, Shorvon SD. Diffusion changes in status epilepticus. Lancet 1997; 350:493–494.

43. Hugg J, Butterworth E, Kuzniecky K. Diffusion mapping applied to mesial temporal lobe epilepsy. Preliminary observations. Neurology 1999; 53:173–176.

44. Wieshmann UC, Clark CA, Symms MR, Barker GJ, Birnie KD, Shorvon SD. Water diffusion in the human hippocampus in epilepsy. Magn Reson Imag 1999; 17:29–36.

45. Eriksson SH, Rugg-Gunn FJ, Symms MR, Barker GJ, Duncan JS. Diffusion tensor imaging in patients with epilepsy and malformations of cortical development. Brain 2001; 124:617–626.

46. Rugg-Gunn FJ, Eriksson SH, Symms MR, Barker GJ, Duncan JS. Diffusion tensor imaging of cryptogenic and acquired partial epilepsies. Brain 2001; 124:627–636.

47. Valk PE, Jagust WJ, Derenzo SE, Huesman RH, Geyer AB, Budinger TF. Clinical evaluation of a high-resolution (2.6-mm) positron emission tomography. Radiology 1990; 176:783–790.

48. Swartz BE, Tomiyasu U, Delgado EA, Mandelkern M, Khonsari A. Neuroimaging in temporal lobe epilepsy: test sensitivity and relationships to pathology and postoperative outcome. Epilepsia 1992; 33:624–634.

49. Ryvlin P, Philippon B, Cinotti L, Froment JC, Le BD, Mauguiere F. Functional neuroimaging strategy in temporal lobe epilepsy: a comparative study of 18FDG-PET and ^{99m}Tc-HMPAO-SPECT. Ann Neurol 1992; 31:650–656.

50. Valk PE, Laxer KD, Barbaro NM, Knezevic S, Dillon WP, Budinger TF. High-resolution (2.6-mm) PET in partial complex epilepsy associated with mesial temporal sclerosis [see comments]. Radiology 1993; 186:55–58.

51. Gaillard WD, Bhatia S, Bookheimer SY, Fazilat S, Sato S, Theodore WH. FDG PET and volumetric MRI in the evaluation of patients with partial epilepsy. Neurology 1995; 45:123–126.

52. Knowlton RC, Laxer KD, Ende G, Hawkins RA, Wong ST, Matson GB, Rowley HA, Fein G, Weiner MW. Presurgical multimodality neuroimaging in electroencephalographic lateralized temporal lobe epilepsy. Ann Neurol 1997; 42:829–837.

53. Ryvlin P, Bouvard S, Le Bars D, De Lamerie G, Gregoire MC, Kahane P, Froment JC, Mauguiere F. Clinical utility of flumazenil-PET versus [^{18}F]fluorodeoxyglucose-PET and MRI in refractory partial epilepsy. A prospective study in 100 patients. Brain 1998; 121:2067–2081.

54. Henry TR, Engel JJ, Mazziotta JC. Clinical evaluation of interictal fluorine-18-fluorodeoxyglucose PET in partial epilepsy. J Nucl Med 1993; 34:1892–1898.

55. Henry TR, Mazziotta JC, Engel J Jr. Interictal metabolic anatomy of mesial temporal lobe epilepsy. Arch Neurol 1993; 50:582–589.

56. Hajek M, Antonini A, Leenders KL, Wieser HG. Mesiobasal versus lateral temporal lobe epilepsy: metabolic differences in the temporal lobe shown by interictal ^{18}F-FDG positron emission tomography [see comments]. Neurology 1993; 43:79–86.

57. Ryvlin P, Guenot M, Isnard J, Sindou M, Comar D, Froment J. The role of the temporopolar cortex in temporal lobe epilepsy. Stereotact Funct Neurosurg 1997; 67:143.

58. Swartz BE, Halgren E, Delgado EA, Mandelkern M, Gee M, Quinones N, Blahd WH, Repchan J. Neuroimaging in patients with seizures of probable frontal lobe origin. Epilepsia 1989; 30:547–558.

59. Henry TR, Sutherling WW, Engel JJ, Risinger MW, Levesque MF, Mazziotta JC, Phelps ME. Interictal cerebral metabolism in partial epilepsies of neocortical origin. Epilepsy Res 1991; 10:174–182.

60. Da Silva EA, Chugani DC, Muzik O, Chugani HT. Identification of frontal lobe epileptic foci in children using positron emission tomography. Epilepsia 1997; 38:1198–1208.

61. Lee N, Radtke RA, Gray L, Burger PC, Montine TJ, DeLong GR, Lewis DV, Oakes WJ, Friedman AH, Hoffman JM. Neuronal migration disorders: positron emission tomography correlations. Ann Neurol 1994; 35:290–297.

62. Juhasz C, Watson C, Chugani D, Muzik O, Shah J, Shah A, Chugani H. Epileptogenicity of 'metabolic borderzones' in human neocortical epilepsy. Neurology 2000; 54(suppl 3):107.

63. Savic I, Ingvar M, Stone ES. Comparison of [^{11}C]flumazenil and [^{18}F]FDG as PET markers of epileptic foci. J Neurol Neurosurg Psychiatry 1993; 56:615–621.

64. Henry TR, Frey KA, Sackellares JC, Gilman S, Koeppe RA, Brunberg JA, Ross DA, Berent S, Young AB, Kuhl DE. In vivo cerebral metabolism and central benzodiazepine-receptor binding in temporal lobe epilepsy. Neurology 1993; 43:1998–2006.

65. Burdette DE, Sakurai SY, Henry TR, Ross DA, Pennell PB, Frey KA, Sackellares JC, Albin RL. Temporal lobe central benzodiazepine binding in unilateral mesial temporal lobe epilepsy. Neurology 1995; 45:934–941.

66. Koepp MJ, Richardson MP, Labbe C, Brooks DJ, Cunningham VJ, Ashburner J, Van Paesschen W, Revesz T, Duncan JS. ^{11}C-flumazenil PET, volumetric MRI, and quantitative pathology in mesial temporal lobe epilepsy. Neurology 1997; 49:764–773.

67. Ryvlin P, Bouvard S, Le Bars D, Mauguiere F. Transient and falsely lateralizing flumazenil-PET asymmetries in temporal lobe epilepsy. Neurology 1999; 53:1882–1885.

68. Juhasz C, Chugani DC, Muzik O, Watson C, Shah J, Shah A, Chugani HT. Electroclinical correlates of flumazenil and fluorodeoxyglucose PET abnormalities in lesional epilepsy. Neurology 2000; 55:825–835.

69. Muzik O, Da Silva EA, Juhasz C, Chugani DC, Shah J, Nagy F, Canady A, Von Stockhausen HM, Herholz K, Gates J, Frost M, Ritter F, Watson C, Chugani HT. Intracranial EEG versus flumazenil and glucose PET in children with extratemporal lobe epilepsy. Neurology 2000; 54:171–179.

70. Juhasz C, Chugani DC, Muzik O, Shah A, Shah J, Watson C, Canady A, Chugani HT. Relationship of flumazenil and glucose PET abnormalities to neocortical epilepsy surgery outcome. Neurology 2001; 56:1650–1658.

71. O'Brien TJ, Brinkmann BH, Mullan BP, So EL, Hauser MF, O'Connor MK, Hung J, Jack CR. Comparative study of ^{99m}Tc-ECD and ^{99m}Tc-HMPAO for peri-ictal SPECT: qualitative and quantitative analysis. J Neurol Neurosurg Psychiatry 1999; 66:331–339.

72. Shen W, Lee BI, Park HM, Siddiqui AR, Wellman HH, Worth RM, Markand ON. HIPDM-SPECT brain imaging in the presurgical evaluation of patients with intractable seizures. J Nucl Med 1990; 31:1280–1284.

73. Marks DA, Katz A, Hoffer P, Spencer SS. Localization of extratemporal epileptic foci during ictal single photon emission computed tomography. Ann Neurol 1992; 31:250–255.

74. Kuzniecky R, Mountz JM, Thomas F. Ictal ^{99m}Tc HMPAO brain single-photon emission computed tomography in electroencephalographic nonlocalizable partial seizures. J Neuroimag 1993; 3:100–102.

75. Ho SS, Berkovic SF, Newton MR, Austin MC, McKay WJ, Bladin PF. Parietal lobe epilepsy: clinical features and seizure localization by ictal SPECT. Neurology 1994; 44:2277–2284.

76. Newton MR, Berkovic SF, Austin MC, Rowe CC, McKay WJ, Bladin PF. SPECT in the localisation of extratemporal and temporal seizure foci. J Neurol Neurosurg Psychiatry 1995; 59:26–30.

77. Koh S, Jayakar P, Resnick T, Alvarez L, Liit RE, Duchowny M. The localizing value of ictal SPECT in children with tuberous sclerosis complex and refractory partial epilepsy. Epileptic Disord 1999; 1:41–46.

78. Spanaki MV, Spencer SS, Corsi M, MacMullan J, Seibyl J, Zubal IG. Sensitivity and specificity of quantitative difference SPECT analysis in seizure localization. J Nucl Med 1999; 40:730–736.

79. Sturm JW, Newton MR, Chinvarun Y, Berlangieri SU, Berkovic SF. Ictal SPECT and interictal PET in the localization of occipital lobe epilepsy. Epilepsia 2000; 41:463–466.

80. Zubal IG, Spencer SS, Imam K, Seibyl J, Smith EO, Wisniewski G, Hoffer PB. Difference images calculated from ictal and interictal technetium-^{99m}-HMPAO SPECT scans of epilepsy. J Nucl Med 1995; 36:684–689.

81. O'Brien TJ, O'Connor MK, Mullan BP, Brinkmann BH, Hanson D, Jack CR, So EL. Subtraction ictal SPET co-registered to MRI in partial epilepsy: description and technical validation of the method with phantom and patient studies. Nucl Med Commun 1998; 19:31–45.

82. O'Brien TJ, So EL, Mullan BP, Hauser MF, Brinkmann BH, Bohnen NI, Hanson D, Cascino GD, Jack CR Jr, Sharbrough FW. Subtraction ictal SPECT co-registered to MRI improves clinical usefulness of SPECT in localizing the surgical seizure focus. Neurology 1998; 50:445–454.

83. Houston AS, Kemp PM, Macleod MA. A method for assessing the significance of abnormalities in HMPO brain SPECT images. J Nucl Med 1994; 35:239–244.

84. Urenjak J, Williams SR, Gadian DG, Noble M. Specific expression of N-acetylaspartate in neurons, oligodendrocyte-type-2 astrocyte progenitors, and immature oligodendrocytes in vitro. J Neurochem 1992; 59:55–61.

85. McIntosh J, Cooper J. Studies on the function of N-acetyl-aspartic acid in brain. J Neurochem 1965; 12:825–835.

86. Tsai G, Coyle JT. N-acetylaspartate in neuropsychiatric disorders. Prog Neurobiol 1995; 46:531–540.

87. Davies S, Gotoh M, Richards D, Obrenovitch T. Hypoosmolarity induces an increase in extracellular N-acetylaspartate concentration in rat striatum. Neurochem Res 1998; 23:1021–1025.

88. Hugg JW, Laxer KD, Matson GB, Maudsley AA, Weiner MW. Neuron loss localizes human temporal lobe epilepsy by in vivo proton magnetic resonance spectroscopic imaging. Ann Neurol 1993; 34:488–794.

89. Vainio P, Usenius JP, Vapalahti M, Partanen K, Kalviainen R, Rinne J, Kauppinen RA. Reduced N-acetylaspartate concentration in temporal lobe epilepsy by quantitative ^{1}H MRS in vivo. Neuroreport 1994; 5:1733–1736.

90. Ng TC, Comair YG, Xue M, So N, Majors A, Kolem H, Luders H, Modic M. Temporal lobe epilepsy: presurgical localization with proton chemical shift imaging. Radiology 1994; 193:465–472.

91. Ende G, Laxer KD, Knowlton RC, Matson GB, Weiner MW. Quantitative ^{1}H-SI shows bilateral metabolite changes in unilateral TLE patients with and without hippocampal atrophy. Proc SMR Third Meeting 1995; 144.

92. Hetherington H, Kuzniecky R, Pan J, Mason G, Morawetz R, Harris C, Faught E, Vaughan T, Pohost G. Proton nuclear magnetic resonance spectroscopic imaging of human temporal lobe epilepsy at 4.1 T. Ann Neurol 1995; 38:396–404.

93. Connelly A, Jackson GD, Duncan JS, King MD, Gadian DG. Magnetic resonance spectroscopy in temporal lobe epilepsy. Neurology 1994; 44:1411–1417.

94. Cross JH, Connelly A, Jackson GD, Johnson CL, Neville BG, Gadian DG. Proton magnetic resonance spectroscopy in children with temporal lobe epilepsy. Ann Neurol 1996; 39:107–113.

95. Cendes F, Caramanos Z, Andermann F, Dubeau F, Arnold DL. Proton magnetic resonance spectroscopic imaging and magnetic resonance imaging volumetry in the lateralization of temporal lobe epilepsy: a series of 100 patients. Ann Neurol 1997; 42:737–746.

96. Kuzniecky R, Hugg JW, Hetherington H, Butterworth E, Bilir E, Faught E, Gilliam F. Relative utility of ^{1}H spectroscopic imaging and hippocampal volumetry in the lateralization of mesial temporal lobe epilepsy. Neurology 1998; 51:66–71.

97. Connelly A, Van Paesschen W, Porter DA, Johnson CL, Duncan JS, Gadian DG. Proton magnetic resonance spectroscopy in MRI-negative temporal lobe epilepsy. Neurology 1998; 51:61–66.

98. Woermann FG, McLean MA, Bartlett PA, Parker GJ, Barker GJ, Duncan JS. Short echo time single-voxel ^{1}H magnetic resonance spectroscopy in magnetic resonance imaging–negative temporal lobe epilepsy: different biochemical profile compared with hippocampal sclerosis. Ann Neurol 1999; 45:369–376.

99. Incisa della Rocchetta A, Gadian DG, Connelly A, Polkey CE, Jackson GD, Watkins KE, Johnson CL, Mishkin M, Vargha KF. Verbal memory impairment after right temporal lobe surgery: role of contralateral damage as revealed by ^{1}H magnetic resonance spectroscopy and T2 relaxometry. Neurology 1995; 45:797–802.

100. Martin RC, Sawrie S, Hugg J, Gilliam F, Faught E, Kuzniecky R. Cognitive correlates of ^{1}H MRSI-detected hippocampal abnormalities in temporal lobe epilepsy. Neurology 1999; 53:2052–2058.

101. Sawrie SM, Martin RC, Gilliam FG, Faught RE, Maton B, Hugg JW, Bush N, Sinclair K, Kuzniecky RI. Visual confrontation naming and hippocampal function: a neural network study using quantitative ^{1}H magnetic resonance spectroscopy. Brain 2000; 123:770–780.

102. Cendes F, Stanley JA, Dubeau F, Andermann F, Arnold DL. Proton magnetic resonance spectroscopic imaging for discrimination of absence and complex partial seizures. Ann Neurol 1997; 41:74–81.

103. Maton B, Londono A, Sawrie S, Knowlton R, Martin R, Kuzniecky R. Postictal stability of proton magnetic resonance spectroscopy imaging (^{1}H-MRSI) ratios in temporal lobe epilepsy. Neurology 2001; 42:651–659.

104. Rango M, Spagnoli D, Tomei G, Bamonti F, Scarlato G, Zetta L. Central nervous system trans-synaptic effects of acute axonal injury: a ^{1}H magnetic resonance spectroscopy study. Magn Reson Med 1995; 33:595–600.

105. Hugg JW, Kuzniecky RI, Gilliam FG, Morawetz RB, Fraught RE, Hetherington HP. Normalization of contralateral metabolic function following temporal lobectomy demonstrated by ^{1}H magnetic resonance spectroscopic imaging. Ann Neurol 1996; 40:236–239.

106. Cendes F, Andermann F, Dubeau F, Matthews PM, Arnold DL. Normalization of neuronal metabolic dysfunction after surgery for temporal lobe epilepsy. Evidence from proton MR spectroscopic imaging. Neurology 1997; 49:1525–1533.

107. Garcia PA, Laxer KD, Van der Grond J, Hugg JW, Matson GB, Weiner MW. Proton magnetic resonance spectroscopic imaging in patients with frontal lobe epilepsy. Ann Neurol 1995; 37:279–281.

108. Stanley JA, Cendes F, Dubeau F, Andermann F, Arnold DL. Proton magnetic resonance spectroscopic imaging in patients with extratemporal epilepsy. Epilepsia 1998; 39:267–273.

109. Li LM, Cendes F, Bastos AC, Andermann F, Dubeau F, Arnold DL. Neuronal metabolic dysfunction in patients with cortical developmental malformations: a proton magnetic resonance spectroscopic imaging study. Neurology 1998; 50:755–759.

110. Kuzniecky R, Hetherington H, Pan J, Hugg J, Palmer C, Gilliam F, Faught E, Morawetz R. Proton spectroscopic imaging at 4.1 Tesla in patients with malformations of cortical development and epilepsy. Neurology 1997; 48:1018–1024.

111. Kuzniecky R, Elgavish GA, Hetherington HP, Evanochko WT, Pohost GM. In vivo ^{31}P nuclear magnetic resonance spectroscopy of human temporal lobe epilepsy. Neurology 1992; 42:1586–1590.

112. Hugg J, Laxer K, Matson G, Maudsley A, Husted C, Weiner M. Lateralization of human focal epilepsy by ^{31}P magnetic resonance spectroscopic imaging. Neurology 1992; 42:2001–2018.

113. Laxer KD, Hubesch B, Sappey-Marinier D, Weiner MW. Increased pH and inorganic phosphate in temporal seizure foci demonstrated by [^{31}P]MRS. Epilepsia 1992; 33:618–623.

114. Chu WJ, Hetherington HP, Kuzniecky RJ, Vaughan JT, Twieg DB, Faught RE, Gilliam FG, Hugg JW, Elgavish GA. Is the intracellular pH different from normal in the epileptic focus of patients with temporal lobe epilepsy? A ^{31}P NMR study. Neurology 1996; 47:756–760.

115. Chu WJ, Hetherington HP, Kuzniecky RI, Simor T, Mason GF, Elgavish GA. Lateralization of human temporal lobe epilepsy by ^{31}P NMR spectroscopic imaging at 4.1 T. Neurology 1998; 51:472–479.

116. Garcia PA, Laxer KD, Van der Grond J, Hugg JW, Matson GB, Weiner MW. Phosphorus magnetic resonance spectroscopic imaging in patients with frontal lobe epilepsy. Ann Neurol 1994; 35:217–221.

117. Ogawa S. Brain magnetic resonance imaging with contrast dependent on blood oxygenation. Proc Natl Acad Sci USA 1990; 87:9868–9872.

118. Fox P, Raichle M. Focal physiological uncoupling of cerebrl blood flow and oxidative metabolism during somatosensory stimulation in human subjects. Proc Natl Acad Sci USA 1986; 83:1140–1144.

119. Seeck M, Lazeyras F, Michel C, Banke O, Gericke C, Ives J, Delavelle J, Golay X, Haenggeli C, De Tribolet N, Landis T. Non-invasive epileptic focus localization using

EEG-triggered functional MRI and electromagnetic tomography. Electroencephalogr Clin Neurophysiol 1998; 106:508–512.

120. Krakow K, Allen P, Lemieux L, Symms M, Fish D. Methodology: EEG-correlated fMRI. Adv Neurol 2000; 38:187–201.

121. Goldman R, Stern J, Engel JJ, Cohen M. Acquiring simultaneous EEG and functional MRI. Clin Neurophysiol 2000; 111:1974–1980.

122. Lazeyras F, Blanke O, Zimine I, Delavelle J, Perrig S, Seeck M. MRI, ¹H-MRS, and functional MRI during and after prolonged nonconvulsive seizures activity. Neurology 2000; 55:1677–1682.

123. Rao SM, Binder JR, Bandettini PA, Hammeke TA, Yetkin FZ, Jesmanowicz A, Lisk LM, Morris GL, Mueller WM, Estkowski LD. Functional magnetic resonance imaging of complex human movements. Neurology 1993; 43:2311–2318.

124. Jack C, Thompson R, Butts R. Sensory motor cortex: correlation of presurgical mapping with functional MR imaging and invasive cortical mapping. Radiology 1994; 190:85–92.

125. Rao SM, Binder JR, Hammeke TA, Bandettini PA, Bobholz JA, Frost JA, Myklebust BM, Jacobson RD, Hyde JS. Somatotopic mapping of the human primary motor cortex with functional magnetic resonance imaging. Neurology 1995; 45:919–924.

126. Yetkin FZ, Mueller WM, Hammeke TA, Morris GL 3rd, Haughton VM. Functional magnetic resonance imaging mapping of the sensorimotor cortex with tactile stimulation. Neurosurgery 1995; 36:921–925.

127. Puce A. Comparative assessment of sensorimotor function using functional magnetic resonance imaging and electrophysiological methods. J Clin Neurophysiol 1995; 12:450–459.

128. Yousry TA, Schmid UD, Jassoy AG, Schmidt D, Eisner WE, Reulen HJ, Reiser MF, Lissner J. Topography of the cortical motor hand area: prospective study with functional MR imaging and direct motor mapping at surgery. Radiology 1995; 195:23–29.

129. Conesa G, Pujol J, Deus J, Lopez-Obarrio L, Gabarros A, Marnov A, Rodriguez R, Navarro R, Capdevila A, Isamat F. EPI functional MRI: a useful tool for preoperative rolandic fissure localization. Front Radiat Ther Oncol 1999; 33:23–27.

130. Kido D, LeMay M, Levinson A, Benson W. Computed tomographic localization of the precentral sulcus. Radiology 1980; 135:373–377.

131. Sobel D, Gallen C. Locating the central sulcus: comparison of MR anatomic and magnetoencephalographic functional methods. Am J Neuroradiol 1993; 14:915–926.

132. Chapman PH, Buchbinder BR, Cosgrove GR, Jiang HJ. Functional magnetic resonance imaging for cortical mapping in pediatric neurosurgery. Pediatr Neurosurg 1995; 23:122–126.

133. Righini A, de Divitiis O, Prinster A, Spagnoli D, Appollonio I, Bello L, Scifo P, Tomei G, Villani R, Fazio F, Leonardi M. Functional MRI: primary motor cortex localization in patients with brain tumors. J Comput Assist Tomogr 1996; 20:702–708.

134. Schad LR, Bock M, Baudendistel K, Essig M, Debus J, Knopp MV, Engenhart R, Lorenz WJ. Improved target volume definition in radiosurgery of arteriovenous malformations by stereotactic correlation of MRA, MRI, blood bolus tagging, and functional MRI. Eur Radiol 1996; 6:38–45.

135. Mueller WM, Yetkin FZ, Hammeke TA, Morris GL 3rd, Swanson SJ, Reichert K, Cox R, Haughton VM. Functional magnetic resonance imaging mapping of the motor cortex in patients with cerebral tumors. Neurosurgery 1996; 39:515–520; discussion 520–511.

136. Maldjian J, Atlas SW, Howard RS, 2nd, Greenstein E, Alsop D, Detre JA, Listerud J, D'Esposito M, Flamm ES. Functional magnetic resonance imaging of regional brain activity in patients with intracerebral arteriovenous malformations before surgical or endovascular therapy. J Neurosurg 1996; 84:477–483.

137. Achten E, Jackson GD, Cameron JA, Abbott DF, Stella DL, Fabinyi GC. Presurgical evaluation of the motor hand area with functional MR imaging in patients with tumors and dysplastic lesions. Radiology 1999; 210:529–538.

138. Binder JR, Swanson SJ, Hammeke TA, Morris GL, Mueller WM, Fischer M, Benbadis S, Frost JA, Rao SM, Haughton VM. Determination of language dominance using functional MRI: a comparison with the Wada test. Neurology 1996; 46:978–984.

139. Bahn MM, Lin W, Silbergeld DL, Miller JW, Kuppusamy K, Cook RJ, Hammer G, Wetzel R, Cross D 3rd. Localization of language cortices by functional MR imaging compared with intracarotid amobarbital hemispheric sedation. AJR. AJR 1997; 169:575–579.

140. Yetkin FZ, Swanson S, Fischer M, Akansel G, Morris G, Mueller W, Haughton V. Functional MR of frontal lobe activation: comparison with Wada language results. Am J Neuroradiol 1998; 19:1095–1098.

141. Benson R, FitzGerald D, LeSueur L, Kennedy D, Kwong K, Buchbinder B, Davis T, Weisskoff R, Talavage T, Logan W, Cosgrove G, Belliveau J, Rosen B. Language dominance determined by whole brain functional MRI in patients with brain lesions. Neurology 1999; 52:798–809.

142. Lehericy S, Cohen L, Bazin B, Samson S, Giacomini E, Rougetet R, Hertz-Pannier L, Le Bihan D, Marsault C, Baulac M. Functional MR evaluation of temporal and frontal language dominance compared with the Wada test. Neurology 2000; 54:1625–1633.

143. Gaillard W, Hertz-Pannier L, Mott S, Barnett A, LeBihan D, Theodore W. Functional anatomy of cognitive development: fMRI of verbal fluency in children and adults. Neurology 2000; 54:180–185.

144. Detre J, Maccotta L, King D, Alsop D, Glossser G, D'Esposito, Zarahn E, Aguirre G, French J. Functional MRI lateralization of memory in temporal lobe epilepsy. Neurology 1998; 50:926–932.

145. Killgore WD, Casasanto DJ, Yurgelun-Todd DA, Maldjian JA, Detre JA. Functional activation of the left amygdala and hippocampus during associative encoding. Neuroreport 2000; 11:2259–2263.

146. Binder J, Bellgowan P, Swanson S. fMRI activation asymmetry predicts side of seizure focus in temporal lobe epilepsy. Neuroimage 2000; 11:155.

11
Magnetoencephalography in Clinical Epilepsy

William W. Sutherling
Huntington Medical Research Institutes,
Epilepsy and Brain Mapping Program,
and Huntington Hospital
Pasadena, California, U.S.A.

Massoud Akhtari
Huntington Medical Research Institutes,
and Epilepsy and Brain Mapping Program
Pasadena, California,
and University of New Mexico,
Albuquerque, New Mexico, U.S.A.

Adam N. Mamelak
Huntington Medical Research Institutes,
Epilepsy and Brain Mapping Program,
and Huntington Hospital
Pasadena, California
and City of Hope Medical Center
Durate, California, U.S.A.

John Mosher
Los Alamos National Laboratory
Los Alamos, New Mexico,
and University of Southern California
Los Angeles, California, U.S.A.

Deborah Arthur
Huntington Medical Research Institutes
Pasadena, California, U.S.A.

Nancy Lopez, Jeri E. Nichols, and Joy Sarafian
Epilepsy and Brain Mapping Program
Pasadena, California, U.S.A.

Richard Leahy
University of Southern California
Los Angeles, California, U.S.A.

Warren Merrifield

Huntington Medical Research Institutes,
Pasadena, and Loma Linda University,
Loma Linda, California, U.S.A.

Rachelle Padilla

Epilepsy and Brain Mapping Program
and Huntington Hospital
Pasadena, California U.S.A.

Ross Eto

Huntington Hospital
Pasadena, California, U.S.A.

Edward Flynn

University of New Mexico,
Albuquerque, and Los Alamos National Laboratory
Los Alamos, New Mexico, U.S.A.

INTRODUCTION AND BACKGROUND

Medically Intractable Epilepsy

About 1% of the population has epilepsy (1), and up to a third of epileptic patients have disabling seizures that cannot be controlled by medications (2–5). Half of the patients with intractable epilepsy are good surgical candidates (6–9). Focal excision abolishes seizures in 70% with temporal lobe epilepsy and in 50% with neocortical foci (10,11). Localization of the seizure is essential for surgery (8,11–16). Intracranial electrodes (iEEG) allow 36% more patients to have surgery compared with scalp EEG (7). Recordings from iEEG have led to improved surgical results (8,9,11,17,18). However, iEEG has two principal disadvantages: invasiveness and sampling error. Epilepsy surgery does not completely control seizures in 15–20% (7,17,19) despite iEEG, probably owing to sampling error since iEEG may record a spread pattern. Sampling error is inherent owing to the risk of iEEG, which increases with more electrode coverage (12). Noninvasive protocols allow ~70% of temporal lobe patients to have surgery. Focal temporal lobe seizure onsets on video EEG, with concordant ipsilateral PET or MRI, localize with accuracy, which is equivalent to intracranial depth electrodes but without the risk (9,13,16,20).

Presurgical localization is usually based on seizure recording from costly inpatient monitoring. Seizure spread can create ambiguity necessitating invasive recordings for definitive localization. There is more information in spikes than used today in most surgical centers. Spikes are present on routine outpatient recordings and do not require long-term inpatient monitoring. Spikes help quantify the epileptogenic zone for surgical removal (21–23).

MEG in Epilepsy

There are several studies with large-array or whole-head MEG systems, on a large combined number of patients. Knowlton et al. (24) studied 22 patients with a

37-channel MEG. Wheless et al. (25) studied 58 patients with two 37-channel systems. Lamusuo et al. (26) studied nine patients who had complicated partial epilepsy with a whole-scalp MEG array. Otsubo and Snead studied children with a whole-scalp MEG array (27–29). All found MEG useful; i.e., MEG helped predict seizure zones and improve localization for epilepsy surgery.

The degree of MEG prediction is, however, controversial. Wheless found MEG localized successful surgery in 52% of patients (N = 44), whereas Knowlton found accurate MEG localization in 86% (N = 14). This difference is significant (chi-square, $P = .03$). This difference could be explained by spike propagation or signal-to-noise ratio (SNR). MEG detects ECoG spikes only during synchronous activation of an extended area of cortex when multiple ECoG electrodes are involved. Estimates from EEG simultaneous with ECoG strips have indicated $\sim 6\,cm^2$ (30). Synchronous cortical activity over $\sim 2\,cm^2$ to $3\,cm^2$ is required to produce a detectible extracranial spike in the MEG (31) when MEG was compared to simultaneous recording from large ECoG grids where the area could be quantified over the cortical surface. This is due to detection sensitivity and SNR. The MEG is better suited than EEG to extracranial-intracranial correlations than EEG owing to minimal effect of the volume conductor on MEG (32), allowing simultaneous MEG to iEEG with grids. The MEG is better in extratemporal epilepsy than in temporal epilepsy (25), consistent with findings in the EEG for specificity of spikes (33). These large studies have shown that MEG has nonredundant utility compared with routine EEG analysis, but remains inferior to iEEG localization. The next step is to directly compare the same event in MEG and iEEG to determine why MEG localization is not identical to iEEG localization.

Spikes

Interictal spikes have unexploited information. Near the zone of seizure origin they have several characteristics. First, when 90% of spikes occur in one area, this overlaps the seizure zone and predicts good outcome (34,35). Second, spikes on depth EEG have different propagation in temporal lobe epilepsy compared to frontal lobe epilepsy (36,37). Although interhemispheric spike analysis is used in EEG (38,39) to lateralize the epileptogenic zone in partial seizures, and in MEG to lateralize acquired childhood epileptic aphasia (40), there has been little work on propagation within a hemisphere or lobe as an aid to diagnosis. Robust spike propagation occurs in MEG (41). Spatiotemporal modeling reveals more sources than single dipoles (42). Advanced multiple source modeling would be expected to maximize this information.

Third, the sharpest spike is nearest the seizure zone (34). Sharpness correlates with epileptogenicity (43). Such a correlation is not surprising since temporal dispersion with increasing distance from an initiating source occurs owing to different conduction velocities in different-size axons (44). Electrical activity is more synchronous (shorter duration and sharper waveform) at the source (45). The sharpest spike is composed of a small initial spike phase, followed by a blunter sharp wave. The initial sharpest component of the sharpest spike is most localizing owing to the discharge of the initiating synchronous cortical region, before the later sharp wave and slow wave extend into the inhibitory surround (45). But the initial, sharpest spike is small, buried in background, and difficult to localize visually or with a single-dipole model, owing to low SNR, which impedes dipole searches.

Fourth, stability of occurrence or constant repetition rate across wake-sleep states characterizes the spike nearest the seizure zone (46). This is not surprising since partial disconnection from thalamic input occurs in some animal models of epilepsy (47). Since MEG is restricted to brief sessions, more prolonged video EEG (outpatient or inpatient) is necessary to assess autonomy, and EEG source localization methods become more important.

Realistic Models

The model of the source affects localization accuracy. Signal-to-noise ratio can be improved to detect smaller, sharper initial spikes using such advanced models as *r*ecursively *ap*plied *mu*ltiple *si*gnal *c*lassification (RAP-MUSIC), which separates the signal from the noise subspace (48), increasing SNR. More realistic modeling may therefore improve detection sensitivity of MEG, and has been used successfully by several investigators (49,50). Propagation is best assessed with the more realistic spatiotemporal dipole model.

The model of the volume conductor also significantly affects localization accuracy of dipole and extended source models (51,52). Several mathematical and geometrical models of the human head as a volume conductor have been developed to correlate extracranially measured magnetic fields (MEG) and electric potentials (EEG) to their intracranial generators. Models such as single and multiple spherical shells, boundary element model (BEM), and finite element model (FEM) are among the most widely used (53–62). Skull effects dominate in volume conductor models. Recent detailed studies of conductivity have revealed the complexity of the skull's electrical properties (63,64). Inclusion of the results of such studies in the volume conductor model may improve the localizations from extracranial electric and magnetic measurements.

EEG

Although EEG is less accurate than MEG for spatial localization (48,65), and the sensors are more difficult to co-register with MRI, EEG has several complementary advantages. First, it is used routinely in all comprehensive epilepsy centers in the United States. Also, it is less expensive than the MEG since it records only the voltage differences produced by scalp currents between two sites on the head, although recording of this easily obtainable quantity increases the complexity of the volume conductor necessary to analyze it. Further, recording of epileptic activity usually is easier to obtain in EEG: seizures and a large spike sample across wake-sleep states to assess autonomy.

EEG measures the same current orientations as iEEG. EEG also measures more of the cerebral cortex than MEG, while it concurrently increases the complexity of the source model required for analysis. The EEG combined with MEG gives more accurate localizations than MEG or EEG alone (60,66). More realistic volume conductor models are especially important to improve accuracy of the EEG and are essential to combine the MEG and EEG for localization (54,67).

Central Fissure

The precise localization of central fissure (CF) is important to avoid hand weakness in surgery (68–70). Localization of CF requires electrophysiological techniques since visual identification of CF can be inaccurate (71). Cortical stimulations are useful but time-consuming, and require patient cooperation. Intraoperative somatosensory-evoked responses (SERs) to median nerve stimulation are accurate but may not identify CF owing to location outside the operative field. MEG reliably localizes CF preoperatively for surgery (72–74). Further MEG mapping of the thumb (75) may allow more complete resections of epilepsy and tumors below the hand area. Since digit SERs have a smaller SNR than those of the median nerve, more advanced models such as RAP-MUSIC are promising.

There is a neuroscientific controversy on the sources of the N20. Wood (71,76) found N20 in postcentral gyrus. Allison (77) found N20 and the P25 in the postcentral gyrus. Desmedt (78) found N20 on precentral and postcentral gyrus. Recently, others (79) found sources in precentral and postcentral gyrus for stimulation of median nerve. Combined MEG and EEG modeling is the most sensitive noninvasive technique for radial and tangential sources. ECoG modeling is the most sensitive to gyri. Source models of combined MEG and EEG may allow more precise localization and separation of activity on postcentral than on precentral gyrus.

Language

Using whole-head MEG, some have shown that MEG single dipoles lateralize and delimit language cortex (80–82) confirmed by the Wada test (83) and cortical stimulations (84).

Conclusion and Questions

The MEG is a useful, complementary addition to the EEG in the epileptologist's diagnostic armamentarium. There remain several questions on the utility of the MEG. How accurate are the localizations? How confident can MEG distinguish two distinct sources overlapping in time? How many channels are needed? How reproducible is MEG? How closely does the MEG approximate intracranial recordings such as electrocorticography (ECoG)?

RECENT MEG STUDIES

MEG Localization Accuracy; Phantom Studies; One Dipole and Two Dipoles Overlapping in Time

We quantified the localization error in MEG for a dry dipole phantom for one dipole and two dipoles. We found that the MEG method analyzed with realistic modeling, gives accurate localizations for one dipole and for two dipoles overlapping in time.

The dry phantom consisted of two plastic semicircles fitted together at a right angle to mimic a sphere (Neuromag, Helsinki; 4D Imaging, San Diego). Small wire current dipoles were embedded in the plastic, tangential to the radii. This is used routinely as a calibration phantom. We tested a single-dipole source and a two-dipole source at multiple locations, using RAP-MUSIC from in the NIMH-funded

Table 1. Dry Phantom 1 Dipole (mm)

No.	X	Y	Z	X′	Y′	Z′	Error
14	0.0	−27.0	47.6	−0.7	−27.5	47.8	0.88
25	0.0	32.5	56.3	0.2	32.5	56.1	0.28
26	0.0	27.5	47.6	0.0	27.6	47.5	0.14
14	0.0	−27.5	47.6	0.0	−27.5	46.3	1.30
15	0.0	−22.5	39.0	−0.2	−22.2	37.9	1.16
16	0.0	−17.5	30.3	−0.3	−17.7	29.5	0.88
1	56.3	0.0	32.5	56.3	−0.8	31.4	1.36
2	47.6	0.0	27.5	47.6	−0.8	26.7	1.13
4	30.3	0.0	17.5	30.5	−0.5	16.7	0.96
5	32.5	0.0	56.3	32.1	−0.6	55.0	1.49
6	27.5	0.0	47.6	27.5	−0.5	46.6	1.12
						Mean	**0.97**
						SEM	0.40

BrainStorm software developed as shareware for scientists. The phantom was attached mechanically to the bottom of the dewar inside the space for the head in a 100-SQUID 68 sensor channel whole-cortex neuromagnetometer (CTF Systems, VSM Inc, Vancouver, Canada). The neuromagnetometer used 68 sensor first derivative coaxial gradiometers and 19 reference channels to produce a synthetic third derivative 68-sensor array, which were flux-transformed to dc-SQUIDs. Coil parameters were baseline 5 cm and diameter 2 cm. Channel noise was 5–7 femto T per root Hz.

Table 1 shows that for one-dipole activation, mean localization error was 1.0 mm (SE 0.4), with 95% confidence that the actual location was <2 mm from the estimated location. Table 2 shows that for two dipoles, overlapping in time but offset by 100 msec, mean error was 1.7 mm (SE 0.6) for each, with 95% confidence that each of the dipoles were within 3 mm of estimate.

With perfectly synchronous activations of identical waveforms, errors were larger. Such synchrony may not be relevant to human cortex owing to delays from finite conduction speed of corticocortical association, U-fibers (85). Even in 3 Hz generalized spike-and-wave discharges in primary generalized absence epilepsy (classic "petit mal"), the prototype of generalized epileptic activity, interhemispheric conduction delays are 15–20 msec (86).

Source configurations with two dipoles on the same radius also gave larger errors. This problem, anticipated theoretically, has been approached historically in at least two ways. First, experimental design can help. For instance, the auditory P300 has components from superficial and deep structures, which overlap in time and space, the primary auditory cortex, the hippocampus, and the lateral neocortex. These structures are in the same temporal lobe and, during some parts of the activity, within similar radii. Investigators have addressed this problem by studying the visual P300, where the primary cortical response is in another lobe (occipital), and a later response is in the medial temporal lobe (87). In this case, the fields of the earlier and later responses have less overlap. Thus, innovative experimental design may be able to help avoid situations, where larger localization errors result from coradial sources.

Table 2. Dry Phantom 2 Dipoles (mm)

No.	X	Y	Z	X′	Y′	Z′	Error
25	0.0	32.5	56.3	0.5	33.3	55.1	1.53
26	0.0	27.5	47.6	0.4	28.8	47.6	1.36
25	0.0	32.5	56.3	0.5	32.6	53.9	2.45
27	0.0	22.5	39.0	0.3	23.4	39.1	0.95
13	0.0	−32.5	56.3	1.0	−31.5	58.2	2.37
14	0.0	−27.5	47.6	−0.6	−26.4	47.2	1.32
						Mean	**1.66**
						SEM	0.56

Additional studies with the 68-sensor channel MEG system have shown only slightly larger mean errors of localization when the experiments were repeated in a saline-filled sphere phantom with one dipole. In that case, the mean localization error was 1.4 mm (SE 0.9 mm) (88).

Second, combined MEG and EEG methods may help. For instance, comparison of the timing of an EEG component at the sphenoidal electrode (89) versus the timing of a component at a lateral scalp electrode may help distinguish deep and superficial sources (85,90). The additional sensitivity of an EEG electrode contract recording extracranially but directly under the foramen ovale can thus add complementary sensitivity and spatial specific information to address the problem of coradial, temporally overlapping sources, which are superficial and deep.

MEG Localization Accuracy; Median Nerve Somatosensory-Evoked Field (SEF) from Central Fissure (CF); Required Number of Channels and Reproducibility

We compared the localizations of the median SER from a 68-channel neuro-magnetometer to the localization from a 150-channel neuromagnetometer. The 68-channel localizations were made in 1998. The 150-channel localizations were made in 2001. The two laboratories were in different cities, about 2000 miles apart. The difference was 2.1 mm, within 1 SD of the inherent error of MEG phantom dipole localization and coregistration (1.4 mm; SD 0.9) (88,91). Localizations from the FDA-approved single moving dipole model were applied to the SER. The latencies of the best-fitting dipoles were slightly different in the two studies, but within experimental error for the more stable P30m (P1m). The localization from each lab was coregistered onto the subject's MRI. Figure 1 shows the superimposed MEG localizations of the P30m (P1m) peak of the left median nerve SER in a normal control subject from the 68-channel and from the 150-channel neuromag-netometer. Table 3 shows the measured distances and differences in localization between the two MEG systems.

The three MRI views in the top row of Figure 1 show the close agreement of the two localizations in three planes. There are two P30m dipoles for each study (total of four dipoles), reflecting the two repetitions of 500 trials during each, separate study. The inserts show enlargements of the region of interest (ROI). The parameters were digitization rate 1250 Hz, band pass 0.1 Hz to 300 Hz, 250 msec

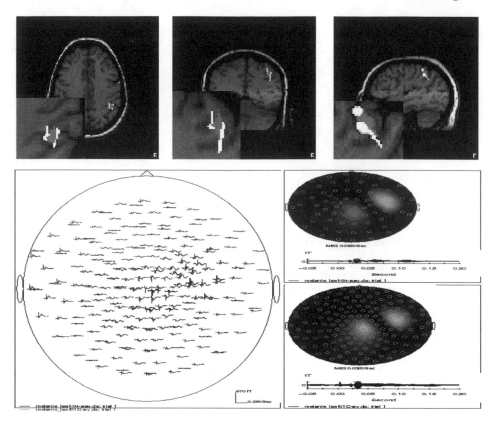

Figure 1. Comparison of median nerve somatosensory-evoked response (SER) dipole localizations using two different whole-cortex neuromagnetometers: 68-sensor channel and 150-sensor channel. (Top) MSI images of SER dipoles superimposed on MRI at sagittal, axial, and coronal slices containing dipole locations. At left is the sagittal view. The insert enlargement shows the 68-sensor neuromagnetometer dipole locations as darker, shaded balls with tails, and the 150-sensor neuromagnetometer dipole locations as lighter, white balls with tails. Two dipoles are shown from the results of each neuromagnetometer, at 20 msec and 30 msec after the shock stimulus of the contralateral median nerve at the wrist slightly above motor threshold. The tails point in the direction of positive current flow, with the ball positive and the end of the tail negative. The superposition of the results of the two neuromagnetometers shows minimal difference in the two localizations, and this was within the phantom experimental error. (Bottom left) The waveforms of the 68-sensor system are darker, black, and those of the 150-sensor system are lighter, gray. (Bottom right) The topographical isocontour maps at 32 msec are shown with the 68-sensor system above. Calibrations: waveforms 670 femtoTesla, 250 msec; map time tics are at 25 msec.

sweep with a 50-msec prestimulus baseline, with a subsequent high-pass filter to eliminate low frequencies and later activity, which were not of interest in this study. The electrical stimuli were delivered to the median nerve at the wrist to give a reliable thumb twitch at 3.1 Hz, to avoid 60-Hz line frequency.

The original, averaged waveforms of the SERs are coregistered on the head diagram at lower left of the figure, to show the similar spatial pattern of the two

Table 3. Reproducibility of Median SEF Dipole Localizations with 68 and 150 Channels

Tr	Peak	Lat	Res	Ampl	X	Y	Z	Lat	Res	Ampl	X	Y	Z
		100-SQUID, 68 sensor channel MEG						180-SQUID, 150 sensor channel MEG					
1	N20m	22.4	2.29	20.75	6.14	39.85	81.62	20.8	6.44	18.59	6.66	39.64	84.07
2	N20m	22.4	9.66	19.87	6.01	35.79	84.05	20.8	4.14	15.28	6.27	37.49	85.05
1	P30m	32.0	4.65	36.26	3.43	41.67	83.21	31.2	3.59	31.04	2.01	38.98	85.19
2	P30m	32.0	3.06	35.18	4.99	40.22	82.64	31.2	2.82	28.57	4.24	39.77	85.12
					ΔX	ΔY	ΔZ	**ΔXYZ**					
1	N20m				0.52	−0.21	−2.45						
2	N20m				0.26	1.70	−1.00						
1	P30m				−1.42	−2.69	−1.98						
2	P30m				−0.75	−0.45	−2.48						
Mean diff (mm): 68 vs 150					**0.34**	**0.412**	**−1.97**	**−2.1**		**SD 1.84**			

separate studies. The waveforms clearly show the peaks of both the N20m and the P30m. The two maps of the P30m are similar. The early deflection in the waveforms near the left ear (left of the diagram) for the 150-channel system is also seen in the time series under the isocontour map to the right. This occurs very soon after the stimulus, is too early for brain activity, and likely reflects artifact from current of the electrical stimulus to the median nerve. This artifact is easily distinguished from the later brain activity, does not affect localization of the later brain activity, and is seen in many MEG and EEG systems.

Table 3 shows that the mean Euclidean distance between coregistered localizations of the two systems (ΔXYZ) was 2.1 mm (SD 1.84), with the largest error vertically, on the z-axis. This difference is within one standard deviation of the localization error in the saline-filled sphere phantom (88,91), and similar to the 2 to 3-mm error in a phantom study on a 122-channel whole-head system (92). Thus, within the error limits derived from phantom studies in two whole-cortex neuromagnetometers, there was no detectable difference in localization of the early dipolar components of the median SER between the 68-channel system and the 150-channel system. This confirms the results of a theoretical study, which predicts no significant difference between 64 channels and 128 channels for localization of one dipole and multiple dipole cortical sources (48).

The comparison of the 68-channel localization to the localization from another system with 150 channels was facilitated by the ease of data transfer and superimposition in the same programs on the same MRI, feasible in MEG studies. The accurate localization of the superficial, focal currents producing the early components of the SER is one of the most difficult tests of a localization method. A superficial source has the highest spatial frequency of topographical map isocontours (93).

MEG Localization Accuracy; The Epileptic Seizure Compared on Simultaneous MEG and ECoG

Figure 2 shows an explanatory diagram of simultaneous MEG and ECoG recording of an electrically induced focal afterdischarge seizure in the frontal lobe of a patient undergoing evaluation for epilepsy surgery. The MEG and ECoG localizations are

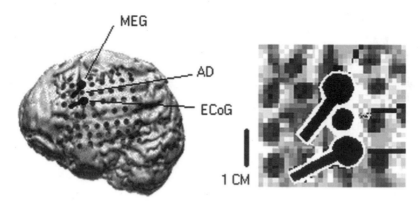

Figure 2. Epileptic seizure afterdischarge on simultaneous MEG and ECoG in a patient with intractable complex partial epilepsy undergoing evaluation for surgery. (Left) Reconstructed cortex from MRI with subdural grid electrodes indicated as black dots. Patient faces to left of the page. Two larger black dots with tails show the MEG dipole on the top and the ECoG dipole on the bottom. (Right) Enlargement of dipole area, showing the two dipoles on either side of the subdural electrode where the afterdischarge was induced. The MRI reconstruction at left appears grainy, likely owing to the usually observed subdural fluid, which surrounds a subdural grid. Distance center-to-center of the subdural grid electrodes was 1 cm. The enlargement at right shows the actual pixels of the MRI reconstruction.

within ~1 cm of the center of the subdural ECoG electrode where the afterdischarge was induced. This finding occurred repeatedly during the afterdischarge with no significant difference between the MEG error (mean 8.5 mm, SE 1.5) and ECoG error (mean 10.4 mm, SE 0.3) ($P = .15$, Student's t-test, 2-tailed) (88). This finding raised a fundamental question. If the MEG and ECoG can both record the same event with a similar SNR, are their localizations identical? Usually ECoG has been thought to be superior to noninvasive electrophysiological methods in both specificity and sensitivity. This study suggests, however, that with similar sensitivities the MEG and ECoG can have equivalent localization specificity. Further work along this line is warranted owing to the great impact this may have in reducing the workload to perform epilepsy presurgical evaluations. This is especially important in the increasing number of patients who are not candidates for "skip" directly from noninvasive recording to focal excisional surgery in epilepsy centers. These patients now require invasive recording with ECoG or depth electrodes to localize and quantify the zone of seizure origin (13,20).

ACKNOWLEDGMENTS

This work was supported by Public Health Service research grant RO1 NS20806 from the Epilepsy Branch, National Institute of Neurological Diseases and Stroke, shared instrumentation grant S10 RR13276 from the National Center for Research Resources, research grant RO1 MH53213 from the National Institutes of Mental Health, and by Huntington Medical Research Institutes, Huntington Hospital, and S. Robert and Denise Zeilstra. John Castillo, Michael Emmanuelson, and Sukvinder

Puri gave helpful assistance with the MRI studies. CTF Corporation and VSM Inc gave helpful technical assistance with the neuromagnetometer. Neuroscan, Inc, and Steve Sands, PhD, gave helpful assistance in the simultaneous MEG and ECoG recordings and analysis.

REFERENCES

1. Hauser W. Incidence and prevalence. In: Engel J, Pedley TA, eds. Epilepsy: A Comprehensive Textbook. Philadelphia: Lippincott-Raven, 1997:47–57.
2. Aicardi J, Shorvon S. Intractable epilepsy. In: Engel J, Pedley TA. eds. Epilepsy: A Comprehensive Textbook. Philadelphia: Lippincott-Raven, 1997:1325–1337.
3. Milner B. Psychological aspects of focal epilepsy and its neurosurgical management. Adv Neurol 1975; 8:299–321.
4. Brown W. Structural substrates of seizure foci in the human temporal lobe (a combined electrophysiological optical microscopic ultra structural study). In: Brazier M, ed. Epilepsy: Its Phenomena in Man. New York: Academic Press, 1973:339–374.
5. Lhatoo SD, Johnson AL, Goodridge DM, MacDonald BK, Sander JW, Shorvon SD. Mortality in epilepsy in the first 11 to 14 years after diagnosis: multivariate analysis of a long-term, prospective, population-based cohort. Ann Neurol 2001; 49:336–344
6. Ward A. Perspectives for surgical therapy of epilepsy. In: Ward A, Penry JK, Purpura D, eds. Epilepsy. New York: Raven Press, 1983:371–390.
7. Spencer S. Depth electroencephalography in section of refractory epilepsy for surgery. Ann Neurol 1981; 9:207–214.
8. Sutherling W. Identifying and referring patients with epilepsy for surgery. Clin Ther 1985; 7:266–271.
9. Engel J, Wieser H, Spencer D. Overview: surgical therapy. In: Engel J, Pedley TA, eds. Epilepsy: A Comprehensive Textbook. Philadelphia: Lippincott-Raven, 1997:1673–1676.
10. Rasmussen T. Surgery of frontal lobe epilepsy. In: Purpura D, Penry JK, Walter RD, eds. Neurosurgical Management of the Epilepsies. New York: Raven Press, 1975:197–206.
11. Sutherling W, Risinger M, Crandall P, Becker D, Baumgartner C, Cahan L, Barth D, Levesque M. Focal functional anatomy of dorsolateral fronto-central seizures. Neurology 1990; 20:87–98.
12. Crandall P. Development in direct recordings from epileptogenic regions in the surgical treatment of partial epilepsies. In: Brazier M, ed. Epilepsy: Its Phenomena in Man. New York: Academic Press, 1973:287–310.
13. Engel J, Levesque M, Crandall P, Shewmon D, Rausch R, Sutherling W. The epilepsies. In: Grossman R, ed. Principles of Neurosurgery. New York: Raven Press, 1991:319–358.
14. Engel J. Surgical Treatment of the Epilepsies, 2nd ed. New York: Raven Press, 1993.
15. Wieser H. Selective amygdalohippocampectomy: indications, investigative technique and results. Adv Tech Stand Neurosurg 1986; 13:39–133.
16. Engel J, Rausch R, Lieb J, Kuhl D, Crandall P. Correlation of criteria used for localizing epileptic foci in patients considered for surgical therapy of epilepsy. Ann Neurol 1981; 9:215–224.
17. Cahan L, Sutherling W, McCullough M, Rausch R, Engel J, Crandall P. Review of the 20-year UCLA experience with surgery for epilepsy. Cleve Clin Q 1984; 51:313–318.
18. Otsubo H, Shirasawa A, Chitoku S, Rutka JT, Wilson SB, Snead OC 3rd. Computerized brain-surface voltage topographic mapping for localization of intracranial spikes from electrocorticography. Technical note. J Neurosurg 2001; 94:1005–1009.
19. Van Buren J, Ajmone-Marsan C, Mutsuga N, Sadowsky D. Surgery of temporal lobe epilepsy. In: Purpura D, Penry JK, Walter RD, eds. Neurosurgical Management of the Epilepsies. Raven Press, 1975:155–196.

20. Sutherling W, Levesque M, Peacock W, Shields D, Shewmon A. Presurgical evaluation. In: Lueders H, ed. Epilepsy Surgery. New York: Raven Press, 1992:792–795.
21. Sutherling W, Crandall P, Cahan L, Barth D. The magnetic field of epileptic spikes agrees with intracranial localizations in complex partial epilepsy. Neurology 1988; 38:778–786.
22. Rose D, Smith P, Sato S. Magneto-encephalography and epilepsy research. Science 1987; 238:329–335.
23. Nakasato N, Levesque M, Barth D, Baumgartner C, Rogers R, Sutherling W. Comparisons of MEG, EEG, and ECoG source localization in neocortical partial epilepsy in humans. Electroenceph Clin Neurophysiol 1994; 171:171–178.
24. Knowlton R, Laxer K, Aminoff M, Roberts T, Wong S, Rowley H. Magnetoencephalography in partial epilepsy: clinical yield and localization accuracy. Ann Neurol 1997; 42:622–631.
25. Wheless J, Willmore L, Breier J, Kataki M, Smith J, King D, Meador K, Park Y, Loring D, Clifton G, Baumgartner J, Thomas A, Constantinou J, Papanicolaou A. A comparison of magneto-encephalography, MRI, and V-EEG in patients evaluated for epilepsy surgery. Epilepsia 1999; 40:931–941.
26. Lamusuo S, Forss N, Ruottinen H-M, Bergman J, Makela J, Mervaala E, Solin O, Rinne J, Ruotsalainen U, Ylinen A, Vapalahti M, Hari R, Rinne J. [^{18}F]FDG-PET and whole-scalp MEG localization of epileptogenic cortex. Epilepsia 1999; 40:921–930.
27. Minassian B, Otsubo H, Weiss S, Elliott I, Rutka JT, Snead OC. Magnetoencephalographic localization in pediatric epilepsy surgery: comparison with invasive intracranial electroencephalography. Ann Neurol 1999; 46:627–633.
28. Otsubo H, Sharma R, Elliott I, Holowka S, Rutka JT, Snead OC 3rd. Confirmation of two magnetoencephalographic epileptic foci by invasive monitoring from subdural electrodes in an adolescent with right frontocentral epilepsy. Epilepsia 1999; 40:608–613.
29. Otsubo H, Snead OC 3rd. Magnetoencephalography and magnetic source imaging in children. J Child Neurol 2001; 16:227–235.
30. Cooper R, Winter A, Crow H, Walter W. Comparison of subcortical, cortical and scalp activity using chronically indwelling electrodes in man. Electroenceph Clin Neurophysiol 1965; 8:217–228.
31. Baumgartner C, Barth D, Levesque M, Crandall P, Sutherling W. Detection sensitivity of spontaneous magnetoencephalography spike recordings in frontal lobe epilepsy. Epilepsia 1989; 30:665.
32. Barth D, Sutherling W, Broffman J, Beatty J. Magnetic localization of a dipolar current source implanted in a sphere and a human cranium. Electroenceph Clin Neurophysiol 1986; 63:260–273.
33. Ajmone-Marsan C. Clinical electrographic correlations of partial seizures. In: JA W, ed. Modern Perspectives in Epilepsy. Montreal: Eden Press, 1978:76–98.
34. Lieb J, Engel J, Gevins A, Crandall P. Surface and deep EEG correlates of surgical outcome in temporal lobe epilepsy. Epilepsia 1981; 22:515–538.
35. Blum D. Prevalence of bilateral partial seizure foci and implications for electroencephalographic telemetry monitoring and epilepsy surgery. Electroencephalogr Clin Neurophysiol 1994; 91(5):329–336.
36. Buser P, Bancaud J, Talairach J. Depth recordings in man in temporal lobe epilepsy. In: Brazier M, ed. Epilepsy: Its Phenomena in Man. New York: Academic Press, 1973:67–97.
37. Buser P, Bancaud J. Unilateral connections between amygdala and hippocampus in man. Electroenceph Clin Neurophysiol 1983; 55:1–12.
38. Tukel K, Jasper H. The electroencephalogram in parasagittal lesions. Electroenceph Clin Neurophysiol 1952; 4:481–494.
39. Jasper H. The ten-twenty electrode system of the International Federation. Electroenceph Clin Neurophysiol 1958; 367–380.

40. Landau W, Kleffner F. Syndrome of acquired aphasia with convulsive disorder in children. Neurology 1957; 7:523–530.
41. Barth D, Sutherling W, Engel J, Beatty J. Neuromagnetic evidence of spatially distributed sources underlying epileptiform spikes in the human brain. Science 1984; 223:293–296.
42. Barth D, Baumgartner C, Sutherling W. Neuromagnetic field modeling of multiple brain regions producing interictal spikes in human epilepsy. Electroenceph Clin Neurophysiol 1989; 73:389–402.
43. Frost J, Kellaway P, Hrachovy R, Glaze D, Mizrahi E. Changes in epileptic spike configuration associated with attainment of seizure control. Ann Neurol 1986; 20:723–731.
44. Erlanger J, Gasser H. Electrical Signs of Nervous Activity. Philadelphia: University of Pennsylvania Press, 1937.
45. Prince D. Mechanisms of epileptogenesis in brain-slice model systems. In: Ward A, Penry JK, Purpura D, eds. Epilepsy. New York: Raven Press, 1983:29–52.
46. Rossi G. Problems of analysis and interpretation of electro cerebral signals in human epilepsy: a neurosurgeon's view. In: Brazier M, ed. Epilepsy: Its Phenomena in Man. New York: Academic Press, 1973:259–285.
47. Purpura D, Penry J, Tower D, Woodbury D, Walter R. Experimental Models of Epilepsy. New York: Raven Press, 1972.
48. Mosher J, Spencer M, Leahy R, Lewis P. Error bounds for EEG and MEG dipole source localization. Electroenceph Clin Neurophysiol 1993; 86:303–320.
49. Dale A, Sereno M. Improved localization of cortical activity by combining EEG and MEG with MRI cortical surface reconstruction: a linear approach. J Cogn Neurosci 1993; 5:162–176.
50. Halgren E. Human evoked potential. In: Boulton A, Baker G, Vanderwolf C, eds. Neuromethods. Clifton, NJ: Humana Press, 1990.
51. Stinstra JG, Peters MJ. The volume conductor may act as a temporal filter on the ECG and EEG. Med Biol Eng Comput 1998; 36:711–716.
52. Van den Broek SP, Reinders F, Donderwinkel M, Peters MJ. Volume conduction effects in EEG and MEG. Electroencephalogr Clin Neurophysiol 1998; 106:522–534.
53. Buchner H, Knoll G, Fuchs M, Rienacker A, Beckmann R, Wagner M, Silny J, Pesch J. Inverse localization of electric dipole current sources in finite element models of the human head. Electroencephalogr Clin Neurophysiol 1997; 102:267–278.
54. Fuchs M, Drenckhahn R, Wischmann HA, Wagner M. An improved boundary element method for realistic volume-conductor modeling. IEEE Trans Biomed Eng 1998; 45:980–997.
55. Yan Y, Nunez P, Hart R. Finite-element model of the human head: scalp potentials due to dipole sources. Med Biol Eng Comput 1991; 29:475–481.
56. Hamalainen M, Sarvas J. Realistic conductivity geometry model of the human head for interpretation of neuromagnetic data. IEEE Trans Biomed Eng 1989; 36(2):165–171.
57. Sarvas J. Basic mathematical and electromagnetic concepts of the biomagnetic inverse problem. Phys Med Biol 1987; 32(1):11–22.
58. Grynszpan F, Gezelowitz D. Model studies of magnetocardiogram. Biophys J 1973; 13(9):911–925.
59. Stok C. The inverse problem in EEG and MEG with application to visual evoked responses. PhD thesis, State University, Leiden, Netherlands, 1986.
60. Stok C. The influence of model parameters on EEG/MEG single dipole source estimation. IEEE Trans Biomed Eng 1987; 34:289–296.
61. Mejis J, Peters M, Oosterom V. Computation of MEG's and EEG's using a realistically shaped multicompartment model of the head. Med Biol Eng Comput 1985; 23:36–37.
62. Barnard AC, Duck IM, Lynn MS. The application of electromagnetic theory to electrocardiology. I. Derivation of the integral equations. Biophys J 1967; 7:443–462.

63. Akhtari M, Bryant H, Mamelak A, Heller L, Shih J, Mandelkern M, Matlachov A, Ranken D, Best E, Sutherling W. Conductivities of three-layer human skull. Brain Topogr 2000; 13:1–4.

64. Akhtari M, Bryant H, Mamelak A, Heller L, Shih J, Mandelkern M, Matlachov A, Ranken D, Best E, DiMauro M, Sutherling W. Conductivities of three-layer live human skull. Brain Topogr 2002; 14:151–167.

65. Cuffin B, Cohen D. Comparison of the magnetoencephalogram and electroencephalogram. Electroenceph Clin Neurophysiol 1979; 47:132–146.

66. Ebersole J, Squires K, Gamelin J. Simultaneous MEG and EEG provide complementary dipole models of temporal lobe spikes. Epilepsia 1993; 34:143. (Abstract.)

67. Fuchs M, Wagner M, Wischmann HA, Kohler T, Theissen A, Drenckhahn R, Buchner H. Improving source reconstructions by combining bioelectric and biomagnetic data. Electroencephalogr Clin Neurophysiol 1998; 107:93–111.

68. Spencer D, Spencer S, Mattson R, Williamson P, Novelly R. Access to the posterior medial temporal lobe structures in the surgical treatment of temporal lobe epilepsy. Neurosurgery 1984; 15:667–671.

69. Shapiro W. Intra-cranial neoplasms. In: Rosenberg R, Grossman RG, eds. The Clinical Neurosciences. New York: Churchill Livingston, 1983:233–283.

70. Spetzler R, Martin N. A proposed grading system for arterio-venous malformations. J Neurosurg 1986; 65:476–483.

71. Wood C, Spencer D, Allison T, McCarthy G, Williamson P, Goff W. Localization of human sensorimotor cortex during surgery by cortical surface recordings of somatosensory evoked potentials. J Neurosurg 1988; 68:99–111.

72. Sutherling W, Crandall P, Darcy T, Becker D, Levesque M, Barth D. The magnetic and electric fields agree with intra-cranial localizations of somatosensory cortex. Neurology 1988; 38:1705–1714.

73. Sobel D, Gallen C, Schwartz B, Waltz T, Copeland B, Yamada S, Hirschkoff E, Bloom F. Locating the central sulcus: comparison of MR anatomic and magnetoencephalographic functional methods. Am J Neuroradiol 1993; 14:915–925.

74. Gallen C, Sobel D, Lewine J, Sanders J, Hart B, Davis L, Orrison WJ. Neuromagnetic mapping of brain function. Radiology 1993; 187:863–867.

75. Sutherling W, Levesque M, Baumgartner C. Cortical sensory representation of the human hand: size of finger regions and non-overlapping digit somatotophy. Neurology 1992; 42:1020–1028.

76. Wood C, Cohen D, Cuffin B, Yarita M, Allison T. Electrical sources in the human somatosensory cortex: identification by combined magnetic and electric potential recordings. Science 1985; 227:1051–1053.

77. Allison T, McCarthy G, Wood C, Darcey T, Spencer D, Williamson P. Human cortical potentials evoked by stimulation of the median nerve. I. Cytoarchitectonic areas generating short-latency activity. J Neurophysiol 1989; 62:694–710.

78. Desmedt J, Cheron G. Somatosensory evoked potentials to finger stimulations in healthy octogenarians and in young adults: wave forms, scalp topography and transit times of parietal and frontal components. Electroenceph Clin Neurophysiol 1980; 50:404–425.

79. Huang M, Aine C, Davis L, Butman J, Christner R, Weisend M, Stephen J, Meyer J, Silveri J, Herman M, Lee R. Sources on the anterior and posterior banks of the central sulcus identified from magnetic somatosensory evoked responses using multi-start spatio-temporal localization. Hum Brain Mapping 2000; 11:59–76.

80. Breier J, Simos P, Zouridakis G, Wheless J, Willmore L, Constantinou J, Maggio W, Papanicolaou A. Language dominance determined by magnetic source imaging: a comparison with the Wada procedure. Neurology 1999; 53:938–945.

81. Papanicolaou A, Simos P, Breier J, Zouridakis G, Willmore L, Wheless J, Constantinou J, Maggio W, Gormley W. Magneto encephalographic mapping of the language-specific cortex. J Neurosurg 1999; 90:85–93.

82. Simos P, Papanicolaou A, Breier J, Wheless J, Constantinou J, Gormley W, Maggio W. Localization of language-specific cortex by using magnetic source imaging and electrical stimulation mapping. J Neurosurg 1999; 91:787–796.

83. Wada J, Rasmussen T. Intra-carotid injection of sodium amytal for the lateralization of cerebral speech dominance: experimental and clinical observations. J Neurosurg 1960; 17:266–282.

84. Ojemann G, Ojemann J, Lettich E. An electrical stimulation mapping investigation in 117 patients. J Neurosurg 1989; 71:316–326.

85. Sutherling W, Barth D. Selective EEG electrode triggering of averaged magnetic data reduces the constraints of the inverse problem of neuromagnetic localization: a principle of relativity in the nervous system due to finite conduction delays. Phys Med Biol 1987; 32:143–144.

86. Lueders H, Daube J, Johnson J, Klass D. Computer analysis of generalized spike-and-wave complexes. Epilepsia 1980; 21:183.

87. Rogers R, Basile L, Taylor S, Akhtari M, Paya M, Sutherling W, Papanicolaou A. Laterality of hippocampal responses to infrequent and unpredictable omissions of visual stimuli. Brain Topogr 1996; 9:15–20.

88. Sutherling W, Akhtari M, Mamelak A, Mosher J, Arthur D, Sands S, Weiss P, Lopez N, DiMauro M, Flynn E, Leahy R. Dipole localization of human induced focal afterdischarge seizure in simultaneous magnetoencephalography and electrocortico-graphy. Brain Topogr 2001; 14:101–116.

89. Pampliglione G, Kerridge J. EEG abnormalities from the temporal lobe studied with sphenoidal electrodes. J Neurol Neurosurg Psychiatry 1956; 19:117 129.

90. Sutherling W, Barth D. Neocortical propagation in temporal spike foci on MEG. Ann Neurol 1989; 25:373–381.

91. Sutherling W. Localization precision of whole cortex neuromagnetometer system for human epilepsy studies. Poster #1.238. Annual Meeting of the American Epilepsy Society, Philadelphia, 2001.

92. Leahy RM, Mosher JC, Spencer ME, Huang MX, Lewine JD. A study of dipole localization accuracy for MEG and EEG using a human skull phantom. Electroencephalogr Clin Neurophysiol 1998; 107:159 173.

93. Romani G, Leoni R. Localization of cerebral sources by neuromagnetic measurements. In: Weinberg H, Stroink G, Katila T, eds. Biomagnetism: Applications and Theory. New York: Pergamon Press, 1984:205–220.

12

Nonsurgical Ablation of Epileptic Tissue

Ara J. Deukmedjian,[1] William A. Friedman,[1] and Steven N. Roper[1,2]
[1]*University of Florida*
Gainesville, Florida, U.S.A.
[2]*Gainesville VA Medical Center*
Gainesville, Florida, U.S.A.

INTRODUCTION

This chapter will discuss "nonsurgical" ablation of epileptic tissue with respect to currently implemented techniques used to treat epileptic tissue or lesions frequently associated with seizures such as cerebral vascular malformations and tumors. Focal intracranial radiation is by far the most common of these techniques and will continue to play a major role in the treatment of seizures either directly or as a "side-effect" of treatment directed towards achieving other therapeutic goals such as AVM obliteration and tumor control. Hence, a firm understanding of the principles of stereotactic radiosurgery is necessary to appreciate its use in the treatment of these central nervous system disorders.

Stereotactic radiosurgery (SRS) is a way of treating brain disorders with the precise delivery of a single, high dose of radiation in a 1-day session. Treatment involves the use of focused ionizing radiation (IR) beams delivered to a specific area of the brain to treat structural and functional neurological disease. Radiosurgery was defined in 1951 by Lars Leksell, the father of stereotactic radiosurgery, as "the delivery of a single, high dose of radiation to a small and critically located intracranial volume through an intact skull." Radiosurgery gained popularity as a "noninvasive" technique for treatment of surgically inaccessible lesions and creating therapeutic lesions in critical areas of the brain to treat functional disorders. Recent attention has been directed towards its role in the treatment of epileptogenic tissue.

Radiosurgery requires the use of IR to exert its effect on tissues. IR is a form of high-energy electromagnetic radiation. Ionizing refers to the ability of the radiation to excite and eject electrons away from atoms by overcoming the binding energy holding the electrons to the nucleus of the atom. There are two basic types of IR: photon beam and particle beam. Both γ-rays and x-rays are forms of photon beam radiation. Gamma-rays are produced by the spontaneous decay of radioactive isotopes and x-rays are generated by the linear accelerator (LINAC) through collision of high-energy electrons with a metal target. Gamma-rays and x-rays exert their effect on tissues through indirect ionization. In this process, electrons within the tissue being irradiated absorb photon beam energy. This absorbed energy allows the excited electron to overcome the binding energy of the nucleus, freeing it to react with other molecules in the tissue and form free radicals. Conversely, particle beam radiation, which includes protons, helium nuclei, and neutrons, exerts its ionizing effect directly on target molecules in tissue, resulting in cellular damage. This effect is actually accomplished through a process whereby highly reactive intermediate molecules are generated from tissue oxygen and water. The intermediate molecules are believed to cause most of the cellular damage induced by particle beam radiation.

Radiation-absorbed dose, the amount of energy absorbed per unit mass of tissue, is expressed in grays (Gy). One Gy is equal to 1 joule of energy absorbed per kilogram tissue. In older literature, radiation dose was specified in rads (100 rads = 1 Gy). The effect on tissue of the energy deposited by radiation depends on the relative biological effectiveness (RBE) of the radiation. For γ-rays and x-rays the RBE is 1.0, and for protons it is 1.1.

There are three basic forms of stereotactic radiosurgery represented by three different technological instruments: LINAC, gamma knife (GK), and the cyclotron. Each instrument operates differently and has a different source of radiation; however, the basic stratagem of radiosurgery remains the same across the three techniques: delivery of a high dose of radiation to a focal region of the brain in a single fraction with minimal irradiation of the surrounding normal brain. Radiotherapy, on the other hand, is the application of radiation over a series of sessions or "fractions." Fractionating means taking the prescribed dose and dividing it into smaller amounts given over a longer period of time. The main reason for fractionation is to minimize the negative acute effects of radiation on surrounding tissue, sparing normal brain. However, it is important to bear in mind that radiation dose to tissue is cumulative and independent of time.

LINAC radiosurgery (Fig. 1) is able to focus multiple noncoplanar, conformal beams of high-dose radiation, x-rays, to specific areas within the head. The LINAC accelerates electrons to very high speeds before they collide with a heavy metal target (e.g., tungsten) releasing x-rays. The x-rays are focused into beams directed at a target stereotactically positioned at the arc's isocenter with a high degree of accuracy.

The GK (Fig. 2) delivers a single, high dose of ionizing (photon beam) γ-radiation emanating from 201 radioactive cobalt-60 sources positioned uniformly about an isocenter. The 201 individual beams simultaneously intersect at an intracranial target previously defined by advanced imaging techniques with a high degree of accuracy. The effect of the radiation on tissue is the same as that of the LINAC.

Finally, particle beam radiation is used as a form of SRS at select centers across the United States. This type of radiation includes helium nuclei, protons, and neutrons. Massive cyclotrons that use enormous amounts of energy are used to accelerate these particles. The Bragg Peak describes the unaltered dose-depth distribution curve for proton beam radiation in tissue characterized by the low entrance dose, sharply defined high-dose region (Bragg Peak) at the target, and lack

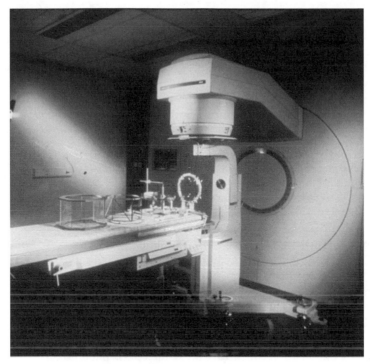

Figure 1. Linear accelerator (LINAC) and the headframes used to position the patient for treatment. (Courtesy of David A. Peace, MS,CMI.)

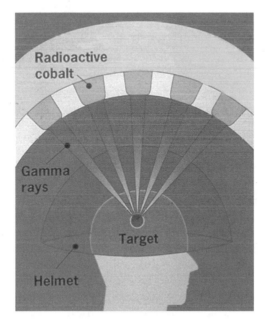

Figure 2. Gamma knife collimator helmet diagram demonstrating the 201 cobalt sources focused at the beam's isocenter. (Courtesy of Elekta Instruments, Inc.)

of exit dose. In practice, the dose distribution curve is flatter and broader to accommodate the geometry of the target. The proton's penetration through tissue is a function of the proton beam's energy and the tissue density through which the beam passes. Protons slow down when they interact with matter. When their velocity slows down enough, they release the bulk of their energy in a sharp burst (ionization), followed by a rapid decline in their dose energy. The rapid fall-off of dose beyond the target theoretically allows the normal surrounding brain to remain unaffected by the radiation, a feature shared by photon beam radiation strategies as well.

Stereotactic MRI and CT have allowed better definition of the target margin for precise conformal dose planning. Several techniques can be used to help shape the radiation dose to fit the target volume including arc weighting, beam size, and multiple isocenters. Multiple isocenters are used to conform the dose to an irregularly shaped target in three dimensions, minimizing radiation exposure to surrounding brain tissue. The ability to carefully place and shape the radiation dose allows the treatment of patients with intracranial disorders that are too difficult or dangerous to treat with conventional surgical procedures, and there is no recovery period. The actual radiation treatment only takes ~10–15 min per isocenter, with most patients being treated on an outpatient basis.

Other advantages of stereotactic radiosurgery over conventional microsurgery stem from the noninvasive nature of this treatment modality. There is no risk of postoperative complications such as wound infection, pneumonia, or deep venous thrombosis. There is no risk from undergoing general anesthesia. The procedure is done with local anesthetic only during head ring application. Hospital-associated costs are significantly less for SRS. Lunsford et al. found hospital charges to be reduced by as much as 65% for SRS compared to microsurgical treatment of the same types of lesions (1). Stereotactic radiosurgery offers advanced computerized treatment planning, which facilitates the design of complex treatment plans to precisely treat the entire volume of the target which is often not possible with microsurgery. Patients are able to resume normal activities the day after treatment.

TISSUE EFFECTS OF RADIATION

DNA damage from IR is mediated through the formation of free radicals and peroxides, and by direct damage from charged particles. The hydroxyl radical, $OH^{\cdot}$, is an example of one such molecule formed by the effects of IR on cellular water. The passage of an energetic charged particle through a cell produces a region of dense ionization along its track. The ionization of water and other cell components can damage DNA molecules near the particle path, but a "direct" effect of proton beam radiation is breaks in DNA strands. DNA fragmentation is both time and dose dependent (2,3). Single-strand breaks (SSB) are quite common, and double-strand breaks (DSB) are less common; however, both can be repaired by built-in cell mechanisms. "Clustered" DNA damage, areas where both SSB and DSB occur, can lead to cell death. Both the yield and the spatial distribution of DSB are influenced by radiation quality (4). Underlying this observation is the interaction of particle tracks with the higher-order chromosomal structures within cell nuclei. The frequency distributions of fragments induced by the charged particles were shifted toward smaller sizes with respect to that induced by comparable doses of gamma rays (5). Hence, DSB were two times greater for proton beam radiation than equivalent dose γ-ray treatment. The most important process for the survival of a tumor cell following IR is the repair of DNA double-strand breaks.

Cellular responses to IR include: activation of signal transduction enzymes (6); stimulation of DNA repair, most notably DNA double strand break repair; activation of transcription factors and subsequent IR-inducible transcript and protein changes; cell cycle checkpoint delays in G1, S, and G2 required for repair or for programmed cell death of severely damaged cells (7); activation of caspases needed for programmed cell death; and stimulation of IR-inducible proteins that may mediate bystander effects influencing signal transduction, DNA repair, angiogenesis, the immune response, late responses to IR, and possibly adaptive survival responses (8). IR induces the release of mitochondrial cytochrome c into the cell's cytosol by oncogene and tumor suppressor gene regulation, chromosomal deletions, and point mutations, all of which can lead to apoptosis (9,10). These changes can be detected in vitro as early as 6–10 h postirradiation (11). Both neurons and vascular endothelium undergo p53-dependent radiation induced apoptosis (12,13).

Histological changes seen in blood vessels that have been irradiated include early endothelial degeneration and proliferation with impaired microcirculation and neuronal loss (14,15), proliferation of thick-walled capillaries, and perivascular hemorrhages. Later changes include thrombosis of dilated capillaries, medial degeneration, and fibrinoid necrosis with hyalinization of vessel walls (16,17), ectasia and thinning of vessel walls, white matter pathology ranging from demyelination to coagulative necrosis (18), perivascular monocytes, and dystrophic calcifying microangiopathy (18) (Fig. 3). The quality and degree of histopathologic changes seen depend on several parameters including target volume, IR dose, vessel

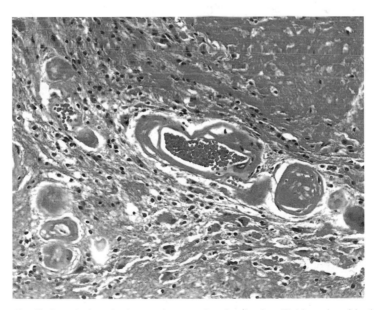

Figure 3. Radiation induced tissue changes in the brain. Evident in this histological preparation is pronounced hyalinization and occlusion of vessels, gliosis and inflammatory response. (Courtesy of Anthony Yachnis, MD.)

diameter, and time. The abnormal vessels of an arteriovenous malformation (AVM) are more radiosensitive than normal cerebral vessels of similar caliber (19). Finally, inflammatory mediators probably play a key role in radiation induced tissue injury as well. In vitro studies of irradiated endothelial cells revealed increased platelet (20) and polymorphonuclear leukocyte adhesion (21).

Radiation has been found to cause cortical atrophy, white matter injury, and, in its most severe form, radiation necrosis. These effects are believed to be a result of a combination of both direct cellular damage and secondary ischemia from vascular compromise (22). As discussed earlier, there is a propensity for radiated vessels to occlude, resulting in ischemic tissue injury downstream. The occlusion is a result of both thrombosis and endothelial proliferation within the microcirculation (23). Not surprisingly, there is an appreciable decrease cerebral blood flow 12–18 months after radiation with doses as low as 15 Gy (24,25).

The temporal (26) and histological (27) characteristics of cerebral radiosurgical lesions have been described in a cat model. Maximum tissue edema occurred between 3.5 and 4.5 weeks after radiation and could be appreciated on T2-weighted MR imaging. Lesion size remains constant over time and at different doses (75, 100, 125, and 150 Gy to the 84% isodose) with a 1-cm collimator. Early on, necrosis and edema predominate but give way to progressive cavitation and perilesional vascular proliferation followed by gliosis. At higher doses, the lesions contained hemorrhage and coagulative necrosis, findings that were not appreciated in the low-dose lesions. Primates receiving 150 Gy single-dose SRS with an 8-mm collimator demonstrated well-demarcated, focal cerebral radionecrosis 2 months after being irradiated (28).

In summary, IR affects tissue by altering a variety of cellular processes including the regulation of genes and signal transduction pathways. Cells may undergo apoptosis or necrosis, dedifferentiation, or an alteration of phenotypic expression. Vascular changes may result in ischemic effects at sites remote from the area of direct injury. Local inflammatory response is initiated by endothelial damage. Dose of radiation, time since treatment, and degree of tissue radiosensitivity determine the overall effect of IR on a particular region in the brain. Recent studies have demonstrated that a physiologic effect on tissue can be achieved in the absence of radiation-induced necrosis (29,30). This finding is important for treatment of regions of the brain where maintaining functional viability posttreatment is desirable—for example, in eloquent neocortex or the hippocampus.

VASCULAR MALFORMATIONS

Vascular malformations associated with epilepsy include AVMs and cavernous malformations. Both of these lesions are believed to be congenital and can present in childhood or later. They are both commonly treated with surgery and many centers use a "combined" approach for the treatment of AVMs that includes the use of endovascular embolization and SRS. Radiosurgery is especially useful for patients with AVMs in deep brain locations and critical lobar areas.

Cavernous malformations (CM) account for 5–10% of all central nervous system vascular malformations (31,32). They are most easily recognized by their characteristic appearance on magnetic resonance imaging and are not seen on angiography (33,34). These lesions are composed of abnormally dilated, thin-walled vascular channels with no intervening brain parenchyma (35,36). CM may present with seizure, hemorrhage, neurological deficit, and headache. The most common presenting symptom is seizure (37,38). In one series, 40% of patients with supratentorial CM had medically refractory epilepsy (39). A mesiotemporal location is associated with more severe forms of epilepsy. Surgical excision of the CM has highly variable success rates for seizure control ranging from 20% to 80% (40–44). In cases of good concordance between the electroclinical data and the location of the CM, complete lesionectomy led to the disappearance of seizures in 86% of patients with chronic forms of epilepsy (39). Patients with untreated CM will continue to have seizures (45).

Radiosurgery has been used successfully to treat seizures associated with CM. The first report of successful treatment of seizures associated with CM came out of Japan in 1995 (46). Kida et al. (46) used gamma knife surgery (GKS) to treat 20 symptomatic patients with CMs of whom seven presented with seizures. Seizure control was significantly improved in all. In 1995 Regis et al. (47) performed a retrospective review of CM treated at five centers from 1991–1997. There were 49 patients that presented with seizures followed for an average of 24 months. The mean duration of epilepsy prior to treatment was 7.5 years. All patients were treated with GKS and a mean marginal dose of 19.17 Gy. Fifty-three percent became seizure-free during this time period with combined medical and radiosurgical treatment. Forty-nine percent were Engel's class IA, and 4% class IB. Another 20% had a significant reduction in seizure frequency, and no improvement in seizure frequency was seen in 27%. The complication rates were low, with one patient experiencing a hemorrhage after GKS and another with postradiation edema and aphasia. Approximately 50% of the lesions treated were in the temporal lobe, and 30% in the frontal lobe. Factors associated with failure to make patients seizure-free were mesiotemporal location of the CM and a history of complex partial seizures. Only 14% of those patients with mesiotemporal lesions became seizure-free, and only 28% of those with a history of complex partial seizures were seizure-free. Seventy-seven percent of patients with simple partial seizures became seizure-free, and 86% of patients with CM located in the lateral temporal cortex became seizure-free. Of those patients that responded well to GKS, most became seizure-free within the first 9 months after radiosurgery.

Other studies have confirmed these results. Zhang et al. (48) treated 28 patients with seizures associated with CM using GKS and a mean marginal dose of 20.3 Gy. Over a mean follow-up period of 4.2 years, 18 of the 28 patients had a significant decrease in their seizure frequency. Similarly, patients with CM and epilepsy treated at the Harvard cyclotron with proton beam radiosurgery experienced a significant reduction in seizure frequency (38%); however, only one patient became seizure-free (49). The mean marginal dose used on those patients was lower, 15 Gy, and may account for the difference in seizure-free outcome. This group reported a 16% incidence of permanent neurological deficit. Only one patient experienced radiation-induced complications.

Management of intracranial cavernous malformations should take into account the natural history of these lesions with respect to hemorrhage as well the location of the lesion. Lesions that present with hemorrhage have an increased risk of rehemorrhage if left untreated. In a prospective study of the natural history of these lesions in 122 patients, the annual rate of hemorrhage was 0.6% for CM that had not previously hemorrhaged. In contrast, the rehemorrhage rate was significantly higher, at 4.5% (45). In another retrospective analysis of the natural history of these lesions, the first-time hemorrhage rate was found to be 1.4% per lesion per year, and the rehemorrhage rate 3.8% per person per year (50). SRS has been shown to confer a protective effect toward rehemorrhage; however, it is a delayed effect evident several years after treatment, during which time the patient is at risk for rehemorrhage (51). Lesionectomy combined with appropriate medical management of seizures has been reported to result in excellent seizure outcomes in most patients with few seizures over a short preoperative course (52–54).

In summary, for surgically accessible symptomatic cavernous malformations, microsurgery and observation remain the treatment modalities of choice, especially for those that present with hemorrhage. The use of SRS for intracranial CMs is considered by most experts to be highly controversial at best. For patients presenting with seizures and multiple hemorrhages with a deep-seated cavernous malformation, SRS may be considered by some experts to be a viable alternative to surgery.

AVM

AVMs are the most common cerebral vascular malformation encountered. Histologically, they are composed of abnormal tangles of dilated vessels without a normal intervening capillary bed. There is abnormal intervening brain parenchyma and one or more dilated, arteriolized draining veins. They create a local physiologic shunt from arterial to venous system through a disorganized tangle of thin-walled vascular channels called a nidus. AVMs are prone to thrombosis and hemorrhage. The surrounding brain parenchyma is abnormally edematous and gliotic as a result of the chronic ischemic state.

Cerebral AVM prevalence is estimated to be 10.3/100,000 population (55). AVMs most commonly present with hemorrhage in both adult and pediatric populations. An unruptured AVM has approximately a 2–3% risk of bleeding per year, with about a 1% risk of death per year. The mortality rate of the first hemorrhage is ~10% (56). Seizures are the second most common presenting symptom after hemorrhage, and they occur in 13%–35% of symptomatic patients with AVMs (57–63). The estimated risk of occurrence of seizures in patients harboring AVMs is 1.5% per person-year (64).

The gold standard in diagnosis of intracranial AVMs is cerebral angiography (65). MRI and contrast-enhanced CT scans are helpful in 3D stereotactic planning of the radiosurgical treatment to maximize nidus coverage and minimize normal brain irradiation. The primary goal in most SRS treatment protocols is angiographic obliteration of the AVM nidus. Incomplete obliteration of the nidus provides no protection against hemorrhage (66). SRS can treat carefully selected AVMs up to 30 cc achieving angiographic obliteration with an acceptable risk (67). Repeat SRS for incomplete AVM obliteration has been found efficacious with an acceptably low risk (68).

The results of SRS treatment on seizures associated with AVMs have been encouraging with seizure-free rates of 59-88% after treatment (57,58,60–62,69,70). In one series the best results with regard to seizure-free outcome were seen in the patients treated with SRS using both stereotactic MRI and cerebral angiography for 3D dose-target planning. Conventional angiography provides only 2D information about nidus shape. Combining stereotactic MRI or CT data into the dose plan adds another dimension of accuracy to targeting and hence better results.

The median marginal doses used for treatment in most studies range from 12.5–22 Gy. In some studies, patients whose AVMs received the higher median marginal doses (20 Gy) had better seizure free outcomes (60,62,71). The SALT group, using LINAC radiosurgery and a mean marginal dose of 25 Gy, reported seizure "control" in 47/47 patients that presented with seizures (71). In an early review of GKS treatment of AVMs at the Karolinska Institute in Sweden, 59 of the 247 patients treated had seizures of which 88% became seizure-free, 21% off medication (70). The Pittsburgh group reported an 85% seizure-free outcome off medication in 15 pediatric patients treated with GKS with a mean marginal dose of 20 Gy and mean AVM volume of 3.6 cc (62). At the University of Florida LINAC was used to treat 33 patients with AVMs and seizures resulting in a 59% seizure-free outcome. Radiosurgery was most effective for generalized tonic-clonic and complex partial seizure disorders. Interestingly, 40% of the seizure free patients in this study did not have angiographic occlusion of their AVMs. In two other studies, 30% (57) and 32% (60) of the seizure-free patients did not have complete angiographic occlusion of their AVMs.

This brings up a very important question. Is angiographic obliteration of an AVM necessary to achieve a seizure-free outcome? Based on the studies performed to date, angiographic obliteration of the AVM nidus is not correlated with seizure-free outcome (57,58,60 62). In fact, in most studies the seizure remission occurred within the first year of treatment, well before the radiographic disappearance of the AVM nidus, which takes 1 2 years in most cases (72,73). Other prognostic factors for seizure outcome include duration of epilepsy and total number of seizures experienced by the patient prior to treatment with SRS. Patients with fewer than five pretreatment seizures and a short (<6 months) duration of epilepsy were more likely to become seizure-free (60).

The risk of symptomatic post-radiosurgical sequelae for treatment of cerebral AVM is estimated to be 9–11% based on a multicenter review of 1255 treated leslons published by Flickinger et al. in 1999 (74). The median number of isocenters was two, median marginal dose was 19 Gy, and median AVM volume was 5.7 cc. In 30% of these patients, posttreatment MRI revealed T2 changes in the brain surrounding the AVM; however, the majority of these patients were asymptomatic. Symptomatic postradiation injury occurred in 10% of patients and included parenchymal injury (6.4%), cranial neuropathy (1.5%), de novo seizures (1.8%), and porencephalic cyst formation (0.4%). Post-SRS symptom resolution rate was found to be 58% in another study (75). The highest resolution rates were for headache and seizures, and the use of steroids did not affect the chance of symptom resolution (74). The risk of developing a permanent neurological injury was dependent on dose of radiation, location of AVM, volume of AVM, and a history of pervious radiation (74,76,77).

There is no single definitive study that elucidates the mechanism by which radiosurgery manifests its antiepileptic effect in patients with AVMs. Most researchers in this area agree that it is the physiologically deranged neural tissue surrounding the AVM's nidus that is responsible for initiation of epileptiform activity. It is uncertain as to whether it is the byproducts of hemorrhage, gliosis, or vascular insufficiency from steal, or some combination of all three that predispose this tissue to epileptic discharges. One theory proposes a predisposed hypersensitivity of adjacent epileptogenic tissue to irradiation resulting in destruction of that tissue along with the lesion (78). Another theory was founded on the observation that elimination of the AVM results in normalization of perfusion to the ischemic brain after occlusion of the vessels responsible for the "steal" (79). Yet another study revealed an alteration in neuronal somatostatin receptors in response to irradiation which led to a reduced epileptogenic potential for the cell (80).

The role of SRS in the treatment of cerebral AVMs is still being defined. One recent study has shown that microsurgical resection of the AVM nidus may be superior to SRS for small, highly selected (<3 cm diameter) lesions when comparing posttreatment hemorrhage rate and Glasgow outcome scores (81). However, these results are highly controversial and may have been subject to selection bias. SRS is widely used to treat AVMs that are in surgically inaccessible or eloquent locations where the risk of craniotomy-induced neurological morbidity is deemed too high. Some institutions are currently utilizing a "multimodality" approach to the treatment of these lesions and achieving good outcomes with low complication rates (82). Preliminary seizure-free rates for multimodality treatment of AVMs are excellent, as seen in a study from Boston with 90% seizure-free rate in children posttreatment. Some experienced clinicians would argue that all cerebral AVMs should be referred to facilities that are capable of providing patients with comprehensive state-of-the-art diagnostic and therapeutic modalities, including the capability to treat AVMs with an combination of microsurgery, stereotactic radiosurgery, and endovascular embolization.

BRAIN TUMORS

Seizures occur in 15–95% of all primary brain tumors on presentation (83). They are most frequently associated with low-grade gliomas (65–95%) and less commonly with malignant gliomas (15–25%). In tumor-associated epilepsy, seizure control following craniotomy and resection has been reported in 82–91% of cases (84–86). Radiation has also been used to successfully treat seizures associated with brain tumors. One study reported the effects of GKS in 23 patients with medically intractable epilepsy attributable to a cerebral lesion. Mean seizure duration was 11.6 years, and these patients were treated with a mean marginal dose of 22.9 Gy (87). At follow-up, 52% were seizure-free (25% of these were off medications) and another 9% had a significant reduction in seizure frequency. The remaining 39% had no change in seizure frequency. Epilepsy associated with metastatic tumors to the brain has been shown to respond to SRS as well (88). In this study, five of 23 patients with metastatic renal cell carcinoma had seizures associated with their brain tumors. These patients received a median dose of 22 Gy to the tumor margin, and all five patients became seizure-free off medications 4–6 months after radiosurgery. Schrottner et al. found three factors that determined favorable seizure outcome in patients with tumor-induced medically refractory epilepsy (89). Better seizure outcomes were experienced in those patients who received >10 Gy of irradiation outside the tumor margin, had temporally located tumors, and had a seizure history <2.5 years.

Two earlier studies highlighted the effectiveness of IR on seizures in patients with low-grade gliomas who were treated with iodine-125 interstitial brachytherapy. In the first study, 80 patients with low-grade gliomas and seizures were treated with carbamazepine and 60 Gy of interstitial radiation (90). Carbamazepine alone controlled seizures in only 28% of the patients. The combination of radiation and carbamazepine led to seizure control in 79% of patients at 6 months after treatment. These patients showed an increase in benzodiazepine receptor density in tissue surrounding the tumor on SPECT after radiation treatment. In another study using a similar treatment protocol (91), 40% of patients with seizures became seizure-free, and the other 60% had a significant reduction in seizure frequency.

Conventional fractionated radiation therapy for low-grade gliomas has yielded limited success with seizure control. In one study, five adults with medically intractable epilepsy were treated with 54–66 Gy of focal IR to the tumor (92). One patient became seizure-free and two others experienced a reduction in seizure frequency of >90% that persisted for up to 1.5 years. The seizure-free patient relapsed as the tumor progressed. In another study, of four patients with chronic seizures and frontal gliomas, three of the patients became seizure-free after conventional radiation during 4 years of follow-up (93). Chalifoux et al. reported a seizure-free rate of 55% in patients that received conventional fractionated radiotherapy (dose range 30–66 Gy) for high grade primary brain tumors; however, all relapsed as tumor growth progressed (94).

In summary, IR has been clearly shown to be beneficial in the treatment of seizures and medically refractory epilepsy associated with brain tumors. However, when indicated, surgical resection has been proven to afford patients with a greater degree of seizure control when combined with appropriate medical therapy (95–97). It is important to keep in mind that SRS does not ameliorate symptoms of mass effect and should not be considered as a primary form of treatment for lesions presenting with symptoms of intracranial hypertension and herniation.

THERAPEUTIC EFFECT OF CEREBRAL IRRADIATION ON EPILEPSY IN ANIMAL MODELS

Focal cerebral irradiation has successfully reduced seizures in certain animal models of chronic epilepsy (98). Gaffey et al. (99) demonstrated restriction of the spread of epileptic discharges in cats by proton beam focal irradiation. Barcia-Salorio et al. used a cobalt-induced cat epilepsy model to study the effects of gamma irradiation on electrographic neocortical seizures (100). By 3 weeks postradiation, the animals ceased having behavioral manifestations of seizures, and by 6 months the EEG recordings returned to normal. In another study, chronic stimulus-induced electrographic seizures in rats were treated with 10 Gy and 40 Gy of focal LINAC-based irradiation to the hippocampus. The rats treated with 40 Gy demonstrated an increased seizure threshold and decreased duration of after-discharges compared to controls 3 months after radiosurgery (101).

Mori et al. found that increasing the dose of focal irradiation stepwise from 20 Gy to 100 Gy to the hippocampal target in kainic acid–induced seizures in rats would result in higher percentages of rats that became seizure free by EEG (102,103). No histopathological changes were noted for the 20-, 40-, and 60-Gy-treated rats during blinded posttreatment evaluation of the hippocampal tissue, implying that seizures can be controlled at subnecrotic doses. Behavioral effects of irradiation to the hippocampal focus were studied in these rats as well using a Morris water maze. The epileptic rats that received focal hippocampal irradiation performed significantly better than their nonirradiated counterparts and no differently from the control (naive) rats (103). Chen et al. demonstrated that a single, bilateral, subnecrotic dose of focal gamma radiation to the ventral hippocampus significantly decreased the incidence of spontaneous behavioral and electrographic seizures in rats with chronic limbic epilepsy (30). There was a functional increase in seizure threshold of hippocampal neurons radiated at 40 Gy as evidenced by a reduced susceptibility to penicillin-induced epileptiform activity in hippocampal slices with a concomitant preservation of synaptically driven neuronal firing.

Several papers have reported an antiepileptic effect of radiation at subnecrotic doses (absence of coagulative necrosis) with preservation of normal tissue histology (102,103), signifying the potential of SRS to treat the underlying tissue pathophysiology while allowing preservation of function. Biochemical evidence for differential functional effects of IR was presented by Regis et al. (29) in a paper that summarized the results of comparative radioisozyme labeling for cholinergic and GABAergic systems in rat striatum. They found that single-fraction gamma irradiation reduced levels of glutamic acid decarboxylase (transiently), choline acetyl transferase, and excitatory amino acids while increasing levels of glycine. These neurochemical changes may play a role in the antiepileptic effects associated with IR.

MESIAL TEMPORAL LOBE EPILEPSY

As early as the 1960s some clinicians were performing selective hippocampal and amygdala ablation using a radiofrequency lesion. This technique involves the use of a stereotactic head-frame to guide an electrode to an intracranial target and produce a radiofrequency lesion with a thermocoagulator powered by a generator (Fig. 4). This technique has been used by surgeons to treat medically intractable temporal lobe epilepsy (TLE) (104–109). The seizure-free outcome for stereotactic amygdalotomy and/or hippocampotomy ranged from 11% to 63% in these published series. In contrast, temporal lobectomy in carefully selected patients results in seizure-free outcomes in 70–90% of patients with intractable temporal lobe seizures (110).

Stereotactic radiosurgery to treat medically intractable TLE was first reported by Barcia-Salorio et al. (111) and shortly thereafter in a 29-year-old Finnish male in 1992 by Heikkinen et al. (112). Seven months after the LINAC based treatment of the mesiotemporal structures the Finnish man became seizure-free. Regis et al. pursued GKS treatment of mesiotemporal structures in patients with medically refractory TLE (113), and they have published their results in 25 patients (114). Two-year follow-up was available in 16 patients with intractable TLE treated with a dose of 20–25 Gy to the 50% isodose line which encompassed the anterior hippocampus, amygdala, anterior parahippocampal gyrus and entorhinal cortex. Eighty-one percent of the patients were seizure-free at a median latent interval of 10.5 months. The posttreatment MRI revealed a necrotic target with an enhancing rim at 11 months. Three patients had visual field deficits (two were "asymptomatic"), and three patients experienced transient headaches, nausea, and emesis.

Other authors have reported the incidence of optic neuropathy is zero in patients that have received a radiation dose of 10 Gy or less to their visual apparatus (115,116). Visual-field deficits after surgical temporal lobectomy are commonly underreported, as most patients are asymptomatic (117). The most common visual-field disturbance found in postresective patients undergoing formal perimetry testing

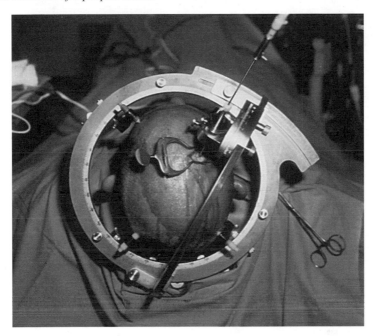

Figure 4. Patient positioned for stereotactic radiofrequency lesioning (for pallidotomy). Pictured here is a standard stereotactic head-ring with lesioning electrode visible in upper right. (Courtesy of David A. Peace, MS,CMI.)

after anterior temporal lobectomy was a homonymous superior quadrant deficit in 69–83% (117–119). A typical MRI-based dose plan for MTLE from the University of Florida demonstrates the targeted structures (Fig. 5). The preliminary results of SRS for TLE are comparable to surgical outcomes for seizure control and the low rate of complications combined with the added benefit of avoiding a major surgical procedure and lengthy hospitalization make this treatment modality quite promising. Before standards of care can be set regarding the use of SRS to treat TLE, further trials should be implemented, and long-term follow-up for seizure outcome, delayed complications, and quality of life must be analyzed. There is an ongoing U.S. multicenter trial for the treatment of TLE with SRS in phase 1 evaluation. It will be several years before any definitive data regarding the efficacy of this modality will become available; however, resective surgery currently offers patients with medically refractory TLE a safe and proven means to an improved quality of life.

EXTRATEMPORAL IDIOPATHIC FOCAL EPILEPSY

The treatment of extratemporal idiopathic focal epilepsy with IR has been reported, though infrequently, in the medical literature. The largest clinical study published to date involved the treatment of 11 patients with medically intractable extratemporal onset epilepsy (78). All of the patients had standard "phase 1" monitoring and invasive subdural electrode monitoring through "burr holes" followed by a second invasive procedure involving stereotactic placement of depth electrodes around the seizure focus to define its margins for the SRS treatment plan. Of the 11 patients that

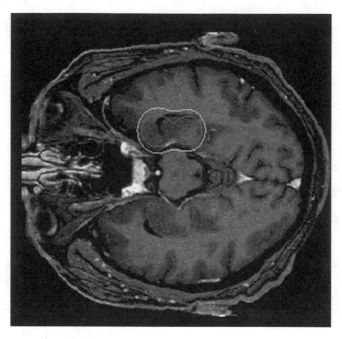

Figure 5. MRI based LINAC dose plan for SRS treatment of mesial temporal lobe epilepsy. Inner circle represents prescription dose and outer circle is the 50% isodose line. (Courtesy of William Friedman, MD.)

received the 10–20 Gy isodose to their focus and had adequate follow-up (mean of 75 months), 36% became seizure-free and another 45% had improvement of their seizures. Seizures began to improve after a period of 2.5 months to 1 year posttreatment for all patients except two, one of whom had immediate improvement. Fractionated stereotactic radiotherapy was successfully used to treat a single male with posttraumatic focal epilepsy localized by magnetic source imaging (MSI) (120). He received seven daily fractions of 3 Gy, and after 9 months he became seizure-free with no change in his seizure medication schedule. The development of clinical applications for MSI technology for seizure onset localization is still in its infancy; however, this technique may have more widespread clinical use in the future (121). Another potential application of SRS to the treatment of epilepsy was illustrated by Pendl et al. when their group performed stereotactic radiosurgical corpus callosotomies in two patients with Lennox-Gastaut syndrome and another patient with multifocal epilepsy (122). None were rendered seizure-free; however, all had significantly improved seizure frequency and severity at 3–12 months follow-up.

HYPOTHALAMIC HAMARTOMAS

Hypothalamic hamartomas (123) typically present in childhood with brief gelastic fits (124,125) that evolve into more complex seizure types (126–128). A review of the literature on the treatment of the lesions with radiofrequency lesioning or SRS reveals that some patients respond with a reduction in seizure frequency or, less commonly, cessation after treatment (129). Microsurgery for these lesions produces similar results but with greater risk for perioperative complications (130,131), making SRS an acceptable alternative in appropriate cases.

In summary, stereotactic radiosurgery has been used successfully to treat seizures associated with a variety of intracranial lesions as well as nonlesional epilepsy. Definitive conclusions cannot be made regarding the physiological mechanism by which it exerts its antiepileptic effect on tissue. Nor is it possible at this time to draw any conclusions about the most appropriate doses or target volume necessary to provide the optimal therapeutic effect. Although incipient as a tool to treat epilepsy, SRS has shown promise and the potential to provide clinicians with a noninvasive technique for resective therapy.

REFERENCES

1. Lunsford LD, Flickinger J, Lindner G, Maitz A. Stereotactic radiosurgery of the brain using the first United States 201 cobalt-60 source gamma knife. Neurosurgery 1989; 24(2):151–159.
2. Gajdusek C, Onoda K, London S, Johnson M, Morrison R, Mayberg M. Early molecular changes in irradiated aortic endothelium. J Cell Physiol 2001; 188(1):8–23.
3. Raicu M, Vral A, Thierens H, De Ridder L. Radiation damage to endothelial cells in vitro, as judged by the micronucleus assay. Mutagenesis 1993; 8(4):335–339.
4. Prise KM, Pinto M, Newman HC, Michael BD. A review of studies of ionizing radiation-induced double-strand break clustering. Radiat Res 2001; 156(5):572–576.
5. Belli M, Cherubini R, Dalla VM, Dini V, Esposito G, Moschini G. DNA fragmentation in mammalian cells exposed to various light ions. Adv Space Res 2001; 27(2):393–399.
6. Szumiel I. Ionizing radiation-induced cell death. Int J Radiat Biol 1994; 66(4):329–341.
7. Rubin DB, Drab EA, Bauer KD. Endothelial cell subpopulations in vitro: cell volume, cell cycle, and radiosensitivity. J Appl Physiol 1989; 67(4):1585–1590.
8. Leskov KS, Criswell T, Antonio S, Li J, Yang CR, Kinsella TJ et al. When x-ray-inducible proteins meet DNA double strand break repair. Semin Radiat Oncol 2001; 11(4):352–372.
9. Canman CE, Kastan MB. Induction of apoptosis by tumor suppressor genes and oncogenes. Semin Cancer Biol 1995; 6(1):17–25.
10. Peltenburg LT. Radiosensitivity of tumor cells. Oncogenes and apoptosis. Q J Nucl Med 2000; 44(4):355–364.
11. Langley RE, Bump EA, Quartuccio SG, Medeiros D, Braunhut SJ. Radiation-induced apoptosis in microvascular endothelial cells. Br J Cancer 1997; 75(5):666–672.
12. Mayberg MR, London S, Rascy J, Gajdusek C. Inhibition of rat smooth muscle proliferation by radiation after arterial injury: temporal characteristics in vivo and in vitro. Radiat Res 2000; 153(2):153–163.
13. Wood KA, Youle RJ. The role of free radicals and p53 in neuron apoptosis in vivo. J Neurosci 1995; 15(8):5851–5857.
14. Reinhold HS, Keyeux A, Dunjic A, Jovanovic D, Maisin JR. The influence of radiation on blood vessels and circulation. XII. Discussion and conclusions. Curr Top Radiat Res Q 1974; 10(1):185–198.
15. Hopewell JW. The late vascular effects of radiation [letter]. Br J Radiol 1974; 47(554):157–158.
16. Nilsson A, Wennerstrand J, Leksell D, Backlund EO. Stereotactic gamma irradiation of basilar artery in cat. Preliminary experiences. Acta Radiol Oncol Radiat Phys Biol 1978; 17(2):150–160.
17. Hopewell JW, Wright EA. The nature of latent cerebral irradiation damage and its modification by hypertension. Br J Radiol 1970; 43(507):161–167.

18. Valk PE, Dillon WP. Radiation injury of the brain. Am J Neuroradiol 1991; 12(1):45–62.
19. Schneider BF, Eberhard DA, Steiner LE. Histopathology of arteriovenous malformations after gamma knife radiosurgery. J Neurosurg 1997; 87(3):352–357.
20. Rubin DB, Drab EA, Ts'ao CH, Gardner D, Ward WF. Prostacyclin synthesis in irradiated endothelial cells cultured from bovine aorta. J Appl Physiol 1985; 58(2):592–597.
21. Dunn MM, Drab EA, Rubin DB. Effects of irradiation on endothelial cell–polymorphonuclear leukocyte interactions. J Appl Physiol 1986; 60(6):1932–1937.
22. O'Connor MM, Mayberg MR. Effects of radiation on cerebral vasculature: a review. Neurosurgery 2000; 46(1):138–149.
23. Kamiryo T, Lopes MB, Berr SS, Lee KS, Kassell NF, Steiner L. Occlusion of the anterior cerebral artery after gamma knife irradiation in a rat. Acta Neurochir (Wien) 1996; 138(8):983–990.
24. Keyeux A. The influence of radiation on blood vessels and circulation. Chapter IX. Blood flow and permeability in the central nervous system. Curr Top Radiat Res Q 1974; 10(1):135–150.
25. Keyeux A, Brucher JM, Ochrymowicz-Bemelmans D, Charlier AA. Late effects of X irradiation on regulation of cerebral blood flow after whole-brain exposure in rats. Radiat Res 1997; 147(5):621–630.
26. Blatt DR, Friedman WA, Bova FJ, Theele DP, Mickle JP. Temporal characteristics of radiosurgical lesions in an animal model. J Neurosurg 1994; 80(6):1046–1055.
27. Spiegelmann R, Friedman WA, Bova FJ, Theele DP, Mickle JP. LINAC radiosurgery: an animal model. J Neurosurg 1993; 78(4):638–644.
28. Lunsford LD, Altschuler EM, Flickinger JC, Wu A, Martinez AJ. In vivo biological effects of stereotactic radiosurgery: a primate model. Neurosurgery 1990; 27(3):373–382.
29. Regis J, Kerkerian-Legoff L, Rey M, Vial M, Porcheron D, Nieoullon A. First biochemical evidence of differential functional effects following gamma knife surgery. Stereotact Funct Neurosurg 1996; 66(suppl 1):29–38.
30. Chen ZF, Kamiryo T, Henson SL, Yamamoto H, Bertram EH, Schottler F. Anticonvulsant effects of gamma surgery in a model of chronic spontaneous limbic epilepsy in rats. J Neurosurg 2001; 94(2):270–280.
31. New PF, Ojemann RG, Davis KR, Rosen BR, Heros R, Kjellberg RN. MR and CT of occult vascular malformations of the brain. AJR 1986; 147(5):985–993.
32. McCormick WF, Nofzinger JD. "Cryptic" vascular malformations of the central nervous system. J Neurosurg 1966; 24(5):865–875.
33. Sage MR, Blumbergs PC. Cavernous haemangiomas (angiomas) of the brain. Australas Radiol 2001; 45(2):247–256.
34. Ide C, De Coene B, Baudrez V. MR features of cavernous angioma. JBR BTR 2000; 83(6):320.
35. Wong JH, Awad IA, Kim JH. Ultrastructural pathological features of cerebrovascular malformations: a preliminary report. Neurosurgery 2000; 46(6):1454–1459.
36. Zabramski JM, Henn JS, Coons S. Pathology of cerebral vascular malformations. Neurosurg Clin North Am 1999; 10(3):395–410.
37. Robinson JR, Awad IA, Little JR. Natural history of the cavernous angioma. J Neurosurg 1991; 75(5):709–714.
38. Maraire JN, Awad IA. Intracranial cavernous malformations: lesion behavior and management strategies. Neurosurgery 1995; 37(4):591–605.
39. Casazza M, Broggi G, Franzini A, Avanzini G, Spreafico R, Bracchi M. Supratentorial cavernous angiomas and epileptic seizures: preoperative course and postoperative outcome. Neurosurgery 1996; 39(1):26–32.
40. Cohen DS, Zubay GP, Goodman RR. Seizure outcome after lesionectomy for cavernous malformations. J Neurosurg 1995; 83(2):237–242.

41. Dodick DW, Cascino GD, Meyer FB. Vascular malformations and intractable epilepsy: outcome after surgical treatment. Mayo Clin Proc 1994; 69(8):741–745.
42. Giulioni M, Acciarri N, Padovani R, Galassi E. Results of surgery in children with cerebral cavernous angiomas causing epilepsy. Br J Neurosurg 1995; 9(2):135–141.
43. Schroeder HW, Gabb MR, Runge U. Supratentorial cavernous angiomas and epileptic seizures: preoperative course and postoperative outcome. Neurosurgery 1996; 39(6):1271.
44. Acciarri N, Giulioni M, Padovani R, Galassi E, Gaist G. Surgical management of cerebral cavernous angiomas causing epilepsy. J Neurosurg Sci 1995; 39(1):13–20.
45. Kondziolka D, Lunsford LD, Kestle JR. The natural history of cerebral cavernous malformations. J Neurosurg 1995; 83(5):820–824.
46. Kida Y, Kobayashi T, Tanaka T. Treatment of symptomatic AOVMs with radiosurgery. Acta Neurochir Suppl (Wien) 1995; 63:68–72.:68–72.
47. Regis J, Bartolomei F, Kida Y, Kobayashi T, Vladyka V, Liscak R. Radiosurgery for epilepsy associated with cavernous malformation: retrospective study in 49 patients. Neurosurgery 2000; 47(5):1091–1097.
48. Zhang N, Pan L, Wang BJ, Wang EM, Dai JZ, Cai PW. Gamma knife radiosurgery for cavernous hemangiomas. J Neurosurg 2000; 93(suppl 3):74–77.
49. Amin-Hanjani S, Ogilvy CS, Candia GJ, Lyons S, Chapman PH. Stereotactic radiosurgery for cavernous malformations: Kjellberg's experience with proton beam therapy in 98 cases at the Harvard Cyclotron. Neurosurgery 1998; 42(6):1229–1236.
50. Kim DS, Park YG, Choi JU, Chung SS, Lee KC. An analysis of the natural history of cavernous malformations. Surg Neurol 1997; 48(1):9–17.
51. Kondziolka D, Lunsford LD, Flickinger JC, Kestle JR. Reduction of hemorrhage risk after stereotactic radiosurgery for cavernous malformations. J Neurosurg 1995; 83(5):825–831.
52. Cappabianca P, Alfieri A, Maiuri F, Mariniello G, Cirillo S, De Divitiis E. Supratentorial cavernous malformations and epilepsy: seizure outcome after lesionectomy on a series of 35 patients. Clin Neurol Neurosurg 1997; 99(3):179–183.
53. Cohen DS, Zubay GP, Goodman RR. Seizure outcome after lesionectomy for cavernous malformations. J Neurosurg 1995; 83(2):237–242.
54. Dodick DW, Cascino GD, Meyer FB. Vascular malformations and intractable epilepsy: outcome after surgical treatment. Mayo Clin Proc 1994; 69(8):741–745.
55. Berman MF, Sciacca RR, Pile-Spellman J, Stapf C, Connolly ES Jr, Mohr JP. The epidemiology of brain arteriovenous malformations. Neurosurgery 2000; 47(2):389–396.
56. Wilkins RH. Natural history of intracranial vascular malformations: a review. Neurosurgery 1985; 16(3):421–430.
57. Falkson CB, Chakrabarti KB, Doughty D, Plowman PN. Stereotactic multiple arc radiotherapy. III. Influence of treatment of arteriovenous malformations on associated epilepsy. Br J Neurosurg 1997; 11(1):12–15.
58. Steiner L, Lindquist C, Adler JR, Torner JC, Alves W, Steiner M. Clinical outcome of radiosurgery for cerebral arteriovenous malformations. J Neurosurg 1992; 77(1):1–8.
59. Sutcliffe JC, Forster DM, Walton L, Dias PS, Kemeny AA. Untoward clinical effects after stereotactic radiosurgery for intracranial arteriovenous malformations. Br J Neurosurg 1992; 6(3):177–185.
60. Kurita H, Kawamoto S, Suzuki I, Sasaki T, Tago M, Terahara A. Control of epilepsy associated with cerebral arteriovenous malformations after radiosurgery. J Neurol Neurosurg Psychiatry 1998; 65(5):648–655.
61. Eisenschenk S, Gilmore RL, Friedman WA, Henchey RA. The effect of LINAC stereotactic radiosurgery on epilepsy associated with arteriovenous malformations. Stereotact Funct Neurosurg 1998; 71(2):51–61.
62. Gerszten PC, Adelson PD, Kondziolka D, Flickinger JC, Lunsford LD. Seizure outcome in children treated for arteriovenous malformations using gamma knife radiosurgery. Pediatr Neurosurg 1996; 24(3):139–144.

63. Nataf F, Merienne L, Schlienger M, Lefkopoulos D, Meder JF, Touboul E. Cerebral arteriovenous malformations treated by radiosurgery: a series of 705 cases. Neurochirurgie 2001; 47(2–3 Pt 2):268–282. (In French.)

64. Brown RD Jr, Wiebers DO, Forbes G, O'Fallon WM, Piepgras DG, Marsh WR. The natural history of unruptured intracranial arteriovenous malformations. J Neurosurg 1988; 68(3):352–357.

65. Mehta MP, Petereit D, Turski P, Gehring M, Levin A, Kinsella T. Magnetic resonance angiography: a three-dimensional database for assessing arteriovenous malformations. Technical note. J Neurosurg 1993; 79(2):289–293.

66. Karlsson B, Lax I, Soderman M. Risk for hemorrhage during the 2-year latency period following gamma knife radiosurgery for arteriovenous malformations. Int J Radiat Oncol Biol Phys 2001; 49(4):1045–1051.

67. Pan DH, Guo WY, Chung WY, Shiau CY, Chang YC, Wang LW. Gamma knife radiosurgery as a single treatment modality for large cerebral arteriovenous malformations. J Neurosurg 2000; 93(suppl 3):113–119.

68. Maesawa S, Flickinger JC, Kondziolka D, Lunsford LD. Repeated radiosurgery for incompletely obliterated arteriovenous malformations. J Neurosurg 2000; 92(6):961–970.

69. Heikkinen ER, Konnov B, Melnikov L, Yalynych N, Zubkov Y, Garmashov Y. Relief of epilepsy by radiosurgery of cerebral arteriovenous malformations. Stereotact Funct Neurosurg 1989; 53(3):157–166.

70. Lindquist C, Kihlstrom L, Hellstrand E. Functional neurosurgery—a future for the gamma knife? Stereotact Funct Neurosurg 1991; 57(1–2):72–81.

71. Schlienger M, Atlan D, Lefkopoulos D, Merienne L, Touboul E, Missir O. LINAC radiosurgery for cerebral arteriovenous malformations: results in 169 patients. Int J Radiat Oncol Biol Phys 2000; 46(5):1135–1142.

72. Lunsford LD, Kondziolka D, Flickinger JC, Bissonette DJ, Jungreis CA, Maitz AH. Stereotactic radiosurgery for arteriovenous malformations of the brain. J Neurosurg 1991; 75(4):512–524.

73. Colombo F, Pozza F, Chierego G, Francescon P, Casentini L, De Luca G. Linear accelerator radiosurgery of cerebral arteriovenous malformations: current status. Acta Neurochir Suppl (Wien) 1994; 62:5–9.

74. Flickinger JC, Kondziolka D, Lunsford LD, Pollock BE, Yamamoto M, Gorman DA. A multi-institutional analysis of complication outcomes after arteriovenous malformation radiosurgery. Int J Radiat Oncol Biol Phys 1999; 44(1):67–74.

75. Flickinger JC, Kondziolka D, Maitz AH, Lunsford LD. Analysis of neurological sequelae from radiosurgery of arteriovenous malformations: how location affects outcome. Int J Radiat Oncol Biol Phys 1998; 40(2):273–278.

76. Karlsson B, Lax I, Soderman M. Factors influencing the risk for complications following gamma knife radiosurgery of cerebral arteriovenous malformations. Radiother Oncol 1997; 43(3):275–280.

77. Lax I, Karlsson B. Prediction of complications in gamma knife radiosurgery of arteriovenous malformation. Acta Oncol 1996; 35(1):49–55.

78. Barcia-Salorio JL, Barcia JA, Hernandez G, Lopez-Gomez L. Radiosurgery of epilepsy. Long-term results. Acta Neurochir Suppl (Wien) 1994; 62:111–113.

79. Guidetti B, Delitala A. Intracranial arteriovenous malformations. Conservative and surgical treatment. J Neurosurg 1980; 53(2):149–152.

80. Elomaa E. Focal irradiation of the brain: an alternative to temporal lobe resection in intractable focal epilepsy? Med Hypotheses 1980; 6(5):501–503.

81. Pikus HJ, Beach ML, Harbaugh RE. Microsurgical treatment of arteriovenous malformations: analysis and comparison with stereotactic radiosurgery. J Neurosurg 1998; 88(4):641–646.

82. Hoh BL, Ogilvy CS, Butler WE, Loeffler JS, Putman CM, Chapman PH. Multimodality treatment of nongalenic arteriovenous malformations in pediatric patients. Neurosurgery 2000; 47(2):346–357.

83. DeAngelis LM. Brain tumors. N Engl J Med 2001; 344(2):114–123.

84. Berger MS, Ghatan S, Haglund MM, Dobbins J, Ojemann GA. Low-grade gliomas associated with intractable epilepsy: seizure outcome utilizing electrocorticography during tumor resection. J Neurosurg 1993; 79(1):62–69.

85. Fried I, Kim JH, Spencer DD. Limbic and neocortical gliomas associated with intractable seizures: a distinct clinicopathological group. Neurosurgery 1994; 34(5):815–823.

86. Kirkpatrick PJ, Honavar M, Janota I, Polkey CE. Control of temporal lobe epilepsy following en bloc resection of low-grade tumors. J Neurosurg 1993; 78(1):19–25.

87. Whang CJ, Kwon Y. Long-term follow-up of stereotactic gamma knife radiosurgery in epilepsy. Stereotact Funct Neurosurg 1996; 66(suppl 1):349–356.

88. Schoggl A, Kitz K, Ertl A, Dieckmann K, Saringer W, Koos WT. Gamma knife radiosurgery for brain metastases of renal cell carcinoma: results in 23 patients. Acta Neurochir (Wien) 1998; 140(6):549–555.

89. Schrottner O, Eder HG, Unger F, Feichtinger K, Pendl G. Radiosurgery in lesional epilepsy: brain tumors. Stereotact Funct Neurosurg 1998; 70(suppl 1):50–56.

90. Warnke PC, Berlis A, Weyerbrock A, Ostertag CB. Significant reduction of seizure incidence and increase of benzodiazepine receptor density after interstitial radiosurgery in low-grade gliomas. Acta Neurochir Suppl (Wien) 1997; 68:90–92.

91. Rossi GF, Scerrati M, Roselli R. Epileptogenic cerebral low-grade tumors: effect of interstitial stereotactic irradiation on seizures. Appl Neurophysiol 1985; 48(1–6):127–132.

92. Rogers LR, Morris HH, Lupica K. Effect of cranial irradiation on seizure frequency in adults with low-grade astrocytoma and medically intractable epilepsy. Neurology 1993; 43(8):1599–1601.

93. Goldring S, Rich KM, Picker S. Experience with gliomas in patients presenting with a chronic seizure disorder. Clin Neurosurg 1986; 33:15–42.

94. Chalifoux R, Elisevich K. Effect of ionizing radiation on partial seizures attributable to malignant cerebral tumors. Stereotact Funct Neurosurg 1996; 67(3–4):169–182.

95. Jorge CL, Nagahashi-Marie SK, Pedreira CC, Rosemberg S, Valerio RM, Valente KD. Clinical characteristics and surgical outcome of patients with temporal lobe tumors and epilepsy. Arq Neuropsiquiatr 2000; 58(4):1002–1008.

96. Rossi GF, Pompucci A, Colicchio G, Scerrati M. Factors of surgical outcome in tumoural epilepsy. Acta Neurochir (Wien) 1999; 141(8):819–824.

97. Britton JW, Cascino GD, Sharbrough FW, Kelly PJ. Low-grade glial neoplasms and intractable partial epilepsy: efficacy of surgical treatment. Epilepsia 1994; 35(6):1130–1135.

98. Kitchen N. Experimental and clinical studies on the putative therapeutic efficacy of cerebral irradiation (radiotherapy) in epilepsy. Epilepsy Res 1995; 20(1):1–10.

99. Gaffey CT, Montoya VJ, Lyman JT, Howard J. Restriction of the spread of epileptic discharges in cats by means of Bragg peak, intracranial irradiation. Int J Appl Radiat Isot 1981; 32(11):779–784.

100. Barcia-Salorio JL, Vanaclocha V, Cerda M, Ciudad J, Lopez-Gomez L. Response of experimental epileptic focus to focal ionizing radiation. Appl Neurophysiol 1987; 50(1–6):359–364.

101. Sun B, DeSalles AA, Medin PM, Solberg TD, Hoebel B, Felder-Allen M. Reduction of hippocampal-kindled seizure activity in rats by stereotactic radiosurgery. Exp Neurol 1998; 154(2):691–695.

102. Mori Y, Kondziolka D, Balzer J, Fellows W, Flickinger JC, Lunsford LD. Effects of stereotactic radiosurgery on an animal model of hippocampal epilepsy. Neurosurgery 2000; 46(1):157–165.

103. Maesawa S, Kondziolka D, Dixon CE, Balzer J, Fellows W, Lunsford LD. Subnecrotic stereotactic radiosurgery controlling epilepsy produced by kainic acid injection in rats. J Neurosurg 2000; 93(6):1033–1040.

104. Narabayashi H, Mizutani T. Epileptic seizures and the stereotaxic amygdalotomy. Confin Neurol 1970; 32(2):289–297.

105. Schwab RS, Sweet WH, Mark VH, Kjellberg RN, Ervin FR. Treatment of intractable temporal lobe epilepsy by stereotactic amygdala lesions. Trans Am Neurol Assoc 1965; 90:12–19.

106. Vaernet K. Stereotaxic amygdalotomy in temporal lobe epilepsy. Confin Neurol 1972; 34(1):176–183.

107. Flanigin HF, Nashold BS. Stereotactic lesions of the amygdala and hippocampus in epilepsy. Acta Neurochir (Wien) 1976; 23(suppl):235–239.

108. Mempel E, Witkiewicz B, Stadnicki R, Luczywek E, Kucinski L, Pawlowski G. The effect of medial amygdalotomy and anterior hippocampotomy on behavior and seizures in epileptic patients. Acta Neurochir Suppl (Wien) 1980; 30:161–167.

109. Nadvornik P, Sramka M, Gajdosova D, Kokavec M. Longitudinal hippocampectomy. A new stereotaxic approach to the gyrus hippocampi. Confin Neurol 1975; 37(1–3):245–248.

110. Engel J Jr. Surgery for seizures. N Engl J Med 1996; 334(10):647–652.

111. Barcia-Salorio JL, Barcia JA, Roldan P, Hernandez G, Lopez-Gomez L. Radiosurgery of epilepsy. Acta Neurochir Suppl (Wien) 1993; 58:195–197.

112. Heikkinen ER, Heikkinen MI, Sotaniemi K. Stereotactic radiotherapy instead of conventional epilepsy surgery. A case report. Acta Neurochir (Wien) 1992; 119(1–4):159–160.

113. Regis J, Peragui JC, Rey M, Samson Y, Levrier O, Porcheron D. First selective amygdalohippocampal radiosurgery for 'mesial temporal lobe epilepsy.' Stereotact Funct Neurosurg 1995; 64(suppl 1):193–201.

114. Regis J, Bartolomei F, Rey M, Genton P, Dravet C, Semah F. Gamma knife surgery for mesial temporal lobe epilepsy. Epilepsia 1999; 40(11):1551–1556.

115. Leber KA, Bergloff J, Pendl G. Dose-response tolerance of the visual pathways and cranial nerves of the cavernous sinus to stereotactic radiosurgery. J Neurosurg 1998; 88(1):43–50.

116. Leber KA, Bergloff J, Langmann G, Mokry M, Schrottner O, Pendl G. Radiation sensitivity of visual and oculomotor pathways. Stereotact Funct Neurosurg 1995; 64(suppl 1):233–238.

117. Egan RA, Shults WT, So N, Burchiel K, Kellogg JX, Salinsky M. Visual field deficits in conventional anterior temporal lobectomy versus amygdalohippocampectomy. Neurology 2000; 55(12):1818–1822.

118. Guenot M, Krolak-Salmon P, Mertens P, Isnard J, Ryvlin P, Fischer C. MRI assessment of the anatomy of optic radiations after temporal lobe epilepsy surgery. Stereotact Funct Neurosurg 1999; 73(1–4):84–87.

119. Jensen I, Seedorff HH. Temporal lobe epilepsy and neuro-ophthalmology. Ophthalmological findings in 74 temporal lobe resected patients. Acta Ophthalmol (Copenh) 1976; 54(6):827–841.

120. Stefan H, Hummel C, Grabenbauer GG, Muller RG, Robeck S, Hofmann W. Successful treatment of focal epilepsy by fractionated stereotactic radiotherapy. Eur Neurol 1998; 39(4):248–250.

121. Smith JR, King DW, Park YD, Lee MR, Lee GP, Jenkins PD. Magnetic source imaging guidance of gamma knife radiosurgery for the treatment of epilepsy. J Neurosurg 2000; 93(suppl 3):136–140.

122. Pendl G, Eder HG, Schroettner O, Leber KA. Corpus callosotomy with radiosurgery. Neurosurgery 1999; 45(2):303–307.

123. Paillas JE, Roger J, Toga M, Soulayrol R, Salamon G, Dravet C. Hamartoma of the hypothalamus. Clinical, radiological and histological study. Results of excision. Rev Neurol (Paris) 1969; 120(3):177–194. (In French.)

124. Munari C, Kahane P, Francione S, Hoffmann D, Tassi L, Cusmai R. Role of the hypothalamic hamartoma in the genesis of gelastic fits (a video-stereo-EEG study). Electroencephalogr Clin Neurophysiol 1995; 95(3):154–160.

125. Berkovic SF, Andermann F, Melanson D, Ethier RE, Feindel W, Gloor P. Hypothalamic hamartomas and ictal laughter: evolution of a characteristic epileptic syndrome and diagnostic value of magnetic resonance imaging. Ann Neurol 1988; 23(5):429–439.

126. Regis J, Bartolomei F, De Toffol B, Genton P, Kobayashi T, Mori Y. Gamma knife surgery for epilepsy related to hypothalamic hamartomas. Neurosurgery 2000; 47(6):1343–1351.

127. Kitajima K, Ikeda A, Terada K, Shibasaki H, Kimura J. A case of hypothalamic hamartoma manifesting gelastic seizure and multifocal independent seizure foci. Rinsho Shinkeigaku 1998; 38(4):305–310. (In Japanese.)

128. Parrent AG. Stereotactic radiofrequency ablation for the treatment of gelastic seizures associated with hypothalamic hamartoma. Case report. J Neurosurg 1999; 91(5):881–884.

129. Unger F, Schrottner O, Haselsberger K, Korner E, Ploier R, Pendl G. Gamma knife radiosurgery for hypothalamic hamartomas in patients with medically intractable epilepsy and precocious puberty. Report of two cases. J Neurosurg 2000; 92(4):726–731.

130. Cascino GD, Andermann F, Berkovic SF, Kuzniecky RI, Sharbrough FW, Keene DL. Gelastic seizures and hypothalamic hamartomas: evaluation of patients undergoing chronic intracranial EEG monitoring and outcome of surgical treatment. Neurology 1993; 43(4):747–750.

131. Machado HR, Hoffman HJ, Hwang PA. Gelastic seizures treated by resection of a hypothalamic hamartoma. Child Nerv Syst 1991; 7(8):462–465.

13
Special Treatments in Epilepsy

James W. Wheless
University of Texas–Houston
Houston, Texas, U.S.A.

INTRODUCTION

Seizure disorders represent a frequently occurring neurologic problem. Antiepileptic drugs (AEDs) are the primary treatment modality and provide good seizure control in most patients. However, more than 25% of children and adults with seizure disorders have either intractable seizures or suffer significant adverse effects secondary to medications. A limited number will benefit from surgical therapy. The shortcomings of antiepileptic drug therapy have allowed alternative treatments to emerge. In this chapter, I will review three specific and unique treatments of special interest to the epileptologist (pyridoxine, acetazolamide, and magnesium sulfate).

PYRIDOXINE (VITAMIN B$_6$)

History

The relationship between vitamin B$_6$ and convulsions has attracted general interest, especially in light of the role of vitamin B$_6$ in gamma-aminobutyric acid (GABA) metabolism (see Table 1 and Fig. 1) (1,2). Vitamin B$_6$ deficiency (3) and dependency (4) were described first ~50 years ago and are well known among the vitamin B$_6$-related convulsions. In 1968 Hansson and Hagberg (5) reported efficacy of high-dose pyridoxine in some epileptic children. These seizures were called vitamin B$_6$ responsive seizures (5,6), indicating they were neither vitamin B$_6$ dependent or deficient in etiology.

Mechanism of Action

Vitamin B$_6$ (as pyridoxal phosphate) is the coenzyme for glutamate decarboxylase and GABA transaminase, the enzymes that regulate GABA in the central nervous

Table 1. Pyridoxine-Associated Seizure Disorders

Condition	B$_6$ level	Age of onset	Family history	Response to AEDs	Response of seizures to B$_6$	Seizure recurrence after stopping B$_6$	Interictal EEG	Duration of treatment	Genetics
I. B$_6$ deficiency	Decreased	1–4 months	Negative	Poor	Good, physiologic dose (1.0–5.0 mg)	(−)	Normal	Brief (single dose)	None known, all acquired
II. B$_6$ dependency	Normal	Neonatal (siblings with similar problem or SE in infancy)	Positive	Poor	Good, pharmacologic dose (10–50 mg/d)	(+)	Abnormal	Indefinite	Autosomal-recessive transmission (chromosome 5q31)
III. B$_6$ responsiveness	Normal	2–14 months	Negative	Poor	Good, pharmacologic dose (20–400 mg/kg/d)	(−)	Abnormal	Brief (weeks to months)	None known

AEDs, antiepileptic drugs; SE, status epilepticus.

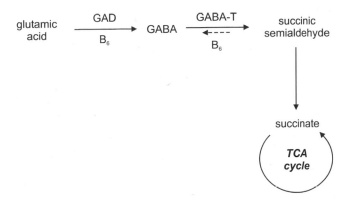

Figure 1. GABA metabolism.

system. Rats treated with semicarbazide had inhibition of glutamic acid decarboxylase, a subsequent decrease in GABA levels, and development of seizures. This sequence was competitively reversed by pyridoxine, demonstrating its critical role in GABA metabolism (7) and its presumed effect in treating pyridoxine-deficient seizures. Mice lacking tissue nonspecific alkaline phosphatases develop seizures due to defective metabolism of pyridoxal 5'-phosphate, and have decreased brain GABA levels (8). This mutant seizure phenotype can be rescued by the administration of pyridoxine. Additionally, the crucial role pyridoxine has in the central nervous system is evident from the fact it is a cofactor for >100 enzymatic reactions. These pyridoxine-dependent enzymes are involved in the metabolism of amino acids, neurotransmitters (dopamine, serotonin, GABA, and norepinephrine), as well as sphingolipids and polyamines (9). There exists experimental evidence for B_6 acting as a modulator of steroid activity, which may explain its efficacy in treating infantile spasms (10).

The pathogenic mechanism in pyridoxal-dependent seizures is not known but disturbed GABA synthesis due to a mutation affecting GAD activity has been proposed. A defect in GAD that would reduce pyridoxal phosphate (PLP) binding and enzyme activity would result in low GABA and high glutamate levels, a combination that favors seizures. The possibility that pyridoxine-dependent seizures are not a discrete disease of single etiology (due to insufficient activation of GAD) is supported by a report of normal CSF GABA levels and low glutamate levels (11). Neonatal seizures due to pyridoxine deficiency or dependency have low cerebrospinal fluid (CSF) GABA levels, which improve after treatment with vitamin B_6 (12–14). Baumeister et al. (15) examined CSF levels of glutamate and GABA in a patient with pyridoxine dependency while on and off vitamin B_6 treatment. GABA levels were normal, but off vitamin B_6, the glutamate level was markedly elevated and required higher doses of pyridoxine to normalize than did the EEG. The imbalance of excitatory (glutamate) to inhibitory (GABA) neurotransmitters may explain the seizures and the cognitive difficulties. A child with vitamin B_6-dependent seizures had reduced glutamic acid decarboxylase and GABA levels in the frontal and occipital cortices (16). A boy with pyridoxine-responsive West syndrome had CSF GABA levels examined before and during treatment with high-dose vitamin B_6 (17). The low GABA levels normalized with treatment, the hypsarrhythmia resolved, and B_6 was withdrawn. The authors hypothesize that pyridoxine-responsive West syndrome may be due to a developmental change of GABA metabolism that responds to high-dose pyridoxine therapy. This was presumed to be due to abnormal cofactor binding (1). However genetic linkage studies do not implicate mutations in GAD genes as the primary causative factor in pyridoxine-dependent seizures (18–20).

As a consequence of these observations, attention has been focused on pyridoxine. Biochemical studies have not demonstrated abnormalities in the metabolism or transport of pyridoxine or its active form, pyridoxal phosphate (PLP). PLP binds to and dissociates from GAD in a cycle that alternately activates and inactivates GAD. One hypothesis is that a mutation of a protein involved in this PLP cycle could cause the alteration of metabolism that leads to a change in GABA levels. This has yet to be proven or rejected.

Reports of pyridoxine dependency occurring in multiple family members suggested that this was a genetic condition, with a recessive pattern of inheritance (20–29). Results of genetic linkage analysis in four families with consanguineous parents identified the locus for pyridoxine-dependent epilepsy to chromosome 5q31 (20). Further work is needed to understand the relationship of this to the clinical symptoms and treatment.

Pyridoxine Deficiency

The requirement for pyridoxine was first noted in the 1930s and 1940s after removal from the diet caused convulsions and a hypochromic, microcytic anemia in chicks, swine, calves, and ducks (30,31). However, little was known about man's requirement until Snyderman gave two infants a pyridoxine-deficient diet (3). One developed seizures, which were promptly relieved by the intravenous administration of 50 mg pyridoxine.

Subsequently, a considerable number of infants were reported between 1951 and 1954 that developed convulsions, which were abruptly alleviated when given 5–10 mg of pyridoxine (32). In each instance the child had received a commercial food formula with inadequate amounts of vitamin B_6 (32–36). These observations led to a report in the Journal of the American Medical Association in 1951, warning that convulsions in infancy could be produced by pyridoxine deficiency (37). Prompt treatment was associated with immediate cessation of symptoms and no residual findings (35,38), although if prompt treatment is not given the prognosis for mental development is poor. In recent years isoniazid poisoning has caused a relative pyridoxine deficiency by inhibiting the activity of brain pyridoxal-5'-phosphate. In this clinical setting, children present in refractory convulsive status epilepticus which is responsive to intravenous pyridoxine administration.

Pyridoxine-Dependent Seizures

Pyridoxine dependency is a rare cause of generalized seizures in children first reported ~50 years ago (4). It is an autosomal-recessive disorder with variable penetrance, which typically presents in neonates as generalized seizures or status epilepticus, unresponsive to standard antiepileptic drug therapy. However, seizures stop immediately following parenteral pyridoxine. Lifelong therapy with pyridoxine is required to prevent seizure recurrence. There has been only one report of

Table 2. Pyridoxine-Dependent Seizures: Clinical Features

	Typical	Atypical
Onset	Before birth or shortly after (first 2–3 days)	After neonatal period, up to age 3 years
Response to pyridoxine	Rapid	Yes, some patients respond only to larger doses
Response to AEDs	None	Rapid response
Seizure recurrence after B$_6$ withdrawal	Yes, within 3–5 days	Yes, may take up to 6 months

long-term follow-up, which suggested that the prognosis for complete seizure control is excellent (21).

Knowledge about this condition comes from case reports and small clinical series. However, from these there appears to be a consistent constellation of features. The typical presentation is that of neonatal seizures beginning before birth or in the first 2 days of life that are intractable to antiepileptic drugs (AEDs) and that, when pyridoxine is administered, stop completely (4,23,24,26,27,39–43) (see Table 2). The seizures are frequent and brief. All seizure types have been described and multiple seizure types are usual, particularly clonic and generalized tonic (21,26,39,41).

Atypical (later onset or onset beyond infancy) presentations do not follow this classic pattern, and may occur in up to 35% of affected children (21,22,28,44–48). Children may present up to age 3 years, have initial seizures only occurring during febrile illnesses, or experience bouts of status epilepticus; the initial seizures may be partially or completely controlled with standard AEDs, but later become difficult to control (6,28,45). Prolonged seizure-free intervals (up to 6 months) may occur without pyridoxine. Rarely, high-dose pyridoxine may be required; however, in others small doses (1 mg) can control the seizures, allowing multivitamin supplements to confuse the diagnosis (49).

The EEG findings in untreated patients have not been specifically described. The EEG can be normal before seizure onset. In typical (i.e., neonatal) pyridoxine-dependent seizures the background may be normal or diffusely slow, but normal sleep patterns are lacking (25). Superimposed paroxysmal features include focal or multifocal spikes or sharp waves, or burst suppression patterns (21,24,25,41,50). In a small number of late-onset patients the interictal EEG is normal, and high voltage slow activity is less prominent.

Early-onset seizures are not the only clinical manifestation of this condition. Over half of the infants present with an encephalopathy that is not secondary to the seizure activity. This is characterized by hyperalertness, irritability, tremulousness, abnormal cry, feeding difficulties and vomiting, and an exaggerated startle respond which can trigger seizures (25,27,39). Meconium staining, hypotonia, and difficulties at birth can lead to a misdiagnosis of hypoxic-ischemic encephalopathy (44). In contrast, most children with the late-onset form are normal or mildly delayed before seizure onset. Mothers of those with early-onset pyridoxine-dependent seizures may have abnormal episodic fetal movements, beginning at 20 weeks' gestation, lasting 15–20 min, and occurring one or more times a day (25,26). The use of pyridoxine in pregnancy is advantageous to babies with pyridoxine-dependent seizures. In addition to treating the seizures, the neurodevelopmental outcome is normal in cases in which mothers take pyridoxine during pregnancy.

The diagnosis of pyridoxine-dependent seizures is based on confirming that the seizures stop after pyridoxine administration and recur when it is withdrawn. When performing a trial of pyridoxine the doses used vary from 5 to 100 mg, although 100 mg was commonly used in more recent reports. Both oral and intravenous routes are effective, but the latter yields a more rapid onset. The EEG reveals an initial disappearance of spikes followed by slow activity (21). Rarely, the pyridoxine trial may cause severe electrocerebral suppression lasting hours (21,47,51). Patients with a short-lived response, or no initial response and then a response to subsequent doses have been reported (51). As a result, Gospe recommended that an initial dose of 100 mg be given, and if no improvement is seen, this can be repeated every 10 min to a total of 500 mg (43). In late-onset forms, a dose of 100–200 mg is given daily for 1 week. The seizure control should improve by the second day, but complete control may take the whole week. A lack of response to this regimen or seizure recurrence while receiving pyridoxine probably excludes the diagnosis.

Not only does the administration of pyridoxine stop the seizures, but typically the child will sleep for hours, and remain hypotonic and less responsive. This is primarily seen in the typical form. The second part of establishing the diagnosis of pyridoxine-dependent seizures is demonstration of seizure recurrence with pyridoxine withdrawal and resolution of seizures when pyridoxine is restarted. There is no definitive test for diagnosis other than a trial of withdrawal. Employing the criteria outlined above for diagnosis affirms that this is a rare condition, with epidemiologic studies showing a prevalence of 1:20,000 to 1:700,000 (26,40,44,52). After stopping pyridoxine, in typical cases, the clinical sequence consists of a prodrome of altered behavior and irritability, with seizure recurrence typically within five days. If the trial is performed later in infancy or childhood, it may take 6 weeks or more before seizures recur (1,41,53). The best age at which to perform a withdrawal trial is not known. Some authors recommend the preschool years, with the parents having 100 mg liquid pyridoxine on hand to use as a rescue agent. Intercurrent illnesses have been reported to precipitate seizures, and increasing the daily dose by 100 mg for the duration of the illness has been recommended (26,47).

Maintenance doses of 50–100 mg/d have typically been proposed. However, a recent report suggests that while the seizures may respond to these doses, higher doses (15–18 mg/kg/d, up to 500 mg/d) may improve the cognitive outcome, and that the daily dose should be based on the later (26,40,47). This dose is unlikely to produce a sensory neuropathy; a finding confirmed using similar doses for the treatment of homocystinuria (40,54).

The prognosis is determined by several factors. Untreated patients die, usually in status epilepticus, typically within the first days to months of life (39). In treated patients, a poorer prognosis has been associated with onset in the neonatal period, initial responsiveness to routine AEDs, persistently abnormal EEG background, and a delay in treatment of over 1 week in the early-onset form (21). Antenatal pyridoxine might positively influence outcome, and the maintenance dose may have some influence (25,40). Specific difficulties are often encountered even with early treatment. Limited formal neuropsychologic testing has been reported. Baxter noted normal nonverbal skills, although below average, and impairment of expressive verbal skills even with early treatment (26,40). Additionally, some children show a marked articulatory dysphasia. These findings are less pronounced in children with late-onset forms. Neuroimaging studies, primarily magnetic resonance imaging (MRI), show abnormalities of white matter and brain structure (26,29,47,48,55). The most common finding is hypoplasia of the posterior portion of the corpus callosum (53). Also reported are cerebellar hypoplasia with a mega cisterna magna and, rarely, hydrocephalus.

Pyridoxine-Responsive Seizures (Infantile Spasms)

The finding that cerebrospinal fluid GABA levels were significantly lower in children with infantile spasms than in controls led to initial trials with vitamin B_6 (56). Initial reports suggested efficacy in some patients and led to larger open-label prospective trials (57–63) (see Table 3). These children had a variable age of onset of seizures, no signs or symptoms of vitamin B_6 deficiency, cryptogenic or symptomatic seizures, and a response to high-dose pyridoxine without the need for indefinite treatment (hence the term B_6-responsive seizures). Typically, spasms were completely suppressed and the EEG normalized or dramatically improved within 3–4 weeks of initiation of vitamin B_6 therapy. While cryptogenic patients responded best, symptomatic patients with various etiologies also responded. Additionally, follow-up studies have suggested that their mental and seizure outcomes were more favorable in children with vitamin B_6–responsive West syndrome than those with vitamin B_6–nonresponsive West syndrome, regardless of etiology (61). Pyridoxine therapy can be discontinued after 1 year of age if the child's EEG does not exhibit epileptiform discharges.

Clinical features and laboratory data cannot predict which children with infantile spasms will respond to pyridoxine. Accordingly, some authors suggest high-dose (200–400 mg/d) vitamin B_6 treatment for 2 weeks should be tried in all cases of West syndrome.

Unfortunately, no standard treatment protocols have evaluated initial and subsequent drug therapy for infantile spasms. Several surveys of the treatment of infantile spasms have been performed over the last 8 years (60,64–67) (see Table 4). The disparities in treatment protocols, in populations that have no known pharmacogenomic differences to account for differing drug responses, further supports the need for comparative sequential treatment protocols in West syndrome.

Adverse Events

The adverse event profile of vitamin B_6 is only partially established, as many of the authors do not mention side effects, and all of the studies are open-label. Intravenous B_6 administration has been associated with apnea, lethargy, pallor, decreased responsiveness and hypotonia (21,24,25,39,47). These reactions may occur immediately and persist for hours. Rarely, these same side effects have followed the initial oral dose (49,68) or intramuscular administration (22,23). These symptoms are usually mild, but exceptionally have resulted in intubation and mechanical ventilation (69). The pathophysiology of these events is felt to be a burst of GABA release from accumulated substrate and exaggeration of its physiological effect (68). As a result, some authors have suggested that it would be prudent to

Table 3. Efficacy of Vitamin B$_6$ in Infantile Spasms

Author	Number of patients	Age (months) of patients	Success rate	Dose B$_6$ (mg/kg/d)	Comments
French et al. (1965) (63)	15	1–54	Four had EEG normalize and spasms resolve within 2 weeks (one improved immediately = B$_6$ dependency)	0.1–1 mg/kg IV single dose, then 8–14 mg/kg/d PO	10 symptomatic. Open label EEG monitored
Blennow et al. (1986) (57)	3	6, 7, 14.5	100% seizure-free by day 5–6 of treatment	200–400 mg PO	2 symptomatic, 1 cryptogenic. B$_6$ initial treatment for 3–4 weeks, then placed on standard AEDs. Open label, EEG improved in all
Ohtsuka et al. (1987) (62)	118	—	15 (12.7%) seizure-free (5 cryptogenic), within first 2–16 days	30–400 mg/d PO	104 symptomatic. Open label, EEG monitored. B$_6$ 1st treatment. Long-term follow-up shows 12/15 continued seizure-free and EEG improved

Ito et al. (1991) (58)	20	1–14 (mean 7.2)	Three of 13 seizure-free on B$_6$ (only 1 had improved EEG), 3 of 4 improved or seizure-free on B$_6$ + VPA as initial treatment; 7 of 9 B$_6$ failures improved or seizure-free with addition of VPA	20–50 mg/d PO	18 symptomatic. Open label, EEG monitored. Only 1 patient maintained seizure-free on B$_6$. ACTH given to treatment failures and was most effective
Pietz et al. (1993) (59)	17	2.5–13 (mean 7.2)	5 of 17 improved with B$_6$ (noted in 1st week) and by 4 weeks were seizure-free	300 PO	All symptomatic. Open label, EEG monitored. ACTH given to treatment failures and was the most effective
Ito (1998) (60)	39	—	14 of 36 seizure-free (all symptomatic)	15–50 PO	36 symptomatic. Open label, EEG monitored. VPA initiated with B$_6$. ACTH given to failures and was effective in 80%
Ohtsuka et al. (2000) (61)	216	2–13	30 (13.6%) seizure-free (8 cryptogenic) (occurred within first 20 days)	30–400 mg/d PO	191 symptomatic. Open label, EEG monitored. B$_6$ 1st treatment. (Includes patients from 1987 series)

VPA, valproate.

Table 4. Surveys of the Treatment of Infantile Spasms by Child Neurologists

Author	Country	Number of respondents	First choice (symptomatic)	First choice (cryptogenic)	Pyridoxine as 1st choice
Bobele et al. (1994) (66)	USA	462	ACTH (88%), VPA (8.1%)	(No differentiation made)	0
Appleton (1996) (65)	United Kingdom, Ireland	38	Vigabatrin (76%), ACTH (13%)	Vigabatrin (45%), ACTH (37%)	1 (2.6%)
Ohashi et al. (1995) (64)	Japan	45 institutions	Pyridoxine (71%), VPA (8%), ACTH (2%)	(No differentiation made)	71%
Ito (1998) (60)	Japan	129 institutions	Pyridoxine (67.4%), B$_6$+VPA (9.3%), ACTH (4.7%)	Pyridoxine (70.5%), B$_6$+VPA (9.3%), ACTH (5.4%)	67.4–70.5%

administer the first dose in an environment with full resuscitation facilities at hand (68).

Loss of appetite (71%), periods of restlessness and crying (59%), vomiting (47%), apathy (29%), and hemorrhagic gastritis (6%) have been reported during high-dose vitamin B_6 therapy for infantile spasms (59). Laboratory abnormalities reported during therapy for infantile spasms consist of rare elevations of serum transaminases (AST, ALT) with doses >400 mg/d, rapidly recovering by decreasing the dose (62).

Long-term pyridoxine use can produce a sensory neuropathy, which has been documented both experimentally in rats, guinea pigs, dogs (70–72), and humans (73), and described clinically in humans (74,76). Depending on the daily dose and duration of administration, a distal neuropathy, neuronopathy, and diffuse axonopathy have all been described after experimental pyridoxine intoxication. The dose required to produce toxicity to the dorsal root ganglia, with subsequent degeneration of the peripheral sensory nerves was initially reported to be 2000–6000 mg/d (76). However, later reports indicated daily doses of 200–500 mg could be neurotoxic in adults (75,77). In all cases, the effects were dose dependent and at least partially reversible upon discontinuation of pyridoxine.

Prospective studies of adults taking 100–300 mg/d of pyridoxine showed no clinical or electrophysiologic evidence of neuropathy (78,79). Vitamin B_6–associated neuropathy appears to be very rare in children. Only a single report evaluated and documented unchanged sensory nerve conduction velocities in three children treated with high-dose vitamin B_6 for infantile spasms (57). Only one case of sensory neuropathy associated with high-dose (2000 mg/d), long-term pyridoxine therapy (for pyridoxine-dependent epilepsy) has been reported (80). A single child had a paradoxical increase in neonatal seizures after intravenous treatment with pyridoxine (81).

ACETAZOLAMIDE

History

Acetazolamide (N-[5-(aminosulfonyl)-1,3,4-thiadiazol-2-yl]acetamide) is an unsubstantiated sulfonamide that was synthesized in 1950 (82) and first used to treat epilepsy in 1952 (83). Acetazolamide inhibits the enzyme carbonic anhydrase (CA) (see Fig. 2), with subsequent generation of carbon dioxide and water. Carbonic anhydrase activity was first discovered in the early 1930s in red blood cells, and has subsequently been found in the central nervous system, eyes, adrenal cortex, pancreas, and gastric mucosa.

Early open-label reports confirmed acetazolamide's effectiveness in most seizure types (84–91); however, this was limited by the development of tolerance (84,91–93). There have been no prospective, controlled clinical trials of acetazolamide to establish its efficacy against specific seizure types or in epilepsy syndromes. As a result, acetazolamide's use in epilepsy is empiric, and guidelines for its use are lacking.

Pharmacokinetics

Acetazolamide is absorbed mainly in the duodenum and upper jejunum. Absorption is rapid with peak levels achieved in 2–4 h after oral ingestion of 5–10 mg/kg.

$$CO_2 + H_2O \xleftrightarrow{\text{carbonic anhydrase}} H_2CO_3 \xleftrightarrow{\hspace{2cm}} H^+ + HCO_3^-$$

Figure 2.   Chemistry of carbonic anhydrase.

At higher doses the absorption is erratic. The time-release formulation reaches a plateau at 3.5 h and is maintained for 10 h.

Acetazolamide is 90–95% protein bound. The percentage of protein binding is dose dependent. Acetazolamide diffuses into tissue water as the free form, where it binds to and inhibits CA. In the tissue, its concentration is higher than in plasma. The highest concentrations are found in that tissue that contains the highest amounts of CA (i.e., erythrocytes, glia). After 24 h, 90% of the drug is bound to CA. The volume of distribution is 0.2 L/kg. Acetazolamide is completely excreted in the urine without metabolism. The renal half-life is 10–15 h, but the enzyme-inhibitor complex has a slow dissociation constant. Thus, acetazolamide has an effective half-life of several days (94).

In children, acetazolamide doses range from 8 to 36 mg/kg/d (91,93), typically divided into two or three doses. Acetazolamide is usually initiated at one-third of the total daily dose, and increased by this same amount weekly, as needed. In adults, the usual dose varies from 10 to 20 mg/kg/d (95), with occasional benefit at doses up to 30 mg/kg/d. In some patients, increasing the dose overcomes the tolerance developed at lower doses. Patients with compromised renal function may need a reduced dose because the ability to clear unbound acetazolamide is directly related to creatinine clearance. Plasma acetazolamide levels are less than erythrocyte concentrations, and in most studies, no relationship between plasma levels and efficacy has been found.

Mechanism of Action

Brain CA is located in glial cells and myelin (96). Specifically, the carbonic anhydrase II isoenzyme is localized in the cytoplasm of oligodendrocytes and astrocytes, and the cytoplasm of the myelin sheath.

Carbonic anhydrase is involved in the transfer of H^+, HCO_3^-, or both from neurons to glial cells. Interruption of this process by acetazolamide leads to CO_2 accumulation in neurons. Development of tolerance to the anticonvulsant effect of acetazolamide is the primary limitation to its therapeutic use. This results from the induction of both increased amount and activity of carbonic anhydrase in glial cells (94).

Acetazolamide inhibits CA in the brain by >99%, leading to CO_2 accumulation, which appears to cause the anticonvulsant effect. This is the only known mechanism of action of this drug and is believed to mediate its activity (94).

The accumulation of CO_2 is sufficient to prevent the tonic extensor component of maximal electroshock-induced seizures (a measure of spread of seizure activity and efficacy against generalized toxic-clonic seizures) (97–101). At higher doses, acetazolamide inhibits erythrocyte CA, causing further CO_2 accumulation, which may contribute to its anticonvulsant effect. The degree of inhibition of brain CA correlates with acetazolamide's anticonvulsant effect in mice (102–105). Nephrectomy does not alter the anticonvulsant activity, proving it is not secondary to the systemic acidosis produced from renal CA inhibition (103). Doses of acetazolamide greater than those which produce complete CA inhibition do not increase the anticonvulsant activity. Mutant mice, deficient in CA II enzyme, have a reduced seizure susceptibility to flurothyl-, pentylenetetrazol-, and audiogenic-induced seizures (106). These data provide supporting evidence of the role of CA in seizure generation. The increased extracellular concentration of protons may block the N-methyl-D-aspartate receptor (107). In animal models, acetazolamide has been shown to protect against seizures induced by various methods: audiogenic seizures (104,108), pentylenetetrazol- and picrotoxin-induced seizures (95), and maximal electroshock (97–101), suggesting a broad spectrum of clinical efficacy in the treatment of human epilepsy.

Clinical Use

Acetazolamide has been used over the last 50 years to treat a variety of seizure types or epilepsy syndromes. Unfortunately, trial designs using modern methods have not been performed. Most patients have acetazolamide used as adjunctive therapy, after failing standard AEDs (83,86,91–93). Many of the early studies were performed before modern seizure classification, and all but one (91) was open label. However, given these limitations, all but one (109) suggested that, at least in the short term, acetazolamide was effective in the treatment of various types of epilepsy. Over time, most patients appear to develop tolerance to its antiepileptic effect. This could be observed after 2–8 weeks (84,91), but one study showed no loss of seizure control over 2–3 years, questioning the role of tolerance in these patients (90).

Partial Seizures

Forsythe et al. (90) performed an open-label, long-term trial, assessing the effectiveness of adjunctive therapy with acetazolamide in the treatment of 54 children with carbamazepine-resistant epilepsy. Patients who responded were followed for at least 2 years. Fifty percent (7/14) of children with "temporal lobe" epilepsy (i.e., complex partial seizures) were seizure free for 2 years, 67% (6/9) at the end of 3 years, and 100% (2/2) at the end of 4 years.

Eight years later, Oleos et al. (87) performed a similar study, using adjunctive acetazolamide therapy in 48 refractory partial seizure patients. The patients, ages 6–64 years (average age 28 years), were on monotherapy with carbamazepine. This was an open-label, retrospective review. Twenty-one patients (44%) had a >50% reduction in seizure frequency, and three were seizure-free for more than 3 months. The mean time on treatment was 9.6 months. With this length of follow-up, tolerance was not a problem.

Generalized Seizures

Lombroso and Forsythe (93) reported a seizes of 277 patients treated with acetazolamide, of whom 91 had absence seizures and 80 were less than 12 years old (i.e., most had childhood-onset absence epilepsy) (93). All had failed at least one AED, and in 48, acetazolamide monotherapy was used. This is the easiest group to judge the effect of acetazolamide alone. At the end of 3 months, nine (19%) had at least a 99% seizure reduction, and 20 (42%) had a 90% or more seizure reduction. At 1 year, eight (17%) of the patients continued to be at least 99% absence-free, while 12 (25%) continued to have at least a 90% reduction in seizure frequency.

In the same series reported by Lombroso and Forsythe were 19 patients with only generalized tonic-clonic (GTC) seizures (93). However, most were under age 12 years and failed prior AEDs, making it unlikely they had primary generalized epilepsy. In 15, acetazolamide was used as adjunctive therapy. At the end of 3 months, seven (37%) had their seizures decreased by at least 99% and 12 (67%) had at least a 90% improvement. However, by 2 years only two patients continued to have at least a 99% improvement. The same authors noted that acetazolamide helped decrease GTC seizures in patients who also had absence or myoclonic seizures, often associated with photic sensitivity and generalized spike and slow wave discharges. This suggests that acetazolamide might be useful in the treatment of GTC seizures seen in primary generalized epilepsy. Resor and Resor reported the use of chronic acetazolamide monotherapy in 51 patients with juvenile myoclonic epilepsy (JME) unresponsive to valproate (85). Among the 51 they could isolate the effect of acetazolamide on the GTC seizures of JME in 31. Fourteen patients (45%) were seizure-free or had a single provoked GTC seizure (2/14; 1 due to sleep deprivation, 1 due to antihistamines) on acetazolamide monotherapy for 10–70 months (average 41 months). Acetazolamide appeared less effective in controlling myoclonus. Initially, all 31 patients reported complete control of myoclonus; however, only four remained seizure-free, although the myoclonus was improved in all. This suggests that even when acetazolamide completely controls the GTC seizures of JME, most patients develop a degree of tolerance to its antimyoclonic effect.

Catamenial Epilepsy

Tolerance to acetazolamide's anticonvulsant effect limits use of this medicine. However, alternate-day or cyclical dosing has been suggested to reduce the development of tolerance. It was hypothesized that intermittent dosing would allow this drug to be a useful adjunct in the treatment of catamenial seizures, without development of tolerance.

Ansell and Clark report the initial use of acetazolamide to treat catamenial epilepsy (84). The drug was initiated 2 days prior to their menses, and a benefit was seen in two patients over a 3-month period. Lim et al. retrospectively analyzed the efficacy, safety profile, and tolerability of acetazolamide in catamenial epilepsy in the modern era (89). Eleven women took the drug continuously, and nine intermittently. Eight women (40%) reported their catamenial seizures decreased by 50% or more, with no significant difference in effectiveness noted between continuous and intermittent dosing. Response rates were similar in generalized or focal epilepsy. A loss of efficacy over 6–24 months was reported in three (15%) women. This study suggests acetazolamide is a useful adjunct in the treatment of catamenial epilepsy, but a double-blind, prospective study is needed.

Side Effects

Acetazolamide is a well-tolerated AED. Side effects are mostly mild or transient. All of the adverse effects are thought to be related to inhibition of CA, with the exception of hypersensitivity reactions. There are only rare reports of sulfonamide-type hypersensitivity reactions to acetazolamide, and cross-sensitivity to acetazol-amide is uncommon even in patients with a history of allergy to sulfa drugs (110).

Dyspepsia occurs in at least 90% of patients (95). Acetazolamide eliminates the tingle of carbonated beverages, giving them a flat taste. The effect is specific for CA inhibitors, and is localized to the taste buds, which contain CA. Anorexia is common, and in many patients, a pleasant surprise. Renal nephrolithiasis has been reported, although the incidence varies from 2–3% to 43% in adults, and appears much lower in children (95). Encouraging fluid intake and, when indicated, specific therapy based on the stone composition can minimize recurrence. The most common adverse effects are transient, mild polyuria, hypokalemia, paresthesias, irritability, anorexia, headache, nausea, diarrhea, and drowsiness (88).

Acetazolamide causes a metabolic acidosis by inhibition of renal CA in the proximal tubular epithelium with resultant bicarbonate diuresis and loss of sodium and potassium. A normal anion gap hypochloremic acidosis may be found on routine serum chemistries, although this is usually asymptomatic. However, Futagi et al. reported suppression of growth in children receiving acetazolamide as adjunctive therapy (111). They speculated this was related to the metabolic acidosis. Rarely, acetazolamide-associated blood dyscrasias (thrombocytopenia and aplastic anemia) have occurred (88). However, most of these occurred in patients being treated for glaucoma, and in one study the median age of patients who developed aplastic anemia was 71 years (112). To date, aplastic anemia has not been associated with acetazolamide's use in epilepsy. If periodic blood counts are checked, it appears sufficient to do this for the first 6 months to detect hematologic reactions to acetazolamide. Acetazolamide is teratogen i.e., in animals, and in some species acetazolamide has caused forelimb abnormalities. In humans, this has not been reported.

MAGNESIUM

History

Magnesium is second only to potassium in abundance as an intracellular cation. Tetany and convulsions, subsequent to experiemental magnesium deficiency, were first shown to occur in rats in 1932 (113) and subsequently in other animals (114–117). In 1934, Hirschfielder first reported the association of seizures and magnesium depletion in man (118).

However, scientific documentation of the relationship between convulsions and hypomagnesemia in man was not possible until the development of the multichannel flame spectrometer (119). This allowed simple, accurate, and rapid measurement of magnesium levels, correlation with clinical symptoms, and reversal of symptoms upon treatment with parenteral magnesium sulfate.

As early as 1906, magnesium sulfate was injected intrathecally to prevent eclamptic seizures (120,121). Subsequently, reports of intramuscular magnesium sulfate controlling convulsions associated with tetanus led to a similar regimen being used in 1926 to prevent recurrent seizures in women with eclampsia (122). Lazard, following up on his initial observations (123), administered magnesium sulfate intravenously to over 500 women with pre-eclampsia and eclampsia at the Los Angeles General Hospital (124). All of these early studies used small doses of magnesium. Later authors used larger doses given intramuscularly (125), but

Pritchard (126), then Zuspan (127), popularized the current protocol using intramuscular and intravenous treatment.

Mechanism of Action

The pathophysiology of hypomagnesemic seizures and the beneficial role magnesium has in the treatment of pre-eclampsia and eclampsia are not clearly known. First, I will review the proposed pathophysiology in hypomagnesemic seizures.

Hypomagnesemia may diminish the normal magnesium block of the N-methyl-D-aspartate (NMDA) subtype of glutamate receptors, triggering neuronal depolarization (128,129). The NMDA glutamate receptor is a voltage-dependent, ligand-gated channel that modulates flux of Ca^{2+} and Na^+. Magnesium ordinarily inhibits cation flux by means of a voltage-dependent block of the ion channel, preventing it from contributing to the excitatory postsynaptic potential (130–132). At resting membrane potetial ($\sim -70\,mV$), ambient extracellular concentrations of magnesium block the NMDA-receptor ion channel and prevent current flow, even when the glutamate and glycine binding sites are occupied (133). It has been hypothesized that hypomagnesemia removes the inhibitory influence this electrolyte has on glutamate-activated depolarizations, increasing neuronal excitability and seizure susceptibility. Supportive of this hypothesis is the observation that low levels of extracellular magnesium induce epileptiform activity in the rat hippocampal slice model (129,134–136). These epileptiform events closely resemble the electrographic pattern associated with tonic-clonic seizures.

Although excellent results have been obtained in treating pre-eclampsia and eclampsia with magnesium sulfate, the physiologic basis for the use of large doses in modern obstetrics remains unclear. However, it is suspected that magnesium is superior to traditional AEDs because mechanisms other than anticonvulsant properties enhance its therapeutic benefit for women with pre-eclampsia. I will first review the animal and then the human experiments that have been performed to verify or refute its anticonvulsant action, and then discuss other possible mechanisms.

First, investigations in the intact animal have demonstrated that the blood-brain barrier offers considerable resistance to changes in the brain and cerebrospinal fluid magnesium concentrations (137). As a result, intravenous administration of magnesium raises the magnesium content of brain tissue only slightly. However, other authors have argued that since acute convulsions may cause significant alterations in the blood-brain barrier permeability, additional research on convulsing animals is necessary to understand the effect of magnesium. Borges and Gucer demonstrated diminished epileptiform activity and seizures in animals given intravenous magnesium sulfate (138). The epileptiform activity was induced by topical application of penicillin G to the motor cortex in anesthetized cats and dogs and in awake primates. This animal model is felt to be predictive of efficacy against partial seizures in humans. Magnesium was able to directly suppress neuronal burst firing and interictal EEG spike generation at serum levels below those producing paralysis. However, subsequently, Koontz and Reid disputed these findings (139). They studied the effect of parental magnesium sulfate on established penicillin-induced seizure foci in anesthetized cats. Control animals were infused normal saline. Analysis of the electroencephalogram recordings demonstrated no significant difference in epileptic spike activity between the control and the magnesium sulfate groups (139). In both groups maximum spike frequency occurred ~30 min after application of penicillin and declined rapidly thereafter. The discrepancy between the two studies was felt to be due to a lack of controls by Borges and Gucer (138).

An investigation of thresholds for electroshock convulsions (felt to be predictive of efficacy in partial seizures with or without secondary generalization) and pentylenetetrazol-induced seizures (felt to predictive of efficacy in human absence seizures) in mice failed to show significant attenuation of the electrographic seizures, despite serum levels of magnesium sufficient to cause neuromuscular blockade in the mice (140).

Disruption of the blood-brain barrier may be important for the entry and efficacy of magnesium. Hallack et al. (141) demonstrated that sustained, elevated, serum magnesium concentrations increased magnesium concentrations in the cortex and hippocampus of rats, and induction of hippocampal seizure activity further elevated CSF magnesium concentrations. Additionally, the threshold for hippocampal seizure in the magnesium sulfate treatment group was increased significantly more (34% vs. 3.5%) than the control group. Once in the extracellular space of the brain, magnesium has been shown to antagonize depolarizations and seizures mediated by the N-methyl-D-aspartate subtype of glutamate receptor (32,142,143). These studies demonstrate that magnesium does have a central inhibitory action and that this action maybe at least partially mediated by suppression of the NMDA receptor. This counters the long-standing argument that magnesium sulfate has no central anticonvulsant activity. However, these same authors then compared the effect of magnesium sulfate versus phenytoin for seizure preventions in amygdala-kindled rats (144). Although kindled seizures are unrelated to eclamptic seizures, this study was performed to provide information regarding magnesium sulfate's effect in a model of partial seizure activity. Phenytoin significantly reduced seizure duration, duration of postictal depression, and behavioral seizure stage. Magnesium sulfate had no effect on any of the seizure parameters assessed.

This result may be explained by the magnesium's being more effective at reducing seizure activity when it acts as an NMDA antagonist. The outcome may reflect a difference in NMDA receptor distribution (i.e., relatively few in the amygdala) and/or subunit combination. Alternatively, this could be explained because excitotoxicity in hippocampal and cortical neurons depends only slightly on extracellular magnesium (145). The magnesium block of the ligand-gated calcium channel is voltage dependent and is present at physiologic levels of magnesium. During a seizure (i.e., continuous depolarization), elevated serum magnesium levels may not effectively block this channel.

Magnesium sulfate was given by intravenous infusion to treat a man with myoclonic status epilepticus (146). Over 3 days, the serum magnesium was increased from 1.5 to 14.2 mEq/L. CSF magnesium was elevated by the infusion only to 3.5 mgEq/L (normal is 2–2.5 mEq/L), reflecting the difficulty in elevating CSF levels. Despite magnesium-related neuromuscular blockade and cessation of visible myoclonus, the electroencephalogram revealed ongoing epileptiform activity at the baseline frequency. While magnesium was ineffective in this case of myoclonic epilepsy, this may not bear directly on the controversy over the use of magnesium sulfate in eclampsia, a condition with a different pathophysiology.

How magnesium sulfate acts as an anticonvulsant in pre-eclampsia remains controversial. Some believe this agent acts primarily by neuromuscular blockade. However, magnesium also has a central depressant effect. The abnormal electroencephalograms commonly found in pre-eclampsia or eclampsia may not be altered by therapeutic blood levels of magnesium (147). In addition, eclamptic seizures are occasionally seen in patients with confirmed therapeutic magnesium serum levels. Recent studies suggest that independently of any possible anticonvulsant efficacy, magnesium may have several other, potentially beneficial mechanisms of action.

Watson et al. investigated the action of magnesium sulfate on prostaglandin I2 (prostacyclin) (148). This is based on the observation that in advanced stages, pre-eclampsia is characterized pathologically by microvascular occlusions consisting of platelet and fibrin thrombi. Prostaglandin production may be relatively deficient during pre-eclampsia. Magnesium sulfate amplified release of prostacyclin and enhanced the antiaggregatory effect of intact human umbilical vein endothelial cells using serum levels achieved in treating pre-eclampsia (148). These results provide a physiologic basis for the use of large amounts of magnesium sulfate in pre-eclampsia.

Other mechanisms proposed for the action of magnesium sulfate in pre-eclampsia include opposition of calcium-dependent arterial vasoconstriction by antagonizing the increase in the intracellular calcium concentration caused by ischemia. Belfort and Moise evaluated the effect of intravenous magnesium sulfate (or placebo) on maternal brain blood flow in pre-eclampsia using Doppler ultrasonography (149). They showed that magnesium vasodilates the smaller-diameter intracranial vessels distal to the middle cerebral artery, and hypothesized that the drug may exert its main effect in the prophylaxis and treatment of eclampsia by relieving cerebral ischemia. This improved perfusion would prevent cell damage, cerebral edema, and possibly convulsions. The effect of magnesium sulfate may be multiple in eclamptic patients, including a depressant effect on the central nervous system, induction of hypotension, and changes in the renin-angiotensin system. These multiple sites of action may explain its efficacy, rather than viewing it as pure anticonvulsant. It has been argued that an eclamptic seizure is like any other seizure and therefore should be treated as such, but the efficacy of magnesium sulfate suggests that this assumption may not be correct. Ultimately, once the exact cascade of pathophysiologic events in pre-eclampsia is understood, then specific, targeted therapy will be advocated.

Clinical Efficacy

Hypomagnesemia

Symptomatic hypomagnesemia is rare in childhood (150,151). Hypomagnesemia occurs as a result of (1) abnormal gastrointestinal absorption; (2) renal wasting, of a genetic or acquired origin; and (3) primary hypomagnesemia (152–159). Neurologic disturbances constitute the most prominent clinical manifestations. These include confusional states, focal or generalized tonic-clonic seizures, and increased neuromuscular irritability with hyperreflexia, tremors, tachycardia, and myoclonic jerks (128,129,150). Phenomenologically, the magnesium-deficiency tetany syndrome is indistinguishable from hypocalcemic injury. Additionally, the neurologic manifestations of hypomagnesemia most frequently occur in association with hypocalcemia. Serum chemistries, magnesium, calcium, and albumin levels are necessary for differentiation. Hypomagnesemic seizures are usually generalized tonic-clonic, although partial seizures have been reported (119,150,151,156–158,160). Seizures usually are associated with serum magnesium levels <1.0 mg/dL (157,160), but seizures have occurred at 1.4 mg/dL (150).

Parenteral or oral preparations of magnesium sulfate can correct hypomagnesemic seizures. For oral administration, an isotonic, 4% solution is prepared, avoiding an osmotic cathartic effect. No established therapeutic regimen exists in the pediatric literature. Bappal et al. used magnesium sulfate (10 mg/kg IM) to stop ongoing seizures, and then a maintenance dose of 130 mg/kg/d given in three divided doses (161). To treat neonatal hypomagnesemic convulsions, 200 mg/kg is given IV or by IM administration (162). To acutely correct hypomagnesemia, the Harriet Lane Handbook recommends magnesium sulfate 25–50 mg/kg IV or IM every 4–6 h, followed by a maintenance oral dose of 30–60 mg/kg/d (163).

Pre-eclampsia/Eclampsia

Eclampsia is one of the dreaded complications of pregnancy as it carries high morbidity and mortality to the baby and mother. Pre-eclampsia and eclampsia represent a continuum of an acute hypertensive disorder peculiar to women (164). Pre-eclampsia is characterized by gestational hypertension in association with proteinuria, generalized edema, or both, and occurs after 20 weeks' gestation. Other causes of hypertension and seizures must be excluded (165). Eclampsia is defined by the appearance of seizures or coma. Yearly, about 200,000 maternal deaths are attributed to eclampsia worldwide, and it remains the leading cause of maternal death in the United States (165).

Pre-eclampsia is a multisystem disorder (166). One mechanism is thought to be vasospasm, with a secondary hypertensive encephalopathy and failure of cerebral blood pressure autoregulation. The exact cause of eclamptic seizures remains unclear. A number of pathological changes, including breakdown of the blood-brain barrier, vascular spasm, ischemia, and hypertensive encephalopathy, have been reported. The neuropathologic hallmarks of eclampsia are petechial hemorrhages and microinfarcts in cerebral cortex, subcortical hemorrhages, cerebral edema, small subarachnoid hemorrhage and multiple 3- to 5-mm hemorrhages in the corona radiata, caudate nucleus, or brainstem (167–169).

The treatment of pre-eclampsia is directed at decreasing elevated blood pressure, preventing seizures, preventing brain edema, and delivering a viable baby (169). The treatment of seizures and eclampsia has provided a controversy for obstetricians and neurologists (170–173). Numerous open-label, retrospective studies have documented the efficacy of magnesium sulfate in the treatment of severe pre-eclampsia or eclamptic seizures (126,174,175). Recently, prospective, randomized, large trials in the United States and the United Kingdom have compared magnesium sulfate to phenytoin or diazepam as therapy for the prevention of eclampsia (176) or for the management of eclampsia (177,178). Magnesium sulfate was found to be superior to phenytoin for the prevention of eclampsia in hypertensive pregnant women (176). The findings of this study were complemented by the Eclampsia Trial Collaborative Group (177). They reported that women receiving magnesium were half as likely to have recurrent seizures as women receiving diazepam and one-third as likely as women receiving phenytoin. Both studies reinforced the finding of seizure occurrence being associated with substantially increased maternal morbidity, and established the scientific validity of magnesium sulfate as a treatment regimen.

Subsequently, a case-controlled evaluation of magnesium sulfate's efficacy in pre-eclampsia (179) and Cochrane reviews of magnesium sulfate's efficacy in eclampsia (180,181) have been performed. All conclude there is compelling evidence in favor of magnesium sulfate for the treatment of eclampsia. Eclampsia appears to be distinguished from other forms of seizures in that it is better controlled by magnesium sulfate than by conventional AEDs (i.e., diazepam or phenytoin). This knowledge may offer opportunities to explore the pathogenesis of eclampsia.

Side Effects

Serious toxic symptoms can develop with magnesium overdosage, especially if renal function is compromised. Signs and symptoms of magnesium toxicity are dose dependent, typically occurring at magnesium concentrations $>4\,mEq/L$ (the normal serum Mg^{2+} concentration is $1.5–2.5\,mEq/L$). Depression of blood pressure is observed with serum levels of $3–5\,mEq/L$ (157). Loss of knee and ankle deep tendon reflexes occurs at magnesium levels of $8–10\,mEq/L$. Somnolence and slurred speech may also be seen. Generalized muscular paralysis, including respiratory muscles, occurs when the levels rise above $10\,mEq/L$, and coma at levels between 12 and 15 mEq/L. Cardiac arrest can occur at levels of $15\,mEq/L$. It is imperative to monitor the patient's clinical status, urine output, and serum levels of magnesium periodically. Magnesium toxicity should be identified promptly and remedial measures instituted. Administration of $10–20\,cc$ of 10% calcium gluconate intravenously is helpful in combating the respiratory and cardiac toxicity of magnesium. Loop diuretics may hasten the urinary excretion when renal function is normal. In the setting of renal failure, dialysis may be required.

Hypermagnesemia causes a myasthenic syndrome and blocks transmission in sympathetic ganglion (170). Administration of magnesium sulfate to a woman with myasthenia gravis will precipitate a myasthenic crisis. Hypermagnesemia potentiates neuromuscular blocking agents during anesthesia; hence, reduced doses must be used in toxemia patients treated with magnesium sulfate.

In pre-eclampsia, the load of magnesium transferred to the fetus depends on peak maternal levels and the duration of maternal hypermagnesemia. A serum level should be performed in the neonate and appropriate supportive care provided. Rarely, it may take up to 1 week for neonatal magnesium levels to become normal. Fetal morbidity has been shown to be reduced in randomized studies comparing magnesium sulfate to either phenytoin or benzodiazepines (176,177,180–182). The risk of cerebral palsy is lower among babies born to mothers given magnesium sulfate for eclampsia than in those not given magnesium sulfate (183).

CONCLUSION

Of these three agents—vitamin B_6, acetazolamide, and magnesium—the last has had the most thorough clinical evaluation to date. For all three, there is a clear need for future double-blind, controlled trials to establish their roles in the treatment of epilepsy, using the criteria established for evidence-based medicine. In the interim, however, magnesium sulfate appears to have a unique and important role in the treatment of pre-eclampsia. In women with an established seizure disorder, a traditional AED will also be a necessary part of their treatment regimen.

Vitamin B_6–dependent seizures should be considered in all infants and children with intractable epilepsy that begins prior to age 3 years. They should have an appropriate trial of vitamin B_6; if a patient responds to a challenge, vitamin B_6 should be withdrawn and reinitiated at a convenient time to document seizure recurrence and clinical response. It is important to firmly establish the diagnosis of pyridoxine-dependent seizures and to convince the family of an affected patient that lifelong supplementation is required, as it is a treatable disorder. Further, a controlled trial of vitamin B_6 in the treatment of infantile spasms is necessary to define a logical treatment sequence for this difficult-to-treat seizure disorder.

Acetazolamide continues to be a useful adjunctive AED, although its use may be limited now by the emergence of two other agents possessing carbonic anhydrase activity (i.e., zonisamide and topiramate). Acetazolamide's niche may ultimately be in the treatment of catamenial epilepsy. However, double-blind, prospective studies are needed to define the exact role of intermittent acetazolamide therapy.

All of the three agents reviewed in this chapter provide special insights into the complex neurochemistry and pathophysiology of epilepsy. This fact alone, combined with their potential therapeutic utility, justifies further investigation and understanding of their precise roles in the treatment of special populations with epilepsy.

REFERENCES

1. Jakobs C, Jaeken J, Gibson KM. Inherited disorders of GABA metabolism. J Inher Metab Dis 1993; 16(4):704–715.
2. Minns R. Vitamin B_6 deficiency and dependency. Dev Med Child Neurol 1980; 22:795–799.
3. Snyderman SE, Carretero R, Holt LE. Pyridoxine deficiency in the human being. Fed Proc 1950; 9:372–373.
4. Hunt AD, Stockes J, McCrory WW. Pyridoxine dependency: report of a case of intractable convulsions in an infant controlled by pyridoxine. Pediatrics 1954; 13.140–145.
5. Hansson O, Hagberg B. Effect of pyridoxine treatment in children with epilepsy. Acta Soc Med Uppsala 1968; 73:35–43.
6. Ekelund H, Gamstorp J, Von Studnitz W. Apparent response of impaired mental development, minor motor epilepsy and ataxia to pyridoxine. Acta Pediatr Scand 1969; 58:572–576.
7. Killiam KF, Bain JA. Convulsant hydrazides. I. In vitro and in vivo inhibition of vitamin B_6 enzymes by convulsant hydrazides. J Pharmacol Exp Ther 1957; 119:255–262.
8. Waymire KG, Mahuren JD, Jaje JM, Guilarte TR, Coburn SP, MacGregor GR. Mice lacking tissue non-specific alkaline phosphatase die from seizures due to defective metabolism of vitamin B-6. Nat Genet 1995; 11(1):45–51.
9. Dakshinamurti K, Paulose CS, Viswanathan M, Siow YL, Sharma SK. Neurobiology of pyridoxine. Ann NY Acad Sci 1990; 585:128–144.
10. Cake MH, DiSorbo DM, Litwack G. Effect of pyridoxal phosphate on the DNA binding site of activated glucocorticoid receptor. J Biol Chem 1978; 253:4886–4891.
11. Goto T, Matsuo N, Takahashi T. CSF glutamate/GABA concentrations in pyridoxine-dependent seizures: etiology of pyridoxine-dependent seizures and the mechanisms of pyridoxine action in seizure control. Brain Dev 2001; 23:24–29.

12. Kurleman NG, Loscher W, Dominick HC, Palm GD. Disappearance of neonatal seizures and low CSF GABA levels after treatment with vitamin B_6. Epilepsy Res 1987; 1:152–154.

13. Kurlemann G, Menges EM, Palm DG. Low level of GABA in CSF in vitamin B_6–dependent seizures. Dev Med Child Neurol 1991; 33:749–750.

14. Kurlemann G, Ziegler R, Gruneberg M, Bomelburg T, Ullrich K, Palm DG. Disturbance of GABA metabolism in pyridoxine-dependent seizures. Neuropediatrics 1992; 23:257–259.

15. Baumeister FAM, Gsell W, Shin YS, Egger J. Glutamate in pyridoxine-dependent epilepsy: neurotoxic glutamate concentration in the cerebrospinal fluid and its normalization by pyridoxine. Pediatrics 1994; 94(3):318–321.

16. Lott IT, Coulomb T, Di Paolo RV, Richardson EP, Levy HL. Vitamin B_6–dependent seizures: pathology and chemical findings in brain. Neurology 1978; 28:47–54.

17. Kurlemann G, Deufel T, Schuierer G. Pyridoxine-responsive West syndrome and gamma-aminobutyric acid. Eur J Pediatr 1997; 156(2):158–159.

18. Battaglioli G, Rosen DR, Gospe SM, Martin DL. Glutamate decarboxylase is not genetically linked to pyridoxine-dependent seizures. Neurology 2000; 55:309–311.

19. Kure S, Sakata Y, Miyabayashi S. Mutation and polymorphic marker analysis of 65k- and 67k-glutamate decarboxylase genes in two families with pyridoxine-dependent epilepsy. J Hum Genet 1998; 43:128–131.

20. Cormier-Daire V, Dagoneau N, Nabbout R, Burglen L, Penet C, Soufflet C, Desguerre I, Munnich A, Dulac O. A gene for pyridoxine-dependent epilepsy maps to chromosome 5q31. Am J Hum Genet 2000; 67:991–993.

21. Mikati MA, Trevathan E, Krishnamoorthy KS, Lombroso CT. Pyridoxine-dependent epilepsy: EEG investigations and long-term follow-up. Electroencephalogr. Clin Neurophysiol 1991; 78:215–221.

22. Bankier A, Turner M, Hopkins IJ. Pyridoxine dependent seizures: a wider clinical spectrum. Arch Dis Child 1983; 58:415–418.

23. Garty R, Yonis Z, Braham J, Steinitz K. Pyridoxine-dependent convulsions in an infant. Arch Dis Child 1962; 37:21–24.

24. Waldinger C, Berg RB. Signs of pyridoxine dependency manifest at birth in siblings. Pediatrics 1963; 32:161–168.

25. Nabbout R, Soufflet C, Plouin P, Duloc O. Pyridoxine dependent epilepsy: a suggestive electroclinical pattern. Arch Dis Child 1999; 81:F125–F129.

26. Baxter P, Griffiths P, Kelly T, Gardner-Medwin D. Pyridoxine dependent seizures: demographic, clinical, radiological, and psychometric features and effect of dose on intelligence quotient. Dev Med Child Neurol 1996; 38:998–1006.

27. Scriver CR. Vitamin B_6 dependency and infantile convulsions. Pediatrics 1960; 26:62–74.

28. Coker SB. Postneonatal vitamin B_6–dependent epilepsy. Pediatrics 1992; 90(2):221–223.

29. Jardim LB, Pires RF, Martins CES, Vargas CR, Vizioli J, Kliemann FAD, Giugliani R. Pyridoxine-dependent seizures associated with white matter abnormalities. Neuropediatrics 1994; 25:259–261.

30. Snyderman SE, Holt LE, Carretero R, Jacobs K. Pyridoxine deficiency in the human infant. Am J Clin Nutr 1952; 53(1):200–207.

31. Tower DB. Neurochemical aspects of pyridoxine metabolism and function. Am J Clin Nutr 1956; 4:329–345.

32. Bessey OA, Adam DJD, Bussey DR, Hansen AE. Vitamin B_6 requirements in infants. Fed Proc 1954; 13:451.

33. Coursin DB. Convulsive seizures in infants with pyridoxine-deficient diets. JAMA 1954; 154:406–408.

34. Molony CJ, Parmelee AH. Convulsions in young infants as a result of pyridoxine (vitamin B_6) deficiency. JAMA 1954; 154(5):405–406.

35. Coursin DB. Vitamin B_6 deficiency in infants. A follow-up study. Am J Dis Child 1955; 90:344–348.

36. Bessey OA, Adam DJD, Hansen AE. Intake of vitamin B_6 and infantile convulsions: a first approximation of requirements of pyridoxine in infants. Pediatrics 1957; 20:33–40.

37. Pyridoxine hydrochloride (vitamin B_6): a status report. Report of the Council on Pharmacy and Chemistry. JAMA 1951; 147(4):322–325.

38. Scriver CR, Hutchison JH. The vitamin B_6 deficiency syndrome in human infancy: biochemical and clinical observations. Pediatrics 1963; 31:240–250.

39. Haenuggeli CA, Girandin E, Paunier L. Pyridoxine-dependent seizures, clinical therapeutic aspects. Eur J Pediatr 1991; 150:452–455.

40. Baxter P. Pyridoxine-dependent and pyridoxine-responsive seizures. Dev Med Child Neurol 2001; 43:416–420.

41. Crowell GF, Roach ES. Pyridoxine-dependent seizures. Am Fam Physician 1983; 27(3):183–187.

42. Gordon N. Pyridoxine dependency: an update. Dev Med Child Neurol 1997; 39:63–65.

43. Gospe SM. Current perspectives on pyridoxine-dependent seizures. J Pediatr 1998; 132(6):919–923.

44. Baxter P. Epidemiology of pyridoxine dependent and pyridoxine responsive seizures in the UK. Arch Dis Child 1999; 81:431–433.

45. Goutieres F, Aicardi J. Atypical presentations of pyridoxine-dependent seizures: a treatable cause of intractable epilepsy in infants. Ann Neurol 1985; 17:117–120.

46. Krishnamoorthy KS. Pyridoxine-dependency seizures: report of a rare presentation. Ann Neurol 1983; 13:103–104.

47. Tanaka R, Okumura M, Arima J, Yamakura S, Momoi T. Pyridoxine-dependent seizures: report of a case with atypical clinical features and abnormal MRI scans. J Child Neurol 1992; 7:24–28.

48. Shih JJ, Kornblum H, Shewmon DA. Global brain dysfunction in an infant with pyridoxine dependency: evaluation with EEG, evoked potentials, MRI, and PET. Neurology 1996; 47:824–826.

49. Grillo E, Da Silva RJM, Barbato JH. Pyridoxine-dependent seizures responding to extremely low-dose pyridoxine. Dev Med Child Neurol 2001; 43:413–415.

50. Pettit RE. Pyridoxine dependency seizures: report of a case with unusual features. J Child Neurol 1987; 2:38–40.

51. Bass NE, Wyllie E, Cohen B, Joseph SA. Pyridoxine-dependent epilepsy: the need for repeated pyridoxine trials and the risk of severe electrocerebral suppression with intravenous pyridoxine infusion. J Child Neurol 1996; 11(5):422–424.

52. Ebinger M, Schultze C, Konig S. Demographics and diagnosis of pyridoxine-dependent seizures. J Pediatr 1999; 134:795–796.

53. Yoshikawa H, Abe T, Oda Y. Pyridoxine-dependent seizures in an older child. J Child Neurol 1999; 14(10):687–690.

54. Mpofu C, Alani SM, Whitehouse C, Fowler B, Wraith JE. No sensory neuropathy during pyridoxine treatment in homocystinuria. Arch Dis Child 1991; 66:1081–1082.

55. Gospe SM, Hecht ST. Longitudinal MRI findings in pyridoxine-dependent seizures. Neurology 1998; 51:74–78.

56. Ito M, Mikawa H, Taniguchi T. Cerebrospinal fluid GABA levels in children with infantile spasms. Neurology 1984; 34:235–238.

57. Blennow G, Starck L. High dose B_6 treatment in infantile spasms. Neuropediatrics 1986; 17:7 10.

58. Ito M, Okuno T, Hattori H, Fujii T, Mikawa H. Vitamin B_6 and valproic acid in treatment of infantile spasms. Pediatr Neurol 1991; 7:91–96.

59. Pietz J, Benninger C, Schafer H, Sontheimer D, Mittermaier G, Rating D. Treatment of infantile spasms with high-dosage vitamin B_6. Epilepsia 1993; 34(4):757–763.

60. Ito M. Antiepileptic drug treatment of West syndrome. Epilepsia 1998; 39(suppl 5): 38–41.

61. Ohtuska Y, Ogino T, Asano T, Hattori J, Ohta H, Oka E. Long-term follow-up of vitamin B$_6$-responsive West syndrome. Pediatr Neurol 2000; 23(3):202–206.

62. Ohtsuka Y, Matsuda M, Ogino T, Kobayaski K, Ohtahara S. Treatment of the West syndrome with high-dose pyridoxal phosphate. Brain Dev 1987; 9:418–421.

63. French JH, Grueter BB, Druckman R, O'Brien D. Pyridoxine and infantile myoclonic seizures. Neurology 1965; 15(2):101–113.

64. Ohashi N, Watanabe K, Aso K. The treatment of West syndrome by child neurologists in Japan. Psychiatry Clin Neurosci 1995; 49(3):S244–S245.

65. Appleton RE. The treatment of infantile spasms by paediatric neurologists in the UK and Ireland. Dev Med Child Neurol 1996; 38(3):278–279.

66. Bobele GB, Bodensteiner JB. The treatment of infantile spasms by child neurologists. J Child Neurol 1994; 9:432–435.

67. Ito M, Seki T, Takuma Y. Current therapy for West syndrome in Japan. J Child Neurol 2000; 15(6):424–428.

68. Kroll J. Pyridoxine for neonatal seizures: an unexpected danger. Dev Med Child Neurol 1985; 27:369–382.

69. Heeley A, Puch RJP, Clayton BE, Shepherd J, Wilson J. Pyridoxal metabolism in vitamin B$_6$ responsive convulsions of early infancy. Arch Dis Child 1978; 53:794–802.

70. Xu Y, Sladky JT, Brown MJ. Dose-dependent expression of neuronopathy after experimental pyridoxine intoxication. Neurology 1989; 39:1077–1083.

71. Antopol W, Tarlov IM. Experimental study of the effects produced by large doses of vitamin B$_6$. J Neuropathol Exp Neurol 1942; 1:330–336.

72. Kinke G, Schaumburg HH, Spencer PS, Suter J, Thomann P, Hess R. Pyridoxine megavitaminosis produces degeneration of peripheral sensory neurons (sensory neuronopathy) in the dog. Neurotoxicology 1981; 2(1):13–24.

73. Berger AR, Schaumburg HH, Schroeder C, Apfel S, Reynolds R. Dose response, coasting, and differential fiber vulnerability in human toxic neuropathy: a prospective study of pyridoxine neurotoxicity. Neurology 1992; 42:1367–1370.

74. Dalton K, Dalton JT. Characteristics of pyridoxine overdose neuropathy syndrome. Acta Neurol Scand 1987; 76:8–11.

75. Parry GJ, Bredesen DE. Sensory neuropathy with low-dose pyridoxine. Neurology 1985; 35:1466–1468.

76. Schaumburg H, Kaplan J, Windebank A, Vick N, Rasmus S, Pleasure D, Brown MJ. Sensory neuropathy from pyridoxine abuse: a new megavitamin syndrome. N Engl J Med 1983; 309:445–448.

77. Berger A, Schaumberg HH. More on neuropathy from pyridoxine abuse. N Engl J Med 1984; 311:986–987.

78. Bernstein AL, Lobitz CS. A clinical and electrophysiologic study of the treatment of painful diabetic neuropathies with pyridoxine. In: Leklem JE, Reynolds RD, eds. Clinical and Physiological Application of Vitamin B$_6$. Current Topics in Nutrition and Disease, Vol 19. New York: Alan R. Liss 1988:415–423.

79. Del Tredici AM, Berstein AL, Chinn K. Carpal tunnel syndrome and vitamin B$_6$ therapy. In: Reynolds RD, Leklem JE, eds. Vitamin B$_6$: Its Role in Health and Disease. Current Topics in Nutrition and Disease, Vol 13. New York: Alan R. Liss 1985:459–462.

80. McLachlan RS, Brown WF. Pyridoxine dependent epilepsy with iatrogenic sensory neuropathy. Can J Neurol Sci 1995; 22:50–51.

81. Hammen A, Wagner B, Berkhoff M, Donati F. A paradoxical rise of neonatal seizures after treatment with vitamin B$_6$. Eur J Paediatr Neurol 1988; 2:319–322.

82. Roblin RO, Clapp JW. The preparation of heterocyclic sulfonamides. J Am Chem Soc 1950; 72:4890–4892.

83. Bergstrom WH, Garzdi RF, Lombroso C, Davidson DT, Wallace WM. Observations on metabolic and clinical effects of carbonic-anhydrase inhibitors in epileptics. Am J Dis Child 1952; 84:771–772.

84. Ansell B, Clark E. Acetazolamide in treatment of epilepsy. BMJ 1956; 1:650–654.

85. Resor SR, Resor LD. Chronic acetazolamide monotherapy in the treatment of juvenile myoclonic epilepsy. Neurology 1990; 40:1677–1681.

86. Golla F, Hodge RS. Control of petit mal by acetazolamide. J Ment Sci 1957; 103:214–217.

87. Oleos KS, Penry JK, Cole DL, Howard G. Use of acetazolamide as an adjunct to carbamazepine in refractory partial seizures. Epilepsia 1989; 30(1):74–78.

88. Reiss WG, Oleos KS. Acetazolamide in the treatment of seizures. Ann Pharmacother 1996; 30:514–519.

89. Lim LL, Foldvary N, Mascha E, Lee J. Acetazolamide in women with catamenial epilepsy. Epilepsia 2001; 42(6):746–749.

90. Forsythe WI, Owens JR, Toothill C. Effectiveness of acetazolamide in the treatment of carbamazepine resistant epilepsy in children. Dev Med Child Neurol 1981; 23:761–769.

91. Millichap JG. Anticonvulsant action of Diamox in children. Neurology 1956; 6:552–559.

92. Lombroso CT, Davidson DT, Gross-Bianchi ML. Further evaluation of acetazolamide (Diamox) in treatment of epilepsy. JAMA 1956; 16:268–272.

93. Lombroso CT, Forythe I. A long-term follow-up of acetazolamide (Diamox) in the treatment of epilepsy. Epilepsia 1959/1960; 1:493–500.

94. Woodbury DM. Carbonic anhydrase inhibitors. In: Glaser GH, Penry JK, Woodbury DM, eds. Advances in Neurology. Antiepileptic Drugs, Vol 27. Mechanisms of Action. New York: Raven Press, 1980:617–634.

95. Resor SR, Resor LD, Woodbury DM, Kemp JW. Other antiepileptic drugs: acetazolamide. In: Levy RII, Mattson RH, Meldrum BS, eds. Antiepileptic Drugs, 4th ed. New York: Raven Press, 1995:969–985.

96. Sapirstein VS, Strocchi P, Gilbert JM. Properties and functions of brain carbonic anhydrase. Ann NY Acad Sci 1984; 429:481–493.

97. Woodbury DM, Esplin DW. Neuropharmacology and neurochemistry of anticonvulsant drugs. Proc Assoc Res Nerv Ment Dis 1969; 37:24–56.

98. Woodbury DM, Kailer R. The role of carbon dioxide in the nervous system. Anesthesiology 1960; 21:686–703.

99. Millichap JG. Development of seizure patterns in newborn animals. Significance of brain carbonic anhydrase. Proc Soc Exp Biol Med 1957; 96:125–129.

100. Millichap JG. Seizure patterns in young animals. II. Significance of brain carbonic anhydrase. Proc Soc Exp Biol Med 1958; 97:606–611.

101. Millichap JG, Balter M, Hernandez P. Development of susceptibility to seizures in young animals. III. Brain water, electrolyte and acid-base metabolism. Proc Soc Exp Biol Med 1958; 99:6–11.

102. Anderson RE, Howard RA, Woodbury DM. Correlation between effects of acute acetazolamide administration to mice on electroshock seizure threshold and maximal electroshock seizure patterns, and on carbonic anhydrase activity in subcellular fraction of brain. Epilepsia 1986; 27:504–509.

103. Millichap JG, Woodbury DM, Goodman LS. Mechanism of the anticonvulsant action of acetazolamide, a carbonic anhydrase inhibitor. J Pharmacol Exp Ther 1955; 115:251–258.

104. Gray WD, Maren TH, Sisson GM, Smith FH. Carbonic anhydrase inhibition. VII. Carbonic anhydrase inhibition and anticonvulsant effect. J Pharmacol Exp Ther 1957; 121:160–170.

105. Gray WD, Rauth CE. The anticonvulsant action of inhibitors of carbonic anhydrase: site and mode of action in rats and mice. J Pharmacol Exp Ther 1967; 156(2):383–396.

106. Velisek L, Moshe SL, Xu SG, Cammer W. Reduced susceptibility to seizures in carbonic anhydrase II deficient mutant mice. Epilepsy Res 1993; 14(2):115–121.

107. Traynelis FS, Cull-Candy SG. Proton inhibition of N-methyl-D-aspartate receptors in cerebellar neurons. Nature 1990; 345:347–350.

108. Engstrom FL, White HS, Kemp JW, Woodbury DM. Acute and chronic acetazolamide administration in DBA and C57 mice: effects of age. Epilepsia 1986; 27:19–26.

109. Livingston S, Peterson D, Boks L. Ineffectiveness of Diamox in the treatment of childhood epilepsy. Pediatrics 1956; 17:541.

110. Stock JG. Sulfonamide hypersensitivity and acetazolamide. Arch Ophthalmol 1990; 108:634–635.

111. Futagi Y, Otani K, Abe J. Growth suppression in children receiving acetazolamide with antiepileptic drugs. Pediatr Neurol 1996; 15:323–326.

112. Keisu M, Wiholm BE, Ost A, Mortimer O. Acetazolamide associated aplastic anemia. J Intern Med 1990; 228:627–632.

113. Kruse HD, Orent ER, McCollum EV. Studies on magnesium deficiency in animals. I. Symptomatology resulting from magnesium deficiency. J Biol Chem 1932; 96:519–539.

114. Orent ER, Kruse HD, McCollum EV. Studies on magnesium deficiency in animals. II. Species variation in symptomatology of magnesium deprivation. Am J Physiol 1932; 101:454–461.

115. Roine P, Booth AN, Elvehjem CA, Hart EB. Importance of potassium and magnesium in nutrition of guinea pig. Proc Soc Exp Biol Med 1949; 71:90.

116. Barron GP, Brain SO, Pearson PB. Histological manifestations of magnesium deficiency in rat and rabbit. Proc Soc Exp Biol Med 1949; 70:220–223.

117. Blaxter KL, Rook JAF, MacDonald AM. Experimental magnesium deficiency in calves: clinical and pathological observations. J Comp Pathol Ther 1954; 64:157–175.

118. Hirschfelder AD. Clinical manifestations of high and low plasma magnesium; dangers of epson salt purgation in nephritis. JAMA 1934; 102:1138–1141.

119. Vallee Bl, Wacker WEC, Ulmer DD. The magnesium-deficiency tetany syndrome in man. N Engl J Med 1960; 262(4):155–161.

120. Horn E. To tilfaelde af eclampsia gravidarum behandlet med sulfas magnesicus injeceret: rygmarvens subarachnoidalrum. Med Rev 1906; 32:264–272.

121. Alton BH, Lincoln GC. The control of eclampsia convulsions by intraspinal injections of magnesium sulphate. Am J Obstet Gynecol 1925; 9:167–177.

122. Dorsett L. The intramuscular injection of magnesium sulphate for the control of convulsions in eclampsia. Am J Obstet Gynecol 1926; 11:227–231.

123. Lazard EM. A preliminary report on the intravenous use of magnesium sulphate in puerperal eclampsia. Am J Obstet Gynecol 1925; 9:178–188.

124. Lazard EM. An analysis of 575 cases of eclamptic and preeclamptic toxemias treated by intravenous injections of magnesium sulphate. Am J Obstet Gynecol 1933; 26:647–656.

125. Eastman NJ, Steptoe PP. The management of pre-eclampsia. Can Med Assoc J 1945; 52:562–568.

126. Pritchard JA. The use of magnesium ion in the management of eclamptogenic toxemias. Surg Gynecol Obstet 1955; 100:131–140.

127. Zuspan FP. Treatment of severe pre-eclampsia and eclampsia. Clin Obstet Gynecol 1966; 9:954–972.

128. Avoli M, Louvel J, Pumain R. Seizure-like discharges induced by lowering (Mg^{2+}) in the human epileptogenic neocortex maintained in vitro. Brain Res 1987; 417:199–203.

129. Mody I, Lambert JD, Heinemann U. Low extracellular magnesium induces epileptiform activity and spreading depression in rat hippocampal slices. J Neurophysiol 1987; 57:869–888.

130. Dingledine R, McBain CJ. Excitatory: amino acid neurotransmitters. In: Siegel CJ, ed. Basic Neurochemistry. New York: Raven Press, 1994:367–387.

131. Nowak L, Bregestovski P, Ascher P. Magnesium gates glutamate-activated channels in mouse central neurons. Nature 1984; 307:462–465.

132. Mayer ML, Westbrook GL, Guthrie PB. Voltage-dependent block by Mg of NMDA responses in spinal cord neurons. Nature 1984; 309:261–263.

133. Goldman RS, Finkbeiner SM. Therapeutic use of magnesium sulfate in selected cases of cerebral ischemia and seizure. N Engl J Med 1988; 319(18):1224–1225.

134. Dreier JP, Heinemann U. Regional and time dependent variations of low Mg^{2+} induced epileptiform activity in rat temporal cortex slices. Exp Brain Res 1991; 87:581–596.

135. Herron CE, Lester RAJ, Coan EJ, Collingridge GL. Intracellular demonstration of an N-methyl-D-aspartate receptor-mediated component of synaptic transmission in the rat hippocampus. Neurosci Lett 1985; 60:19–23.

136. Walther H, Lambert JDC, Jones RSG, Heinemann H, Hammon B. Epileptiform activity in combined slices of the hippocampus, subiculum and entorhinal cortex during perfusion with low Mg^{++} medium. Neurosci Lett 1986; 69:156–161.

137. Hilmy MI, Somjen GG. Distribution and tissue uptake of magnesium related to its pharmacological effects. Am J Physiol 1968; 214(2):406–413.

138. Borges LF, Gucer G. Effect of magnesium on epileptic foci. Epilepsia 1978; 19:81–91.

139. Koontz WL, Reid KH. Effect of parenteral magnesium sulfate on penicillin-induced seizure foci in anesthetized cats. Am J Obstet Gynecol 1985; 153:96–99.

140. Krauss GL, Kaplan P, Fisher RS. Parenteral magnesium sulfate fails to control electroshock and pentylenetetrazol seizures in mice. Epilepsy Res 1989; 4(3):201–206.

141. Hallak M, Berman RF, Irtenkauf SM, Evans MI, Cotton DB. Peripheral magnesium sulfate enters the brain and increases the threshold for hippocampal seizures in rats. Am J Obstet Gynecol 1992; 167:1605–1610.

142. Cotton DB, Hallak M, Janusz C, Irtenkauf SM, Serman RF. Central anticonvulsant effects of magnesium sulfate on N-methyl-D-aspartate-induced seizures. Am J Obstet Gynecol 1993; 168:974–978.

143. Cotton DB, Janusz CA, Berman RF. Anticonvulsant effects of magnesium sulfate on hippocampal seizures: therapeutic implications in pre-eclampsia-eclampsia. Am J Obstet Gynecol 1992; 166:1127–1136.

144. Standley CA, Irtenkauf SM, Stewart L, Mason B, Colton DB. Magnesium sulfate versus phenytoin for seizure prevention in amygdala-kindled rats. Am J Obstet Gynecol 1994; 171:948–951.

145. Lipton SA, Rosenberg PA. Excitatory amino acids as a final common pathway for neurologic disorders. N Engl J Med 1994; 330(9):613–622.

146. Fisher RS, Kaplan PW, Krumholz A, Lesser RP, Rosen SA, Wolff MR. Failure of high-dose intravenous magnesium sulfate to control myoclonic status epilepticus. Clin Neuropharmacol 1988; 11(6):537–544.

147. Sibai BM, Spinnato JA, Watson DL, Lewis JA, Anderson GD. Eclampsia. IV. Neurological findings and future outcome. Am J Obstet Gynecol 1985; 152:184–192.

148. Watson KV, Moldow CF, Ogburn PL, Jacob HS. Magnesium sulfate: rationale for its use in pre-eclampsia. Proc. Natl Acad Sci USA 1986; 83:1075–1078.

149. Belfort MA, Moise KJ. Effect of magnesium sulfate on maternal brain blood flow in pre-eclampsia: a randomized, placebo-controlled study. Am J Obstet Gynecol 1992; 167:661–666.

150. Fishman RA. Neurological aspects of magnesium metabolism. Arch Neurol 1965; 12:562–569.

151. Tsau Y, Tsai W, Lu FL, Tsai W, Chen C. Symptomatic hypomagnesemia in children. Acta Paediatr Sin 1998; 39:393–397.

152. Muldowney FP, McKenna TJ, Kyle LA, Freaney R, Swan M. Parathormone-like effect of magnesium replenishment in steatorrhea. N Engl J Med 1970; 282:61–68.

153. Dudin KI, Teebi AS. Primary hypomagnesemia. Eur J Pediatr 1987; 146:303–305.

154. Evans RA, Carter JN, George CRP. The congenital magnesium-losing kidney. Q J Med 1981; 197:39–52.

155. Bettinelli A, Bianchetti MG, Girardin E, Caringella A, Cecconi M, Appianci AC, Pavanello L, Gastaldi R, Isimbaldi C, Lama G. Use of calcium excretion values to distinguish two forms of primary renal tubular hypokalemic alkalosis: Bartter and Gitelman syndromes. J Pediatr 1992; 120:38–43.

156. Nuytten D, Van Hess J, Meulemaws SA, Carton H. Magnesium deficiency as a cause of acute intractable seizures. J Neurol 1991; 238:262–264.

157. Rude RK, Singer FR. Magnesium deficiency and excess. Annu Rev Med 1981; 32:245–259.

158. Ahsan SK, Al-Swoyan S, Hanif M, Ahmad M. Hypomagnesemia and clinical implications in children and neonates. Indian J Med Sci 1998; 52:541–547.

159. Martin HE. Clinical magnesium deficiency. Ann NY Acad Sci 1969; 162:891–900.

160. Chutkow JG, Meyers S. Chemical changes in the cerebrospinal fluid and brain in magnesium deficiency. Neurology 1968; 18:963–974.

161. Bhasker B, Raghupathy P, Nair TM, Ahmed SR, De Silva V, Bhuyan BC, Al Khusaiby SM. External hydrocephalus in primary bypomagnesemia: a new finding. Arch Dis Child 1999; 81(6):505–507.

162. Morgan JD, Painter MJ. Neonatal seizures. In: Swaiman KF, Ashwal S, eds. Pediatric Neurology: Principles and Practice. St. Louis: Mosby 1999:183–190.

163. Siberry GK, Iannone R. The Harriet Lane Handbook, 15th ed. St. Louis: Mosby 2000:762.

164. Ramin KD. The prevention and management of eclampsia. Obstet Gynecol Clin North Am 1999; 26(3):489–503.

165. Kaplan PW. Neurologic issues in eclampsia. Rev Neurol (Paris) 1999; 155(5):335–341.

166. Bolte AC, Van Geijn HP, Dekker GA. Management and monitoring of severe pre-eclampsia. Eur J Obstet Gynecol Reprod Biol 2001; 96:8–20.

167. Kenny L, Baker PN. Maternal pathophysiology in pre-eclampsia. Bailleres Best Pract Res Clin Obstet Gynaecol 1999; 13(1):59–75.

168. Thomas SV. Neurological aspects of eclampsia. J Neurol Sci 1998; 155(1):37–43.

169. Donaldson JO. Eclampsia. In: Donaldson JO, ed. Neurology of Pregnancy, 2nd ed. (Major Problems in Neurology, Vol 19). Philadelphia: W.B. Saunders, 1988:269–310.

170. Donaldson JO. Does magnesium sulfate treat eclamptic convulsions? Clin Neurophysiol 1986; 9(1):37–45.

171. Dinsdale HB. Does magnesium sulfate treat eclamptic seizures? Yes. Arch Neurol 1988; 45:1360–1361.

172. Kaplan PW, Lesser RP, Fisher RS, Repke JT, Hanley DF. No, magnesium sulfate should not be used in treating eclamptic seizures. Arch Neurol 1988; 45:1361–1364.

173. Sankar R, Licht EA. Magnesium sulfate versus phenytoin for the prevention of eclampsia. N Engl J Med 1995; 333(13):1638.

174. Sibai BM, Spinnato JA, Watson DL, Hill GA, Anderson GD. Pregnancy outcome in 303 cases with severe pre-eclampsia. Obstet Gynecol 1984; 64:319–325.

175. Pritchard JA, Cunningham FG, Pritchard SA. The Parkland Memorial Hospital protocol for treatment of eclampsia: evaluation of 245 cases. Am J Obstet Gynecol 1984; 148:951–960.

176. Lucas MJ, Leveno KJ, Cunningham FG. A comparison of magnesium sulfate with phenytoin for the prevention of eclampsia. N Engl J Med 1995; 333(4):201–205.

177. Eclampsia Trial Collaborative Group. Which anticonvulsant for women with eclampsia? Evidence from the collaborative Eclampsia Trial. Lancet 1995; 345:1455–1463.

178. Sawhney H, Sawhney IM, Mandal R, Subramanyam AV, Vasishta K. Efficacy of magnesium sulphate and phenytoin in the management of eclampsia. J Obstet Gynaecol Res 1999; 25(5):333–338.

179. Abi-Said D, Annegers JF, Combs-Cantrell D, Suki R, Frankowski RF, Willmore LJ. A case-controlled evaluation of treatment efficacy: the example of magnesium sulfate prophylaxis against eclampsia in patients with pre-eclampsia. J Clin Epidemiol 1997; 50(4):419–423.

180. Duley L, Henderson-Smart D. Magnesium sulphate versus diazepam for eclampsia (Cochrane Review). In: The Cochrane Library. Oxford Update Software, Issue 2, 2001 (CD000127).

181. Duley L, Henderson-Smart D. Magnesium sulphate versus phenytoin for eclampsia (Cochrane Review). In: The Cochrane Library. Oxford Update Software, Issue 2, 2001 (CD000128).

182. Anthony J, Johanson RB, Duley L. Role of magnesium sulfate in seizure prevention in patients with eclampsia and pre-eclampsia. Drug Saf 1996; 15(3):188–199.

183. Nelson KB, Grether JK. Can magnesium sulfate reduce the risk of cerebral palsy in very low birth weight infants. Pediatrics 1995; 95:263–269.

14
The Ketogenic Diet: Scientific Principles Underlying Its Use

Kristopher J. Bough
Emory University
Atlanta, Georgia, U.S.A.

Carl E. Stafstrom
University of Wisconsin
Madison, Wisconsin, U.S.A.

INTRODUCTION

The ketogenic diet (KD) is a high-fat, low-carbohydrate, low-protein diet that was initially formulated in the early 1920s as a treatment for intractable epilepsy (1). Physicians in the 1920s and 1930s were well aware of the diet's effectiveness; at that time, phenobarbital was the only other epilepsy treatment in widespread use. With the discovery of phenytoin in 1935, and other anticonvulsants in subsequent decades, the KD was used much less commonly. However, over the past decade, the KD has reemerged as a viable alternative to standard anticonvulsants in the treatment of refractory epilepsy, especially in children. The history of the KD, including its origin and the reasons for the recent resurgence in its use, are reviewed in detail elsewhere (2–6).

Now that the KD has again found a place among epilepsy treatments, the time is ripe to understand the scientific principles underlying its use. Much of the KD protocol is based on lore, passed on from generation to generation, rather than on rigorously tested principles. Since its inception, little has changed in the formulation or administration of the KD. Although there is no longer any question that the KD "works", to optimize its clinical usefulness we must understand its mechanism of action more clearly. At present, the KD remains "a treatment in search of an explanation" (7). The optimal use of the KD in the future, including possible modifications of diet composition and utilization, will depend on new information based on sound experimentation and principles. Some such data can be obtained through clinical studies, while other information requires experiments in animals. There is a burgeoning interest among laboratory scientists to determine how the KD works.

Keeping with the spirit of this volume, our goals for this chapter are to briefly review clinical aspects of KD, summarize recent clinical and animal data that may bear on KD mechanisms, and synthesize this information into clinically useful guidelines for clinicians using the diet. We do not intend this discussion to be a "guidebook" for KD use, as such resources already exist (5). Rather, we hope to raise clinically relevant questions that will encourage further research, and thus improve the effectiveness and usefulness of the KD.

Clinical Aspects of Ketogenic Diet Use

The KD was formulated to mimic the physiology of fasting. The term "ketogenic" refers to the physiological condition in which fats are preferentially metabolized and ketone bodies are produced in the liver. During treatment, ketones, rather than glucose, become the primary source of metabolic fuel for the brain. Somehow, this conversion to fats as the primary cerebral energy source creates an anticonvulsant effect (8). The hypotheses to explain this anticonvulsant effect will be explored in more detail in subsequent sections.

The "classic" KD is based on the consumption of long-chain saturated triglycerides (LCTs) with a fat:[carbohydrate + protein] ratio of 4:1, by weight. That is, for every gram of combined protein and carbohydrate, 4 g of fat is consumed. Each meal must be planned in accordance with this ratio. In the 4:1 KD, ~90% of daily calories are derived from fat sources. Just enough protein is provided to ensure growth (~1 g/kg body weight); somewhat more or less protein may be required in rapidly growing infants and adolescents, respectively. Other ratios are sometimes employed, e.g., 3:1, based on the patient's age and metabolic needs. It is important to realize that the KD is not a fad diet, but rather a rigid medical regimen that must be adhered to strictly to ensure an optimum effect. The importance of a dietician experienced with the KD cannot be overemphasized.

Alternative KDs, based on different fat types, have also been used with similar efficacy. For example, a KD that was composed of medium-chain triglycerides (MCTs) as the fat constituent was intended to make the diet more palatable by allowing more carbohydrates (9). The MCT diet induces more pronounced ketonemia (plasma concentration of ketone bodies) for a given amount of fat. The MCT diet ratio of fat:[carbohydrate + protein] is on the order of 1.2:1. However, experience with the MCT diet revealed that it was associated with unpleasant gastrointestinal side effects such as diarrhea (10). Therefore, although both types of KD are effective in controlling seizures, the classic KD is used most often today.

The KD regimen is implemented gradually over a period of ~5 days (5). Initially, the child is fasted for 24–48 h, while hospitalized. Even during the fasting phase, seizures often decrease (11), an observation that may have mechanistic implications. Once fasting has produced sufficient ketosis, the KD is advanced in one-third increments of the full diet, over 3 days. During the fast and initiation of the KD, acute metabolic side effects must be screened for (e.g., hypoglycemia, vomiting, dehydration) (12), hence the need for hospitalization during this period.

The KD protocol must be adhered to rigidly; individual ingredients of the diet must be carefully weighed each day, and each meal must conform to the prescribed ratio. If carbohydrates are reintroduced (e.g., "sneaking" a cookie or lollipop), ketosis is lost, and breakthrough seizures can occur rapidly (in <1 h) (13).

The requirement of strict compliance, the difficulty of preparation, and the narrow food choices have limited widespread use of the KD, especially in children capable of making their own food choices. For these reasons, the KD has most commonly been used as an *alternative* treatment for epilepsy, despite its established efficacy. The KD's effectiveness as a first- or second-line treatment in epilepsy is unknown.

The long-term goal is to maintain the KD for 2 years, although this is an arbitrary target. Some children obtain long-lasting benefit from much shorter use, while many remain on the KD for several years. Compliance with the KD is generally related to its effectiveness. Patients who remain on the diet for 1 year or longer experience good seizure control and tend to be free of significant side effects (5). Reasons for earlier discontinuation include the lack of KD effectiveness, difficulty in its preparation, and intercurrent illnesses that interfere with its administration. These three factors are interrelated; i.e., parents find the diet more restrictive to administer if seizures are not well controlled (14).

The KD is the treatment of choice for certain inborn errors of metabolism, such as deficiencies of the glucose transporter (GLUT-1) (15,16) and pyruvate dehydrogenase (E_1) (17,18). Both disorders result in cerebral energy failure and consequent epilepsy. In GLUT-1 deficiency, the protein required for the transport of glucose into the CNS is dysfunctional, and in this situation, ketone bodies generated by the diet can provide an alternative source of energy. Children with GLUT-1 deficiency often present with seizures and developmental delay; KD treatment improves both the seizures and the developmental outcome. In pyruvate dehydrogenase (PDH) deficiency, the KD provides an alternative source for brain acetyl-CoA and enhances tricarboxylic acid (TCA) cycle activity (19).

Efficacy of the KD

The KD is a time-tested anticonvulsant treatment. Despite early skepticism about whether a high-fat diet could improve seizure control, especially in refractory patients, there is now little doubt as to the effectiveness of the KD. The KD's success rate in controlling refractory seizures is at least as good as, or often better than, that of most of the new antiepileptic medications (20). In general, half of all patients treated with the KD will exhibit at least a 50% reduction in seizure frequency, as documented in both U.S. and international series (21–29). In general, gender and seizure type do not affect outcome (25,26,30), but some epilepsy types may respond preferentially (see section on clinical question). Interestingly, the KD's success rate is similar now to when it was first introduced (24). Perhaps most importantly, the KD can often be discontinued without a concomitant loss of seizure control (5,14). This observation suggests that the KD may be both anticonvulsant (stops seizures) and antiepileptic (retards the development of the epileptic state).

Treatment with a KD has several advantages over more traditional pharmacotherapy. The KD effectively controls multiple types of epilepsy and works when other medications fail. At diet onset, a typical patient will have been treated with as many as seven antiepileptic drugs (AEDs) (25). With KD treatment, AEDs can typically be reduced or even discontinued. According to anecdotal reports, behavioral function and mental capacity may improve (21–24). A recent prospective study documented improved attention span, developmental quotient, and social functioning in a cohort of children on the KD for 1 year (31). These behavioral improvements can sometimes be as important to a family as better seizure control. The need for fewer sedative anticonvulsants may account for some of this cognitive improvement. A reduction in medications can also reduce the financial costs and occurrence of side effects arising from AED polypharmacy (2).

Integrating Clinical and Basic Science Understanding of the KD

Despite 80 years of clinical use, we still do not understand how the diet works. Few studies have carefully examined key aspects of treatment, and even fewer have investigated the mechanisms underlying anticonvulsant or antiepileptic actions of the KD. Many clinical questions remain about the optimal use of the KD, including diet composition (i.e., classic vs. MCT), the need for calorie or fluid restriction, optimal age at diet onset, and duration of diet treatment.

To approach the plethora of questions remaining about the KD and its elusive mechanism of action, animal studies must be utilized. In the laboratory, variables such as seizure type, age of seizure onset, age of KD initiation, duration of KD, and composition of KD can be controlled to a greater extent than in human studies. Unfortunately, laboratory investigations to date have employed a bewildering variety of methodologies (32). Generalizations from such an array of studies have proven difficult and numerous fundamental questions remain. In this chapter, we highlight some important questions about the KD and discuss what we might glean from a better understanding of these variables in terms of KD mechanisms.

OVERVIEW OF KETONES AND CEREBRAL METABOLISM

The first step in understanding how the KD may work as an antiepileptic treatment is to understand how ketosis occurs. We summarize this broad subject here. For further details, the reader is referred to comprehensive reviews of this topic (33–36).

The KD was originally formulated to mimic the effects of fasting, as it had been known since biblical times that fasting had a beneficial effect on epilepsy. Ever since then, it has been assumed that fasting and the KD share a common mechanism in alleviating seizures, although this assumption has not been rigorously tested. Whether the antiepileptic effectiveness of fasting or the high-fat diet is related to the level of ketosis is a lingering controversy.

As seen in Figure 1A, dietary fats are ordinarily broken down in the liver into two-carbon acetyl-CoA molecules, in a process called β-oxidation. Acetyl-CoA molecules enter the tricarboxylic acid (TCA) cycle, producing energy via generation of adenosine triphosphate (ATP). However, under conditions of fasting, starvation, or the high-fat KD, acetyl-CoA cannot readily enter the TCA cycle because of low availability of the TCA rate-limiting substrate oxaloacetate and the rate-limiting enzyme α-ketoglutarate dehydrogenase (which have been diverted to gluconeogenesis) (19). Instead, acetyl-CoA molecules are used to synthesize the four-carbon ketone bodies β-hydroxybutyrate (BHB) and acetoacetate (AcAc) (as well as the volatile ketone, acetone, which is exhaled). Therefore, both fasting and the KD produce ketosis, i.e., elevated blood levels of BHB and AcAc (37,38). The liver lacks the enzymes necessary to break down ketone bodies, so BHB and AcAc are exported in the circulation to tissues where they can be utilized for energy, such as muscle and brain.

A) Liver: ketogenesis

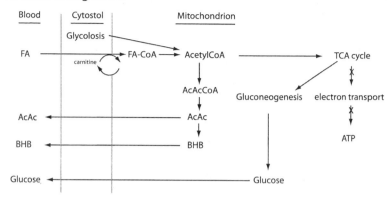

B) Brain: ketone body oxidation and utilization

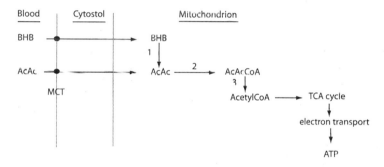

Figure 1. Schematic summary of ketogenesis and ketone body utilization by the liver and brain (A) Ketogenesis in the liver. Fatty acids from the circulation enter hepatocytes, then cross the inner mitochondrial membrane by either diffusion (short- and medium-chain FA) or via carnitine transport (long-chain FA). Under conditions of fasting or the high-fat, low-carbohydrate ketogenic diet, carbohydrate substrate is lacking, so FA are metabolized. Since oxaloacetate (a TCA cycle intermediate) is diverted to gluconeogenesis, the TCA is not actively involved in energy generation (X'd arrows). Acetyl-CoA molecules are therefore not funneled into the TCA, but instead are used for ketone body synthesis (AcAc, BHB). The ketones are exported into the circulation, since the liver lacks the enzymes required to metabolize AcAc and BHB. (B) In the brain, BHB and AcAc enter neurons via monocarboxylic acid transport system. In mitochondria, BHB and AcAc are broken down (by enzymes 1, 2, and 3) into acetyl-CoA molecules that can then enter the TCA cycle for energy production. (C) TCA cycle and GABA shunt. In ketosis, α-KG is increased (40), and GABA synthesis from glutamate (via enzyme 4) is favored (36). In addition, the GABA shunt, bypassing normal oxidative metabolism, facilitates GABA production. *Abbreviations*: FA, fatty acid; CoA, coenzyme A; TCA, tricarboxylic acid; AcAc, acetoacetate; BHB, β-hydroxybutyrate; ATP, adenosine triphosphate; AcCoA, acetyl-CoA; MCT, monocarboxylic acid transport protein; OA, oxaloacetate; asp, aspartate; α-KG, α-ketoglutarate; glut, glutamate; GABA, γ-aminobutyric acid; SSA, succinic semialdehyde; 1, BHB dehydrogenase; 2, succinyl-CoA transferase (3-ketoacid CoA-transeferase); 3, acetoacetyl-CoA thiolase; 4, glutamic acid decarboxylase.

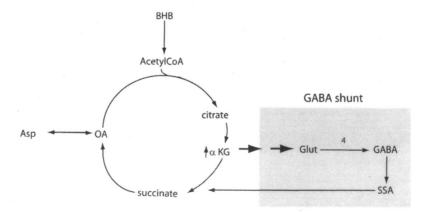

Figure 1. Continued.

The brain has a very high metabolic rate. Although it comprises only 2% of body weight, the brain accounts for 20% of basal oxygen consumption in adults and up to 50% in children. Oxygen is used to oxidize carbohydrates for energy production. Ordinarily, the brain is an obligate consumer of glucose as its energy source, and there is no arteriovenous concentration difference for ketone bodies. However, when carbohydrates are restricted, as in fasting, starvation, or the KD, the brain can no longer use glucose exclusively. There is a shift in metabolism whereby the brain preferentially oxidizes ketone bodies derived from fats, instead of carbohydrates, as the primary fuel source (33,39,40).

Therefore, under conditions of fasting or high fat/low carbohydrate intake, the brain can utilize ketones as the main oxidizable substrate for cerebral metabolism (Fig. 1B) (33,41). Ketones from the circulation are transported across the blood-brain barrier by facilitated diffusion, using a monocarboxylate transport system (42,43). This transport system is induced by fasting and may be crucial to the mechanism of the KD, especially as it pertains to the age dependency of its efficacy. However, even adult animals can upregulate brain monocarboxylate transporter levels when placed on the KD (44). In humans, both fasting and intravenous BHB infusion increase brain BHB levels, as measured by ^{1}H magnetic resonance spectroscopy (45,46).

Neurons and glia possess the requisite enzymes to break down BHB and AcAc into acetyl-CoA fragments (BHB dehydrogenase and 3-oxoacid-CoA transferase, respectively). Acetyl-CoA molecules can, in turn, enter the TCA cycle and produce energy (Fig. 1B) (33). These enzymes are regulated developmentally, with maximal expression early in life, consistent with the higher utilization of ketones by the brain in children as opposed to adults (47–50). Although the brain can metabolize ketones if deprived of its usual carbohydrate fuels, cerebral activity may be optimal only if some glucose is present (51–53).

It has been assumed that the brain itself is not ketogenic; i.e., the brain does not possess the synthetic machinery to produce ketones for energy. However, a recent study showed that cortex, brainstem, and primary cultures of cortical astrocytes do express enzymes responsible for ketogenesis, especially early in development (before weaning) (54). Absence of one such mitochondrial enzyme, 3-hydroxy-3-methyl-glutaryl-coA synthase, leads to hypoketonemia in patients (55).

Changes in cerebral energetics induced by the KD favor an increase in "energy charge," i.e., a relative increase in the ATP/ADP ratio resulting from metabolic alterations in the enzymes involved in glycolysis and the TCA cycle (40,41,56). Greater availability of brain energy was hypothesized to produce an anticonvulsant effect. This hypothesis of an increase in energy charge has been supported by recent experiments in patients with Lennox-Gastaut syndrome; using ^{31}P spectroscopic imaging, it was shown that KD treatment was associated with an improvement in energy metabolism (57).

In addition to alteration of TCA cycle activity by ketosis, the synthesis or function of gamma-aminobutyric acid (GABA) may also be modified. GABA is the main inhibitory neurotransmitter in the brain and is synthesized from glutamate via the action of glutamate decarboxylase (Fig. 14.1C). In ketosis, α-ketoglutarate, the precursor of glutamate, is increased, thereby enhancing the synthesis of GABA via the "GABA shunt" (36,58). Whole-brain GABA levels are unchanged on the KD (59), but regional differences have been reported (60). Enhanced GABA accumulation or function at the receptor level could lead to reduced cortical excitability. At the same time, the rate of glutamate conversion to aspartate, which has an excitatory role, is reduced (36). These observations could explain in part how the KD suppresses seizures.

CLINICAL QUESTIONS CONCERNING KETOGENIC DIET EFFICACY

Is the KD Equally Effective Across All Types of Epilepsy?

Clinically, the KD has been used to treat numerous seizure types. Early studies were limited by failure to adequately describe seizure types and epilepsy syndromes, at least in terms of modern classification. Recent prospective reports have found no consistent correlation between efficacy and seizure type (25,26,30). Nonetheless, it is noteworthy that some differences may exist. For example, Livingston states that despite the lack of "an absolute relationship between the type of epilepsy and . . . a satisfactory response to the KD," the best results were observed in children with myoclonic epilepsy (23). In a prospective evaluation of 106 consecutive children who stayed on the KD for 6 months, about half (43–60%) of all patients with myoclonic, atonic/drop, or atypical absence seizures exhibited a >90% reduction in the number of seizures (25). Seizures in children with Lennox-Gastaut syndrome (tonic, myoclonic, atypical absence) are notoriously difficult to control, and yet such children often benefit from the KD. In addition to generalized seizures, partial seizures (with or without secondary generalization) also respond to the KD. In Freeman's study, 63% of children with partial seizures had a ≥50% seizure reduction (25). In another study, 27% of children with partial seizures had a ≥50% seizure reduction (61). Therefore, many epilepsy types appear to respond to the KD.

Despite widely discrepant methodologies, laboratory evidence—like clinical findings—indicates that the KD is effective against a variety of seizure types (Table 1). The correlation between human epilepsies and animal epilepsy models is inexact, and is based principally on both the clinical semiology of the seizures and their responsiveness to anticonvulsant drugs (62). In general, seizures in animals

Table 1. Animal Models of the Ketogenic Diet—Seizure Types

Model	Analogous human seizure type	Selected references
Electroshock (maximal and threshold models)	Generalized (tonic, tonic-clonic)	56,63,64,69,70,78,112,113
Pentylenetetrazole	Generalized (myoclonic)	63,73,78
Flurothyl	Generalized (myoclonic, tonic-clonic)	65,72
Kindling	Partial complex with secondary generalization	74
Kainic acid	Partial complex with secondary generalization	108,109
EL (genetic; stress/ handling-induced)	Partial complex with secondary generalization	114

induced by electroshock (causing tonic limb extension) represent a model of generalized tonic seizures, while the chemoconvulsant pentylenetetrazole (PTZ) models generalized myocolonic seizures. Kindling, kainic acid, and the genetic EL mouse mimic partial onset seizures. As seen in Table 1, the KD affords some protection across generalized and partial seizure models (see Ref. 32 for a detailed review). However, some studies failed to show a protective effect of the KD, particularly against status epilepticus induced by kainic acid or maximal electro-convulsive shock (63,64).

How might observed differences in animal models translate to differences in KD clinical efficacy? The relative efficacy of the KD in some models over others suggests that different brain regions might be affected more profoundly than others, and this could relate to localized differences in the function of GABA or other neurotransmitters (65). It remains unclear, however, whether seizure etiology plays a role in KD effectiveness in patients. For instance, a genetic susceptibility (e.g., a channelopathy) might respond very differently to KD treatment than would an acquired pathology (e.g., mesial temporal sclerosis) or cortical dysplasia. There are scarce data about KD responsiveness in different etiological subgroups. To complicate matters, many children have multiple seizure etiologies and seizure types. An improved understanding of KD efficacy in relation to seizure type and its cognate region of epileptogenicity or pathology will help us select appropriate KD candidates and administer the KD more effectively. Such information may also provide clues as to underlying mechanisms.

Despite differences in KD protocols in the various laboratory experiments, these data collectively show that the KD can increase the resistance to multiple seizure types by increasing seizure threshold (either chemical or electroconvulsive). The response of most seizure types to the KD implies that the diet exerts a general suppressant effect on neuronal excitability. The enhanced response of some particular seizure types (e.g., generalized epilepsies) suggests that the mechanism of KD action may have additional, specific pathophysiological actions on seizure initiation or propagation. For now, we recommend that the KD be considered for any patient with refractory epilepsy.

Does Age at Diet Onset Affect KD Efficacy?

Clinically, the KD is very effective in controlling intractable seizures in children. It is believed that the age at which the KD is begun determines responsiveness. In a large study of 1001 patients, the greatest success with the KD was in the 2- to 5-year-old age group (23). Freeman reported similar results for this age group, concluding that the efficacy of the KD was particularly prominent in this age range because these children were able to produce the most pronounced levels of ketonemia and adhered to the diet's exacting regimen most closely (25). Prospective clinical studies report that 50–54% children aged 3–16 years exhibited a >50% reduction in the number of seizures after 1 year (25,26,30).

However, recent studies attest to the KD's effectiveness across a wider age range. In 32 infants <2 years of age, 55% of exhibited a >50% reduction in the number of seizures (66). The KD appears to be effective in adults as well (67). Of 11 patients aged 19–45 years with refractory epilepsy, the KD produced a sustained ketosis and afforded a seizure reduction of >50% in six of the patients (68).

Compliance with the KD regimen directly affects its efficacy. In 150 children, the relationship among age, compliance with the KD regimen (i e., tolerance), and KD efficacy was examined (25). Sixty-eight percent of all children less than 5 years old remained on the diet for 1 year, whereas 49% of children 6–16 years old were still on the diet after the same time. The authors concluded that retention time on the diet was not principally affected by age at onset; rather, the most common reason why the diet was discontinued was lack of efficacy. If there was significant seizure control, the diet was more likely to be continued. However, it follows that if older children are less likely to be protected from seizures with a KD, they are then also less likely to continue on the diet. Therefore, it is difficult to tease apart how these three inextricably linked variables are related—i.e., to remove the more behavioral and psychological aspects of compliance from the physiological variables of age and KD responsiveness.

Experimentally, compliance issues can be circumvented, and the effect of age is an independent, controllable variable. To date, only a few animal studies have directly investigated the effects of age at diet onset on KD efficacy. Despite various diet types, duration of diet treatments, and seizure testing methods, all of the studies concluded that animals started on the diet at a younger age exhibited a greater level of seizure protection than those that started the diet at an older age (69–72). However, adult animals also exhibit an elevated seizure threshold (56,73,74). Therefore, while we may conclude that the efficacy of the KD is somewhat better at early ages, there is no reason to withhold its use in appropriately selected adult patients.

Is KD Efficacy Related to Ketonemia?

Ketonemia is an obvious consequence of the KD. Therefore, it would seem like a simple matter to determine the relationship between ketonemia and seizure control. However, this relationship has been difficult to establish. While several clinical studies have described positive correlations between ketonemia and seizure control, it is not clear whether ketosis is *sufficient* to explain seizure control. For children maintained on the KD for 3 or 6 months, the threshold BHB level for seizure control was about 4 mmol/L (75). However, correlation values at earlier and later time points are not known. Furthermore, it is unclear whether there is an inverse correlation between seizure frequency and BHB levels.

Of the 1001 patients treated by Livingston, only those that exhibited both pronounced ketonemia throughout treatment and appreciable loss of body weight during the fasting period responded favorably to the KD (23). Huttenlocher studied the relationship between BHB and seizure control using the MCT diet (13). Children with the highest plasma BHB concentrations had the greatest degree of seizure control. In addition, if ketosis was lost, seizures returned rapidly. A KD-fed 4-year-old boy developed a breakthrough seizure 45 min after ketosis was eliminated by intravenous glucose infusion (13). Others have reported similar results; even slight deviation from the KD regimen by increasing carbohydrates can result in loss of seizure control (76). Since hypoglycemia is infrequently found in KD-treated patients, it was concluded that the anticonvulsant effects of the KD were mediated by the action of BHB, AcAc, or both in the brain (5). Serum glucose is in the normal range in children on the KD, suggesting that the antiseizure effect is independent of glucose concentration and may be more related to the level of ketones or some other factor.

The possibility has been raised that acetone, a volatile ketone body, may be involved in the KD mechanism. When the concentration of ketone bodies in the brain was studied by ^{1}H magnetic resonance spectroscopy, there was a significant reduction of N-acetyl aspartate and creatine concentrations in gray matter in KD-treated epileptic patients compared to untreated patients with epilepsy and healthy controls (77). There was also a significant concentration of acetone in KD-treated epileptic patients versus controls, but no detectable BHB or AcAc levels. In rats, breath acetone has been successfully monitored, and correlates with systemic ketosis (78). Given the poor correlation of urinary ketones with serum ketone levels, the possibility that breath acetone could provide a reliable measure of serum ketones is intriguing.

Findings from all of the above clinical reports, however, are taken from human patients of various ages. Given that age at diet onset and ketonemia are negatively correlated (10,23,71), the effects of ketonemia may have been masked by the effects of age on KD efficacy (as discussed above). Indeed, experimental studies show that when age is controlled for, ketonemia is not positively correlated with the efficacy of the KD. In 270 rats maintained on KDs of various ratios (i.e., 1:1 to 9:1), rats fed diets of higher ketogenic ratios (i.e., larger proportion of fats by weight) had elevated levels of ketonemia, but failed to show a positive correlation to PTZ seizure threshold (79). In another study, the same investigators found that neither BHB nor age significantly influenced PTZ seizure threshold. Instead, body weight and ketogenic diet ratio (i.e., diet type) markedly affected seizure protection in rats (80).

The effects of qualitatively different KDs were studied in rats (81). For animals maintained on any of the three different types of KD (based on different types of fats), significantly fewer rats exhibited seizures after PTZ than did control-fed animals. Ketone levels for the different dietary groups were markedly different and did not correlate with seizure thresholds, however, leading to the conclusion that ketonemia and seizure control were not correlated.

Other data also indicate a lack of correlation between ketonemia and seizure control. Clinical reports (22,82,83) and experimental results (56) indicate that the KD does not become maximally efficacious for at least 10 days after KD initiation.

Conversely, ketonemia develops within 48–72 h of fasting and the KD regimen is begun (30,82). These findings indicate that ketonemia may be *necessary but not sufficient* for KD-induced seizure control (7,84). Hence, it seems clear that ketonemia is not necessarily the best predictor of KD success.

Of course, it is possible that the concentration of ketone bodies in the blood may not accurately reflect their concentration in the brain. Since ketone bodies are transported across the blood-brain barrier by a family of monocarboxylate transporter proteins (MCT-1 and -2), transport could be saturated as high concentrations of ketone bodies approach V_{max} (43). To more appropriately evaluate KD efficacy it would be better to consider correlative measurements of brain levels of ketones (45,77).

In summary, it seems clear that some "threshold level" of ketosis is required and must be maintained for the KD to be maximally effective. Whether seizure control correlates with ketone levels remains a vexing question. The clinical goal should be to maintain serum ketonemia, with the assumption that brain ketone levels are proportionate.

Does Calorie Restriction Affect KD Efficacy?

Ever since the KD was designed, some degree of calorie restriction has been part of the protocol. The scientific rationale underlying this practice is that calorie restriction enhances the ketotic state. Fasting (the most radical form of calorie restriction) improves seizures (41,85). Therefore, the question arises as to whether calorie restriction alone is *sufficient* to afford seizure protection.

Typically, children on the KD are restricted to 75% of the recommended daily allowance (RDA) for their ideal weight and height, but this is flexible, and depends on the child's basal metabolic rate, age, and activity level. This caloric intake allows linear growth to occur, but prevents the child from gaining significant weight. There is clinical evidence that calorie restriction is not *required* for seizure protection, and KDs have been administered successfully using diets with and without calorie restriction. However, calorie restriction facilitates ketosis and may have an antiseizure effect independent of ketosis.

In laboratory models of the KD, a variety of calorie regimens have been investigated. Whether rats are fed diets that are hypocaloric (71), eucaloric (56), "slightly more" than eucaloric (81), or even ad libitum (74), the KD has been shown to increase the resistance to seizures induced by various means. However, calorie restriction by itself also significantly increases seizure threshold experimentally. Rats maintained on a normal, calorie-restricted diet exhibited a significantly elevated PTZ seizure threshold compared to animals fed the same normal diet ad libitum (63,86). Furthermore, rats maintained on a calorie-restricted KD exhibited a significantly elevated PTZ seizure threshold compared to animals fed a ketogenic ad libitum diet. PTZ seizure thresholds for the respective diet treatments could be ranked in the following manner: ketogenic calorie restricted > normal calorie restricted > ketogenic ad libitum > normal ad libitum (63). These data suggest that calorie restriction can significantly influence seizure threshold and may augment the effects of KD treatment.

Additionally, there is accumulating evidence that calorie restriction reduces brain damage following excitotoxic and metabolic insults (87–89). The mechanism by which calorie restriction reduces the likelihood of seizures may relate to an effect on blood glucose (86). The energy demands during a seizure are met primarily through glycolysis, so less glucose availability from glycolysis could allow less generation and maintenance of paroxysmal activity. Notably, in children on the KD, blood glucose levels are typically normal (5,30).

It is unknown why calorie resxtriction is so important to the KD effect. Perhaps calorie restriction facilitates and maintains the metabolic state induced by KD by ensuring that gluconeogenesis is limited during KD treatment. Although the potential adverse effects of restricting calories during a child's critical periods of growth and development must be weighed against the benefits of seizure control and improved long-term outcome, calorie restriction seems to be an important variable in the successful administration of the diet. It should be noted that ingestion of excess calories of any type might result in gluconeogenesis and decreased KD efficacy.

Does Diet Type Affect KD Efficacy?

A persistent clinical and research question is whether variation in lipid composition or ratio relates to degrees of KD efficacy. Fats are essential for the development of ketosis. In clinical use, the optimal quantity and type of fat have not been delineated. Typically, a KD includes fats of all chain lengths, most often in the form of heavy cream and butter. The fats in the classic KD consist of a mixture of animal- and plant-derived fats; fatty acids of varying chain lengths are likely to be included, but no attempt is made to specify fat type or chain length. An exception, of course, is the MCT diet, where oils containing triglycerides of medium chain length are the main source of fat. In the classic KD, long-chain saturated fatty acids likely predominate. Therefore, the classic KD may have a relative dearth of long-chain polyunsaturated fatty acids (PUFAs). This distribution of fats is important because of the critical roles played by PUFAs in brain development and in the modulation of excitability (90–92). Given the effects of PUFAs on the excitability of several types of excitable tissue, including neurons (93) and cardiac myocytes (94), it is possible that a KD with a higher PUFA content might improve the diet's effectiveness.

Clinical studies have shown that both the MCT and classic KD both confer similar levels of seizure control (10,30). In a clinical study, there was a positive correlation between plasma lipids and seizure control in epileptic children treated with the KD (82). The temporal elevation of plasma lipids peaked as KD-induced seizure control became maximal (i.e., 10–12 days). These data led to the conclusion that lipids are positively associated with seizure control.

Experimental studies in rats have yielded similar findings. Young rats (postnatal day 20) were fed a variety of qualitatively different types of diets, including butter, flaxseed oil, MCT, and a mixture of fat types, or a control diet (81). The butter, flaxseed oil, and MCT KDs all resulted in similar levels of seizure protection, although the mixed diet did not. In another study from the same laboratory, fatty acid profiles were similar in the brains of rats fed any of the above fat combinations (95). The authors concluded that qualitative differences (i.e., different sources of fats) in the KD do not markedly affect seizure control.

Increasing the dietary ratio of fats:[carbohydrates + proteins], however, can improve seizure control clinically (5) and experimentally (79,80). Higher diet ratios produce greater levels of ketonemia (79), but, as discussed above, there was no correlation between ketonemia and KD efficacy.

In general, these findings indicate that increasing the diet ratio (the quantity of fats, not the type of fat) has a greater influence on KD efficacy. However, the prospect that specific fat types (e.g., PUFAs) may be clinically efficacious is suggested by a recent clinical trial (96). In five patients, enrichment of the diet with omega-3 fatty acids reduced seizure frequency and intensity over a 6-month period. This study involved institutionalized adolescents and young adults, and did not include a control group or a washout period. Nevertheless, these intriguing results support laboratory investigations (92) and lend credence to the idea that alteration of dietary fats can lead to seizure improvement. There is a pressing need for further research and clinical trials in this area.

What Is the Effect of Other AEDs on KD Efficacy?

In the clinical setting, the KD is often used as the last resort for medically refractory epilepsy. Most patients beginning the KD have had exhaustive trials of AEDs. For example, in a large prospective study, the 150 children had previously been on an average of more than six medications (25). If the KD was successful, many children were able to discontinue or at least reduce their AEDs, with a corresponding decrease in sedation and other side effects. However, few data are available as to which AED, if any, is best utilized in conjunction with the KD.

This question is difficult to decipher clinically, but is approachable in the laboratory. Recently, Bough and colleagues placed rats on the KD plus various combinations of the standard anticonvulsants phenytoin and valproic acid (97). Using the PTZ infusion threshold and maximal electroshock models, they showed that the best seizure protection was obtained with a combination of valproic acid and the ketogenic diet (summarized in Table 2), suggesting a possible synergistic effect. The clinical relevance of these observations remains to be determined, but many children beginning the KD are already on valproic acid. Caution with this combination of treatments is well recognized (98), but this is not an absolute contraindication.

The timing of AED discontinuation, once the KD is working, is another decision that must be made without the benefit of solid clinical data. The goal is to maintain the KD for 2 years or until the patient is seizure-free off medications

Table 2. Effects of Anticonvulsants and the Ketogenic Diet on Seizures in Rats

	Seizure Induction Method	
	Maximal electroshock	Pentylenetetrazole
Valproic acid	Protective	Protective
Ketogenic diet	Not protective	Protective
Phenytoin	Protective	Not protective
Valproic acid + ketogenic diet	Not checked	Better protection than either treatment alone

Source: Ref. 97.

for 1 year (5). The best clinical advice is to ensure that the KD is working, and then slowly wean AEDs, one at a time.

What Are the Complications and Contraindications to Use of the KD?

With this unusual dietary regimen, adverse effects can occur. Some, such as constipation, are readily managed, while others are more serious. In some series, up to 10% of patients develop complications, the most severe of which (including hypoproteinemia and liver toxicity) occurred in children treated concurrently with valproic acid (98). Renal calculi develop in 5–10% of patients (99,100), but fortunately, this problem usually responds well to conservative treatment such as fluids and urine alkalinization. Most of the stones are urate or calcium oxalate; monitoring the urine calcium-to-creatinine ratio is a useful measure as to when more aggressive measures are indicated. Growth must be monitored carefully (101), and children are supplemented with essential vitamins and minerals (5). Other potential complications include pancreatitis (102), cardiac abnormalities (103), and platelet dysfunction (104). However, with careful monitoring, the majority of children do very well on the KD (5).

In addition to those complications, many of which are manageable, it is possible that some children experience severe, idiosyncratic reactions when placed on the KD. Physicians must be especially aware of metabolic disorders that may be worsened by the KD, such as porphyria, pyruvate carboxylase deficiency, carnitine deficiency, fatty acid oxidation disorders, and mitochondrial cytopathies (12). In many of these disorders, which involve alteration in energy regulation, fasting can precipitate severe neurologic dysfunction. Since carnitine is required for transport of long-chain fatty acids across the inner mitochondrial membrane, there is a theoretical concern that carnitine deficiency could be caused by or result from KD use (105). In the clinical setting, symptomatic carnitine deficiency is rarely seen with KD use (106). Before starting the KD, it would be prudent to obtain a metabolic screen, including urine amino and organic acids, serum amino acids, lactate, and carnitine profile (12).

There has been some concern about adverse cognitive effects of the KD, despite the clinical experience being overwhelmingly positive in this regard. Specifically, adults on the KD for weight loss performed poorer on some neuro-cognitive tasks than did nontreated controls (107). Nevertheless, experimentally, kindled rats maintained on the KD performed similarly to controls in both Morris water maze and open-field tests (74). These findings suggest that the KD does not adversely affect spatial learning and memory, nor does it alter an animal's response to novel environments. Other experiments confirm that the KD does not produce neurobehavioral deficits. Rats fed a variety of different KDs (i.e., 3:1, 4:1, 5:1, etc.) performed similarly to ad libitum and calorie-restricted controls in a battery of behavioral tests (79). In comparison to acute administration of VPA and PHT, the KD did not exhibit any neurobehavioral side effects, whereas adverse behavioral changes were seen with high doses of both VPA and PHT (alone or in combination with KD) (97). These data support the conclusion that the KD does not induce cognitive side effects.

Overall, both clinical and experimental findings indicate that the KD is worth considering for cases of intractable epilepsy, once metabolic contraindications are excluded.

Are the Effects of the KD Anticonvulsant, Antiepileptic, or Both?

The anticonvulsant profile of the KD involves a wide spectrum of activity. Although research has focused on the acute effects of ketosis on seizure thresholds, questions with more realistic clinical relevance would be how the KD affects long-term seizure occurrence and whether it alters epileptogenesis (processes by which the brain develops into an epileptic condition).

Clinically, there are anecdotal reports of antiepileptogenicity and long-term efficacy after diet treatment (5,23). Evidence that the KD might be antiepileptogenic, as well as anticonvulsant, comes from the observation that children can be gradually weaned off the KD, and a normal diet can be reintroduced without a concomitant loss of seizure control (5). It is unclear whether this is related to natural spontaneous remission, to some prolonged or permanent effect that outlasts KD treatment, or to some other factor.

Experimentally, the KD may inhibit the development of spontaneous seizures in rats. Two days after kainic acid–induced status epilepticus, rats were put onto a 4:1 KD or a normal diet (108). KD-fed animals exhibited ~75% fewer spontaneous seizures over the ensuing 8 weeks. Compared to controls, KD-fed animals had ~50% less sprouting of hippocampal mossy fibers. These findings suggest that the KD can retard the development of both abnormally reorganized synaptic circuitry (mossy fiber sprouting) and functional sequalae (spontaneous seizures) that are typically seen following kainic acid–induced status epilepticus. However, this protective effect was seen only if the KD was started within 2 weeks after status epilepticus, suggesting that there is a time window of opportunity for KD effectiveness (109).

Additional evidence that the KD can prevent epileptogenesis was found in knockout mice lacking the Kv1.1 potassium channel subunit. In these mice, spontaneous seizures occur during development (110), and histologically, mossy fiber sprouting occurs. Treatment of the mice with an experimental KD suppressed mossy fiber sprouting (111), providing another model in which the KD inhibits the development of the epileptic state.

SUMMARY

The KD appears to induce a unique physiologic and metabolic state that somehow dampens aberrant neuronal excitability and results in seizure control in individuals with refractory epilepsy. We are only beginning to sort out the critical variables involved in understanding how the KD exerts its anticonvulsant, and perhaps antiepileptic, effect. Many clinical questions remain, as discussed throughout this review. An improved understanding of the underlying mechanisms of KD action would not only aid in the development of novel anticonvulsant or antiepileptic treatments but would enhance our understanding of how bioenergetic changes, reflecting altered metabolism, modulate neuronal excitability. Using a combination

Table 3.   Principles and Clinical Applications of the Ketogenic Diet[a]

Principles	Clinical Applications
1. Seizure types	The KD is worth trying in refractory epilepsy, regardless of seizure/epilepsy type, though it may work best in the generalized epilepsies.
2. Optimal age range	The KD is worth trying at any age.
3. Role of ketonemia	It is important to maintain ketosis in any patient on the KD; ketosis is necessary for seizure control, but the correlation is inexact.
4. Fasting	Fasting allows a quicker attainment of ketosis.
5. Calorie restriction	Most practitioners restrict calories to 75% of the RDA, but this guideline is flexible, based on the patient's age, weight, and activity level.
6. Fluid restriction	Fluids are usually limited to 75 cc/kg/d; the role of this mild dehydration in seizure control is unknown.
7. Diet type	a. The classical 4:1 diet is preferred. b. A ratio >4:1 might theoretically afford better seizure control, but this is often impractical. c. At this time, there is insufficient evidence to recommend specific fat types.
8. Contraindications	Before KD initiation, it is recommended that screening be performed for metabolic disorders that may be exacerbated by the KD (see text).
9. Adjunctive medications	a. There are insufficient data to recommend specific adjunctive AEDs. b. There are no data to guide decisions as to when to discontinue AEDs.

[a]Derived from clinical and laboratory studies.

of clinical and laboratory research, we will hopefully improve the KD's utilization and effectiveness. Until such information becomes available, the principles outlined in Table 3 provide general clinical guidelines for using the KD.

ACKNOWLEDGMENT

We thank Steve Kriegler, Ph.D., for assistance with figure preparation.

REFERENCES

1. Wilder RM. The effects of ketonemia on the course of epilepsy. Mayo Clin Proc 1921; 2:307–308.
2. Wheless JW. The ketogenic diet: fa(c)t or fiction. J Child Neurol 1995; 10:419–423.
3. Swink TD, Vining EPG, Freeman JM. The ketogenic diet: 1997. Adv Pediatr 1997; 44:297–329.
4. Prasad AN, Stafstrom CE. Dietary therapy of epilepsy in the nineties: renewed experience with the ketogenic diet. Nutr Res 1998; 18:403–416.
5. Freeman JM, Freeman JB, Kelly MT. The Ketogenic Diet—A Treatment for Epilepsy, 3rd ed. New York: Demos Publications, 2000.

6. Wheless JW, Baumgartner J, Ghanbari C. Vagus nerve stimulation and the ketogenic diet. Neurol Clin North Am 2001; 19:371–407.

7. Stafstrom CE, Spencer S. The ketogenic diet: a therapy in search of an explanation. Neurology 2000; 54:282–283.

8. Schwartzkroin P. Mechanisms underlying the anti-epileptic efficacy of the ketogenic diet. Epilepsy Res 1999; 37:171–180.

9. Huttenlocher PR, Wilbourn AJ, Signore JM. Medium-chain triglycerides as a therapy for intractable childhood epilepsy. Neurology 1971; 21:1097–1103.

10. Schwartz RM, Boyes S, Aynsley-Green A. Metabolic effects of three ketogenic diets in the treatment of intractable epilepsy. Dev Med Child Neurol 1989; 31:152–160.

11. Freeman JM, Vining EPG. Seizures decrease rapidly after fasting: preliminary studies of the ketogenic diet. Arch Pediatr Adolesc Med 1999; 153:946–949.

12. Wheless JW. The ketogenic diet: an effective medical therapy with side effects. J Child Neurol 2001; 16:633–635.

13. Huttenlocher PR. Ketonemia and seizures: metabolic and anticonvulsant effects of two ketogenic diets in childhood epilepsy. Pediatr Res 1976; 10:536–540.

14. Hemingway C, Freeman JM, Pillas DJ, Pyzik PL. The ketogenic diet: a 3- to 6-year follow-up of 150 children enrolled prospectively. Pediatrics 2001; 108:898–905.

15. DeVivo DC, Trifiletti RR, Jacobson RI, Ronen GM, Behmand RA, Harik SI. Defective glucose transport across the blood-brain barrier as a cause of persistent hypoglycorrhachia, seizures, and developmental delay. N Engl J Med 1991; 325:703–709.

16. Boles RG, Seashore MR, Mitchell WG, Kollros PR, Mofidi S, Novotny EJ. Glucose transporter type 1 deficiency: a study of two cases with video-EEG. Eur J Pediatr 1999; 158:978–983.

17. Wexler ID, Hemalatha SG, McConnell J, Buist NRM, Dahl H-IIM, Berry SA, Cedarbaum SD, Patel MS, Kerr DS. Outcome of pyruvate dehydrogenase deficiency treated with ketogenic diets. Neurology 1997; 49:1655–1661.

18. Wijburg FA, Barth PG, Bindoff LA, Birch-Machin MA, Van der Blij JF, Ruitenbeek W, Turnbull DM, Schutgens RB. Leigh syndrome associated with a deficiency of the pyruvate dehydrogenase complex: results of treatment with a ketogenic diet. Neuropediatrics 1992; 23:147–152.

19. Nordli DR, DeVivo DC. The ketogenic diet revisited: back to the future. Epilepsia 1997; 38:743–749.

20. LeFever F, Aronson N. Ketogenic diet for the treatment of refractory epilepsy in children: a systematic review of efficacy. Pediatrics 2000; 105(4):www.pediatrics.org/cgi/content/full/105/4/e46.

21. Peterman MG. The ketogenic diet in epilepsy. JAMA 1925; 84:1979–1983.

22. Helmholz HF, Keith HM. Eight years' experience with the ketogenic diet in the treatment of epilepsy. JAMA 1930; 95:707–709.

23. Livingston S. Dietary treatment of epilepsy. In: Livingston S, ed. Comprehensive Management of Epilepsy in Infancy, Childhood and Adolescence. Springfield, IL: Charles C. Thomas, 1972:378–405.

24. Kinsman SL, Vining EPG, Quaskey SA, Mellits D, Freeman JM. Efficacy of the ketogenic diet for intractable seizure disorders: review of 58 cases. Epilepsia 1992; 33:1132–1136.

25. Freeman J, Vining E, Pillas D, Pryzik P, Casey J, Kelly M. The efficacy of the ketogenic diet—1998: a prospective evaluation of intervention in 150 children. Pediatrics 1998; 102:1358–1363.

26. Vining E, Freeman JM, Ballaban-Gil K, Camfield C, Camfield P, Holmes G, Shinnar S, Shuman R, Trevathan E, Wheless JW. A multicenter study of the efficacy of the ketogenic diet. Arch Neurol 1998; 55:1433–1437.

27. Kaytal NG, Koehler AN, McGhee B, Foley CM, Crumrine PK. The ketogenic diet in refractory epilepsy: the experience of Children's Hospital of Pittsburgh. Clin Pediatr 2000; 39:153–159.

28. Magrath G, MacDonald A, Whitehouse W. Dietary practices and use of the ketogenic diet in the UK. Seizure 2000; 9:128–130.

29. Coppola G, Veggiotti P, Cusmai R, Bertoli S, Cardinali S, Dionisi-Vici C, Elia M, Lispi ML, Sarnelli C, Tagliabue A, Toraldo C, Pascotta A. The ketogenic diet in children, adolescents and young adults with refractory epilepsy: an Italian multicentric experience. Epilepsy Res 2002; 48:221–227.

30. Schwartz RM, Eaton J, Bower BD, Aynsley-Green A. Ketogenic diets in the treatment of epilepsy: short term clinical effects. Dev Med Child Neurol 1989; 31:145–151.

31. Pulsifer M, Gordon J, Vining E, Freeman J. Effects of the ketogenic diet on development and behavior: preliminary report of a prospective study. Dev Med Child Neurol 2001; 43:301–306.

32. Stafstrom CE. Animal models of the ketogenic diet: what have we learned, what can we learn? Epilepsy Res 1999; 37:241–259.

33. Sokoloff L. Metabolism of ketone bodies by the brain. Annu Rev Med 1973; 24:271–279.

34. Robinson AM, Williamson DH. Physiological role of ketone bodies as substrates and signals in mammalian tissues. Physiol Rev 1980; 60:143–187.

35. Sankar R, Sotero de Menezes M. Metabolic and endocrine aspects of the ketogenic diet. Epilepsy Res 1999; 37:191–201.

36. Yudkoff M, Daikhin Y, Nissim I, Lazarow A, Nissim I. Ketogenic diet, amino acid metabolism, and seizure control. J Neurosci Res 2001; 66:931–940.

37. Saudek CD, Felig P. The metabolic events of starvation. Am J Med 1976; 60:117–126.

38. McGarry JD, Foster DW. Regulation of hepatic fatty acid oxidation and ketone body production. Annu Rev Biochem 1980; 49:395–420.

39. Owen OE, Morgan AP, Kemp HG, Sullivan JM, Herrera MG, Cahill J. Brain metabolism during fasting. J Clin Invest 1967; 46:1589–1595.

40. DeVivo DC, Leckie MP, Ferrendelli JS, McDougal DB. Chronic ketosis and cerebral metabolism. Ann Neurol 1978; 3:331–337.

41. DeVivo DC, Malas KL, Leckie MP. Starvation and seizures. Arch Neurol 1975; 32:755–760.

42. Moore T, Lione A, Sugden M, Regen D. Hydroxybutyrate transport in rat brain: developmental and dietary modulations. Am J Physiol 1976; 230:619–630.

43. Pellerin L, Pellegri G, Martin J-L, Magistretti PJ. Expression of monocarboxylate transporter mRNAs in mouse brain: support for a distinct role of lactate as an energy substrate for the neonatal vs. adult brain. Proc Natl Acad Sci USA 1998; 95: 3990–3995.

44. Leino RL, Gerhart DZ, Duelli R, Enerson BE, Drewes LR. Diet-induced ketosis increases monocarboxylate transporter (MCT1) levels in rat brain. Neurochem Int 2001; 38:519–527.

45. Pan JW, Rothman DL, Behar KL, Stein DT, Hetherington HP. Human brain beta-hydroxybutyrate and lactate increase in fasting-induced ketosis. J Cereb Blood Flow Metab 2000; 20:1502–1507.

46. Pan JW, Telang FW, Lee JH, DeGraaf RA, Rothman DL, Stein DT, Hetherington HP. Measurement of beta-hydroxybutyrate in acute hyperketonemia in human brain. J Neurochem 2001; 79:539–544.

47. Hawkins RA, Williamson DH, Krebs HA. Ketone-body utilization by adult and suckling rat brain in vivo. Biochem J 1971; 122:13–18.

48. Dahlquist G, Persson U, Persson B. The activity of D-beta-hydroxybutyrate dehydrogenase in fetal, infant and adult rat brain and the influence of starvation. Biol Neonate 1972; 20:40–50.

49. Kraus H, Schlenker S, Schwedesky D. Developmental changes of cerebral ketone body utilization in human infants. Hoppe-Seylers Z Physiol Chem 1974; 355:164–170.

50. Nehlig A. Age-dependent pathways of brain energy metabolism: the suckling rat, a natural model of the ketogenic diet. Epilepsy Res 1999; 37:211–221.

51. Arakawa T, Goto T, Okada Y. Effect of ketone body (D-3-hydroxybutyrate) on neural activity and energy metabolism in hippocampal slices of the adult guinea pig. Neurosci Lett 1991; 130:53–56.

52. Yang B, Sakurai T, Takata T, Yokono K. Effects of lactate/pyruvate on synaptic plasiticity in the hippocampal dentate gyrus. Neurosci Res 2003; 46:333–337.

53. Izumi Y, Ishii K, Katsuki H, Benz AM, Zorumski CF. Beta-hydroxybutyrate fuels synaptic function during development: histological and physiological evidence in rat hippocampal slices. J Clin Invest 1998; 101:1121–1132.

54. Cullingford TE, Dolphin CT, Bhakoo KK, Peuchen S, Canevari L, Clark JB. Molecular cloning of rat mitochondrial 3-hydroxy-3-methylglutaryl-coA lyase and detection of the corresponding mRNA and of those encoding the remaining enzymes comprising the ketogenic 3-hydroxy-3-methylglutaryl-coA cycle in central nervous system of the suckling rat. Biochem J 1998; 329:373–381.

55. Bouchard L, Robert MF, Vinarov D, Stanley CA, Thompson GN, Morris A. Mitochondrial 3-hydroxy-3-methylglutaryl-CoA synthase deficiency: clinical course and description of causal mutations in two patients. Pediatr Res 2001; 49:326–331.

56. Appleton DB, DeVivo DC. An animal model for the ketogenic diet. Epilepsia 1974; 15:211–217.

57. Pan J, Bebin E, Chu W, Hetherington H. Ketosis and epilepsy:[31]P spectroscopic imaging at 4.1T. Epilepsia 1999; 40:703–707.

58. Erecinska M, Nelson D, Daikhin Y, Yudkoff M. Regulation of GABA level in rat synaptosomes: fluxes through enzymes of the GABA shunt and effects of glutamate, calcium, and ketone bodies. J Neurochem 1996; 67:2325–2334.

59. Al-Mudallal AS, LaManna JC, Lust WD, Harik SI. Diet-induced ketosis does not cause cerebral acidosis. Epilepsia 1996; 37:258–261.

60. Yudkoff M, Daikhin Y, Nissim I, Lazarow A, Nissim I. Brain amino acid metabolism and ketosis. J Neurosci Res 2001; 66:272–281.

61. Maydell BV, Wyllie E, Akhtar N, Kotagal P, Powaski K, Cook K, Weinstock A, Rothner AD. Efficacy of the ketogenic diet in focal versus generalized seizures. Pediatr Neurol 2001; 25:208–212.

62. White HS. Clinical significance of animal seizure models and mechanism of action studies of potential antiepileptic drugs. Epilepsia 1997; 38(suppl 1):S9–S17.

63. Bough KJ, Matthews PJ, Eagles DA. A ketogenic diet has different effects upon seizures induced by maximal electroshock and by pentylenetetrazole infusion. Epilepsy Res 2000; 38:105–114.

64. Thavendiranathan P, Mendonca A, Dell C, Likhodii S, Musa K, Iracleous C, Cunnane SC, Burnham WM. The MCT ketogenic diet: effects on animal seizure models. Exp Neurol 2000; 161:696–703.

65. Szot P, Weinshenker D, Rho JM, Storey TW, Schwartzkroin PA. Norepinephrine isrequired for the anticonvulsant effect of the ketogenic diet. Dev Brain Res 2001; 129:211–214.

66. Nordli DR, Kuroda MM, Carroll J, Koenigsberger DY, Hirsch LJ, Bruner HJ, Seidel WT, DeVivo DC. Experience with the ketogenic diet in infants. Pediatrics 2001; 108:129–133.

67. Barborka CJ. Results of treatment by ketogenic diet in 100 cases. Arch Neurol Psychiatry 1930; 23:904–914.

68. Sirven J, Whedon B, Caplan D, Liporace J, Glosser D, O'Dwyer J, Sperling MR. The ketogenic diet for intractable epilepsy in adults: preliminary results. Epilepsia 1999; 40:1721–1726

69. Uhlemann ER, Neims AH. Anticonvulsant properties of the ketogenic diet in mice. J Pharm Exp Ther 1972; 180:231–238.

70. Otani K, Yamatodani A, Wada H, Mimaki T, Yabuuchi H. Effect of ketogenic diet on convulsive threshold and brain monoamine levels in young mice. No To Hattatsu 1984; 16:196–204.

71. Bough KJ, Valiyil R, Han FT, Eagles DA. Seizure resistance is dependent upon age and caloric restriction in rats fed a ketogenic diet. Epilepsy Res 1999; 35:21–28.

72. Rho J, Kim D, Robbins C, Anderson G, Schwartzkroin P. Age-dependent differences in flurothyl seizure sensitivity in mice treated with a ketogenic diet. Epilepsy Res 1999; 37:233–240.

73. Bough KJ, Eagles DA. A ketogenic diet increases the resistance to pentylenetetrazole-induced seizures in the rat. Epilepsia 1999; 40:138–143.

74. Hori A, Tandon P, Holmes GL, Stafstrom CE. Ketogenic diet: effects on expression of kindled seizures and behavior in adult rats. Epilepsia 1997; 38:750–758.

75. Gilbert DL, Pyzik PL, Freeman JM. The ketogenic diet: seizure control correlates better with serum beta-hydroxybutyrate than with urine ketones. J Child Neurol 2000; 15:787–790.

76. Freeman JM. The ketogenic diet and epilepsy. Nestle Nutr Worksh Ser Clin Perform Prog 2001; 5:307–321.

77. Seymour KJ, Bluml S, Sutherling J, Sutherling W, Ross BD. Identification of cerebral acetone by ^{1}H-MRS in patients with epilepsy controlled by ketogenic diet. MAGMA 1999; 8:33–42.

78. Likhodii SS, Musa K, Cunnane SC. Breath acetone as a measure of systemic ketosis assessed in a rat model of the ketogenic diet. Clin Chem 2002; 48:115–120.

79. Bough KJ, Yao SG, Eagles DA. Higher ketogenic diet ratios confer protection from seizures without neurotoxicity. Epilepsy Res 2000; 38:15–25.

80. Bough K, Chen R, Eagles D. Path analysis shows that increasing ketogenic ratio, but not beta-hydroxybutyrate, elevates seizure threshold in the rat. Dev Neurosci 1999; 21:400–406.

81. Likhodii SS, Musa K, Mendonca A, Dell C, Burnham WM, Cunnane SC. Dietary fat, ketosis, and seizure resistance in rats on the ketogenic diet. Epilepsia 2000; 41:1400–1410.

82. Dekaban AS. Plasma lipids in epileptic children treated with the high fat diet. Arch Neurol 1966; 15:177–184.

83. Dodson WE, Prensky AL, DeVivo DC, Goldring S, Dodge PR. Management of seizure disorders: selected aspects, Part II. J Pediatr 1976; 89:695–703.

84. Vining EPG. Clinical efficacy of the ketogenic diet. Epilepsy Res 1999; 37:181–190.

85. Geyelin H. Fasting as a method for treating epilepsy. Med Rec 1921; 99:1037–1039.

86. Greene AE, Todorova MT, McGowan R, Seyfried TN. Caloric restriction inhibits seizure susceptibility in epileptic EL mice by reducing blood glucose. Epilepsia 2001; 42:1371–1378.

87. Sohal RS, Weindruch RW. Oxidative stress, caloric restriction, and aging. Science 1996; 273:59–63.

88. Bruce-Keller A, Umberger G, McFall R, Mattson M. Food restriction reduces brain damage and improves behavioral outcome following excitotoxic and metabolic insults. Neurology 1999; 45:8–15.

89. Mattson MP, Duan W, Lee J, Guo Z. Suppression of brain aging and neurodegenerative disorders by dietary restriction and environmental enrichment: molecular mechanisms. Mech Ageing Dev 2001; 122:757–778.

90. Uauy R, Peirano P, Hoffman D, Mena P, Birch D, Birch E. Role of essential fatty acids in the function of the developing nervous system. Lipids 1996; 31(suppl): S167–S176.

91. Vreugdenhil M, Bruehl C, Voskuyl RA, Kang JX, Leaf A, Wadman WJ. Polyunsaturated fatty acids modulate sodium and calcium currents in CA1 neurons. Proc Natl Acad Sci USA 1996; 93:12559–12563.

92. Stafstrom CE. Effects of fatty acids and ketones on neuronal excitability: implications for epilepsy and its treatment. In: Mostofsky DI, Yehuda S, Salem N, eds. Fatty Acids—Physiological and Behavioral Functions. Totowa, NJ: Humana Press, 2001:273–290.

93. Xiao Y-F, Li X. Polyunsaturated fatty acids modify mouse hippocampal neuronal excitability during excitotoxic or convulsant stimulation. Brain Res 1999; 846:112–121.

94. Leaf A, Kang J, Xiao Y-F, Billman G, Voskuyl R. Functional and electrophysiologic effects of polyunsaturated fatty acids on excitable tissues: heart and brain. Prostaglandins Leukot Essent Fatty Acids 1999; 60:307–312.

95. Dell CA, Likhodii SS, Musa K, Ryan MA, Burnham WM, Cunnane SC. Lipid and fatty acid profiles in rats consuming different high-fat ketogenic diets. Lipids 2001; 36:373–378.

96. Schlanger S, Shinitzky M, Yam D. Diet enriched with omega-3 fatty acids alleviates convulsion symptoms in epilepsy patients. Epilepsia 2002; 43:103–104.

97. Bough KJ, Eagles DA. Comparison of the anticonvulsant efficacies and neurotoxic effects of valproic acid, phenytoin, and the ketogenic diet. Epilepsia 2001; 42: 1345–1353.

98. Ballaban-Gil K, Callahan C, O'Dell C, Pappo M, Moshe S, Shinnar S. Complications of the ketogenic diet. Epilepsia 1998; 39:744–748.

99. Herzberg GZ, Fivush BA, Kinsman SL, Gearhart JP. Urolithiasis associated with the ketogenic diet. J Pediatr 1990; 117:742–745.

100. Furth SL, Casey JC, Pyzik PL, Neu AM, Docimo SG, Vining EPG, Freeman JM, Fivush BA. Risk factors for urolithiasis in children on the ketogenic diet. Pediatr Nephrol 2000; 15:125–128.

101. Couch S, Schwarzman F, Carroll J, Koenigsberger D, Nordli D, Deckelbaum R, DeFelice AR. Growth and nutritional outcomes of children treated with the ketogenic diet. J Am Diet Assoc 1999; 99:1573–1575.

102. Stewart WA, Gordon K, Camfield P. Acute pancreatitis causing death in a child on the ketogenic diet. J Child Neurol 2001; 16:682.

103. Best TH, Franz DN, Gilbert DL, Nelson DP, Epstein MR. Cardiac complications in pediatric patients on the ketogenic diet. Neurology 2000; 54:2328–2330.

104. Berry-Kravis E, Booth G, Taylor A, Valentino LA. Bruising and the ketogenic diet: evidence for diet-induced changes in platelet function. Ann Neurol 2001; 49:98–103.

105. DeVivo DC, Bohan TP, Coulter DL, Dreifuss FE, Greenwood RS, Nordli DR, et al. L-Carnitine supplementation in childhood epilepsy: current perspectives. Epilepsia 1998; 39:1216–1225.

106. Berry-Kravis E, Booth G, Sanchez AC, Woodbury-Kolb J. Carnitine levels and the ketogenic diet. Epilepsia 2001; 42:1445–1451.

107. Wing R, Vazquez J, Ryan C. Cognitive effects of ketogenic weight-reducing diets. Int J Obes 1995; 19:811–816.

108. Muller-Schwarze AB, Tandon P, Liu Z, Yang Y, Holmes GL, Stafstrom CE. Ketogenic diet reduces spontaneous seizures and mossy fiber sprouting in the kainic acid model. NeuroReport 1999; 10:1517–1522.

109. Su SW, Cilio MR, Sogawa Y, Silveira D, Holmes GL, Stafstrom CE. Timing of ketogenic diet initation in an experimental epilepsy model. Dev Brain Res 2000; 125:131–138.
110. Rho JM, Szot P, Tempel BL, Schwartzkroin PA. Developmental seizure susceptibility of Kv1.1 potassium channel knockout mice. Dev Neurosci 1999; 21:320–327.
111. Rho JM, Robbins CA, Wenzel J, Tempel BL, Schwartzkroin PA. An experimental ketogenic diet promotes long-term survival and reduces synaptic reorganization in the hippocampus of epileptic Kv1.1 null mutant mice. Epilepsia 2000; 41(suppl 7):34.
112. Millichap JG, Jones JD, Rudis BP. Mechanism of anticonvulsant action of the ketogenic diet. Am J Dis Child 1964; 107:593–604.
113. Nakazawa M, Kodama S, Matsuo T. Effects of ketogenic diet on electroconvulsive threshold and brain contents of adenosine nucleotides. Brain Dev 1983; 5:375–380.
114. Todorova MT, Tandon P, Madore RA, Stafstrom CE, Seyfried TN. The ketogenic diet inhibits epileptogenesis in EL mice: a genetic model for idiopathic epilepsy. Epilepsia 2000; 41:933–940.

15
Vagus Nerve Stimulation

Dean K. Naritoku
Southern Illinois University
Springfield, Illinois, U.S.A.

INTRODUCTION

The development of vagus nerve stimulation (VNS) for the treatment of epilepsy has demonstrated well the translation of concepts gained through laboratory research into a clinical therapy. Information gained from clinical research has, in turn, generated important basic research questions resulting in new directions for laboratory studies. In clinical practice, trains of current are applied intermittently to the left vagus nerve using a pacemakerlike device (the Neurocybernetic Prosthesis, Cyberonics, Houston, TX). Randomized, double-blind controlled trials have established its efficacy for partial-onset seizures in human epilepsy, and open-label studies have suggested good efficacy for other seizure types. As will be discussed, laboratory studies have also suggested that modulation of the vagal system may be a therapeutic modality for other neurobiologic disorders, including depression, pain, and memory loss.

PRETRANSLATIONAL RESEARCH

The vagus nerve is a large cranial nerve with nuclei in the medulla of the brain. It conveys of a wide range of functions, including somatic and visceral afferent information, and motor and visceral efferent information, which control diverse functions, including phonation, cardiac autonomic regulation, gastric function, and somatic and visceral sensation. Although the vagal system is regarded as a brainstem system, it projects widely to the forebrain, suggesting it has widespread influence on forebrain function. Of relevance to epilepsy and other neurologic disorders, there are direct projections from the solitary nucleus to the limbic system, via the amygdala, and to other regulatory structures in the brainstem, including the serotonergic and noradrenergic nuclei (Fig. 1) (1,2).

The concept that sensory stimuli may modulate general cortical activity, and even seizures, has been long proposed. Gowers (3) believed that sensory stimuli may prevent seizures, and proposed applying ligatures, i.e., bands of cloth, to various

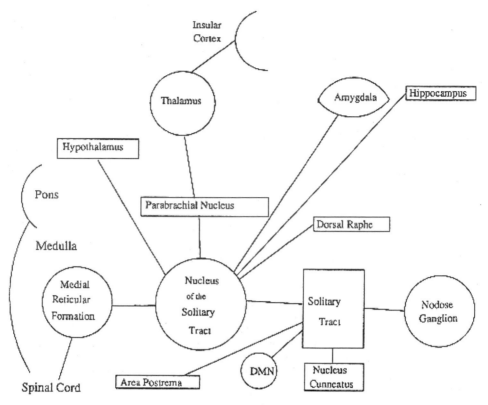

Figure 1. Schematic of efferent projections from the vagal system to the forebrain. The solitary nucleus is the primary afferent nucleus of the vagus nerve. It has widespread projections to the forebrain, either directly or indirectly through thalamic and brainstem monoaminergic nuclei. (From Ref. (1).)

parts of the body of persons with epilepsy. In Chinese medicine, pressure of a thumbnail applied to a patient's philtrum is believed to arrest seizures. Interestingly, a recent extensive review of literature from the 1800s had found carotid compression as a proposed therapy for epilepsy, and invention of devices to provide external compression and/or electrical stimulation of the vagus nerve (4). Penry described how sensory input could change the behavioral manifestations of absence seizures, and noted that these seizures could be arrested by tactile stimulation (5,6).

Neurophysiologic evidence that VNS may affect cortical function may be found in literature dating as far back as 1939, when Bailey and Bremer noted changes in the electrocorticogram of anesthetized cats upon stimulation of severed vagal nerves. Although the electrographic changes were attributed to VNS-induced hypotension, Zanchetti et al. in 1952 (7) demonstrated that this phenomenon could occur in the absence of systemic changes in cats that received spinal de-efferentation. Chase and Nakamura (8,9) demonstrated that different current and frequencies could cause either synchronization or desynchronization of EEG in anesthetized cats (see Fig. 2). Zabarra (10) postulated that the ability of VNS to desynchronize EEG activity could also arrest seizures, since they are presumably caused by hypersynchronous firing of neuronal populations. His initial studies demonstrated

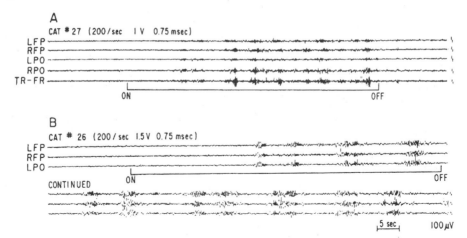

Figure 2. EEG changes with vagus nerve stimulation. The tracings are from an anesthetized cat receiving vagal stimulation. Chase et al. (9) demonstrated that in this preparation, either hypersynchronization or desynchronization could be elicited, depending on the voltage and current used.

dramatically VNS-induced arrest of convulsive activity in canine seizures induced by strychnine (Fig. 3). However, later studies found no acute desynchronization of electrocerebral activity during VNS in *awake* and freely moving rodents (11,12) or during clinical VNS in humans (13). It is therefore possible that the EEG changes described in anesthetized animals may be dependent anesthesia-induced unconsciousness and VNS-induced arousal. A small study of the effects on primates treated with topical brain convulsants attempted to look at long-term effects of VNS on seizures (14). This study suggested that VNS could suppress both ictal and interictal EEG abnormalities. Although the study was not of sufficient size to draw conclusions about efficacy, it was able to demonstrate safety of chronic electrical stimulation. Long-term observational studies in persons with epilepsy and abnormal slowing of EEG background have shown improvement in the frequency of spikes and reduction in slowing in responders (15).

Antiepileptic drug (AED) development has traditionally screened for potential therapies against standardized seizure models, which include administration of pentylenetetrazol (PTZ) or maximal electroshock (16) to mice or rats. Threshold convulsant doses of PTZ induce facial and forelimb convulsive seizures in rodents that are likely limbic in onset, whereas MES induces tonic seizures with hindlimb extension that probably originate in the brainstem. Woodbury and Woodbury demonstrated the ability of VNS to attenuate PTZ and MES-induced seizures (17,18). Interestingly, when VNS was administered early in the PTZ-induced seizure, marked abortive effects are observed, but if the stimulus was presented more than a few seconds after onset, there was little effect on total seizure duration. This suggested that the abortive effect was most effective if presented early. Anecdotal reports from patients receiving VNS, as well as analysis of self-reported data from clinical trials (19), also suggested that seizures may be terminated more readily if given early during the seizure.

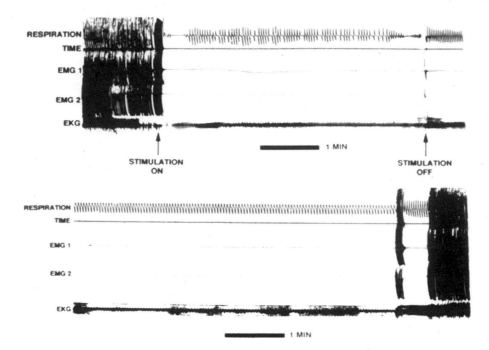

Figure 3. Abortion of strychnine-induced convulsions by vagus nerve stimulation. Zabarra (10) demonstrated the abortion of convulsive behavior using VNS. The tracings show motor (EMG) patterns induced by strychnine. Note the abrupt arrest of convulsive activity with application of VNS.

Other basic research efforts have examined extensively the role of the vagal afferent system in modulating neural systems that have strong implications for its use in other neurologic disorders. VNS acutely attenuates nociceptive pain in animals (20) and appears to inhibit neuronal firing in at least some structures, including the nucleus of the trigeminal nerve (21,22). A recent in vivo study demonstrated increases in slow afterhyperpolarization in cortical pyramidal cells of anesthetized rats (23). However, the effect was maximal with very small stimulation current of 0.1 mA and declined with even slightly higher current of 0.5 mA, raising the question of whether it is a clinically relevant phenomenon. The vagus nerve appears to mediate the effects of peripherally acting agents that modulate memory consolidation. In rats, functional inactivation or severing the vagus nerve blocks enhancement of memory consolidation normally induced by peripherally acting catecholamines, and electrical stimulation of the vagus nerve improves memory consolidation in rats given tasks (24). This effect appears to be mediated by the afferent vagal system, since inactivation of the vagus nerve proximal to the point of stimulation abolishes this effect (25).

TRANSLATION TO CLINICAL PRACTICE

In translating laboratory findings to the clinical setting, there are questions that cannot be answered in advance, which require a "leap of faith" to establish the proof of concept in humans. Key factors include the reliability of the animal model in predicting a response to the new therapy and conversion of dosing to humans. Physiologic differences between species may result in differences in efficacy and toxicity. Finally, interspecies differences raise questions of unseen adverse effects and safety issues. Thus, translation to a human study requires an initial "best guess" about dosing that will demonstrate efficacy with minimal or acceptable adverse effects, and allow resolution of outcomes between treatment groups. Unfortunately, the great expense associated with clinical studies, as well as limitations in research capital, often prohibit additional studies required to determine optimal dosing in humans.

At the time of initial human testing, the abortive effects of VNS on the acute seizure models of PTZ and MES were well established, but effects of VNS on other models of epilepsy were not established. Perhaps an ongoing major criticism of PTZ and MES is that they produce symptomatic seizures, rather than true, spontaneous seizures that define the epileptic state; the "goodness" of animal models of epilepsy has been the subject of recent reviews (26). However, the utility of simple models like PTZ and MES cannot be disputed. These screening methods boast a long track record of identifying successful AEDs, thus validating their utility to predict an antiepileptic effect.

Perhaps unique in medical device development, VNS therapy was subjected to rigorous clinical testing with blinded randomized, controlled clinical trials utilized in modern AED development. Following an initial open-label trial of VNS for epilepsy, there were two large multicenter randomized, double-blind active controlled trials for persons with medically intractable epilepsy with partial-onset seizures.

Although it was clear that VNS exerted an antiseizure effect in experimental models, it was not known what parameters would exert a therapeutic effect in human epilepsy or which parameters would be optimal. Animal studies focused on the abortive effects of VNS in acutely induced seizures. Thus, both induction of experimental seizures and timing of VNS were under direct control of the investigator. In clinical practice, accurate prediction of seizures to provide a "closed-loop" system was impractical with commercially available technology, thus prohibiting automatic application of the stimulus at seizure onset. A commercial pacemakerlike device developed for VNS (Neurocybenetic Prosthesis [NCP; Cyberonics, Houston, TX]) was designed to provide intermittent trains of stimulation at programmable preset intervals (Fig. 4). Other practical considerations included the duration of the nerve-electrode interface. Long-term loss of the interface, along with the potential for difficulty with replacement of the raised the question of whether successful therapy would be limited for mechanical reasons. Subsequent studies have shown a lack of nerve changes at postmortem examination (Cyberonics, data on file), and during electrode replacement (27).

Interestingly, currently established stimulation parameters in humans were selected primarily for practical reasons of patient comfort, safety of nerve stimulation, and battery life. Higher frequencies of 60–100 Hz were not tolerated in pilot clinical trials due to severe pain. More importantly, continuous chronic stimulation could lead to permanent nerve damage, and it was estimated that no more than a 50% duty cycle could be given using the currents and frequencies proposed (28). The high current consumption needed continuous stimulation would make an implantable device less practical, because of the need for frequent battery

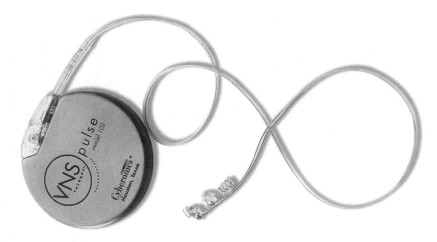

Figure 4. Human vagus nerve stimulator. Shown is the commercially available stimulator approved by the FDA for human use. The device is a pacemakerlike object, with attached leads and spiral elelctrodes that attach to the vagus nerve. (Photo courtesy of Cyberonics, Inc, Houston, TX.)

replacement. Thus, the decision to provide lower frequency, intermittent stimulation on a fixed cycle addressed these pragmatic issues, but represented a potential compromise of efficacy; at the time of clinical trial initiation, it was unclear if VNS would have an anticonvulsant effect if it did not occur during the time of the seizure. The stimulator device was designed so that patients could trigger a stimulus "on demand"; unfortunately, in practice only a minority of patients can trigger the device before loss of consciousness.

In two pivotal trials of VNS for epilepsy, intermittent electrical stimulation using 30-sec trains of current ("high" stimulation; 30 Hz, 500 µS pulse width, 5 min between trains, maximally tolerated current) were compared to "low" stimulation parameters (1 Hz, 130 µS pulse width, 180 min between trains, current set to perceived threshold) in a double-blinded manner. Self-triggering of the device using a magnet was allowed in the "high" group, to provide VNS "on demand," whereas no stimulation occurred with triggering in the "low" group. This demonstrated a significantly greater reduction of seizures efficacy in the "high" group. In both studies, the response rate—i.e., the percentage of patients achieving at least a 50% reduction in seizure frequency—was ~35% in patients receiving the higher stimulation parameters during the blinded phase (first 3 months) (29,30). Continued therapy during the open-label extension demonstrated a response in ~40% of patients. Furthermore, a steady improvement was seen over the following 12 months, suggesting a cumulative effect of VNS (31).

Established functions of the vagal system initially raised apprehensions about safety of VNS in human. In rats, there is a robust slowing of heart rate with stimulation of the left vagus nerve, which results in a relative hypotension. The first stimulation of human vagus nerve was performed with full resuscitation equipment on standby in the operating room, but was accomplished without complications.

Surprisingly, no patients in either of the pivotal trials or in open-label trials experienced significant bradycardia or hypotension (32). Prolonged EKG recording in humans using Holter monitor was performed on each patient prior to VNS and during VNS stimulation during the second pivotal study, and showed a lack of EKG changes. However, in postmarketing experience, rare instances of cardiac asystole have been described (33).

Other concerns included the potential for increased gastric acid secretion. Indeed, prior to the approval of histamine blockers for gastointestinal ulcers, left vagotomy was one of the most commonly performed surgical procedures. Direct measurement of gastric acid production was performed on a small number of patients and showed no increases in acid production. Serum gastrin was measured in all patients in the second pivotal study, and no significant changes occurred (30). These examples of lack of VNS-induced cardiac or gastric abnormalities underscore the unpredictable nature of translational medicine; our understanding of well-established physiologic mechanisms may not hold true in clinical applications, whether they are desired outcomes or adverse effects.

Retrospective studies and case series suggest VNS may also be useful for other seizure types and epilepsy syndromes. VNS appears to be effective for Lennox-Gastaut syndrome (30,34), which is characterized by poor response to medical therapy, multiple seizure types, and intellectual decline. The benign nature of VNS has largely supplanted corpus callosotomy as a surgical adjunct to medical therapy. Other series suggest efficacy against primarily generalized seizures. Overall efficacy may be better in patients with less intractable epilepsy; a postmarketing patient registry maintained by the manufacturer suggests that the response rate may be 50–60% in open label clinical use (35). However, the possibility that differences in data acquisition in an open registry are responsible for the improved numbers cannot be excluded.

TRANSLATION TO THE LABORATORY

The demonstrated efficacy of VNS against partial-onset seizure in humans indicated that VNS alters seizure genesis in forebrain structures. This finding immediately raised the question of which brain structures mediate the anticonvulsant effect and how VNS exerted its anticonvulsant effect. As previously outlined, there were few data to verify an electrophysiologic effect in human forebrain. VNS-induced EEG desynchrony was not demonstrated, and recording of a VNS-evoked potential was unsuccessful (36). There was modest prolongation of the subcortical-cortical (N20) potential in evoked potentials elicited from stimulation of median nerve in patients receiving VNS (37), suggesting a VNS-induced change in somatosensory neurotransmission, but visual or brainstem auditory evoked potentials were unchanged (36,37).

Takaya et al. identified VNS-induced changes in neural transmission in the forebrain by measuring Fos expression in rats receiving VNS with parameters used for epilepsy therapy (38). In this study, VNS induced immunolabeling in amygdala, hypothalamus, cingulate cortex, and hypothalamus in the forebrain, suggesting increases in neuronal activity in these structures. In the hindbrain, there was labeling of trigeminal sensory nucleus, and interestingly, of the A5 nucleus and locus coeruleus, suggesting activation of the noradrenergic system. Although the role of monoamines in epilepsy remains unclear, both serotonin and norepinephrine regulate seizure threshold in animal models (39,40). The production of Fos, which is an early intermediate gene product that promotes further gene transcription, raises the question of whether it may mediate sustained and long-term effects of VNS.

Metabolic mapping studies of the brain have yielded differing results, and likely reflect the conditions under which the studies were performed. Autoradiographic studies in rat, using radiolabeled 2-deoxyglucose, compared sham controls and stimulated anesthetized rats, receiving continuous stimulation for 1 h using anticonvulsant parameters (41). Interestingly, there were no areas of increased uptake. VNS induced no changes in several brain regions, and reductions of glucose uptake in several structures, most notably frontal cortex, hippocampus, and thalamus. In the brainstem, there were reductions of glucose uptake in solitary nucleus, which may be consistent with observations of Easton and colleagues that *inhibition* of the solitary nucleus with microinfusions of drugs is anticonvulsant (42).

An early positron emission tomography (PET) study by Ko et al. (43) utilized patients who had already received VNS for several months. During acute VNS, there were increases in blood flow in ipsilateral thalamus, contralateral parietal cortex, and ipsilateral cerebellum when compared to interstimulation states. However, the design of the study would not account for long-term or sustained changes incurred by the chronic VNS therapy. A more recent PET study by Henry et al. compared VNS-treated patients to their untreated baseline (44). Several areas of blood flow changes occurred during stimulation, but most importantly, increases of thalamic blood flow were correlated with VNS efficacy, suggesting that modulation of thalamic activity may be crucial to VNS effect (44). Interstimulation changes that may have occurred as a consequence of cumulative effects were not measured.

The clinical data also raised important questions about the temporal aspects of VNS with respect to seizure control. By using intermittent 30-sec stimulation at fixed intervals of 5 min, the probability that the stimulus would occur the onset of a seizure (30:300, or 10%) was lower than seizure efficacy observed. Although manual triggering of the device was possible, most patients did not routinely trigger the device. This raised the question of whether VNS exerts preventive, in addition to abortive, antiseizure effects.

The potential for sustained effects of VNS were addressed in laboratory studies by Takaya et al. in the rodent PTZ model (Fig. 5) (45). Animals were pretreated with VNS and stimulation was discontinued *prior* to PTZ administration. The findings verified that the anticonvulsive effects are not limited to the duration of stimulation; i.e., VNS exhibits antiepileptic effects. Increasing the duration of VNS stimulation caused progressive increases in seizure latency, with reductions in total number of seizures, seizure duration and seizure severity. These findings suggested that there is a cumulative effect of VNS, at least under acute conditions. This notion is attractive in light of long-term findings in clinical trials which show progressive improvement over the first year of treatment.

VNS appears to retard electrical kindling of the amygdala in rodents and felines, suggesting that it may have antiepileptogenic properties. Naritoku and Mikels demonstrated that the number of amygdalar stimulations required to reach class 5 seizures was increased when VNS was administered prior to each kindling session (46). Furthermore, the threshold current required to trigger an afterdischarge was significantly reduced in control animals, but in not animals treated with VNS,

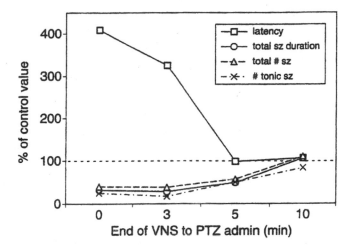

Figure 5. Effects of VNS duration on seizures. Pretreatment with VNS prior to pentylenetetrazol can block the induction of seizures, providing evidence for a sustained effect that persists after the end of stimulation. Shown in the diagram is the decay of the effect on seizure parameters. After 1 h of VNS, the animals were treated with pentylenetetrazol either immediately or 3 min, 5 min, or 10 min after the end of VNS. Note the return to control values by 10 min, suggesting that after an acute stimulation the effects diminish over that time period. (From Ref. 45.)

even after reaching class 5 seizures. VNS also reduced the duration of class 5 seizures once kindling had already been achieved in rodents (47). Fernandez-Guardiola et al. suggested that the effects of VNS on kindling, as well as its anticonvulsant effect, may relate to changes in sleep architecture (48). Malow et al. reported changes in sleep architecture in patients receiving VNS (49). However, changes in sleep cycles would not explain the efficacy of VNS on acutely induced seizures and therefore cannot explain fully the anticonvulsant and anticpileptic effect of VNS.

Laboratory studies have also focused on the potential mediation of VNS effect by the monoaminergic system. Krahl et al. found that by either destroying the serotonergic nuclei or lesioning the locus coeruleus with focal infusions of 6-hydroxydopamine could reverse the effects of VNS on MES-induced seizures (50). The activation of monoaminergic systems by VNS may be an especially important mechanism for clinical application in depression and memory disorders.

AREAS TO BE EXPLORED IN LABORATORY AND CLINICAL SETTINGS

Further research on the mechanisms of VNS is important for its neurobiologic implications. It represents the first approved therapy for brain disorders that clearly modulates large neuronal networks by electrical stimulation. Understanding how these networks are activated and regulated by stimulation will undoubtedly yield information that may allow further exploitation of the vagal network for other applications. Ultimately, information gained from such studies would develop paradigms for studying and utilizing other neural networks.

The efficacy of VNS in multiple seizure models suggests that it may be effective in a wide variety of seizure types in humans. To date, clinical efficacy has been established in partial-onset seizures in humans following two randomized, controlled trials, and against "drop attacks" and atypical absence seizures in open-label studies in patients with the Lennox-Gastaut syndrome. Whether VNS is effective in other types of primarily generalized seizures in humans remains to be studied.

There is a natural tendency to compare and contrast the potential mechanisms of VNS with other forms of neural stimulation, most notably deep brain stimulation (DBS). In current practice, VNS differs greatly from DBS. First, the stimulation paradigms are quite different. In the case of VNS, efficacy can be demonstrated using relatively lower frequencies of 20–30 Hz. In contrast, DBS uses a higher frequency, 100 Hz. Stimulation at 100 Hz may potentially induce a functional blockade of the nucleus, although this is currently under debate. At least some neurons may be able to fire at this rate. A stimulation frequency of 30 Hz clearly does not cause a conduction block of the peripheral vagus nerve, nor would it would be expected to cause a conduction block the afferent nuclei.

Other major differences in VNS compared to DBS are the targets for stimulation. At least for the present time, targets for DBS have been limited to brain nuclei directly involved with the seizure network, as identified by functional imaging of seizures (51). This includes structures such as the anterior nucleus (52) or centromedian nucleus of the thalamus (53). In contrast, the primary afferent system for VNS lies remotely from the sites of seizure genesis in forebrain. Presumably, VNS exerts its action by modulation of epileptic foci through large neuronal networks within the brain.

As with many therapies for epilepsy, VNS may have potential applications in other diseases of the central nervous system. A recent open-label pilot study showed a marked improvement of Hamilton Depression Rating Scores in patients with medically intractable depression (54). A subsequent randomized controlled trial did not show a significant improvement during short-term stimulation because of a high degree of variability (Cyberonics, data on file), but long-term follow up showed significant improvement in depression scores.

The findings of improved memory consolidation following VNS have been extended to human studies. A small randomized, double-blind controlled study performed in patients receiving VNS for intractable epilepsy studied the effects on consolidation of word recognition memory (55). VNS or sham stimulation was given to patients immediately after reading a block of words. There was a significant improvement in recall in patients receiving 0.5 mA stimulation, but not at higher or lower current levels, supporting laboratory findings of both VNS enhancement of memory and an inverted "U" function of response, related to intensity of current. Another study showed a VNS-induced decline, rather than improvement in memory functions in patients with epilepsy (56); however, the mean stimulation current was much higher, and thus consistent with intensity-dependent findings identified in animal and human studies. A small open-label trial of VNS in patients with Alzheimer's disease showed improvements in seven of 10 patients of the Alzheimer's Disease Assessment Scale cognitive subscale and Mini-Mental Exam, suggesting possible use of VNS in this disorder (57).

The use of VNS for pain management remains to be explored. Although there are extensive laboratory data to support use of VNS for pain, at present there are only a few small reports that suggest VNS may be useful in pain syndromes. A recent study measured pain perception in patients with epilepsy and demonstrated reduced nociception during VNS (58). A small retrospective case series in patients who had epilepsy with migraine has suggested VNS may reduce migraine headaches (59).

CONCLUSIONS

VNS represents an excellent example of parallel development and interchange between clinical and basic science. Its value to neurobiologic research extends beyond current applications for neurologic and psychiatric disorders. Understanding the complex interactions between the brainstem vagal system and the forebrain will undoubtedly identify neural mechanisms that may be leveraged for many brain disorders.

REFERENCES

1. Rutecki P. Anatomical, physiological, and theoretical basis for the antiepileptic effect of vagus nerve stimulation. Epilepsia 1990; 31(S2):S1–S6.
2. Schachter SC, Saper CB. Vagus nerve stimulation. Epilepsia 1998; 39(7):677–686.
3. Gowers WR. Epilepsy and Other Chronic Convulsive Diseases. London: J. and A. Churchill, 1881.
4. Lanska DJ. J.L. Corning and vagal nerve stimulation for seizures in the 1880s. Neurology 2002; 58:452–459.
5. Penry JK, Dreifuss FE. Automatisms associated with the absence of petit mal epilepsy. Arch Neurol 1969; 21:142–149.
6. Penry JK, Dreifuss FE. A study of automatisms associated with the absence of patit mal. Epilepsia 1969; 10:417–418.
7. Zanchetti A, Wang SC, Moruzzi G. The effects of vagal afferent stimulation on the EEG pattern of the cat. 1952; 5:357–361.
8. Chase MH, Sterman MB, Clemente CD. Cortical and subcortical patterns of response to afferent vagal stimulation. 1966; 16:36–49.
9. Chase MH, Nakamura Y, Clemente CD, Sterman MB. Afferent vagal stimulation: neurographic correlates of induced EEG synchronization and desynchronization. Brain Res 1967; 5:236–249.
10. Zabarra J. Inhibition of experimental seizures in canines by repetitive vagal stimulation. Epilepsia 1992; 33:1005–1012.
11. McLachlan RS. Suppression of interictal spikes and seizures by stimulation of the vagus nerve. Epilepsia 1993; 34:918–923.
12. Takaya M, Terry WJ, Naritoku DK. Pretreatment with vagus nerve stimulation (VNS) results in a sustained anticonvulsant effect. Epilepsia 1994; 35(S8):6.
13. Hammond EJ, Uthman BM, Reid SA, Wilder BJ. Electrophysiological studies of cervical vagus nerve stimulation in humans. I. EEG effects. Epilepsia 1992; 33:1013–1020.
14. Lockard JS, Congdon WC, DuCharme LL. Feasibility and safety of vagal stimulation in monkey model. Epilepsia 1990; 31(S):20–26.
15. Koo B. EEG changes with vagus nerve stimulation. J Clin Neurophysiol 2001; 18:434–441.
16. Krall RL, Penry JK, White BG, Kupferberg HJ, Swinyard EA. Antiepileptic drug development. II. Anticonvulsant drug screening. Epilepsia 1978; 19:409–428.
17. Woodbury DM, Woodbury JW. Effects of vagal stimulation on experimentally induced seizures in rats. Epilepsia 1990; 31(S):7–19.

18. Woodbury JW, Woodbury DM. Vagal stimulation reduces the severity of maximal electroshock seizures in intact rats: use of a cuff electrode for stimulating and recording. Pacing Clin Electrophysio 1991; 14:94–107.

19. Naritoku D, Willis J, Manon-Espillat R, Group NS. Patient-activated "therapeutic bursts" of stimulation delivered via the vagus nerve. Epilepsia 1992; 33(S3):102.

20. Randich A, Gebhart GF. Vagal afferent modulation of nociception. 1992; 17:77–99.

21. Fromm GH, Sun K. How does vagal nerve stimulation prevent seizures? Epilepsia 1993; 34(S6):52.

22. Bossut DF, Maixner W. Effects of cardiac vagal afferent electrostimulation on the responses of trigeminal and trigeminothalamic neurons to noxious orofacial stimulation. Pain 1996; 65:101–109.

23. Zagon A, Kemeny AA. Slow hyperpolarization in cortical neurons: a possible mechanism behind vagus nerve simulation therapy for refractory epilepsy? Epilepsia 2000; 41:1382–1389.

24. Clark KB, Krahl SE, Smith DC, Jensen RA. Post-training unilateral vagal stimulation enhances retention performance in the rat. Neurobiol Learn Mem 1995; 63:213–216.

25. Clark KB, Smith DC, Hassert DL, Browning RA, Naritoku DK, Jensen RA. Posttraining electrical stimulation of vagal afferents with concomitant vagal efferent inactivation enhances memory storage processes in the rat. Neurobiol Learn Mem 1998; 70:364–373.

26. Loscher W. Animal models of drug-resistant epilepsy. Novartis Found Symp 2002; 243:149–159; discussion 159–166, 180–185.

27. Espinosa J, Aiello MT, Naritoku DK. Revision and removal of stimulating electrodes following long-term therapy with the vagus nerve stimulator. 1999; 51:659–654.

28. Agnew WF, McCreery DB. Considerations for safety with chronically implanted nerve electrodes. Epilepsia 1990; 31(S2):S27–S32.

29. Ben-Menachem E, Mañon-Espaillat R, Ristanovic R. Vagus nerve stimulation for treatment of partial seizures: 1. A controlled study of effect on seizures. Epilepsia 1994; 35:616–626.

30. Handforth A, DeGiorgio CM, Schachter SC. Vagus nerve stimulation therapy for partial-onset seizures: a randomized active-control trial. Neurology 1998; 51:48–55.

31. DeGiorgio CM, Schachter SC, Handforth A. Prospective long-term study of vagus nerve stimulation for the treatment of refractory seizures. Epilepsia 2000; 41:1195–1200.

32. Ramsay RE, Uthman BM, Augustinsson LE. Vagus nerve stimulation for treatment of partial seizures. 2. Safety, side effects, and tolerability. Epilepsia 1994; 35:627–636.

33. Asconape JJ, Moore DD, Zipes DP, Hartman LM, Duffell WH Jr. Bradycardia and asystole with the use of vagus nerve stimulation for the treatment of epilepsy: a rare complication of intraoperative device testing. Epilepsia 1999; 40:1452–1454.

34. Hosain S, Nikalov B, Harden C, Li M, Fraser R, Labar D. Vagus nerve stimulation treatment for Lennox-Gastaut syndrome. J Child Neurol 2000; 15:509–512.

35. Labar DR. Antiepileptic drug use during the first 12 months of vagus nerve stimulation therapy: a registry study. Neurology 2002; 59:S38–S43.

36. Hammond EJ, Uthman BM, Reid SA, Wilder BJ. Electrophysiologic studies of cervical vagus nerve stimulation in humans. II. Evoked potentials. Epilepsia 1992; 33:1021–1028.

37. Naritoku DK, Morales A, Pencek TL, Winkler D. Chronic vagus nerve stimulation increases the latency of the thalamocortical somatosensory evoked potential. Pacing Clin Electrophysiol 1992; 15:1572–1578.

38. Naritoku DK, Terry WJ, Helfert RH. Regional induction of fos immunoreactivity in the brain by anticonvulsant stimulation of the vagus nerve. 1995; 22:53–62.

39. Jobe PC, Daily JW, Reigel CE. Noradrenergic and serotonergic determinants of seizure sisceptibility and secerity in genetically epilepsy-prone rats. 1986; 39:775–782.

40. Jobe PC, Dailey JW, Wernicke JF. A noradrenergic and serotonergic hypothesis of the linkage between epilepsy and affective disorders. Crit Rev Neurobiol 1999; 13:317–356.

41. Terry WJ, Takaya M, Naritoku DK. Regional changes in brain glucose metablism in rats following anticonvulsant stimulation of the vagus nerve. Epilepsia 1996; 37(S5):117.

42. Easton A, Walker B, Gale K. Influence of activity in nucleus tractus solitarius (NTS) on seizure manifestations. Epilepsia 1996; 37(S5):68.

43. Ko D, Heck C, Grafton S. Vagus nerve stimulation activates central nervous system structures in epileptic patients during PET H2(15)O blood flow imaging. Neurosurgery 1996; 39:426–430; discussion 430–431.

44. Henry TR, Votaw JR, Pennell PB. Acute blood flow changes and efficacy of vagus nerve stimulation in partial epilepsy. Neurology 1999; 52:1166–1173.

45. Takaya M, Terry WJ, Naritoku DK. Vagus nerve stimulation induces a sustained anticonvulsant effect. Epilepsia 1996; 37:1111–1116.

46. Naritoku DK, Mikels JA. Vagus nerve stimulation (VNS) is antiepileptogenic in the elecrical kindling model. Epilepsia 1997; 38(S3):220.

47. Naritoku DK, Mikels JA. Vagus nerve stimulation (VNS) attenuates electrically kindled seizures. Epilepsia 1996; 37(S5):75.

48. Fernandez-Guardiola A, Martinez A, Valdes-Cruz A, Magdaleno-Madrigal VM, Martinez D, Fernandez-Mas R. Vagus nerve prolonged stimulation in cats: effects on epileptogenesis (amygdala electrical kindling): behavioral and electrographic changes. Epilepsia 1999; 40:822–829.

49. Malow BA, Edwards J, Marzec M, Sagher O, Ross D, Fromes G. Vagus nerve stimulation reduces daytime sleepiness in epilepsy patients. Neurology 2001; 57:879–884.

50. Krahl SE, Clark KB, Smith DC, Browning RA. Locus coeruleus lesions suppress the seizure-attenuating effects of vagus nerve stimulation. Epilepsia 1998; 39:709–714.

51. Mirski MA, Ferrendelli JA. Anterior thalamic mediation of generalized pentylenetetrazol seizures. Brain Res 1986; 399:212–223.

52. Mirski MA, Rossell LA, Terry JB, Fisher RS. Anticonvulsant effect of anterior thalamic high frequency electrical stimulation in the rat. Epilepsy Res 1997; 28:89–100.

53. Velasco F, Velasco M, Velasco AL, Jimenez F. Effect of chronic electrical stimulation of the centromedian thalamic nuclei on various intractable seizure patterns. I. Clinical seizures and paroxysmal EEG activity. Epilepsia 1993; 34:1052–1064.

54. Sackeim HA, Rush AJ, George MS. Vagus nerve stimulation (VNS) for treatment-resistant depression: efficacy, side effects, and predictors of outcome. Neuropsychopharmacology 2001; 25:713–728.

55. Clark KB, Naritoku DK, Smith DC, Browning RA, Jensen RA. Enhanced recognition memory following vagus nerve stimulation in human subjects. Nat Neurosci 1999; 2:94–98.

56. Helmstaedter C, Hoppe C, Elger CE. Memory alterations during acute high-intensity vagus nerve stimulation. Epilepsy Res 2001; 47:37–42.

57. Sjogren MJ, Hellstrom PT, Jonsson MA, Runnerstam M, Silander HC, Ben-Menachem E. Cognition-enhancing effect of vagus nerve stimulation in patients with Alzheimer's disease: a pilot study. J Clin Psychiatry 2002; 63:972–980.

58. Kirchner A, Birklein F, Stefan H, Handwerker HO. Left vagus nerve stimulation suppresses experimentally induced pain. Neurology 2000; 55:1167–1171.

59. Hord ED, Evans MS, Adamolekun B, Mueed S, Naritoku DK. Effect of vagus nerve stimulation (VNS) on migraine headaches. 10th World Congress on Pain Abstracts 2002.

16

Immunomodulation of Epilepsy

Paul T. Golumbek

Washington University School of Medicine
St. Louis, Missouri, U.S.A.

INTRODUCTION

The nervous system and the immune system possess a number of interesting similarities. Both use well-defined, specialized cell types that communicate through a variety of intercellular mechanisms and develop a specific response to external stimuli. Both demonstrate memory and adapt to historical experiences. Dysfunction in the brain can lead to seizures; dysfunction in the immune system can lead to autoimmunity. This chapter concerns the intersection of those two complex fields.

Why do we believe that the immune system plays a role in epilepsy? With even the most basic background in clinical neurology, one sees many examples of the direct interactions of the immune system and the brain in patients with epilepsy. First, there is an increased incidence of epilepsy after stroke, trauma, or infection; all of these events can release brain antigens, stimulate cytokine release, and result in immune activation. Second, most patients with epilepsy will have a transient worsening of their symptoms with intercurrent illness (1). Such worsening does not necessarily imply a CNS infection, but rather an example of the brain's response to active immune surveillance. In children with simple febrile seizures, infection/inflammation is an integral part of epileptogenesis, but interestingly, prophylaxis against fever is not useful in preventing these seizures (2). This observation implies a more direct effect of the immune system on the brain, rather than simply a temperature-related phenomenon. Third, there are also obvious cases of encephalitis where the immune system is active against infectious agents in the brain. These encephalitic patients often have seizures as an accompaniment.

There are a number of other neurologic diseases, such as ataxia-telangiectasia, multiple sclerosis, Sydenham's chorea, and paraneoplastic syndromes, which seem to have a definite immune component affecting the brain (3–5), yet these syndromes often are not associated with seizures. This chapter will be concerned with those syndromes where the immune system plays some role either in the pathogenesis or modulation of seizures (particularly where no infectious agent is clearly described). By understanding mechanisms of these diseases, we may be able to better control them in the future.

BRIEF REVIEW OF THE IMMUNE SYSTEM

The immune system protects the body against foreign threats from within and from outside the body. These threats can be either intra- or extracellular, or in the form of transformed cancer cells. They are generally protein, carbohydrate, or lipid in nature, but they can even be simple organic or inorganic molecules. The body has developed "humoral" chemical defenses (soluble immunoglobulin and complement). Immunoglobulins are proteins secreted by mature B-cells. There are various types (IgG1–IgG4, IgA, and IgM), each with different functions, and each defined by its conserved/constant portion (Fc fragment). The idiotypic specificity of an immunoglobulin is determined by its antigen-binding portion (Fab), which is encoded by the somatically rearranged portion of the gene. All immunoglobulins are monomeric molecules with two identical Fab sites and one Fc site, except for IgM. IgM is generally of lower affinity and exists as a pentamer (with 10 identical Fab sites). IgG is transferred from mother to child via the placenta. IgA is most abundant in secretions (including saliva, tears, and breast milk) and on mucous membranes such as the gastrointestinal tract. The complement cascade is guided to a target site by surface/chemical properties (i.e., alternate pathway) or by bound Ig (i.e., the classic pathway). There, the complement cascade, composed of multiple serum soluble proteins, is able to form pores in the plasma membranes (lysing the target), increase the efficiency of phagocytosis (opsonization), and attract nearby inflammatory cells to the site. Oligoclonal bands (OCB) in the CSF (absent in concurrent serum samples) indicate intrathecal immunoglobulin synthesis, rather than simple breakdown of the blood-brain barrier.

"Cellular" defenses are also harnessed and honed within the immune system. The simpler cellular defenses (polymorphonuclear cells, granulocytes, microglia/monocytes, and natural killer [NK] cells) can use the humoral components to guide them against a target or may have fixed targeting receptors that have evolved against commonly encountered foes. The more advanced cellular defenses (T-cells and B-cells) go through specialized maturational processes involving gene rearrangements in order to produce unique receptors (T-cell and immunoglobulin receptors, respectively) for each threat. Each mature T-cell or B-cell clone expresses one unique receptor, giving it specificity for a given target.

In a given immune response, there are multiple different clones directed against different parts of a given target. There is a highly complex system of communication utilized by the body in order to initiate, amplify, and later downregulate a coordinated attack of all the above components against a perceived threat. These communications involve direct cell surface-to-cell-surface interactions between immune cells (cognate), as well as secreted prostaglandins and cytokines that can affect nearby cells (noncognate). A host of cytokines are secreted by the brain and by the immune system. Key cognate interactions involve $CD4^+$ T-cell receptors recognizing the combination of a target peptide fragment bound to the class II MHC molecule (HLA-DQ, -DR, or -DP) expressed on the surface of an antigen presenting cell (APC). APCs include macrophages, activated B-cells, dendritic cells, and activated microglia. In addition, important coreceptors are present on T-cells and APCs that must also be engaged for a successful activation and programming. $CD8^+$ T-cell receptors recognize the combination of a target peptide fragment bound to the class I MHC molecule (HLA-A, -B, or -C) that can be expressed by all cells of the body, including the brain.

The expression of MHC molecules in the brain is tightly regulated and is most evident during inflammatory states. Genetic linkage of an MHC gene to a specific epilepsy syndrome is always at least partially causally meaningful, but increased expression of MHC proteins may be a secondary noncausal phenomenon of seizures. Whereas increased risk in identical twins relative to fraternal twins implies some genetic factor, true MHC linkage implies immune involvement of T- or B-cells (and by extension, antigen specificity). The linkage must, of course, be to the MHC gene and not simply to a tightly linked gene.

SPECIFIC EPILEPSY SYNDROMES AND IMMUNE CONSIDERATIONS IMPACTING PATHOGENESIS AND TREATMENT

Some investigators argue that Ohtahara syndrome, infantile spasms/West syndrome (IS/WS), and Lennox-Gastaut syndrome (LGS) represent three distinct entities within a spectrum of age-dependent encephalopathic epilepsy. In this chapter, they will be considered separately, much as they have been treated in the general epilepsy literature. One should note that observations relevant to one syndrome may have ramifications for the others.

Ohtahara Syndrome/Early Infantile Epileptic Encephalopathy

Affected patients present within the first months of life with tonic seizures and have a burst suppression pattern in wake or sleep EEG. They are resistant to most antiepileptic drugs (AEDs) and the neurodevelopmental outcome is universally poor. Owing to their treatment-resistant nature and the relative rarity of this condition, there is very little published on this syndrome. There are scattered reports on individual patients responding to adrenocorticotropic hormone or ACTH (6–9). The clinical response has generally been incomplete and of short duration.

Given the very early onset of Ohtahara syndrome, it is conceivable that maternally transmitted immunoglobulin or T-cells directed against the infant could be important in pathogenesis, but there is no evidence for this in the published literature. If this hypothesis is true, even in part, one might predict several consequences. First, the symptoms should wane as the child's immunoglobulin titers drops with advancing age. Second, there should be siblings affected with similar symptoms. And third, there should be evidence of immune cells on neuropathologic specimens. However, none of these predictions have been confirmed thus far. And although ACTH possesses a multitude of activities, including prominent immuno-suppressive actions, there is insufficient evidence to substantiate an immune mechanism accounting for clinical efficacy. Further, as newborn infants have relatively weak and immature immune systems, direct autoimmune causes of Ohtahara syndrome are less likely.

Infantile Spasms/West Syndrome

Patients with infantile spasms manifest characteristic tonic or flexor spasms that are coincident with high-voltage slow waves and electrodecremental responses on the electroencephalogram (EEG). There is often superimposed low-amplitude fast activity over the slow-wave transients. Spasms occur in clusters and are especially common during transitions between wake and sleep. The EEG background is often described as hypsarrhythmia—i.e., high-voltage, chaotic, asynchronous, and with abundant epileptiform discharges. The combination of IS, mental retardation, and hypsarrhythmia defines West syndrome.

Infantile spasms respond to a number of different medicines including pyridoxine (10), ACTH (11), vigabatrin (12–14), valproic acid (15), glucocorticoids (16), intravenous gammaglobulin or IVIG (17), clonazepam, zonisamide, and topiramate. These treatments can be given alone or in combination (18–21). ACTH is clearly the most studied and generally accepted treatment standard despite the lack of large comparative trials (22–24). Unfortunately, its unfavorable side-effects profile often makes it the second- or third-line drug (25–28). Recently, vigabatrin (VGB) has demonstrated superior efficacy in patients with tuberous sclerosis and concomitant infantile spasms (29–32). All treatments are effective in a fraction of symptomatic IS patients, regardless of the associated underlying cause (33–39), and long-term outcome is better in the treated group when compared to untreated historical controls (40–42).

Historically, several interesting observations regarding ACTH treatment of spasms have been made (43). First, a few patients may respond with as little as one dose of the medication. Second, responders generally experience clinical cessation of seizures as well as normalization of their EEG. When the ACTH is stopped, there is often an enduring change that outlasts the drug treatment. Third, while comparison studies addressing the efficacy of steroids versus ACTH have yielded mixed results (44–48), many believe that a cryptogenic etiology, rapid initiation of treatment, and normal development prior to onset are associated with a better long-term outcome, regardless of treatment employed (40,49). Finally, endogenous ACTH levels are lower in the CNS of patients with IS (50).

MHC studies have been controversial, but peripheral blood lymphocytes of untreated IS patients had elevations in class II MHC. Howitz found no difference in HLA expression in IS patients (51). Hrachovy found a significant increase in the frequency of HLA-DRw52 in the infantile spasm patients (90%) as compared with controls (72%) (52). More recently, Suastegui et al. found a strong association of HLA-DR17 in infantile spasms in the Mexican Mestizos population (50). Levels of the cytokines, IL2, IFNα, and TNFα were elevated in West syndrome patients relative to controls (53).

The case for infantile spasms resulting from autoimmune causes is weak. ACTH, corticosteroids, IVIG, and VGB all have demonstrated immune-modulating effects, but these effects are minimal for VGB. There may be reason to use IVIG when there is strong suspicion of ongoing or prenatal viral insult (54). While IVIG does cross the blood-brain barrier (BBB), no specific mechanism underlying its efficacy could be discerned.

ACTH's intense immune modulating effects are thought to be mediated through corticosteroids that are released from the adrenal glands. Evidence from several studies suggests that this action is not necessary for ACTH to be effective against IS. There is one report of ACTH successfully being used in a child with congenital adrenal hyperplasia with salt wasting (55). This child was unable to mount a cortisol response to ACTH. Other studies showed efficacy of ACTH in a children with adrenal suppression secondary to exogenous steroid administration (55,56). Unfortunately, the search for fragments of ACTH that could suppress IS, while at the same time not stimulating the adrenal glands, has been unsuccessful to date (55,57,58). Interestingly, thyroglobulin releasing hormone (TRH) has also been effective for IS without stimulating corticosteroid release (59). Despite these and other observations, it is still generally believed that ACTH affects the hypothalamic-pituitary-adrenal axis in such a way as to alleviate IS. If ACTH is able to act directly to cause immune suppression, such information has not yet been forthcoming.

Lennox-Gastaut Syndrome

The Lennox-Gastaut syndrome (165) is characterized clinically by difficult-to-control seizures of multiple types (including tonic, atonic, myoclonic, atypical absence, and generalized tonic-clonic), cognitive decline, and interictal slow spike-wave discharges. Often patients with WS are considered together with LGS patients in older clinical studies. This may be a downstream developmental state for those patients with IS/WS who do poorly.

Patients with LGS respond to ACTH (60), IVIG (61), and glucocorticoids, as well as to a number of more standard AEDs, though generally incompletely. Unlike IS patients, LGS patients usually do not have an enduring response to ACTH (60,62,63). However, failure of steroids does not necessarily mean that IVIG will be ineffective (64). A single-blinded clinical trial of IVIG with 10 patients demonstrated a trend toward clinical efficacy, but did not reach statistical significance (17). In five patients treated with IVIG, spasms decreased as CSF Ig levels rose (65). Given the intractability of LGS and long-term difficulties in managing these patients, more intense scrutiny of their immune systems has been undertaken. Immunoglobulins directed at brain tissue has been described, despite a reduced humoral response to foreign antigen (66). Serum levels of IgG and IgM are elevated, and there is a depression in the kappa/lambda ratios of total immunoglobulin (67). Further, there is an increase in the frequency of HLA-DR5 positive and decreased HLA-DR4 cells in these patients relative to normal controls (68).

Unfortunately, none of these abnormalities reproducibly correlate with response to treatment. These changes may indicate a general dysfunction of the immune system that is multifactorial. There is at present insufficient evidence that they are central to the pathogenesis of the disease, but they may exacerbate the clinical symptomatology.

Intractable Epilepsies

This broad and heterogeneous group comprises multiple seizure types and syndromes that cannot be fully controlled with standard AEDs. There is usually a component of cognitive impairment and a high percentage of symptomatic etiologies. Within this group, there have been reports of patients responding to ACTH (69), IVIG (70–72), and steroids (73,74). Usually these responses are not lasting; nevertheless, they show substantial clinical (30–50%) as well as EEG improvement (64,75,76). IVIG may be especially useful for patients who demonstrate relative immunoglobulin deficiencies (77,78). Steroids may be helpful if vasculitis is suspected (73). Dose-response studies have not been helpful in defining treatment algorithms, and this is further limited by the small number of patients with heterogeneous backgrounds who have been studied (79). Double-blind controlled trials of IVIG, while not statistically significant, trend toward positive responses (76). Thus, no immune derangements have been implicated in a causal manner to any specific epileptic syndrome.

Landau-Kleffner Syndrome

Landau-Kleffner syndrome (LKS) is characterized clinically by progressive aphasia with continuous generalized spike-wave discharges during slow-wave sleep. Epilepsy is not a common feature in patients with LKS, but when present, the seizures are infrequent. In general, outcome correlates somewhat with the duration of time (measured in months) that continuous spike-wave discharges are seen during sleep (80). The seizure frequency does not usually correlate with the severity of the aphasia. Patients with LKS appear to respond best to IVIG (81,82), steroids (83–85), or ACTH (84,86,87). Both the aphasia and the EEG can improve with the use of such immunomodulatory agents (82), but not standard AEDs (with the exception of valproic acid).

Four unrelated findings provide some mechanistic insights, although none of the hypotheses generated in such fashion have been substantiated. First, SPECT studies of cerebral blood flow show a decrease in the left temporal lobe (88). Second, the cerebral angiogram may show isolated arteritis, and a patient was reported to have responded to nicardipine (interruption leading to symptom relapse) (89). Third, immunoglobulin binding to endothelial cells in temporal lobe slices were found in half the LKS patients (90). Finally, an elevated IgG index was documented and corrected with response to IVIG (91,92). Taken together, these observations suggest a localized vasculitis or inflammation mediated by the immune system resulting in focal cortical dysfunction. Interestingly, response to steroid treatment did not always correlate with changes seen on SPECT scans (83).

Rasmussen's Encephalitis

Rasmussen's encephalitis (RE) represents an epileptic syndrome with the best-defined autoimmune association (93–95). The clinical presentation is one of AED-resistant, progressive focal epilepsy with unilateral hemispheric cortical dysfunction and atrophy. Most of the brain damage occurs in the first 8–12 months after onset of symptoms (96), and thus a firm diagnosis is often difficult within the first several months after presentation (97). Ultrastructural studies have failed to reveal an obvious viral or immune complex–mediated etiology (98), but intense perivascular cuffing with T-cells (less commonly, B-cells) has been reported (99). Unfortunately, these findings have occurred late in the disease process, and it is unclear whether there might be an inciting virus present at an earlier time.

The major immune treatment options for RE include plasmapheresis (100–103), IVIG (104–108), and/or steroids (82,101,109,110). Intraventricular α-interferon has also been useful, and interestingly, antibodies to GluR3 (a glutamate receptor subunit) bind to α-interferon receptors (111–113). These reports involve small numbers of patients, and, given the tremendous disease variability over time, firm conclusions regarding relative efficacy of these treatments cannot be reached. Nevertheless, while these interventions appear helpful for a short time, the typical scenario is that of disease progression (114), necessitating focal cortical resection or functional hemispherectomy (115–119). Long-term responders though, have been reported (120).

Hemispherectomy does not completely arrest seizures in the affected hemisphere, but it halts the clinical spread of seizures and involvement of the contralateral, unaffected side (121). Resected brain tissue shows a characteristic perivascular astrocytic reaction, inflammatory infiltrate of T-cells, and microglial nodules with neuronal loss (122). Local T-cell clones that have expanded in the brain have been demonstrated as well (123). These $CD8^+$ T-cells are postulated to be cytotoxic (99,124). Neurons demonstrate decreased GABA sensitivity consistent with lessened inhibitory tone (125). In one case, cortical dysplasia was found (which may weaken the brain's defenses to initiation of immune attack or viral infection) (126).

Similar pathology, though bilateral, was noted in rabbits (103) and some mouse strains (120) immunized with GluR3; notably, only the rabbits manifested seizure activity. However, interestingly, mice infected with LP-BM5 virus developed neurodegeneration and autoantibodies to the GluR3 subunit (127). GluR3 is a specific glutamate receptor subunit, one of several that comprise the AMPA (α amino-3-hydroxy-5-methyl-4-isoxazoleproprionic acid) receptor which is permeable to Na^+ and Ca^+ ions, and can be blocked by compounds such as CNQX. The anti-GluR3 immunoglobulin derived from immunized animals, whether sick or well, and from patients with RE, bound to brain slices in a similar distribution (128). These antibodies appear to affect the brain in two distinct ways. Some antibodies, especially those generated by immunization of a particular portion of the GluR3 receptor, are directly able to open the GluR3 channel and thus are believed to cause excitotoxic death and apoptosis (127,129). CNQX is able to block these antibody-mediated channel openings in vitro (130). Other antibodies have not been demonstrated to open the channel but merely bind to it. In human brain, GluR4 (another AMPA receptor subunit) is transcriptionally downregulated in RE (131).

In seemingly unrelated work, in vivo chronic partial isolation of neocortical islands results in epileptogenesis involving layer V pyramidal neurons that showed spontaneous downmodulation of surface GluR1, GluR2, and GluR3 (132). In addition, these anti-GluR3 autoantibodies are also able to direct complement at the site, thus killing predominantly bystander glial cells. The neuron itself is better protected from complement attack by endogenous anticomplement defenses (133).

In most patients with RE, anti-GluR3 immunoglobulin has been demonstrated and IgG/complement complexes are seen in brain pathology (134–136). In addition, immunoglobulin to munc18, an intracellular protein localized to presynaptic terminals, has been found in one patient (137). This may demonstrate epitope spreading, where a well-circumscribed immune attack against one target then stimulates nascent immune responses against topographically nearby unrelated targets, or even distant structurally related targets. Granzyme (from T-cells) may play a role in GluR3 receptor proteolysis necessary for immune response initiation (124,138). HLA-A2, -B44 and -DR4 may also be associated with RE (120).

Rasmussen's encephalitis is a compelling example of apparent autoimmunity to neuronal antigens causing epilepsy and perhaps excitotoxic cell death, but several important questions still remain. Why is this disease unilateral in humans (and bilateral in nonhumans, assuming it is the same disease)? This is difficult to reconcile with any immune-based mechanism, given that we believe the antigen localization and the immune surveillance are bilateral. However, this may relate to the apparent strong anticomplement systems that are present to prevent such an attack from beginning. A second insult such as trauma, infection, sustained seizure, or dysplasia may be necessary to initiate the attack. Since bystander killing is postulated as a key in some pathophysiological scenarios, the spread of the local cell death may require a unique combination of neurons and glial cells, and it is unlikely that the corpus callosum is involved.

A unilaterally expressed target antigen has never been demonstrated in patients with RE. What is the phenotype of patients or animals exposed to only subsets of the proposed effectors (Ig, complement, or CD8$^+$ T-cell)? Why do patients respond to functional hemispherectomy but not lobectomy? By containing the seizures to one hemisphere, kindling of the opposite hemisphere may be prevented. Focal seizures could weaken the local BBB, and might lead to bilateral involvement if not contained. Why are autoantibodies to GluR3 seen in so many patients? If the mechanism is simply complement fixation, then there are many surface antigens that are properly situated for this purpose. Yet, other receptors do not cause these same symptoms in rabbits despite a robust immunoglobulin response. Also, while not all Rasmussen patients have anti-GluR3 antibodies, they may still respond to steroids or cyclophosphamide (134). This may imply other pathogenic immunoglobulins or cellular effectors. It is important to remember that in a mature immune response, there will be a variety of immunoglobulin molecules and multiple T-cell clones that are directed against the target antigen. Multiple B-cell clones have been found in Rasmussen's patients (139). In more recent studies, GluR3 autoantibodies have also been demonstrated in many patients with typical epilepsies (not RE) (140–142). With more detailed knowledge regarding the pathogenesis of RE, more intensive therapy with IVIG may be able to temporarily arrest disease in adult patients (107,120), although centers have reported poor long-term outcomes with this treatment modality; similar observations have been made with plasma exchange.

Systemic Lupus Erythematosis

Systemic lupus erythematosis (SLE) is an autoimmune disease that affects multiple organ systems. It is interesting to note that there is a high rate of seizures seen in patients with SLE. Seizure frequency is associated with elevations in serum anticardiolipin (143) and antiphospholipids (144,145) in these patients. But it should be recalled that anti-phospholipid antibodies are also elevated in non-SLE epilepsy patients (146). It is unclear if these immunoglobulins are causal for the seizure or secondary to seizure activity. Mechanistically, these immunoglobulins might affect the brain's vasculature, or instead act directly on neuronal and/or glial tissue. Interestingly, IgGs from patients with the antiphospholipid antibody syndrome induce depolarization of brain synaptoneurosomes (147). On the other hand, mice immunized with β(2)-glycoprotein-1, a phospholipid, develop hyperactive behavior and deficits in learning and memory, but no seizures (147,148).

Other Epilepsies

Patients with mesial temporal lobe epilepsy have a high frequency of HLA-DQ2, -DR4, and -DR7 associations (149). Surgically resected hippocampal sclerotic tissue had elevated class II MHC on the CA1 and CA3 microglial cells (150). Five patients with idiopathic minor motor seizures had an elevated IgG index (151). In a study of focal epilepsy, patients had decreased IgA, $CD4^+$ T-cells, and elevated IgM and $CD8^+$ T-cells (152). $CD4^+/CD8^+$ ratio and B-cell counts were elevated in a patient with mixed primary and secondarily generalized epilepsy (153). A patient with anti-Hu immunoglobulin and epilepsia partialis continua (EPC) had inflammatory infiltrate and neuronal loss (154). In a small study, patients with childhood partial epilepsy with occipital paroxysms (CPEO) had an increased prevalence of celiac disease (an autoimmune disease of the GI system brought on by gluten sensitivity) (155). Several patients with seizures, encephalopathy, and movement disorder were noted to have oligoclonal bands in their CSF; the symptoms resolved spontaneously (156). While these studies fail to convincingly show causality, they are nevertheless intriguing.

GENERAL INTERACTIONS OF THE NERVOUS SYSTEM AND THE IMMUNE SYSTEM

While the literature to date has failed to provide a causal link between immune dysfunction and the pathogenesis of epilepsy, there has nevertheless been a great deal of study concerning the general effects of epileptic seizures on the immune system. Some of these data may be applicable to virtually any epilepsy syndrome.

Febrile seizures may impair cellular immunity, with elevation of $CD8^+$ T-cells, decrease the $CD4^+/CD8^+$ cell ratio, and impair proliferation of T-cells to PHA (157). Pentylenetetrazole (PTZ)- or electroconvulsive shock (ECS)-induced seizures block the subsequent development of experimental allergic encephalitis (EAE) and decrease skin hypersensitivity reactions (158). Tetanus toxoid-induced seizures upregulate microglial class II MHC levels in the substantia nigra (SN) and the hippocampus; levels in the SN eventually return to baseline, but levels in the the CA1 region of the hippocampus, where neuronal cell loss is observed, remains elevated (159). Kainate-induced seizures upregulate class I MHC and β-2-microglobulin levels in the hippocampus (160). Seizures also alter the expression of voltage gated Na^+ channel subunits (158). Seizures increase local prostaglandin synthesis (161) and microglial MHC levels (162). A study employing a cDNA microarray indicated that kainate upregulated 187 of 4000 genes in the brain, many potentially or directly involved in immune function (163). Electroconvulsive shock leads to formation of immunoglobulin, which binds to brain. In other cases, immunoglobulin to brain neuronal membrane component injected in animals causes epileptiform discharges. Deletion of the gene encoding the cytokine IL-6 reduced the brain inflammatory response and increased oxidative stress and neurodegeneration after kainic acid–induced seizures (164).

Epilepsy has also been associated with a variety of immune system changes; (1) a decrease in the total lymphocyte count (165); (2) depressed $CD4^+$, elevated $CD8^+$ T-cell counts, and depressed $CD4^+/CD8^+$ ratios (166–168); (3) depressed NK cell activity (167); and (4) depressed IgA, and IgM levels (169,170). The immune system defects are heterogeneous, and either hyperactivity and/or hypoactivity can occur through dysregulation of a very complex system (171). The anatomic location of seizure activity may influence immune-mediated derangements (172).

Generalized seizures stimulate secretion of prolactin (PRL) and ACTH. This ACTH release is independent of stress and can be demonstrated in an anesthetized cat (173). Repetitive seizures lead to increased adrenal size and elevated cortisol levels (174). Lithium-pilocarpine-induced seizures had an acute effect on immuno-globulin response to antigen (175). Language-dominant cortical resection caused a decrease in absolute lymphocyte count, total T-cells, and $CD4^+$ and $CD8^+$ T-cells, whereas resection of the nondominant side had the opposite effect (176).

Epilepsy-prone mice and rats both have elevated IgG levels and low IgM levels (177,178); however, epilepsy prone rats demonstrated a depressed immunoglobulin response in vivo to new antigen exposure (179). Different mouse strains exhibit different neurosteroid sensitivity and biosynthesis (168,180).

Multiple cytokines, classically regarded as specific to the immune system, are often produced by glial cells and can affect neuronal membrane excitability. IL-1β possesses multiple actions, including hippocampal neuron hyperpolarization (181), cyclo-oxygenase-2 (Cox-2) upregulation (182), and depression of Ca^{2+} currents in hippocampal CA1 neurons (which can be blocked by an IL-1RA receptor antagonist) (183). IL-2 modulates NMDA receptor-mediated responses (184) and hippocampal firing (181). IL-8 can be manufactured by glial cells, and it decreases Ca^{2+} currents in rat septal neurons (185).

FUTURE AREAS OF EXPLORATION IN THE NEUROIMMUNOLOGY OF EPILEPSY

From an immunologic standpoint, there remains great potential for progress in the prevention, diagnosis, and treatment of epileptic disorders. This is in spite of the enormous complexity of both CNS and immune axes, each of which represents unique challenges. Our two greatest immediate challenges are to establish clinically relevant animal models of specific epileptic syndromes and to embark on prospective, controlled, human clinical trials of immunomodulatory agents (186). Animal models will allow careful analysis of the component parts of the system without the heterogeneous external factors, low numbers, and lack of access to tissue that have plagued many previous clinical endeavors. From such studies, well-blinded and adequately powered clinical trials can be designed successfully, through cooperative efforts involving multiple centers.

If there is autoimmune pathogenesis in an epileptic syndrome, then future progress should allow us to prevent or rapidly diagnose and treat these diseases. If the immune system is dysfunctional because of epilepsy, we need to be able to adequately monitor and treat these defects appropriately. Our tools at this time are rather insensitive but they are improving. The possibility of subclinical immune irritants, like celiac disease, exacerbating neural dysfunction must be identified and rooted out.

As we have learned so much in a short time from the Rasmussen's encephalitis model, we are already able to apply these findings to the clinic. More aggressive immunomodulation may allow us to avoid the need for hemispherectomy in the

Table 1. IVIG Effects on the Immune System

1.	Neutralize idiotypes
2.	Correct idiotype deficiencies
3.	Decrease Fc receptors
4.	Compete for available Fc receptors
5.	Inhibit complement activation
6.	Neutralize superantigens
7.	Supplement antiviral and antitoxin response
8.	Neutralize cytokines (IL1, IL6, TNFα, IFNβ)
9.	Inhibit immunoglobulin synthesis
10.	Increase turnover of immunoglobulin
11.	Inhibit cell adhesion
12.	Stimulate apoptosis of activated B-cells
13.	Inhibit CD5 expression
14.	Antagonize CD4,CD8 and MHC actions
15.	Increase "suppressor" Th2 CD4$^+$ T-cells, in vitro

future. Specific therapy directed against B-cells and T-cells may be needed to prevent progression of disease. Further, enhancement of complement resistance or depletion of complement activity may be helpful.

Accurate assessment of the pathogenesis of LKS may allow better rescue of function and lessen poor long-term outcomes. Nonimmunologic treatment could also be assessed. One of the more novel approaches, for general epilepsy, is the use of immunization against the NR1 subunit of NMDA receptors as a means of suppressing seizure threshold in an animal model (187). This treatment resulted in not only strong antiepileptic activity against kainate induction but also neuroprotection from ischemia. Unfortunately, in this case the effect was short-lived. In an unrelated study, protection against nicotine-induced seizures was afforded by nicotine vaccination (188).

Immunoglobulins directed at specific receptors may aid the design and development of clinical pharmaceuticals. The future possibility of targeting the immune response to destroy epileptic foci or abnormal cells such as cortical tubers must be considered as well. While all of this represents exciting new vistas for epilepsy treatment strategies, we must temper this excitement with the knowledge that through epitope spreading, a therapeutic immunoglobulin response could lead to a more pervasive and pathologic autoimmune attack on the brain. The incredible variation in species- and even strain-specific responses, as demonstrated in RE, and the outbred nature of humans make these endeavors difficult to predict or control. Ultimately the hope is that the immune system can be used as a friend and thwarted as a foe.

REFERENCES

1. Garduno-Espinosa A. Status epilepticus in children. Study of 70 cases. Bol Med Hosp Infant Mex 1990; **47**(8):567–575. (In Spanish.)
2. Uhari M. Effect of acetaminophen and of low intermittent doses of diazepam on prevention of recurrences of febrile seizures. J Pediatr 1995; **126**(6): 991–995.

3. Berron PR. Ataxia telangectasia. Probability of damaging immune mechanisms. Bol Med Hosp Infant Mex 1977; **34**(1):29–46.
4. Van der Merwe PL, Kalis NN. Sydenham's chorea—analysis of 27 patients and a review of the literature. S Afr Med J 1997; **87**(suppl 3):C157–C160.
5. Antoine JC, Honnorat J. Anti-neuronal antibodies and central nervous system diseases: contribution to diagnosis and pathophysiology. Rev Neurol (Paris), 2000; **156**(1): 23–33. (In French.)
6. Yelin K, Alfonso I, Papazian O. Syndrome of Ohtahara. Rev Neurol 1999; **29**(4):340–342. (In French.)
7. Takusa Y. Effect of the ketogenic diet for West syndrome into which early infantile epileptic encephalopathy with suppression-burst was evolved. No To Hattatsu 1995; **27**(5):383–387. (In Japanese.)
8. Chakova L. On a rare form of epilepsy in infants—Ohtahara syndrome. Folia Med 1996; **38**(2):69–73.
9. Campistol J. The Ohtahara's syndrome: a special form of age-dependent epilepsy. Rev Neurol 1997; **25**(138):212–214. (In French.)
10. Pietz J. Treatment of infantile spasms with high-dosage vitamin B6. Epilepsia 1993; **34**(4):757–763.
11. Yanagaki S. A comparative study of high-dose and low-dose ACTH therapy for West syndrome. Brain Dev 1999; **21**(7):461–467.
12. Vigabatrin: new indication. An advance in infantile spasms. Prescrire Int 1998; **7**(34):43–44.
13. Chiron C. Randomized trial comparing vigabatrin and hydrocortisone in infantile spasms due to tuberous sclerosis. Epilepsy Res 1997; **26**(2):389–395.
14. Vigevano F, Cilio MR. Vigabatrin versus ACTH as first-line treatment for infantile spasms: a randomized, prospective study. Epilepsia 1997; **38**(12):1270–1274.
15. Dyken PR. Short term effects of valproate on infantile spasms. Pediatr Neurol 1985; **1**(1):34–37.
16. Hrachovy RA. Double-blind study of ACTH vs prednisone therapy in infantile spasms. J Pediatr 1983; **103**(4):641–645.
17. Van Engelen BG. High-dose intravenous immunoglobulin treatment in cryptogenic West and Lennox-Gastaut syndrome; an add-on study. Eur J Pediatr 1994; **153**(10):762–769.
18. Dreifuss F. Infantile spasms. Comparative trial of nitrazepam and corticotropin. Arch Neurol 1986; **43**(11):1107–1110.
19. Zafeiriou DI, Kontopoulos EE, Tsikoulas IG. Adrenocorticotropic hormone and vigabatrin treatment of children with infantile spasms underlying cerebral palsy. Brain Dev 1996; **18**(6):450–452.
20. Seki T. Combination treatment of high-dose pyridoxal phosphate and low-dose ACTH in children with West syndrome and related disorders. Jpn J Psychiatry Neurol 1990; **44**(2):219–237.
21. Mikati MA, Lepejian GA, Holmes GL. Medical treatment of patients with infantile spasms. Clin Neuropharmacol 2002; **25**(2):61–70.
22. Hancock E, Osborne JP, Milner P. The treatment of West syndrome: a Cochrane review of the literature to December 2000. Brain Dev 2001; **23**(7):624–634.
23. Hancock E, Osborne JP, Milner P. Treatment of infantile spasms. Cochrane Database Syst Rev **2002**(2):CD001770.
24. Hrachovy RA, Frost JD Jr, Glaze DG. High-dose, long-duration versus low-dose, short-duration corticotropin therapy for infantile spasms. J Pediatr 1994 **124**(5 Pt 1): 803–806.
25. Haines ST, Casto DT. Treatment of infantile spasms. Ann Pharmacother 1994; **28**(6):779–791.
26. Ito M. Antiepileptic drug treatment of West syndrome. Epilepsia 1998; **39**(suppl 5):38–41.

27. Ito M, Seki T, Takuma Y. Current therapy for West syndrome in Japan. J Child Neurol 2000; **15**(6):424–428.

28. Watanabe K. Medical treatment of West syndrome in Japan. J Child Neurol 1995; **10**(2):143–147.

29. Riikonen RS. Steroids or vigabatrin in the treatment of infantile spasms? Pediatr Neurol 2000; **23**(5):403–408.

30. Chiron C. Role of physiopathological hypotheses in therapeutic choice in epilepsy in children. Rev Neurol 1997; **153**(suppl 1):S34–S38. (In French.)

31. Nabbout R. A risk-benefit assessment of treatments for infantile spasms. Drug Saf 2001; **24**(11):813–828.

32. Elterman RD. Randomized trial of vigabatrin in patients with infantile spasms. Neurology 2001; **57**(8):1416–1421.

33. Sasaki M. Cerebral white matter lesions in a case of incontinentia pigmenti with infantile spasms, mental retardation and left hemiparesis. No To Hattatsu 1991; **23**(3):278–283. (In Japanese.)

34. Miyazaki M. Infantile spasms with localized cerebral lesion detected by ^{99m}TcHMPAO-SPECT. No To Hattatsu 1994; **26**(3):251–256. (In Japaness.)

35. Kirkham FJ, Ebbing A. Case summary: Katc. Seizure 1994; **3**(suppl A):33–36.

36. Harden CL, Tuchman AJ, Daras M. Infantile spasms in COFS syndrome. Pediatr Neurol 1991; **7**(4):302–304.

37. Escofet C. Infantile spasms in children with Down's syndrome. Rev Neurol 1995; **23**(120):315–317. (In French.)

38. Coulter DL. Continuous infantile spasms as a form of status epilepticus. J Child Neurol 1986; **1**(3):215–217.

39. Abe K. A case of Aicardi syndrome with moderate psychomotor retardation. No To Hattatsu 1990; **22**(4):376–380. (In Japanese.)

40. Luthvigsson P. Epidemiologic features of infantile spasms in Iceland. Epilepsia 1994; **35**(4):802–805.

41. Gaszner A. Low dose ACTH therapy in West syndrome. Orv Hetil 1997; **138**(5):281–283. (In Hungarian.)

42. Riikonen R. Long-term outcome of West syndrome: a study of adults with a history of infantile spasms. Epilepsia 1996; **37**(4):367–372.

43. Snead OC 3rd. How does ACTH work against infantile spasms? Bedside to bench. Ann Neurol 2001; **49**(3):288–289.

44. Baram TZ. High-dose corticotropin (ACTH) versus prednisone for infantile spasms: a prospective, randomized, blinded study. Pediatrics 1996; **97**(3):375–379.

45. Singhi PD. Newer antiepileptic drugs and non surgical approaches in epilepsy. Indian J Pediatr 2000; **67**(1 Suppl):S92–S98.

46. Fonseca LF, Oliveira AL. Infantile spasms: experience in 13 cases. Arq Neuropsiquiatr 2000; **58**(2B):512–517. (In Portuguese.)

47. Dulac O. Epileptic encephalopathy. Epilepsia 2001; **42**(suppl 3):23–26.

48. Schlumberger E, Dulac O. A simple, effective and well-tolerated treatment regime for West syndrome. Dev Med Child Neurol 1994; **36**(10):863–872.

49. Michalowicz R. Analysis of adverse factors affecting the result of therapy for West syndrome in children. Pol Tyg Lek 1994; **49**(4–5):93–95. (In Polish.)

50. Suastegui RA. Contribution of the MHC class II antigens to the etiology of infantile spasm in Mexican Mestizos. Epilepsia 2001; **42**(2):210–215.

51. Howitz P, Platz P. Infantile spasms and HLA antigens. Arch Dis Child 1978; **53**(8):680–682.

52. Hrachovy RA. Serologic HLA typing in infantile spasms. Epilepsia 1988; **29**(6):817–819.

53. Liu ZS. Serum cytokine levels are altered in patients with West syndrome. Brain Dev 2001; **23**(7):548–551.

54. Riikonen R. Infantile spasms: infectious disorders. Neuropediatrics 1993; **24**(5): 274–280.

55. Willig RP, Lagenstein I. Use of ACTH fragments of children with infantile spasms. Neuropediatrics 1982; **13**(2):55–58.

56. Farwell J. Adrenocorticotropic hormone controls infantile spasms independently of cortisol stimulation. Epilepsia 1984; **25**(5):605–608.

57. Pentella K, Bachman DS, Sandman CA. Trial of an ACTH4-9 analogue (ORG 2766) in children with intractable seizures. Neuropediatrics 1982; **13**(2):59–62.

58. Willig RP, Lagenstein I. Therapeutic trial with a fragment of ACTH (ACTH 4–10) in early childhood epilepsy (author's transl). Monatsschr Kinderheilkd 1980; **128**(2): 100–103.

59. Matsumoto A. Clinical effects of thyrotropin-releasing hormone for severe epilepsy in childhood: a comparative study with ACTH therapy. Epilepsia 1987; **28**(1):49–55.

60. Yamatogi Y. Treatment of the Lennox syndrome with ACTH: a clinical and electroencephalographic study. Brain Dev 1979; **1**(4):267–276.

61. Ariizumi M. Immunoglobulin therapy in the West syndrome. Brain Dev 1987; **9**(4): 422–425.

62. Pisani F, Oteri G, Di Perri R. Lennox-Gestaut syndrome: therapeutic aspects. Riv Neurol 1989; **59**(6):217–219. (In Italian.)

63. Renier WO, Le Coultre R. Selected data from childhood epilepsies. ACTH treatment and ketogenic diet: a critical evaluation. Tijdschr Kindergeneeskd 1989; **57**(3):81–86. (In Dutch.)

64. Gross-Tsur V. Intravenous high-dose gammaglobulins for intractable childhood epilepsy. Acta Neurol Scand 1993; **88**(3):204–209.

65. Espinosa Zacarias J. Intravenous treatment with immunoglobulins in epileptic syndromes which are difficult to control. Rev Neurol 2002; **34**(9):816–819. (In French.)

66. Van Engelen BG. A dysbalanced immune system in cryptogenic Lennox-Gastaut syndrome. Scand J Immunol 1995; **41**(2):209–213.

67. Haraldsson A. Light chain ratios and concentrations of serum immunoglobulins in children with epilepsy. Epilepsy Res 1992; **13**(3):255–260.

68. Van Engelen BG. Serologic HLA typing in cryptogenic Lennox-Gastaut syndrome. Epilepsy Res 1994; **17**(1):43–47.

69. Kalra V, Passi GR. Analysis of childhood epileptic encephalopathies with regard to etiological and prognostic factors. Brain Dev 1998; **20**(1):14–17.

70. Barontini F, Maurri S, Amantini A. Epilepsia partialis continua" due to multifocal encephalitis: favourable outcome after immunoglobulin treatment. Ital J Neurol Sci 1994; **15**(3):157–161.

71. Etzioni A. High dose intravenous gamma-globulin in intractable epilepsy of childhood. Eur J Pediatr 1991; **150**(9):681–683.

72. Turkay S. Immune globulin treatment in intractable epilepsy of childhood. Turk J Pediatr 1996; **38**(3):301–305.

73. Akanuma H. A case of severe status epilepticus of frontal lobe origin successfully treated with corticosteroids. Rinsho Shinkeigaku 1998; **38**(5):461–464. (In Japanese.)

74. Sinclair DB. Prednisone therapy in pediatric epilepsy. Pediatr Neurol 2003; 28 (online).

75. Van Engelen BG. Immunoglobulin treatment in epilepsy, a review of the literature. Epilepsy Res 1994; **19**(3):181–190.

76. Duse M. Intravenous immune globulin in the treatment of intractable childhood epilepsy. Clin Exp Immunol 1996; **104**(suppl 1):71–76.

77. Sterio M. Malignant epilepsy in children: therapy with high doses of intravenous immunoglobulin. Med Pregl 1992; **45**(5–6):220–224. (In Russian.)

78. Sterio M. Intravenous immunoglobulin in the treatment of malignant epilepsy in children. Wien Klin Wochenschr 1990; **102**(8):230–233. (In German.)

79. Van Rijckevorsel-Harmant K. Treatment of refractory epilepsy with intravenous immunoglobulins. Results of the first double-blind/dose finding clinical study. Int J Clin Lab Res 1994; **24**(3):162–166.

80. Robinson RO. Landau-Kleffner syndrome: course and correlates with outcome. Dev Med Child Neurol 2001; **43**(4):243–247.

81. Mikati MA. Efficacy of intravenous immunoglobulin in Landau-Kleffner syndrome. Pediatr Neurol 2002; **26**(4):298–300.

82. Lagae LG. Successful use of intravenous immunoglobulins in Landau-Kleffner syndrome. Pediatr Neurol 1998; **18**(2):165–168.

83. Tsuru T. Effects of high-dose intravenous corticosteroid therapy in Landau-Kleffner syndrome. Pediatr Neurol 2000; **22**(2):145–147.

84. Aicardi J. Landau-Kleffner syndrome. Rev Neurol 1999; **29**(4):380–385. (In French.)

85. Santos LH. Landau-Kleffner syndrome: study of four cases. Arq Neuropsiquiatr 2002; **60**(2-A):239–241.

86. Tassinari CA. Encephalopathy with electrical status epilepticus during slow sleep or ESES syndrome including the acquired aphasia. Clin Neurophysiol 2000; **111**(suppl 2): S94–S102.

87. Lerman P, Lerman-Sagie T, Kivity S. Effect of early corticosteroid therapy for Landau-Kleffner syndrome. Dev Med Child Neurol 1991; **33**(3):257–260.

88. Guerreiro MM. Brain single photon emission computed tomography imaging in Landau-Kleffner syndrome. Epilepsia 1996; **37**(1).60–67.

89. Pascual-Castroviejo I. Is cerebral arteritis the cause of the Landau-Kleffner syndrome? Four cases in childhood with angiographic study. Can J Neurol Sci 1992; **19**(1):46–52.

90. Connolly AM. Serum autoantibodies to brain in Landau-Kleffner variant, autism, and other neurologic disorders. J Pediatr 1999; **134**(5):607–613.

91. Mikati MA, Saab R. Successful use of intravenous immunoglobulin as initial monotherapy in Landau-Kleffner syndrome. Epilepsia 2000; **41**(7):880–886.

92. Fayad MN, Choueiri R, Mikati M. Landau Kleffner syndrome: consistent response to repeated intravenous gamma-globulin doses: a case report. Epilepsia 1997; **38**(4):489–494.

93. Aarli JA. Epilepsy and the immune system. Arch Neurol 2000; **57**(12):1689–1692.

94. Andrews PI, McNamara JO. Rasmussen's encephalitis: an autoimmune disorder? Curr Opin Neurobiol 1996; **6**(5):673–678.

95. Levite M. Autoimmune epilepsy. Nat Immunol 2002; **3**(6):500.

96. Bien CG. The natural history of Rasmussen's encephalitis. Brain 2002; **125**(Pt 8):1751–1759.

97. Granata T. Rasmussen's encephalitis: early characteristics allow diagnosis. Neurology 2003; **60**(3):422–425.

98. Park SH, Vinters HV. Ultrastructural study of Rasmussen encephalitis. Ultrastruct Pathol 2002; **26**(5):287–292.

99. Prayson RA, Frater JL. Rasmussen encephalitis: a clinicopathologic and immuno-histochemical study of seven patients. Am J Clin Pathol 2002; **117**(5):776–782.

100. Wiendl H, Neuhaus O, Stefan H. The therapy of Rasmussen encephalitis. Dtsch Med Wochenschr 1999; **124**(31–32):937–939. (In German.)

101. Andrews PI. Plasmapheresis in Rasmussen's encephalitis. Neurology 1996 **46**(1): 242–246.

102. Andrews PI, McNamara JO, Lewis DV. Clinical and electroencephalographic correlates in Rasmussen's encephalitis. Epilepsia 1997; **38**(2):189–194.

103. Rogers SW. Autoantibodies to glutamate receptor GluR3 in Rasmussen's encephalitis. Science 1994; **265**(5172):648–651.

104. Topcu M. Rasmussen encephalitis in childhood. Childs Nerv Syst 1999; **15**(8):395–402; discussion 403.

105. Villani F. Positive response to immunomodulatory therapy in an adult patient with Rasmussen's encephalitis. Neurology 2001; **56**(2):248–250.

106. Caraballo R. Rasmussen syndrome. Rev Neurol 1998; **26**(154):978–983. (In French.)

107. Leach JP. Improvement in adult-onset Rasmussen's encephalitis with long-term immunomodulatory therapy. Neurology 1999; **52**(4):738–742.

108. Wise MS, Rutledge SL, Kuzniecky RI. Rasmussen syndrome and long-term response to gamma globulin. Pediatr Neurol 1996. **14**(2):149–152.

109. Chinchilla D. Reappraisal of Rasmussen's syndrome with special emphasis on treatment with high doses of steroids. J Neurol Neurosurg Psychiatry 1994; **57**(11):1325–1333.

110. Hart YM. Medical treatment of Rasmussen's syndrome (chronic encephalitis and epilepsy): effect of high-dose steroids or immunoglobulins in 19 patients. Neurology 1994; **44**(6):1030–1036.

111. Dabbagh O. Intraventricular interferon-alpha stops seizures in Rasmussen's encephalitis: a case report. Epilepsia 1997; **38**(9):1045–1049.

112. Maria BL. Intraventricular alpha interferon therapy for Rasmussen's syndrome. Can J Neurol Sci 1993; **20**(4):333–336.

113. Gahring LC, Carlson NG, Rogers SW. Antibodies prepared to neuronal glutamate receptor subunit3 bind IFN alpha-receptors: implications for an autoimmune process. Autoimmunity 1998; **28**(4):243–248.

114. Frucht S. Dystonia, athetosis, and epilepsia partialis continua in a patient with late-onset Rasmussen's encephalitis. Mov Disord 2002; **17**(3):609–612.

115. Daszkiewicz P. Rasmussen syndrome—indications for surgical treatment of refractory epilepsy: report of two cases. Neurol Neurochir Pol 2000; **34**(6):1251–1260. (In Polish.)

116. Kalinina LV. Rasmussen's chronic progressive focal encephalitis. Zh Nevropatol Psikhiatr Im S S Korsakova 1996; **96**(2):21–25. (In Russian.)

117. Lilly DJ. Functional hemispherectomy: radical treatment for Rasmussen's encephalitis. J Neurosci Nurs 2000; **32**(2):89–92.

118. Dulac O. Rasmussen's syndrome. Curr Opin Neurol 1996; **9**(2):75–77.

119. Vining EP. Why would you remove half a brain? The outcome of 58 children after hemispherectomy—the Johns Hopkins experience: 1968 to 1996. Pediatrics 1997; **100**(2 Pt 1):163–171.

120. Levite M, Hermelin A. Autoimmunity to the glutamate receptor in mice—a model for Rasmussen's encephalitis? J Autoimmun 1999; **13**(1):73–82.

121. Thomas P. Persistence of ictal activity after functional hemispherectomy in Rasmussen syndrome. Neurology 2003; **60**(1):140–142.

122. Vajtai I, Varga Z. Neuropathology of Rasmussen syndrome. Orv Hetil 1996; **137**(37):2035–2039. (In Hungarian.)

123. Li Y. Local-clonal expansion of infiltrating T lymphocytes in chronic encephalitis of Rasmussen. J Immunol 1997; **158**(3):1428–1437.

124. Bauer J, Bien CG, Lassmann H. Rasmussen's encephalitis: a role for autoimmune cytotoxic T lymphocytes. Curr Opin Neurol 2002; **15**(2):197–200.

125. Gibbs JW 3rd. Physiological analysis of Rasmussen's encephalitis: patch clamp recordings of altered inhibitory neurotransmitter function in resected frontal cortical tissue. Epilepsy Res 1998; **31**(1):13–27.

126. Palmer CA. Rasmussen's encephalitis with concomitant cortical dysplasia: the role of GluR3. Epilepsia 1999; **40**(2):242–247.

127. Koustova E. LP-BM5 virus-infected mice produce activating autoantibodies to the AMPA receptor. J Clin Invest 2001; **107**(6):737–744.

128. He XP. Glutamate receptor GluR3 antibodies and death of cortical cells. Neuron 1998; **20**(1):153–163.

129. Moga D. Parvalbumin-containing interneurons in rat hippocampus have an AMPA receptor profile suggestive of vulnerability to excitotoxicity. J Chem Neuroanat 2002; 23(4):249–253.

130. Levite M. Autoantibodies to the glutamate receptor kill neurons via activation of the receptor ion channel. J Autoimmun 1999; 13(1):61–72.

131. Baranzini SE. Gene expression analysis reveals altered brain transcription of glutamate receptors and inflammatory genes in a patient with chronic focal (Rasmussen's) encephalitis. J Neuroimmunol 2002; 128(1–2):9–15.

132. Kharazia VN, Prince DA. Changes of alpha-amino-3-hydroxy-5-methyl-4-isoxazole-propionate receptors in layer V of epileptogenic, chronically isolated rat neocortex. Neuroscience 2001; 102(1):23–34.

133. Whitney KD, McNamara JO. GluR3 autoantibodies destroy neural cells in a complement-dependent manner modulated by complement regulatory proteins. J Neurosci, 2000; 20(19):7307–7316.

134. Krauss GL. Chronic steroid-responsive encephalitis without autoantibodies to glutamate receptor GluR3. Neurology 1996; 46(1): 247–249.

135. Frassoni C. Labeling of rat neurons by anti-GluR3 IgG from patients with Rasmussen encephalitis. Neurology 2001; 57(2):324–327.

136. Twyman RE. Glutamate receptor antibodies activate a subset of receptors and reveal an agonist binding site. Neuron 1995; 14(4):755–762.

137. Yang R. Autoimmunity to munc-18 in Rasmussen's encephalitis. Neuron 2000; 28(2):375–383.

138. Gahring L. Granzyme B proteolysis of a neuronal glutamate receptor generates an autoantigen and is modulated by glycosylation. J Immunol 2001; 166(3):1433–1438.

139. Baranzini SE. Analysis of antibody gene rearrangement, usage, and specificity in chronic focal encephalitis. Neurology 2002; 58(5):709–716.

140. Bernasconi P. Similar binding to glutamate receptors by Rasmussen and partial epilepsy patients' sera. Neurology 2002; 59(12):1998–2001.

141. Wiendl H. GluR3 antibodies: prevalence in focal epilepsy but no specificity for Rasmussen's encephalitis. Neurology 2001; 57(8):1511–1514.

142. Mantegazza R. Antibodies against GluR3 peptides are not specific for Rasmussen's encephalitis but are also present in epilepsy patients with severe, early onset disease and intractable seizures. J Neuroimmunol 2002; 131(1–2):179–185.

143. Herranz MT. Association between antiphospholipid antibodies and epilepsy in patients with systemic lupus erythematosus. Arthritis Rheum 1994; 37(4):568–571.

144. Liou HH. Anticardiolipin antisera from lupus patients with seizures reduce a GABA receptor-mediated chloride current in snail neurons. Life Sci 1994; 54(15): 1119–1125.

145. Liou HH. Elevated levels of anticardiolipin antibodies and epilepsy in lupus patients. Lupus 1996; 5(4):307–312.

146. Eriksson K. High prevalence of antiphospholipid antibodies in children with epilepsy: a controlled study of 50 cases. Epilepsy Res 2001; 46(2):129–137.

147. Chapman J, Shoenfeld Y. Neurological and neuroendocrine-cytokine interrelationship in the antiphospholipid syndrome. Ann N Y Acad Sci 2002; 966:415–424.

148. Shrot S. Behavioral and cognitive deficits occur only after prolonged exposure of mice to antiphospholipid antibodies. Lupus 2002; 11(11):736–743.

149. Ozkara C. An association between mesial temporal lobe epilepsy with hippocampal sclerosis and human leukocyte antigens. Epilepsia 2002; 43(3):236–239.

150. Beach TG. Reactive microglia in hippocampal sclerosis associated with human temporal lobe epilepsy. Neurosci Lett 1995; 191(1–2):27–30.

151. Benson M, Blennow G, Rosen I. Intrathecal immunoglobulin production and minor motor seizures. Acta Paediatr Scand 1987; 76(1):147–150.

152. Eeg-Olofsson O. Immunological studies in focal epilepsy. Acta Neurol Scand 1988; **78**(5):358–368.

153. Malashkhiia VI. The immunopathology and immunogenetics of some forms of pediatric epilepsy. Zh Nevropatol Psikhiatr Im S S Korsakova 1996; **96**(2):18–20. (In Russian.)

154. Shavit YB. Epilepsia partialis continua: a new manifestation of anti-Hu-associated paraneoplastic encephalomyelitis. Ann Neurol 1999; **45**(2):255–258.

155. Labate A. Silent celiac disease in patients with childhood localization-related epilepsies. Epilepsia 2001; **42**(9):1153–1155.

156. Hartley LM. Immune mediated chorea encephalopathy syndrome in childhood. Dev Med Child Neurol 2002; **44**(4):273–277.

157. Montelli TC. Alterations of cell-mediated immune response in children with febrile seizures. Arq Neuropsiquiatr 1997; **55**(2):193–198.

158. Vlajkovic S, Jankovic BD. Experimental epilepsy: electrically and chemically induced convulsions modulate experimental allergic encephalomyelitis and other immune inflammatory reactions in the rat. Int J Neurosci 1990; **54**(1–2):165–172.

159. Shaw JA, Perry VH, Mellanby J. MHC class II expression by microglia in tetanus toxin-induced experimental epilepsy in the rat. Neuropathol Appl Neurobiol 1994; **20**(4):392–398.

160. Corriveau RA, Huh, GS, Shatz CJ. Regulation of class I MHC gene expression in the developing and mature CNS by neural activity. Neuron 1998; **21**(3):505–520.

161. Bazan NG. The accumulation of free arachidonic acid, diacylglycerols, prostaglandins, and lipoxygenase reaction products in the brain during experimental epilepsy. Adv Neurol 1986; **44**:879–902.

162. Lerner-Natoli M. Sequential expression of surface antigens and transcription factor NFkappaB by hippocampal cells in excitotoxicity and experimental epilepsy. Epilepsy Res 2000; **41**(2):141–154.

163. Tang Y. Genomic responses of the brain to ischemic stroke, intracerebral haemorrhage, kainate seizures, hypoglycemia, and hypoxia. Eur J Neurosci 2002; **15**(12): 1937–1952.

164. Penkowa M. Interleukin-6 deficiency reduces the brain inflammatory response and increases oxidative stress and neurodegeneration after kainic acid-induced seizures. Neuroscience 2001; **102**(4):805–818.

165. Czlonkowska A, Korlak J. Non-specific immunologic reactivity in epilepsy. Neurol Neurochir Pol 1980; **14**(4):353–358. (In Polish.)

166. Eeg-Olofsson O, Prchal JF, Andermann F. Abnormalities of T-lymphocyte subsets in epileptic patients. Acta Neurol Scand 1985; **72**(2):140–144.

167. Wang XL. Studies on lymphocyte subpopulations and NK cell activities in epileptic patients. J Tongji Med Univ 1989; **9**(1):25–28.

168. Fontana A. Immunological abnormalities and HLA antigen frequencies in IgA deficient patients with epilepsy. J Neurol Neurosurg Psychiatry 1978; **41**(7):593–597.

169. Czlonkowska A, Iwinska B. Immune humoral response in epilepsy. Neurol Neurochir Pol 1977; **11**(1):53–58. (In Polish.)

170. Margaretten NC, Warren RP. Reduced natural killer cell activity and OKT4/OKT8 ratio in epileptic patients. Immunol Invest 1986; **15**(2):159–167.

171. Matsuoka H. Immunological study of IgA deficiency during anticonvulsant therapy in epileptic patients. Clin Exp Immunol 1983; **53**(2):423–428.

172. Goldstein KR. Effects of hemispheric lateralization and site specificity on immune alterations induced by kindled temporal lobe seizures. Brain Behav Immun 2002; **16**(6):706–719.

173. Goriacheva TV. The ACTH and cortisol content of the blood in experimental focal epilepsy. Biull Eksp Biol Med 1989; **107**(2):139–142. (In Russian.)

174. Lorenz R. Clinical study: epileptic seizures may modify cytokine secretion in patients suffering from epilepsy and in experimental animals. Neuroendocrinol Lett 2001; **22**(5):330–331.

175. Falter H, Persinger MA, Chretien R. Transient suppression of a secondary humoral response in rats is evoked by lithium-pilocarpine-induced limbic seizures. Pharmacol Biochem Behav 1992; **43**(1):315–317.

176. Meador KJ. Differential immunologic effects of language-dominant and nondominant cerebral resections. Neurology 1999; **52**(6):1183–1187.

177. Green-Johnson JM. Role of norepinephrine in suppressed IgG production in epilepsy-prone mice. Life Sci 1996; **59**(14):1121–1132.

178. Rowland RR. Evidence of immunosuppression in the genetically epilepsy-prone rat. Life Sci 1991; **48**(19):1821–1826.

179. Carr JA. Alterations in spleen norepinephrine and lymphocyte [3H]dihydroalprenolol binding site number in genetically epilepsy-prone rats. Brain Behav Immun 1993; **7**(2):113 120.

180. Finn DA, Roberts AJ, Crabbe JC. Neuroactive steroid sensitivity in withdrawal seizure-prone and -resistant mice. Alcohol Clin Exp Res 1995; **19**(2):410–415.

181. Yao H. Effects of interleukin-1 and interleukin-2 on electrophysiological characteristics of rat hippocampal neurons in culture. Sheng Li Xue Bao 1994; **46**(6):539 545. (In Chinese.)

182. Samad TA. Interleukin-1beta-mediated induction of Cox-2 in the CNS contributes to inflammatory pain hypersensitivity. Nature 2001; **410**(6827):471–475.

183. Plata-Salaman CR, French-Mullen JM. Interleukin-1 beta inhibits Ca^{2+} channel currents in hippocampal neurons through protein kinase C. Eur J Pharmacol 1994; **266**(1):1–10.

184. Ye JH, Tao L, Zalcman SS. Interleukin-2 modulates N-methyl-D-aspartate receptors of native mesolimbic neurons. Brain Res 2001; **894**(2):241–248.

185. Puma C. The chemokine interleukin-8 acutely reduces Ca(2+) currents in identified cholinergic septal neurons expressing CXCR1 and CXCR2 receptor mRNAs. J Neurochem 2001; **78**(5):960–971.

186. Villani F, Avanzini G. The use of immunoglobulins in the treatment of human epilepsy. Neurol Sci 2002; **23**(suppl 1):S33–S37.

187. During MJ. An oral vaccine against NMDAR1 with efficacy in experimental stroke and epilepsy. Science 2000; **287**(5457):1453–1460.

188. Tuncok Y. Inhibition of nicotine-induced seizures in rats by combining vaccination against nicotine with chronic nicotine infusion. Exp Clin Psychopharmacol 2001; **9**(2):228–234.

17

Neurosteroids: Endogenous Modulators of Seizure Susceptibility

Michael A. Rogawski
National Institutes of Health
Bethesda, Maryland, U.S.A.

Doodipala S. Reddy
North Carolina State University College of Veterinary Medicine
Raleigh, North Carolina, U.S.A.

INTRODUCTION

The term *neurosteroid*, as originally conceived in 1981 by Baulieu, referred to steroids that are synthesized locally within the brain either from cholesterol or steroid hormone precursors (1). More recently, the term has been used in reference to steroids that rapidly alter the excitability of neurons by binding to membrane-bound receptors such as those for inhibitory or excitatory neurotransmitters (2). In common usage, neurosteroid is generally understood to mean an endogenous steroid (whether peripherally synthesized or brain derived) that acts on the nervous system in a non-classical fashion, that is, via cellular actions that do not involve steroid nuclear hormone receptors. The term *neuroactive steroid* encompasses naturally occurring neurosteroids and their synthetic analogs with similar biological properties.

Certain synthetic steroids such as alphaxalone have long been recognized to possess sedative and general anesthetic properties and also to protect against seizures in animals and possibly humans (3–9). It has also been documented that some endogenous steroid hormones, notably progesterone, an ovarian steroid, and deoxycorticosterone (DOC), an adrenal steroid, similarly have sedative and anticonvulsant activities (3,4,8,10,11). These effects occur rapidly and do not correspond with classical notions of steroid hormone action in other target tissues. Indeed, steroids like alphaxalone lack classical hormonal activity but rather act as modulators of neuronal excitability in a fashion similar (although not identical) to barbiturates. This observation became of even greater interest when it was discovered that progesterone and DOC serve as precursors for the endogenous neurosteroids, respectively, allopregnanolone (5α-pregnane-3α-ol-20-one) and allotetrahydrodeoxycorticosterone (THDOC, 5α-pregnane-3α,21-diol-20-one) that have similar cellular actions to alphaxalone. Like alphaxalone, these neurosteroids do not interact with nuclear hormone receptors, but rather modulate the activity of ligand-gated ion channels, most notably GABA-A receptors.

In this chapter, we review emerging evidence supporting a role for GABA-A receptor–modulating neurosteroids as endogenous regulators of seizure susceptibility and their possible involvement in several conditions of relevance in clinical epilepsy, such as catamenial epilepsy and stress-induced alterations in seizure susceptibility. In addition, we provide an overview of current efforts to develop neurosteroid-based agents for epilepsy therapy. Our focus is mainly on allopregnanolone, but we also touch upon the more recent but still very limited evidence implicating THDOC and 3α-androstanedione (derived from testosterone) in seizure regulation.

BIOSYNTHESIS AND METABOLISM OF NEUROSTEROIDS

GABA-A receptor–modulating neurosteroids are A-ring-reduced metabolites of the hormonal steroids progesterone, DOC, and testosterone. The hormonal steroid precursors of neurosteroids are mainly synthesized in the gonads, adrenal, and fetoplacental unit. The GABA-A receptor active forms are generated by sequential reduction of the parent steroid by 5α-reductase (5α-R) and 3α-hydroxysteroid oxidoreductase (3α-HSOR; also referred to as 3α-hydroxysteroid dehydrogenase) isoenzymes (Fig. 1). These conversion steps largely occur in peripheral tissues that are rich in the two reducing activities. There are two distinct 5α-R isoenzymes that have different tissue distributions. Type I 5α-R is widely distributed throughout the body, and is most abundant in the liver. The type II isoenzyme is primarily expressed in target tissues for androgens, such as the prostate and seminal vesicles. 3α-HSOR activity is also expressed widely. Since neurosteroids are highly lipophilic and can readily cross the blood-brain barrier, neurosteroids synthesized in peripheral tissues accumulate in the brain and can influence brain function (12,13).

In addition to synthesis in peripheral tissues, there is evidence that the neurosteroid biosynthetic enzymes 5α-R and 3α-HSOR are present in brain (14–17). Thus, the steroids can be formed from their parent hormonal steroids directly in the target organ (18,19). Like the neurosteroids, the parent hormones readily enter the brain so that pools of peripherally synthesized precursors are readily available for local neurosteroid biosynthesis. In humans, mRNA for the type I isoenzyme has been demonstrated in neocortex and subcortical white matter as well as in hippocampal tissue specimens obtained from patients with chronic temporal lobe epilepsy (20). The expression levels are about 100-fold lower than in human liver tissue. 5α-R type II mRNA has not been detected in human brain. Similarly, the type I isoenzyme is the predominant form in rat brain, although the type II form is transiently expressed during late fetal and early postnatal life (21) and can be induced in the male brain by testosterone and by progesterone in the female brain (22).

Three functional 3α-HSOR isoenzymes have been characterized. Although the type II isoenzyme is thought to be the main form active in the biosynthesis of neurosteroids (23), a variety of genes that encode proteins related to 3α-HSOR isoenzymes exist and numerous other steroid-reducing enzymes are also capable of catalyzing the formation of neuroactive tetrahydrosteroids from their 5α-dihydro

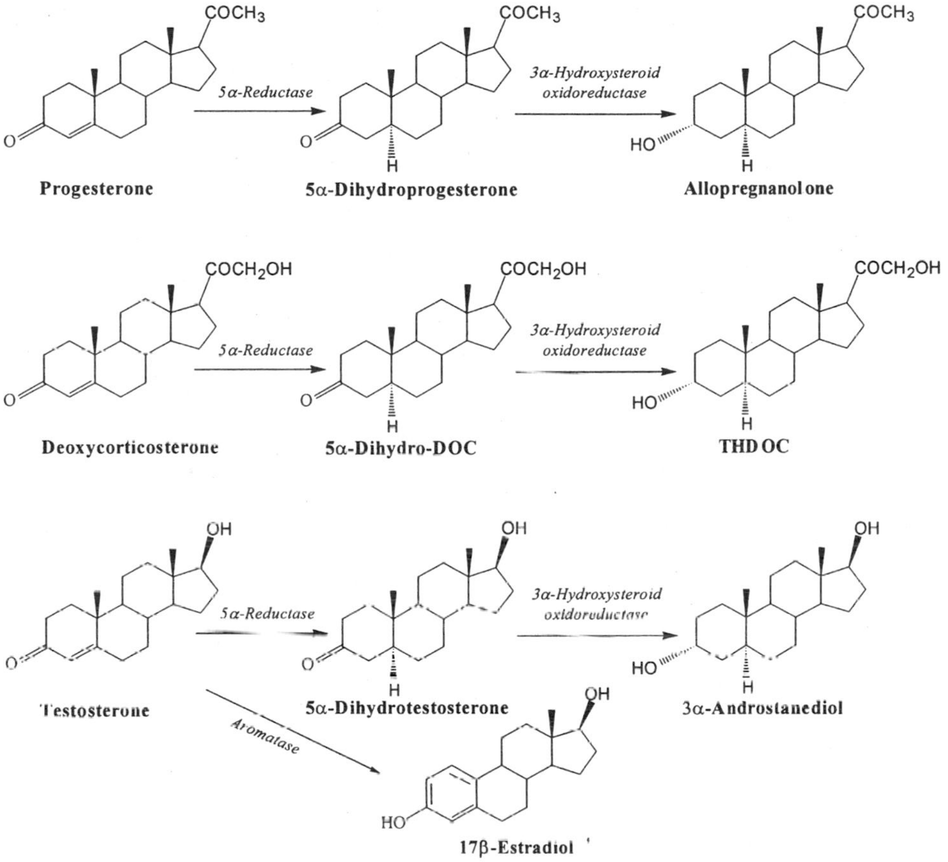

Figure 1. Biosynthetic pathways for the endogenous neurosteroids allopregnanolone allotetrahydrodeoxycorticosterone (THDOC) and 3α-androstanediol.

intermediates. Therefore, the second step in neurosteroid biosynthesis from steroid hormone precursors is likely to be affected by many redundant enzymes. 3α-HSOR activity is found in the pituitary, hypothalamus, and midbrain, and also in limbic structures including the amygdala and hippocampus. Overall, 3α-HSOR activity far exceeds that of the 5α-reductases, so that 5α-reduction is the rate-limiting step in the biosynthesis of neurosteroids (24). 5α-Reductase activity has been identified in both neurons and glial cells (17,25); the cellular localization of the various 3α-HSOR forms has not been determined.

In addition to serving as a site for the conversion of steroid hormones to neurosteroids, there is good evidence that the brain is a steroidogenic organ itself that can synthesize steroid hormones, including progesterone, de novo via classical steroid biosynthetic pathways (26–29). Brain astrocytes and neurons express cytochrome P450 cholesterol side-chain cleavage enzyme (P450$_{SCC}$), which converts cholesterol to pregnenolone, an intermediate necessary for the synthesis of all hormonal steroids (30). Moreover, 3β-hydroxysteroid dehydrogenase, the enzyme required in the further conversion of pregnenolone to progesterone, has been demonstrated in rat brain at the mRNA and protein levels (31). Thus, the enzymes necessary for the in situ synthesis of progesterone from cholesterol are present in brain. Allopregnanolone persists in the brain after adrenalectomy and gonadectomy or after pharmacological suppression of adrenal and gonadal secretions (32), indicating that progesterone synthesized in situ can be converted to allopregnanolone, as is the case for the peripherally synthesized hormone. Additional enzymes that synthesize critical intermediates such as DOC (21-hydroxylase) are probably also present in brain, as well as enzymes that can synthesize dehydroepiandrosterone and various sex steroids including testosterone (15).

Although the enzymatic steps in local neurosteroid biosynthesis have been well characterized, little is known about the regulation of these pathways. The rate-limiting step in the local biosynthesis of neurosteroids is the reaction catalyzed by $P450_{SCC}$, which is located on the inner mitochondrial membrane. The rate of pregnenolone synthesis is controlled not by $P450_{SCC}$ activity itself but rather the rate at which cholesterol is transported to the inner mitochondrial membrane (33). A receptor that is located on the outer mitochondrial membrane participates in the regulation of intramitochondrial cholesterol transport (34). Diazepam-binding inhibitor (DBI), an endogenous 9-kDa (86–amino acid) peptide, binds to this receptor and stimulates steroidogenesis by facilitating cholesterol transport to the inner mitochondrial membrane (35,36). Mitochondrial DBI receptor is a heterooligomeric complex that has high-affinity recognition sites for the isoquinoline carboxamide PK11195, the imidazopyridine alpidem, the benzodiazepine 4'-chlordiazepam and the 2-arylindoleacetamide FGIN-1-27 (37). These agents have been shown to elicit behavioral effects that are at least partly due to increased neurosteroid synthesis (38,39).

Neurosteroid synthesis can be selectively suppressed by agents that inhibit 5α-R or 3α-HSOR. A variety of 5α-R inhibitors have been developed mainly to inhibit the 5α reduction of testosterone to 5α-dihydrotestosterone as a treatment for benign prostatic hyperplasia and male pattern baldness. The most widely available 5α-R inhibitor is finasteride, which is a synthetic 4-azasteroid and a specific inhibitor of type II 5α-reductase in humans, but a nonspecific inhibitor of both the type I and type II isoenzymes in rodents (24,40,41). 3α-HSOR can be inhibited by various nonsteroidal anti-inflammatory agents, including indomethacin (42). However, because 3α-HSOR activity represents a more diverse group of enzymes than 5α-R and this activity is present in excess (that is, it is not rate limiting like 5α-R), it may be more difficult to suppress neurosteroid biosynthesis with 3α-HSOR inhibitors.

NEUROSTEROIDS ARE POSITIVE ALLOSTERIC MODULATORS OF GABA-A RECEPTORS

Neurosteroids and GABA-A Receptors

The neurosteroids allopregnanolone and THDOC are potent positive allosteric modulators of GABA-A receptors which mediate the bulk of synaptic inhibition in the central nervous system. GABA-A receptors are members of the cysteine-cysteine loop transmitter-gated ion channel family that includes glycine, nicotinic, and $5HT_3$ receptors. They are plasma membrane-bound protein complexes that contain recognition sites for the neurotransmitter agonist GABA and various modulators such as benzodiazepines, barbiturates and neurosteroids (Fig. 2). The central core of the receptor complex serves as an ion channel with high selectivity for Cl^-. Upon

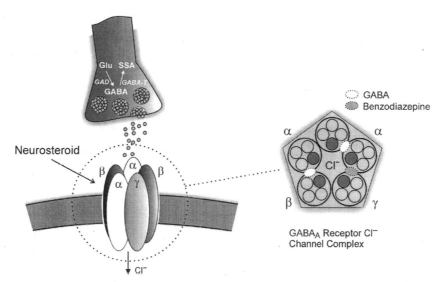

Figure 2. Overview of the inhibitory GABA-ergic synapse –the site of action of neurosteroids. Pathways for GABA biosynthesis and metabolism are schematically illustrated in a presynaptic GABA-ergic nerve terminal. Glutamate (Glu) is converted to GABA by glutamic acid decarboxylase (GAD) and packaged into vesicles. GABA is degraded to succinic semialdehyde (SSA) by 4-aminobutyrate:2-oxoglutarate aminotransferase (GABA-T). The pentameric structure of the GABA-A receptor is illustrated. A typical configuration is believed to be two α subunits, two β subunits, and a γ subunit. Each GABA-A receptor subunit has four transmembrane domains (M1-M4); M2 which forms the pore lining is shown in dark gray. When gated by GABA released from the presynaptic terminal, the GABA receptor permits Cl$^-$ flux. Binding sites for GABA and benzodiazepines are located at subunit interfaces as shown. The binding site for neurosteroids has not yet been delineated but is believed to be distinct from the GABA and benzodiazepine sites.

activation by GABA, the Cl$^-$ channel region of the receptor complex opens, hyperpolarizing the neuron, providing an increase in membrane conductance and effectively shunting the influence of excitatory transmitters such as glutamate (43). GABA-A receptors are believed to be pentameric with the five protein subunits organized like the spokes of a wheel around the ion channel pore. There are seven different classes of subunits, some of which have multiple closely homologous variants (α_{1-6}, β_{1-3}, γ_{1-3}, σ_{1-3}, δ, ϵ, θ); most GABA-A receptors are believed to be composed of α, β, and γ subunits (44).

The first clues to the way in which some steroids affect neural excitability came from work with the steroid anesthetic alphaxolone (3α-hydroxy-5α-pregnane-11,20-dione) (Fig. 3). Alphaxolone was developed as a short acting general anesthetic based upon Selye's original observations on the anesthetic actions of certain steroid hormones (9,45). In 1980, Scholfield reported that alphaxolone exhibited a barbituratelike action to enhance inhibitory postsynaptic responses in guinea pig olfactory cortex slices, suggesting that alphaxolone may modulate GABA-A receptors (46). This was confirmed in studies demonstrating that alphaxolone enhances GABA-evoked responses and at higher concentrations directly activates GABA-A receptors (47,48). These studies were followed by the demonstration that

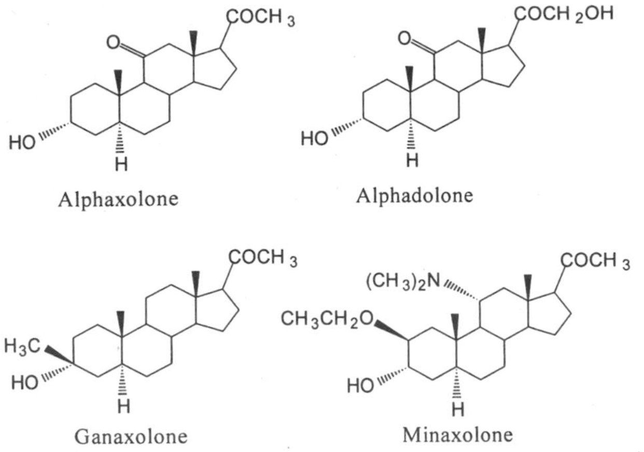

Figure 3. Structures of several synthetic neuroactive steroids. Alphaxalone is often administered as an anesthetic in combination with alphadolone ($3\alpha,21$-dihydroxy-5α-pregnane-11,20-dione-21-acetate) to improve solubility. Alphadolone has about one-half the potency of alphaxolone.

allopregnanolone and THDOC enhance GABA-A receptor responses in a similar fashion (49).

Molecular Physiology of Neurosteroid Action

There is considerable evidence that neurosteroids bind to GABA-A receptors at a site that is distinct from the recognition sites for GABA, benzodiazepines, and barbiturates (50,51). Behavioral studies with selective antagonists also support the view that neurosteroids do not act through "benzodiazepine receptors" (52–54). Like other positive allosteric modulators of GABA-A receptors, neurosteroids enhance the specific binding of [³H]flunitrazepam, a benzodiazepine receptor agonist, and [³H]muscimol, a specific GABA-site agonist, and inhibit the binding of [³⁵S]t-butylbicycloorthobenzoate (TBPS), a cage convulsant and noncompetitive GABA-A receptor antagonist (55–57). Electrophysiological studies have confirmed that neurosteroids act as positive allosteric modulators of GABA-A receptor function (49–50,58–62), and increase the strength of inhibitory postsynaptic potentials (IPSPs) mediated by these receptors (63,64).

Consistent with these studies, neurosteroids potentiate $^{36}Cl^-$ flux stimulated by GABA-A receptor agonists (60,65–67). Neurosteroid enhancement of GABA-A receptor macroscopic currents occurs through increases in both the open frequency and open duration of single GABA-A receptor channels; there is no effect on the single-channel conductance (59,68–70). Kinetic analysis reveals three kinetically distinct open states, and the neurosteroids appear to act primarily by increasing the relative frequency of occurrence of two open states of intermediate and long duration (71). Thus, in the presence of neurosteroids, GABA-A receptors have a greater probability of opening and there is more chloride ion flux so that there is an augmentation of inhibitory GABA-ergic transmission. Studies of near physiological concentrations of THDOC in brain slices have indicated that the effect on inhibitory synaptic transmission occurs mainly through prolongation of the decay rate of inhibitory postsynaptic currents (IPSCs) rather than an augmentation in their amplitude (72).

GABA-A Receptor Modulation by Endogenous Neurosteroids

Concentrations of allopregnanolone as low as 1 nM are active at GABA-A receptors (73,74). This can be compared to serum concentrations, which in women range from 2 to 4 nM, depending on the phase of the menstrual cycle (75). Brain concentrations are typically higher than in the plasma because of local synthesis (76), and are therefore sufficient to have an ongoing modulatory influence on GABA-A receptor–mediated synaptic inhibition. Moreover, in response to stress, brain levels of allopregnanolone rise rapidly by more than twofold (76). Brain and plasma levels of THDOC rise even more dramatically in response to stress. The low nanomolar concentrations of THDOC present in rat serum after stress are also well within the range of concentrations that enhance GABA-activated chloride currents (11,76). Concentrations near this range have also been shown to enhance GABA-A receptor–mediated synaptic inhibition as assessed by effects on IPSCs (72).

At high concentrations, neurosteroids can directly activate GABA-A receptor channels in the absence of GABA (73). In this respect, neurosteroids resemble barbiturates (77). These direct actions, which are picrotoxin and bicuculline sensitive (11,61), could contribute to the sedative and anticonvulsant effects of exogenously administered neuroactive steroids, but are not likely to be relevant to the actions of endogenous neurosteroids which are not present at sufficiently high concentrations.

GABA-A Receptor Subunit Selectivity of Neurosteroids

GABA-A receptor subunits are differentially expressed both temporally and spatially throughout the brain (44,78). Among the more than 2000 subunit combinations that are theoretically possible, as many as 20–30 distinct forms are likely to exist in the mammalian central nervous system. Most GABA-A receptors are believed to be composed of α, β, and γ subunits with a stoichiometry of 2:2:1. The δ, ε, and θ subunits may replace the γ subunit in some receptor subtypes. The diverse GABA-A receptor forms exhibit a range of physiological and pharmacological properties (79–82). Most forms show neurosteroid modulation, although there are moderate differences depending on the presence and type of α or γ subunit (83). The specific α subunit may influence neurosteroid efficacy, whereas the γ subunit type may affect both the efficacy and potency (EC_{50}) for neurosteroid modulation of GABA-A receptors (173,84–87). In contrast, alterations in the type of β subunit do not appear to affect neurosteroid efficacy or potency (88,89). Substitution of the δ subunit, which is expressed in cerebellum, hippocampus, and thalamus, for γ, results in a small enhancement of neurosteroid efficacy (90). This contradicts the results of Zhu et al. (91), who found that the δ subunit inhibits neurosteroid modulation of GABA-A receptors; the reason for the discrepancy is not known. At higher concentrations, neurosteroids positively modulate GABA-activated Cl^- channels assembled as homopentamers of ρ_1 subunits (92,93) (ρ subunits are mainly expressed in the retina and do not coassemble with GABA-A receptor subunits; the receptors they form have been referred to as GABA-C receptors in recognition of their unique pharmacological properties).

Recently, the use of transgenic animals has begun to unravel the contributions of particular GABA-A receptor subtypes to the specific behavioral actions of the benzodiazepines (94). Whether the various in vivo actions of neurosteroids (e.g., sedative, anxiolytic, and anticonvulsant) can similarly be assigned to specific GABA-A receptor isoforms remains to be determined. In a demonstration of the potential utility of transgenic animals in this respect, Mihalek et al. (95) found that the absence of the δ subunit selectively attenuates behavioral responses to neurosteroids. Furthermore, alphaxolone prolongation of the decay (τ) of pharmacologically isolated miniature GABA-A receptor–mediated synaptic currents (mIPSCs) was much smaller in mice lacking the δ subunit compared with wild littermates (96). This corresponds with the observation noted above that the δ subunit enhances neurosteroid potency.

Since the subunit composition of GABA-A receptors may affect neurosteroid sensitivity, "subunit switching," in which the subunit composition of synaptic GABA-A receptors is altered as a result of hormonal or other factors, is a mechanism by which long-term changes in the responsiveness to neurosteroids can occur (97,98) (see section on neurosteroid withdrawal model of catamenial epilepsy). Inasmuch as classical steroid actions involve regulation of gene transcription, this is a potential mechanism for interplay between the genomic and nongenomic actions of steroids. Moreover, it is becoming apparent that factors such as phosphorylation can alter the activity of GABA-A receptors and may also influence neurosteroid modulation (99,100). Protein kinase activity may be affected by the classic genomic actions of many steroids, thus providing another way in which the genomic actions of steroids can influence neurosteroid sensitivity.

Neurosteroid Structure-Activity Relationships

There are strict structural requirements for neurosteroid modulation of GABA-A receptors. In general, steroids that are potent modulators all have a hydrogen bond-donating 3-hydroxy group in the α configuration on the steroid A ring. In addition, they have a hydrogen bond accepting group (typically a keto moiety) on the D ring at either C20 of the pregnane steroid side chain or C17 of the androstane ring system extending in the opposite β direction (50,60,101). The steroid structure forms a framework that rigidly positions these hydrogen bonding groups in three-dimensional space. The strict requirement for a group in the proper stereochemical orientation at C3 which can engage in hydrogen bonding is further emphasized by the observation that esterification and oxidation of the 3α-hydroxy group greatly reduces activity (102). The orientation of the 5-hydroxy group (which determines whether the A ring is in the coplanar *trans* configuration or in the *cis* boat form) is less critical: β-analogs at this position such as pregnanolone (5β-pregnanone-3α-ol-20-one) are only modestly less active in augmenting GABA receptor–mediated $^{36}Cl^-$ uptake and potentiating GABA-activated Cl^- currents than are the corresponding steroids with the 5α-configuration such as allopregnanolone (61,103). Introduction of a 2β-morpholinyl moiety may confer water solubility for pregnane steroids without loss of GABA-A receptor activity (70). Similarly, substitution of the 3β-hydrogen of allopregnanolone with a methyl group as in ganaxolone (Fig. 3) causes a severalfold reduction in binding affinity to GABA-A receptors (104), but this steroid still produces powerful enhancement of responses at GABA-A receptors.

Neurosteroids with partial agonistic activity have also been reported (105), but the extent to which these are useful as neurosteroid antagonists that could serve as tools for elucidating the physiological roles of endogenous steroids is uncertain. For example, 5β-THDOC has limited efficacy as an allosteric modulator of $[^{35}S]$TBPS binding, and has been reported to antagonize the action of allopregnanolone and 5α-THDOC at GABA-A receptors in vitro and in vivo (56,84).

Neurosteroids and GABA-A Receptor Plasticity

There is evidence that chronic exposure and withdrawal from neurosteroids elicits changes in the functional properties of GABA-A receptors (106). For example, chronic treatment with allopregnanolone (2–10 µM for 2–5 days) eliminates neurosteroid potentiation of the binding of $[^3H]$flunitrazepam, $[^3H]$Ro15-1788, and other benzodiazepine site ligands in cultured neurons, a process referred to as "uncoupling" or the loss of the allosteric interaction between neurosteroids and benzodiazepine recognition sites (107–110). In addition, there are decreases in the binding of other GABA receptor ligands including $[^3H]$GABA and TBPS, referred to as heterologous uncoupling. Along with the alterations in radioligand binding, there are corresponding decreases in the efficacy by which GABA and benzodiazepines stimulate $^{36}Cl^-$ influx in neurons that have been chronically exposed to neurosteroids (110). The precise molecular bases for these functional changes in GABA-A receptors and the relevance of these changes for neurosteroid actions in the intact nervous system are not well understood.

In other studies in vivo, withdrawal from chronic allopregnanolone has been reported to upregulate α_4 subunit expression in the hippocampus, leading to alterations in the pharmacology of GABA-A receptors (98,111,112). It has been possible to demonstrate similar changes in α_4 subunit expression in cultured rat cerebellar granule cells upon withdrawal of allopregnanolone (106). Selective increases in α_4 subunit expression are also observed upon withdrawal of benzodiazepines (113). Interestingly, upregulation of the α_4 subunit requires *withdrawal* from chronic exposure to either neuroactive steroids or benzodiazepines; these effects do not occur during the chronic exposure phase. In contrast, in the hypothalamus, there is evidence that chronic neurosteroid exposure (or other hormonal factors) during pregnancy alters the ratio in α_1 and α_2 subunit expression (97,114).

Pregnenolone Sulfate and Dehydroepiandrosterone Sulfate

Although the best-studied action of neurosteroids is positive modulation of GABA-A receptors, some endogenous steroids have inhibitory actions on GABA-A receptors. This mainly occurs with steroids that are sulfated (or alternatively have a hemisuccinate group) at C3 (115). The best-studied examples of such GABA-antagonistic neurosteroids are pregnenolone sulfate (PS) and dehydroepiandrosterone sulfate (DHEAS), which block GABA-A receptors at low micromolar concentrations (116). These steroids act as noncompetitive antagonists of the GABA-A receptor by interacting with a site that is distinct from that at which steroids such as allopregnanolone and THDOC exert their positive modulatory actions (115,117–119). The steroid-negative modulatory action on GABA-A receptors occurs through a reduction in channel opening frequency, although the precise mechanism of block is not well understood (120,121). PS is present in brain at a relatively high concentration compared with many other neurosteroids (126) and is presumably generated by local steroid sulfotransferases since charged steroid sulfates are unlikely to cross the blood-brain barrier.

In addition to effects on GABA-A receptors, sulfated neurosteroids can also interact with excitatory amino acid receptors including AMPA/kainate and NMDA receptors. The effect on NMDA receptors is of particular note in that NMDA receptor responses are enhanced (122–124). This positive modulatory action occurs in a subunit-dependent fashion with the nature of the NR2 subunit in heteromeric NMDA receptors determining the efficacy of the positive modulatory action of PS (125,126). Thus, NMDA receptors composed of the obligatory NR1 subunit and NR2A or NR2B exhibit PS potentiation whereas those containing NR2C or NR2D are actually inhibited. The mechanism of these effects is not well understood but does not involve the glycine modulatory site on NMDA receptors.

Given their abundance in brain, it seems reasonable that PS and DHEAS could function as endogenous neuromodulators (127–129). However, it has yet to be demonstrated that synaptic concentrations are high enough for modulation of synaptic transmission to occur under normal physiological conditions. In any case, it is interesting that PS and DHEAS can antagonize inhibitory neurotransmission through their actions on GABA-A receptors while also potentiating excitatory transmission by effects on NMDA receptors. The steroids therefore have a dual action that could confer proconvulsant activity and, in fact, the steroids do promote seizures as discussed below.

NEUROSTEROIDS ARE POTENT ANTICONVULSANT AGENTS

Anticonvulsant Profile of Neurosteroids

Like benzodiazepines and barbiturates, GABA-A receptor-positive modulating neurosteroids protect against seizures induced in animals by GABA-A receptor antagonists such as pentylenetetrazol (PTZ), bicuculline, picrotoxin, and methyl-6,7-dimethoxy-4-ethyl-β-carboline-3-carboxylate (DMCM) (61,130–133). The spectrum of antiseizure activity of some neurosteroids is summarized in Table 1. The neurosteroids also protect against pilocarpine-induced limbic seizures and status epilepticus, and inhibit status epilepticus–like seizure activity induced by prolonged electrical stimulation of the perforant pathway to the hippocampus (133–135). In addition, they protect against the development of kindled seizures, as do other GABA-A receptor–positive modulators (136–138). Some neurosteroids have also been reported to protect against corneal and PTZ-kindled seizures (137,139). At high (and generally behaviorally toxic) doses, neurosteroids also partially protect mice against maximal electroshock (MES)-, kainate-, and NMDA-induced seizures and mortality (140). In addition, neurosteroids are highly efficacious against cocaine, ethanol, diazepam, and neurosteroid withdrawal seizures (66,141,142), indicating a unique broad-spectrum antiseizure activity. Neurosteroids have differing potencies in various seizure models. In mice, the potency ranking is as

Table 1. Pharmacological Profiles of Neuroactive Steroids and Their Precursors in Animal Seizure Models

Steroid	PTZ	Bicuculline	Pilocarpine	Kindling	MES	Kainic acid	NMDA
Precursors							
Progesterone	+	+	+	+	+	0	0
DOC	+	+	+	+	+	0	0
5α-Dihydro-DOC	++			+	+	0	0
Testosterone	?			−		+	
Naturally occurring							
Allopregnanolone	++	++	++	++	+	0	0
Pregnanolone	++	++	++	++	+	0	0
THDOC	++	++	++	++	+	0	0
5α-Dihydrotestosterone	+	+		+	+	0	0
3α-Androstanediol	++	++		+	+	0	0
17β-Estradiol (chronic)				−	−		
Synthetic analogs							
Alphaxolone	++	++		+	+	0	0
Ganaxolone	++	++		+	+	0	0
Minaxolone	|+	++					
Sulfated derivatives							
Pregnenolone sulfate	−	−				−	−
DHEA sulfate	−	−				−	−

Compilation of results from studies cited in the text. 5α-Dihydro-DOC serves as a precursor for THDOC and has anticonvulsant activity itself (224).
++, Potent anticonvulsant; +, moderately potent anticonvulsant; −, proconvulsant or convulsant; 0, inactive at nonsedative doses; ?, controversial.

follows (most sensitive to least sensitive): pilocarpine > bicuculline > PTZ > kindling > MES.

Several lines of evidence indicate that the anticonvulsant activity of neurosteroids in these animal models is not related to interactions with traditional steroid hormone receptors that regulate gene transcription. First, the anticonvulsant effects of neurosteroids such as allopregnanolone and THDOC occur rapidly (within minutes). Second, A ring-reduced neurosteroids are not known to directly interact with nuclear steroid hormone receptors. Third, studies in progesterone receptor knockout (PRKO) mice, in which the progesterone receptor has been deleted by gene targeting, conclusively demonstrate that the progesterone receptor is not required for the anticonvulsant activity of neurosteroids (143). Interestingly, the progesterone receptor-deficient animals actually have enhanced sensitivity to the anticonvulsant activity of allopregnanolone and the synthetic neuroactive steroid ganaxolone, and in addition show overall reduced seizure susceptibility; the basis for these alterations is unknown. Although allopregnanolone and THDOC do not themselves appear to interact with intracellular steroid hormone receptors, they may nonetheless indirectly affect progesterone receptors through their oxidized metabolites 5α-dihydroprogesterone or 5α-dihydrodeoxycorticosterone, which can be formed by the reverse action of 3α-HSOR (144).

Anticonvulsant Activity of Progesterone

Progesterone has long been known to have anticonvulsant activity in animal seizure models, and in clinical studies progesterone has been found to reduce the frequency of interictal spikes and lessen the risk of seizures (145–147). The anticonvulsant activity of progesterone in rodent models is similar to allopregnanolone and other GABA-A receptor–modulating neurosteroids, although it is less potent and has a more delayed onset of action (148). The ability of progesterone to protect against seizures, at least in the PTZ test, is eliminated by finasteride, indicating that conversion to 5α-reduced neurosteroid metabolites is required. The conventional (genomic) effects of progesterone in target cells are mediated by progesterone receptors, which are intracellular ligand-activated nuclear transcription factors (149). Progesterone receptors are mainly found in reproductive tissues, but are also expressed in brain. They have a nonuniform distribution with high levels in hypothalamus, and moderate levels in neocortex, hippocampus, and limbic areas (150). As noted in the preceding section, nuclear hormone receptors like the progesterone receptor are not believed to mediate the anticonvulsant activity of neurosteroids. There is also strong evidence from studies in PRKO mice that progesterone receptors are not involved in the acute anticonvulsant activity of progesterone (143). As was the case for allopregregnanolone, PRKO mice exhibited enhanced sensitivity to the antiseizure activity of progesterone against PTZ and also kindled seizures. As expected, in the PRKO mice the anticonvulsant effects of progesterone were blocked by finasteride, confirming that conversion to allopregnanolone is required. Although these studies demonstrate that the antiseizure effects of progesterone occur through conversion to allopregnanolone and not via an interaction with progesterone receptors, the possibility that progesterone receptors or other nuclear hormone receptors could play a role in the effects of steroid hormones on seizure susceptibility in some epileptic conditions cannot be excluded (151).

Proconvulsant Effects

As noted previously, the sulfated neurosteroids PS and DHEAS block inhibitory GABA-A receptor responses and also allosterically facilitate excitatory NMDA receptor responses, suggesting that they could be proconvulsant. In fact, acute intracerebroventricular or chronic systemic administration of these steroids reduces the PTZ seizure threshold (152) and intracerebroventricular administration can induce seizures and status epilepticus (153). The seizure-facilitating effects of PS and DHEAS can be blocked by coadministration of allopregnanolone or other related neurosteroids that positively modulate GABA-A receptors, as well as by benzodiazepines and by NMDA receptor antagonists. The overall pharmacological profile suggested that the GABA-A receptor–blocking activity of the sulfated steroids is predominantly responsible for the proconvulsant activity, although the effects on NMDA receptors may also contribute. The possibility that sulphated neurosteroids could have a role in epileptic seizure susceptibility is of interest but has not as yet received experimental support.

It has long been suspected that estrogens can enhance seizure susceptibility and could play a role in seizure exacerbations in women with epilepsy (154). More recently, evidence has accumulated that chronic estrogen treatment has effects on excitatory circuits in the hippocampus that can promote seizure activity (155). In addition, estradiol has been shown to facilitate kindled seizures, decrease the threshold for electroshock-induced seizures, and increase susceptibility to kainate seizures (156–160). These effects of chronic estrogen do not seem to be due to direct modulatory effects on ion channels comparable to the actions of GABA-A receptor modulating neurosteroids. Rather, estrogens could induce slow changes in brain excitability owing to transcriptional effects. In any case, with either acute or chronic estradiol, we have failed to observe dramatic changes in seizure-susceptibility in mice. As noted below, testosterone has also been claimed to have seizure promoting effects that could occur as a result of its conversion by aromatase to estrogen (138,161).

PHYSIOLOGICAL ROLES AND CLINICAL POTENTIAL OF NEUROSTEROIDS

Although it has been amply demonstrated that neurosteroids are powerful modulators of brain excitability, it has been more difficult to demonstrate a physiological role for neurosteroids in normal or pathological brain function. However, in recent years evidence has steadily accumulated suggesting that neurosteroids are critical biochemical mediators in various clinical conditions, such as premenstrual syndrome, fatigue during pregnancy, and depression, especially in the postpartum period (162–164). Regulation of seizure susceptibility is among the clinical situations in which neurosteroids are likely to play a role; the supporting evidence will be discussed in this section. Recognition of the involvement of neurosteroids in brain disorders may provide clues to novel therapeutic approaches. Indeed, during the last decade, many studies have substantiated the promising therapeutic potential of neurosteroids in a wide variety of neurological and psychiatric conditions including anxiety, depression, learning and memory, and sleep disorders (see reviews, 19,165,166). In this section, we also discuss the potential for neurosteroid-based therapies in epilepsy, focusing on the uses of such agents to treat catamenial and stress-related seizure exacerbations, infantile spasms, and ethanol withdrawal seizures.

Catamenial Epilepsy

A hallmark of epilepsy is the unpredictable occurrence of seizures. However, in many women with epilepsy, seizures do not occur randomly but cluster in association with the menstrual cycle. Based on the review of a vast clinical experience, Newmark and Penry (167) defined catamenial epilepsy as epileptic seizures occurring in women of fertile age exclusively or significantly more often during a 7-day period of the menstrual cycle beginning 3 days prior to menstruation and ending 4 days after its onset. With this criterion as a rough guideline, catamenial epilepsy has been reported to occur in 10–72% of women with epilepsy (168,169). Recently, Herzog et al. (170) proposed an extension of the definition of catamenial epilepsy to include periovulatory and luteal forms. In perimenstrual catamenial epilepsy, the most common clinical type, seizures decrease in the midluteal phase, when serum progesterone levels are high, and increase premenstrually, when progesterone levels fall and there is a decrease in the serum progesterone to estrogen ratio (171,172). As early as 1956, Laidlaw proposed that the premenstrual seizure exacerbations are due to withdrawal of the antiseizure effects of progesterone (173). However, only in recent years with the recognition that progesterone is converted to allopregnanolone, a powerful anticonvulsant neurosteroid (see above, section on the anticonvulsant activity of progesterone), have the physiological underpinnings of this concept become clear. With this understanding, it is now apparent why perimenstrual catamenial epilepsy may, at least in part, be attributed to withdrawal of the anticonvulsant action of allopregnanolone.

Neurosteroid Withdrawal Model of Catamenial Epilepsy

Despite the increased awareness and understanding of catamenial epilepsy, there are few specific treatment approaches. The dearth of attention to the development of therapies may be due to the lack of an appropriate animal model. Recently, we described a rat model of perimenstrual catamenial epilepsy (142). Through treatment with gonadotropins, a state of chronically elevated serum progesterone and allopregnanolone was induced in immature female rats, referred to as "pseudo-pregnancy." In pseudopregnancy, secretion of progesterone by the leutinized ovaries occurs in a physiologically appropriate episodic fashion and leads to plasma progesterone levels that are within the physiological range. The magnitude of the increase in serum progesterone is comparable to the six- to eightfold increase that occurs in women during the normal menstrual cycle (75,164). In contrast, the fluctuations in progesterone and allopregnanolone levels in true pregnancy may differ (174). Allopregnanolone was acutely withdrawn by administration of finasteride. On the day following finasteride-induced neurosteroid withdrawal, the animals exhibited increased seizure susceptibility, mimicking the situation in catamenial epilepsy. A similar predisposition to seizures is observed upon abrupt discontinuation of benzodiazepines (175) and ethanol (176), which also have GABA-A receptor–positive modulating properties. Since the fluctuations in neurosteroid levels are similar to those that occur in women during the perimenstrual period, this rat model may replicate the physiological changes that lead to perimenstrual seizure exacerbations and could be useful for the evaluation of therapeutic approaches to the treatment of catamenial epilepsy.

In the development of the rat catamenial epilepsy model, finasteride rather than ovariectomy was used to induce withdrawal from neurosteroids because ovariectomy would be associated with a decrease in estrogens as well as neurosteroids. Ovariectomy would therefore not simulate the reduced ratio of progesterone (and allopregnanolone) to estrogen that is believed to be critical to perimenstrual catamenial epilepsy (177). Nevertheless, ovariectomized pseudo-pregnant animals did exhibit an increase in seizure susceptibility, indicating that maintained estrogen is not required for enhanced seizure reactivity (178).

The basis for the increased seizure susceptibility following neurosteroid withdrawal in pseudopregnant rats is not well understood, but is unlikely to be due to a reduction in the number of GABA-A receptors. Although high doses of progesterone may downregulate GABA-A receptors as assessed with [^{3}H]muscimol binding (179), pregnant rats appear to have increased brain GABA-A receptor densities by [^{3}H]GABA and [^{3}H]flunitrazepam binding (180). As noted above, Smith et al. (111,112) have proposed that progesterone withdrawal is accompanied by alterations in the expression of GABA-A receptor subunits and a consequent change in GABA-A receptor properties that causes reduced inhibition and an overall increase in brain excitability. Specifically, these workers reported increased expression of the GABA-A receptor α_4 subunit that was associated with an acceleration in the decay of GABA-A receptor currents in CA1 hippocampal neurons. However, other investigators have failed to observe any change in the expression of the α_{1-4}, β_{1-3}, and γ_2S GABA-A receptors subunits in rat cerebral cortex and hippocampus during pregnancy or after delivery, which is associated with a large fall in progesterone and allopregnanolone (174). Therefore, the precise nature of any changes in GABA-A receptors that occur following progesterone withdrawal remains to be characterized.

Neurosteroid Replacement Therapy of Catamenial Epilepsy

Using the rat model of perimenstrual catamenial epilepsy discussed in the preceding section, the pharmacological efficacy of neurosteroids was evaluated with the aim of determining whether neurosteroid "replacement" would be an effective approach to protecting against catamenial seizure exacerbations (178). Allopregnanolone and several analogs that act as positive allosteric modulators of GABA-A receptors were tested along with conventional anticonvulsant drugs that are effective in the PTZ model. All neuroactive steroids effectively protected against PTZ-induced seizures. However, there were marked differences between the neuroactive steroids and the other agents in their relative activities in control and withdrawn animals. In all cases, the neuroactive steroids had enhanced anticonvulsant activity in the withdrawn animals, whereas benzodiazepines and valproate exhibited equivalent or reduced anticonvulsant activity. Phenobarbital was similar to the neuroactive steroids in having modestly enhanced activity following neurosteroid withdrawal. These observations suggest that neuroactive steroids may represent a specific treatment approach for perimenstrual catamenial seizure exacerbations due to neurosteroid withdrawal. It is interesting to note that as in the catamenial epilepsy model, the anticonvulsant activity of neurosteroids is also enhanced during withdrawal from chronic ethanol (66,181,234) and diazepam (141).

The molecular mechanisms underlying enhanced neurosteroid anticonvulsant sensitivity following neurosteroid withdrawal are obscure but, like the situation for the overall increase in seizure susceptibility, could be due to changes in the expression of GABA-A receptor subunits associated with withdrawal. There is precedent for reduced benzodiazepine sensitivity following neurosteroid withdrawal and this is likely related to a "switch" in GABA-A receptor subunit expression. Thus, the sedative potency of the benzodiazepine lorazepam in animals is reduced after progesterone or neurosteroid withdrawal (182) and attenuated benzodiazepine sensitivity has been observed clinically in patients with the premenstrual syndrome (183), a condition, like catamenial epilepsy, attributed to fluctuations in endogenous neurosteroids. The reduced potency of benzodiazepines has been ascribed to increased expression of the GABA-A receptor α_4 subunit, which confers diazepam and lorazepam insensitivity (111,112). In the rat catamenial epilepsy model, although there was a similar modest reduction in the potency of diazepam following neurosteroid withdrawal, the anticonvulsant activity of bretazenil, a partial benzodiazepine receptor agonist that does act as a positive allosteric modulator of α_4-containing GABA-A receptors, did not show such reduced activity. This is consistent with the view that neurosteroid withdrawal is associated with increased α_4

subunit expression. However, since the α_4 subunit does not modify the sensitivity of GABA-A receptors to neuroactive steroids and barbiturates (80), it seems unlikely that enhanced α_4 expression accounts for the augmented anticonvulsant activity of neuroactive steroids and phenobarbital following neurosteroid withdrawal. Whether changes in the expression of other subunits could lead to enhanced neuroactive steroid sensitivity remains to be determined. It is interesting that neurosteroid sensitivity is enhanced in human subjects being treated with postmenopausal hormone replacement containing progestagens that are not metabolized to neurosteroids (184). It is conceivable that this effect could occur through a similar mechanism as the enhancement that accompanies neurosteroid withdrawal. However, it has recently been shown that the progestagen medroxyprogesterone acetate, which blocks 3α-HSOR, can enhance the local activity of allopregnanolone by preventing its degradation (through oxidation by 3α-HSOR) to the inactive intermediate 5α-dihydroprogesterone (255). This could also explain the observation that medroxyprogesterone, a steroid that does not have GABA-A receptor modulatory activity, is effective in the treatment of catamenial epilepsy (167).

An additional aspect of GABA-A receptor plasticity seen in the catamenial epilepsy model is manifest as reduced antiseizure sensitivity of benzodiazepines in pseudopregnant animals prior to neurosteroid withdrawal (178). These animals have persistently high neurosteroid levels. Since cross-tolerance to benzodiazepines can occur with chronic neurosteroid exposure (see section below), the reduced benzodiazepine sensitivity likely results from such a cross-tolerance mechanism (185). Again, the molecular basis of this phenomenon is not well understood. However, in cultured neurons, chronic exposure to allopregnanolone does markedly reduce the sensitivity of GABA-A receptors to benzodiazepines (108–110).

Ganaxolone in the Treatment of Catamenial Epilepsy

Although natural progesterone therapy benefits some women with catamenial epilepsy (147,186), it may be associated with undesired hormonal side effects. GABA-A receptor–modulating neurosteroids, which are devoid of such hormonal actions, could provide a rational alternative approach to therapy (54). However, certain obstacles prevent the clinical use of endogenously occurring neurosteroids. Importantly, natural neurosteroids such as allopregnanolone have low bioavailability because they are rapidly inactivated and eliminated by glucuronide or sulfate conjugation at the 3α-hydroxyl group. In addition, the 3α-hydroxyl group of allopregnanolone may undergo oxidation to the ketone, restoring activity at steroid hormone receptors (144). Ganaxolone (CCD 1042; 3α-hydroxy-3β-methyl-5α-pregnane-20-one) (Fig. 3), the 3β-methyl analog of allopregnanolone, is an example of a synthetic neurosteroid congener that overcomes these limitations (137). Like allopregnanolone, ganaxolone is a positive allosteric modulator of GABA-A receptors and is an effective anticonvulsant in the PTZ seizure test as well as in other anticonvulsant screening models (132,137 see Table 2). However, ganaxolone is orally active, and adequate blood levels can be maintained in human subjects with BID or TID dosing (187). In addition, although ganaxolone is extensively metabolized, the potentially hormonally active 3-keto derivative is not formed. Preliminary evidence of the efficacy of ganaxolone in the treatment of human epilepsy is presented below, in the section on clinical experience with neuroactive steroids.

Table 2. The Antiseizure Profile of Ganaxolone

Seizure model	Efficacy	References
PTZ	Potent anticonvulsant	132,137,185,188
TBPS	Potent anticonvulsant	137
Bicuculline	Potent anticonvulsant	137
Flourothyl	Potent anticonvulsant	254
Amygdala kindling	Potent anticonvulsant	D.S. Reddy, unpublished data
Corneal kindling	Potent anticonvulsant	137
PTZ kindling	Potent anticonvulsant	139
Cocaine seizures	Moderate anticonvulsant	132
Strychnine	Inactive	137
Aminophylline	Moderate anticonvulsant	137
N-methyl-D-aspartate	Inactive	132
Maximal electroshock	Inactive at nonsedative doses	137
γ-Hydroxybutyrate	Proconvulsant	257

The potential of ganaxolone in the treatment of perimenstrual seizure exacerbations was evaluated in the rat catamenial epilepsy model (188). Like naturally occurring neurosteroids, the anticonvulsant potency of ganaxolone was enhanced in the period following neurosteroid withdrawal, while the potencies of two reference anticonvulsants diazepam and valproate were reduced. There was no corresponding increase in the motor toxicity of ganaxolone, suggesting that the potentiated anticonvulsant activity of ganaxolone results from specific alterations in the brain mechanisms responsible for seizures and is not due to pharmacokinetic factors. Although the protective index of ganaxolone compares unfavorably with that of many conventional anticonvulsant agents (189), following neurosteroid withdrawal there was an increased separation between the doses of ganaxolone-producing seizure protection and motor side effects, suggesting that the drug may be better tolerated during the perimenstrual period of increased seizure frequency. On the basis of measurements of plasma ganaxolone levels, it was possible to estimate the plasma concentrations associated with seizure protection and motor toxicity. In control and neurosteroid withdrawn animals, the threshold plasma concentrations for seizure protection were 200–250 ng/mL and <100 ng/mL, respectively, and the estimated plasma concentrations producing 50% seizure protection were in the range of 450–550 and 200–250 ng/mL. Thus, ganaxolone protects against the PTZ-induced seizures in neurosteroid withdrawn rats at plasma concentrations that are not anticonvulsant in control animals.

Although motor toxicity was not potentiated in the withdrawn animals, it remains to be determined whether the enhanced potency of ganaxolone generalizes to other behavioral effects of neurosteroids, including their sedative-hypnotic, anxiolytic, and cognitive-impairing effects that may be important determinants of side effects in clinical use. If the side-effects profile is acceptable, neuroactive steroids such as ganaxolone could be uniquely suited for the treatment of catamenial seizure exacerbations. In fact, the steroids may specifically overcome the problem of catamenial "breakthrough" seizures during treatment with conventional anticonvulsants which, if the animal studies are relevant to the clinical situation, may have reduced activity against catamential seizures.

Lack of Tolerance to Neuroactive Steroids

For a neuroactive steroid such as ganaxolone to be of utility in the treatment of catamenial epilepsy, its activity must be maintained with chronic dosing. GABA-A receptor modulating drugs, most notably benzodiazepines such as diazepam, lose activity with chronic dosing due to the development of pharmacodynamic tolerance (190,191). In general, however, anticonvulsant tolerance does not develop to neurosteroids. For example, Kokate et al. (192) demonstrated that the anticonvulsant potency of pregnanolone was not reduced in rats that had received multiple daily doses for up to 2 weeks. In addition, there was no alteration in the pregnanolone plasma concentrations as a result of chronic dosing, demonstrating that there is no induction of metabolism. Because of its longer duration of action, ganaxolone might have a greater liability for tolerance than natural neurosteroids. However, when dosed repeatedly over the course of up to 1 week, tolerance did not develop to the anticonvulsant activity of ganaxolone (185). In addition, tolerance did not develop to the motor toxicity that occurs with higher doses of ganaxolone.

In contrast, there was marked tolerance to diazepam administered according to a similar regimen. Neurosteroids may therefore avoid the problem of tolerance that severely limits the usefulness of anticonvulsants such as benzodiazepines in long-term therapy. Indeed, two recent clinical studies in women with epilepsy (147,186) demonstrated no diminution in the anticonvulsant activity of chronically administered progesterone, which produces anticonvulsant effects via conversion to the neurosteroid allopregnanolone (see above). Similarly, tolerance has not been observed to the anxiolytic and sedative effects of the synthetic neuroactive steroids alphaxolone and 3β-ethenyl-3α-hydroxy-5α-pregnan-20-one (193,194). However, it has been reported that tolerance does occur to the sedative effects of the neuroactive steroid minaxolone (Fig. 3) (195) and the anticonvulsant activity of allopregnanolone when repeatedly administered by intracerebroventricular injections (196).

In the study of Reddy and Rogawski (185) demonstrating lack of tolerance to ganaxolone, it was found that chronic ganaxolone treatment led to cross-tolerance to diazepam. While the molecular basis of this cross-tolerance is not well understood, it could have implications for the clinical use of benzodiaepines. There are fluctuations in endogenous GABA-A receptor-modulating neurosteroids at menarche, during the menstrual cycle, in pregnancy, at menopause, and under stressful circumstances (197,198). In these situations, persistent neurosteroid exposure could lead to reduced benzodiazepine sensitivity and a diminution in clinical efficacy. Reduced benzodiazepine sensitivity has also been associated with *withdrawal* from chronic neurosteroid exposure. Thus, following neurosteroid withdrawal, GABA-A receptor currents have diminished benzodiazepine sensitivity (199), and benzodiazepines exhibit reduced sedative and anticonvulsant actions (111,112,188). Whether neuroactive steroids such as ganaxolone will prove to be superior in clinical situations in which there are fluctuations in neurosteroid levels and reduced benzodiazepine efficacy remains to be determined.

Stress and Seizure Susceptibility

The main focus of attention in studies seeking to understand the importance of neurosteroids in the regulation of seizure susceptibility has been on progesterone-derived allopregnanolone. However, deoxycorticosterone (DOC)-related neurosteroids, which are released in stressful situations, also have central nervous system effects and could affect the propensity for seizures. DOC-related neurosteroids can be considered a component of the hypothalamic-pituitary-adrenal (HPA) axis stress response system. Stress results in the hypothalamic release of corticotropin-releasing hormone (CRH), which liberates adrenocorticotropic hormone (ACTH) from the anterior pituitary. ACTH is generally understood to act by stimulating cortisol synthesis and release from the adrenal zona fasiculata. However, along with cortisol, ACTH also enhances DOC synthesis in the zona glomerulosa. DOC is a weak mineralocorticoid and serves as a precursor of the major mineralocorticoid aldosterone via 11β-hydroxylation to corticosterone by the enzyme CYP11B1 ($P450_{C11}$). However, DOC synthesis in the zona fasciculata is quantitatively greater than in the zona glomerulosa where its synthesis is under the control of ACTH and its secretion correlates with that of cortisol and not aldosterone (200,201). ACTH causes a relatively greater increase in DOC than in cortisol, and DOC synthesis is not suppressed to the same extent as cortisol by exogenous glucocorticoids (201). Thus, in addition to its well-recognized role as a mineralocorticoid precursor, there is substantial evidence that DOC participates in the HPA axis response to acute stress. The neurosteroid THDOC is synthesized from DOC by the same two sequential A-ring reductions that convert progesterone to allopregnanolone. 5α-R isoenzymes first convert DOC to the intermediate 5α-dihydrodeoxycorticosterone, which is then further reduced by 3α-HSOR to form THDOC (Fig. 1). In contrast to allopregnanolone, which is present in the brain even after adrenalectomy and gonadectomy, THDOC appears to be derived nearly exclusively from adrenal sources (76).

Apparently because of enhanced DOC availability, acute stressors such as swimming, foot shock, or carbon dioxide exposure elicit an increase in THDOC concentrations in plasma and brain (11,76,202 207); Plasma levels of THDOC normally fluctuate between 1 and 3 ng/mL, but increase to 6–10 ng/mL within 10–30 min following acute stress and may reach 15–18 ng/mL in pregnant rats. Proconvulsant GABA-A receptor antagonists such as isoniazid or FG7142 also increase brain levels of THDOC in intact but not in adrenalectomized animals (202,203).

THDOC protects against PTZ-induced seizures and is active in several other chemoconvulsant models as well as against amygdaloid kindled seizures in fully kindled rats (4,11) (Table 1). Seizure protection is also conferred by administration of the precursor DOC. Effects of DOC in the rat PTZ seizure threshold test occur with low doses of DOC that are associated with levels of plasma THDOC comparable to those in stressed animals. Moreover, in rats treated with DOC, there is a good correlation between the degree of seizure protection and the plasma THDOC levels achieved. The protective activity of DOC against PTZ seizures is completely blocked by finasteride, which markedly inhibits the rise in plasma THDOC. Indomethacin, an inhibitor of 3α-HSOR (see section on biosynthesis and metabolism of neurosteroids), also significantly reduced the anticonvulsant activity of DOC. Taken together, these results indicate that DOC itself is not anticonvulsant and must be activated by A-ring reduction. In fact, in the seizure models, DOC exhibits a relatively delayed onset and more prolonged duration than THDOC, which is compatible with the possibility that DOC is an inactive precursor that must be metabolically activated.

Stress can profoundly influence seizure control in persons with epilepsy (208–210). Moreover, experimental stress has anticonvulsant effects in animals (211,212). However, until recently, the way in which stress affects seizure susceptibility has been poorly understood. Since THDOC exhibits anticonvulsant activity in a variety of animal seizure models (11) (Table 1), it is attractive to speculate that DOC-derived THDOC could play a physiological role in the modulation of seizures.

Recent studies have confirmed that THDOC can participate in the regulation of seizure susceptibility by stress (11). Experimental stress, such as acute swim stress, raises the threshold for the induction of seizures by PTZ and other GABA-A receptor antagonists within ~10 min (211,213). At the time of seizure protection, swim stress is associated with a threefold elevation in plasma THDOC levels (11). Other stressors including footshock produce similar increases in plasma THDOC levels in adult and also in aged animals (76,205). Moreover, the elevation in seizure threshold and the rise in THDOC were eliminated by pretreatment with the 5α-R inhibitor finasteride, consistent with the possibility that the anticonvulsant effect is mediated by 5α-reduced neurosteroids. The stress-induced increase in seizure threshold and THDOC levels were also abolished in adrenalectomized rats (11,76). Overall, the studies strongly implicate THDOC in the protective effect of stress on seizures. The THDOC responsible for this effect could be synthesized in peripheral tissues and then transported by the circulation to the brain or it could be synthesized locally in the brain. Indeed, because of local biosynthesis, brain neurosteroid levels may be substantially higher than plasma levels after stressful events (76). However, based on the results in adrenalectomized animals, it appears that DOC, the precursor for THDOC synthesis, arises exclusively from the adrenal. Allopregnanolone levels are also moderately enhanced by stress, although the effect is not abolished by adrenalectomy. Therefore, while the acute stress-elicited increase in brain allopregnanolone may contribute to the anticonvulsant effects of stress, THDOC is likely to be a more important factor.

Although there are situations where stress or alerting has been shown to reduce epileptiform manifestations, high stress levels and stressful events are more typically associated with more frequent epileptiform EEG spikes and seizures (210,214). Therefore, it is generally accepted that stress triggers seizures (209). Many neural and hormonal factors likely play a role in the regulation of seizure susceptibility during fluctuations in the level of stress. Indeed, studies with neurosteroid synthesis inhibitors in the swim stress model suggested the existence of endogenous proconvulsant factors that could play a role in the precipitation of seizures by stress (11). The extent of seizure susceptibility during stress may therefore represent a balance between anticonvulsant factors, including neurosteroids, and proconvulsant factors. Stress-induced seizures would therefore occur when the balance is shifted to favor the proconvulsant factors, outweighing the anticonvulsant action of endogenous GABA-A receptor–modulating neurosteroids. The proconvulsant mediators have not yet been identified, but could include glucocorticoids (215,216), CRH (217,218), or even ACTH, which may acutely enhance seizure susceptibility possibly through direct actions on the CNS (214,219,220). Stress is also likely to increase brain levels of pro-convulsant sulfated neurosteroids such as PS and DHEAS, although the extent to which these contribute to the proconvulsant activity of stress has not been defined.

Infantile Spasms

Since the 1950s, ACTH has been known to have beneficial effects in the treatment of infantile spasms and other juvenile epilepsies (221–223). The recognition that ACTH stimulates adrenal DOC synthesis, which leads to enhanced levels of circulating DOC-derived neurosteroids, raises the possibility that the protective activity of ACTH in these epilepsies could, at least in part, be related to neurosteroids (224). Prednisone, a 1,2-reduced steroid that is not biotransformed to neurosteroids, is also well known to have activity in infantile spasms. Therefore, it is unlikely that ACTH effects on neurosteroid synthesis entirely account for its beneficial activity in infantile spasms; stimulation of adrenal glucocorticoids must certainly play a role. However, there is evidence that prednisone is less effective than ACTH (225). The ability of ACTH to stimulate neurosteroid synthesis is one possible explanation for the superiority of ACTH. Treatment with ACTH is still effective against infantile spasms in adrenal-suppressed patients who fail to show a cortisol response to ACTH (226). These studies have been interpreted as indicating that an extra-adrenal mechanism is involved in the anticonvulsant efficacy of ACTH. However, it is notable that DOC synthesis is not suppressed to the same extent as cortisol by exogenous glucocorticoids (201). Although ACTH causes a relatively greater increase in DOC than in cortisol (fourfold for DOC vs. 1.5-fold for cortisol), the glucocorticoid dexamethasone suppresses DOC to a lesser extent than cortisol (41% vs. 95%). Thus, it is conceivable that ACTH may induce an increase in DOC and anticonvulsant neurosteroids even under conditions where the peptide fails to affect cortisol secretion. Given the available evidence, it seems reasonable that neurosteroids could contribute to the anticonvulsant activity of ACTH in infantile spasms and other developmental epilepsies. However, experimental support for this hypothesis is required.

Unfortunately, ACTH has variable and rather undramatic effects on seizure susceptibility in animal models, which has made it difficult to rigorously investigate the hypothesis (227,228). Nevertheless, whether or not the action of ACTH in infantile spasms results to some extent from stimulation of adrenal steroid synthesis leading to increased neurosteroid availability, exogenous neurosteroids—because of their powerful effects on GABA-ergic transmission—would theoretically be expected to have utility as a treatment approach. Indeed, recent clinical trials of ganaxolone support a role for neuroactive steroids in the treatment of infantile spasms (229). Two open-label trials of ganaxolone in infantile spasms have been reported with indications of efficacy in both cases (229). Overall, approximately one-third of 79 patients ages 6 months to 15 years of age with highly refractory infantile spasms showed substantial (>50%) reductions in spasm frequency, with a few subjects becoming spasm-free (229). Detailed information has been provided on 15 children with active refractory infantile spasms who were treated with ganaxolone according to an escalating dosage schedule (230). Many of the children had previously been treated with ACTH or vigabatrin, and all but one were taking conventional antiepileptic drugs throughout the ganaxolone trial. During a 2-month ganaxolone maintenance period, five of these children experienced >50% decrease in spasm frequency (one became spasm-free), five had a 25–50% reduction, and five did not respond. For the high responders, doses ranged from 18 to 36 mg/kg/d, with serum concentrations in the range of 5.0–51.6 ng/mL (15–155 nM). These ganaxolone concentrations are within the range of those that potentiate recombinant GABA-A receptors expressed in *Xenopus* oocytes ($EC_{50} \sim 100$–200 nM) (137). However, they are substantially lower than the threshold concentrations that are protective in the rat PTZ seizure model (750–950 ng/mL) (185,188), indicating that human infantile spasms could be exquisitely sensitive to neuroactive steroids. In any case, appropriately controlled trials will be necessary to confirm the efficacy of neuroactive steroids in pediatric epilepsies.

Ethanol Withdrawal Seizures

There is extensive evidence demonstrating that ethanol affects endogenous neurosteroid levels. This has led to the speculation that neurosteroids could play a role in the behavioral activity of ethanol and in ethanol tolerance and dependence (231,232). Acute ethanol administration causes substantial increases in plasma and brain allopregnanolone concentrations (233). Moreover, there is a good correlation between the time course of the ethanol-induced increase in allopregnanolone levels and various behavioral effects of ethanol, including its anticonvulsant activity. These effects of ethanol are prevented by finasteride, implicating neurosteroids.

Enhanced seizure susceptibility is an important symptom of ethanol withdrawal in humans that is mimicked in laboratory animals. Devaud et al. (66,181,234) have shown that allopregnanolone and THDOC are five- to 15-fold more potent at enhancing the seizure threshold during the period of potentiated seizure susceptibility following withdrawal from chronic ethanol exposure than they are in control animals. Interestingly, this is opposite to the tolerance and cross-tolerance that develops between ethanol and benzodiazepines (235), but as noted previously is similar to the potentiated activity of neurosteroids seen following neurosteroid withdrawal. The ethanol withdrawal–induced changes in neurosteroid activity are unrelated to the changes in endogenous neurosteroids observed following acute ethanol administration since chronic ethanol consumption is not associated with such elevations in allopregnanolone levels (233). In fact, in human alcoholics, Romeo et al. (236) have found markedly decreased levels of allopregnanolone during early withdrawal from ethanol. Thus, although the mechanisms underlying the enhanced activity of neurosteroids in ethanol withdrawal are obscure, the recent experimental work in animals highlights the potential utility of neuroactive steroids in the treatment of alcohol withdrawal seizures.

Seizure Susceptibility in Men

The incidence of epilepsy is ~15% higher in men than in women at all ages and for most seizure types. Although the underlying mechanisms are poorly understood, androgen deficiency is unusually common among men with epilepsy (237). The most important androgen is testosterone. Unlike progesterone, there are few studies that have investigated the effects of testosterone on neuronal excitability and seizures. Interestingly, however, testosterone and its metabolite 3α-androstanediol exhibit anticonvulsant effects in animal seizure models (161,238,239). On the other hand, orchidectomized or castrated male animals show significantly higher incidence of seizures to chemoconvulsants (240,241). In addition, male rats are less susceptile to seizures induced by allylglycine (an inhibitor of GABA synthesis) than are female animals (242). Therefore, changes in testosterone levels in men could potentially influence the occurrence of seizures (243).

3α-Androstanediol (5α-androstan-3α,17β-diol, or 17β-dihydroandrosterone; Fig. 1) is structurally very similar to the progesterone metabolite allopregnanolone (50), and it is tempting to speculate that testosterone-derived 3α-androstanediol could play a role in regulating seizure susceptibility. Like allopregnanolone, 3α-androstanediol is synthesized from testosterone by two sequential A-ring reductions. 5α-Reductase isoenzymes first convert testosterone to the intermediate 5α-dihydrotestosterone, which is then further reduced by 3α-HSOR to form 3α-androstanediol (Fig. 1). Testosterone is also converted to 17β-estradiol by aromatase, which, as noted above, may have long-term proconvulsant actions. 3α-Androstanediol is produced de novo by glial cells in the brain (244,245). In addition, the metabolic conversion of testosterone to 3α-androstanediol could also occur in peripheral tissues that express 5α-reductase and 3α-HSOR activities. This raises the possibility that 3α-androstanediol may mediate the effects of testosterone on seizure susceptibility. Although 3α-androstanediol meets the structural requirements for potent GABA-A receptor modulating activity, its effects on GABA-A receptor function have not been widely investigated. There are, however, studies showing that 3α-androstanediol can alter GABA-stimulated chloride flux and muscimol binding (246–248), supporting the view that it could have activity at GABA-A receptors. 3α-Androstanediol can be converted to androsterone by 17β-hydroxysteroid dehydrogenase present in brain and peripheral tissues. Androsterone is also a GABA-A receptor positive modulator with potency about one-tenth that of allopregnanolone (69); there is evidence that it has anticonvulsant properties (256).

Despite testosterone's antiseizure effects in animals (161), however, it has not been reported to have a beneficial effect on seizures in humans (249). One possible explanation is that enzyme-inducing antiepileptic drugs may enhance the conversion of testosterone to estradiol by aromatase, leading to proconvulsant effects. This possibility is supported by the improved seizure control achieved when testosterone is administered with the aromatase inhibitor testolactone or the antiestrogen clomiphene (249,250). In view of these complexities, the role of testosterone-derived neuroactive steroids in the modulation of seizure susceptibility remains elusive.

Clinical Experience with Neuroactive Steroids

In two open-label studies, natural progesterone therapy has been reported to produce dramatic reductions ($\geq 72\%$) in seizure frequency in women with intractable localization-related epilepsy and catamenial seizure exacerbations (251). In contrast, in published studies of cyclic oral synthetic progestins there was no statistically significant effect on seizure frequency. Since the synthetic progestins are not converted to neurosteroids, it seems likely that the activity of progesterone is related to its ability to form allopregnanolone. Nevertheless, it has been recognized that the open-label trials are open to bias, and a definitive answer regarding the utility of cylic progesterone therapy in catamenial epilepsy awaits the results of an ongoing prospective, randomized, blinded, placebo-controlled study.

Studies with the synthetic allopregnanalone analog ganaxalone also support a role for neurosteroids in epilepsy therapy. A controlled trial in patients with intractable complex partial seizures utilizing an inpatient monotherapy design demonstrated that ganaxolone effectively decreases seizures compared to placebo (252). In other trials, the drug had a favorable safety profile with somnolence, which occurs at higher doses, as the most frequently reported adverse event. As noted previously, open-label data in pediatric patients suggest that ganaxolone may be effective in treating infantile spasms.

In an open-label pilot study, ganaxolone was evaluated for the safety, tolerability, and antiseizure efficacy in two women with catamenial epilepsy (253). Patients received ganaxolone (300 mg/day, PO, BID) starting on the day 21 of the menstrual cycle and continuing through the third full day following the beginning of menstruation. Side effects were mild. During the 4 months of this ganaxolone "pulse" therapy, both patients, who were incompletely controlled with valproate and phenytoin, had a moderate improvement in their catamenial seizures. These promising results warrant further study.

CONCLUSIONS

Although the remarkable GABA-A receptor modulating properties of endogenous neurosteroids have been recognized since 1986 (49), the physiological role of neurosteroids in brain function is still uncertain. Nevertheless, in recent years, evidence has accumulated that neurosteroids could be relevant to several important clinical conditions. Regulation of seizure susceptibility in persons with epilepsy is prominent among these conditions. Hormonal fluctuations in women with catamenial epilepsy, hypogonadism in men, and physiological stress could in part result in alterations in endogenous neurosteroids, which may affect seizure susceptibility.

Synthetic neurosteroids, which lack hormonal properties, have promise in epilepsy therapy. They are particularly likely to be of value in treating hormonally induced fluctuations in seizure susceptibility. In addition, however, they could be useful in a broad range of seizure types, and are of particular promise in infantile spasms.

REFERENCES

1. Baulieu E-E, Robel P, Schumacher M. Neurosteroids: A New Regulatory Function in the Nervous System. Totowa, NJ: Humana Press, 1999.
2. Paul SM, Purdy RH. Neuroactive steroids. FASEB J 1992; 6:2311–2322.
3. Selye H. Anaesthetic effects of steroid hormones. Proc Soc Exp Biol 1941; 46:116–121.
4. Selye H. The antagonism between anesthetic steroid hormones and pentamethylene-tetrazol (Metrazol). J Lab Clin Med 1942; 27:1051–1053.
5. McQuarrie I, Anderson JA, Ziegler MR. Observations on antagonistic effects of posterior pituitary and cortico-adrenal hormones in the epileptic subject. J Clin Endocrinol 1942; 2:406–410.
6. Aird RB. The effect of desoxycorticosterone in epilepsy. J Nerv Ment Dis 1944; 99:501–510.
7. Aird RB, Gordan GS. Anticonvulsive properties of deoxycorticosterone. JAMA 1951; 145:715–719.

8. Gyermek L, Iriarte J, Crabbé P. Steroids. CCCX. Structure-activity relationship of some steroidal hypnotic agents. J Med Chem 1968; 11:117–125.

9. Green CJ, Halsey MJ, Precious S, Wardley-Smith B. Alphaxolone-alphadolone anesthesia in laboratory animals. Lab Anim 1978; 12:85–89.

10. Gyermek L, Genther G, Fleming N. Some effects of progesterone and related steroids on the central nervous system. Int J Neuropharmacol 1967; 6:191–198.

11. Reddy DS, Rogawski MA. Stress-induced deoxycorticosterone-derived neurosteroids modulates $GABA_A$ receptor function and seizure susceptibility. J Neurosci 2002; 42: 3795–3805.

12. Robel P, Baulieu EE. Neurosteroids: biosynthesis and function. Crit Rev Neurobiol 1995; 9:383–394.

13. Schumacher M, Robel P, Baulieu EE. Development and regeneration of the nervous system: a role for neurosteroids. Dev Neurosci 1996; 18:16–21.

14. Li X, Bertics PJ, Karavolas HJ. Regional distribution of cytosolic and particulate 5α-dihydroprogesterone 3α-hydroxysteroid oxidoreductases in female rat brain. J Steroid Biochem Mol Biol 1997; 60:311–318.

15. Mensah-Nyagan AG, Do-Rego JL, Beaujean D, Luu-The V, Pelletier G, Vaudry H. Neurosteroids: expression of steroidogenic enzymes and regulation of steroid biosynthesis in the central nervous system. Pharmacol Rev 1999; 51:63–81.

16. Stoffel-Wagner B, Beyenburg S, Watzka MS, Blumcke I, Bauer J, Schramm J, Bidlingmaier F, Elger CE. Expression of 5α-reductase and 3α-hydroxisteroid oxidoreductase in the hippocampus of patients with chronic temporal lobe epilepsy. Epilepsia 2000; 41:140–147.

17. Petratos S, Hirst JJ, Mendis S, Anikijenko P, Walker DW. Localization of p450scc and 5α-reductase type-2 in the cerebellum of fetal and newborn sheep. Brain Res Dev Brain Res 2000; 123:81–86.

18. Compagnone NA, Mellon SH. Neurosteroids: biosynthesis and function of these novel neuromodulators Front Neuroendocrinol 2000; 21:1–56.

19. Reddy DS, Kulkarni SK. Development of neurosteroid-based novel psychotropic drugs. Progr Med Chem 2000; 37:135–175.

20. Stoffel-Wagner B. Neurosteroid metabolism in the human brain. Eur J Endocrinol 2001; 145:669–679.

21. Poletti A, Negri-Cesi P, Rabuffetti M, Colciago A, Celotti F, Martini L. Transient expression of the 5α-reductase type 2 isozyme in the rat brain in late fetal and early postnatal life. Endocrinology 1998; 139:2171–2188.

22. Matsui D, Sakari M, Sato T, Murayama A, Takada I, Kim M, Takeyama K, Kato S. Transcriptional regulation of the mouse steroid 5α-reductase type II gene by progesterone in brain. Nucleic Acids Res 2002; 30:1387–1393.

23. Khanna M, Qin K-N, Wang RW, Cheng K-C. Substrate specificity, gene structure, and tissue-specific distribution of multiple human 3α-hydroxysteroid dehydrogenases. J Biol Chem 1995; 270:20162–20168.

24. Russell DW, Wilson JD. Steroid 5α-reductase: two genes, two enzymes. Annu Rev Biochem 1994; 63:15266–15272.

25. Melcangi RC, Poletti A, Cavarretta I, Celotti F, Colciago A, Magnaghi V, Motta M, Negri-Cesi P, Martini L. The 5α-reductase in the central nervous system: expression and modes of control. J Steroid Biochem Mol Biol 1998; 65:295–299.

26. Corpechot C, Young J, Calvel M, Wehrey C, Veltz JN, Touyer G, Mouren M, Prasad VV, Banner C, Sjovall J. Neurosteroids: 3α-hydroxy-5α-pregnan-20-one and its precursors in the brain, plasma and steroidogenic glands of male and female rats. Endocrinology 1993; 133:1003–1009.

27. Baulieu E-E, Robel P. Neurosteroids: a new brain function? J Steroid Biochem Mol Biol 1990; 37:395–403.

28. Kulkarni SK, Reddy DS. Neurosteroids: a new class of neuromodulators. Drugs Today 1995; 31:433–455.

29. Mellon SH, Griffin LD, Compagnone NA. Biosynthesis and action of neurosteroids. Brain Res Rev 2001; 37:3–12.

30. Zwain IH, Yen SS. Neurosteroidogenesis in astrocytes, oligodendrocytes, and neurons of cerebral cortex of rat brain. Endocrinology 1999; 140:3843–3852.

31. Guennoun R, Fiddes RJ, Gouezou M, Lombes M, Baulieu EE. A key enzyme in the biosynthesis of neurosteroids, 3β-hydroxysteroid dehydrogenase/$\triangle^5$-$\triangle^4$-isomerase (3β-HSD), is expressed in rat brain. Brain Res Mol Brain Res 1995; 30: 287–300.

32. Cheney DL, Uzunov D, Costa E, Guidotti A. Gas chromatographic-mass fragmentographic quantitation of 3α-hydroxy-5α-pregnan-20-one (allopregnanolone) and its precursors in blood and brain of adrenalectomized and castrated rats. J Neurosci 1995; 15:4641–4650.

33. Krueger KE, Papadopoulos V. Mitochondrial benzodiazepine receptors and the regulation of steroid biosynthesis. Annu Rev Pharmacol Toxicol 1992; 32:211–237.

34. Costa E, Guidotti A. Diazepam binding inhibitor (DBI): a peptide with multiple biological actions. Life Sci 1991; 49:325–344.

35. Guarneri P, Papadopoulos V, Pan B, Costa E. Regulation of pregnenolone synthesis in C6-2B glioma cells by 4′-chlorodiazepam. Proc Natl Acad Sci USA 1992; 89:5118–5122.

36. Papadopoulos V, Guarneri P, Krueger KE, Guidotti A, Costa E. Pregnenolone biosynthesis in C6-2B glioma cell mitochondria: regulation by a mitochondrial diazepam binding inhibitor receptor. Proc Natl Acad Sci USA 1992; 89:5113–5117.

37. Kozikowski AP, Ma D, Brewer J, Sun S, Costa E, Romeo E, Guidotti A. Chemistry, binding affinities, and behavioral properties of a new class of "antineophobic" mitochondrial DBI receptor complex (mDRC) ligands. J Med Chem 1993; 36:2908–2920.

38. Auta J, Romeo E, Kozikowski A, Ma D, Costa E, Guidotti A. Participation of mitochondrial diazepam binding inhibitor receptors in the anticonflict, antineophobic and anticonvulsant action of 2-aryl-3-indoleacetamide and imidazopyridine derivatives. J Pharmacol Exp Ther 1993; 265:649–656.

39. Reddy DS, Kulkarni SK. Role of GABA-A and mitochondrial diazepam binding inhibitor receptors in the anti-stress activity of neurosteroids in mice. Psychopharmacology 1996; 128:280–292.

40. Celotti F, Melcangi RC, Martini L. The 5α-reductase in the brain: molecular aspects and relation to brain function. Front Neuroendocrinol 1992; 13:163–215.

41. Azzolina B, Ellsworth K, Andersson S, Geissler W, Bull HG, Harris GS. Inhibition of rat 5α-reductases by finasteride: evidence for isozyme differences in the mechanism of inhibition. J Steroid Biochem Mol Biol 1997; 61:55–64.

42. Penning TM, Sharp RB, Krieger NR. Purification and properties of 3α-hydroxysteroid dehydrogenase from rat brain cytosol. Inhibition by nonsteroidal anti-inflammatory drugs and progestins. J Biol Chem 1985; 260:15266–15272.

43. Mody I, DeKoninck Y, Otis TS, Soltesz I. Bridging the cleft at GABA synapses in the brain. Trends Neurosci 1994; 17:517–525.

44. McKernan RM, Whiting PJ. Which GABA$_A$-receptor subtypes really occur in the brain? Trends Neurosci 1996; 19:139–143.

45. Child KJ, Currie JP, Dis B, Dodds MG, Pearce DR, Twissell DJ. The pharmacological properties in animals of CT1341—a new steroid anaesthetic agent. Br J Anaesth 1971; 43:2–13.

46. Scholfield CN. Potentiation of inhibition by general anaesthetics in neurones of the olfactory cortex in vitro. Pflügers Arch 1980; 383:249–255.

47. Harrison NL, Simmonds MA. Modulation of the GABA receptor complex by a steroid anaesthetic. Brain Res 1984; 323:287–292.

48. Cottrell GA, Lambert JJ, Peters JA. Modulation of GABA$_A$ receptor activity by alphaxolone. Br J Pharmacol 1987; 90:491–500.

49. Majewska MD, Harrison NL, Schwartz RD, Barker JL, Paul SM. Steroid hormone metabolites are barbiturate-like modulators of the GABA receptor. Science 1986; 232:1004–1007.

50. Gee KW, Bolger MB, Brinton RE, Coirini H, McEwen BS. Steroid modulation of the chloride ionophore in rat brain: structure-activity requirements, regional dependence and mechanism of action. J Pharmacol Exp Ther 1988; 246:803–812.

51. Turner DM, Ransom RW, Yang JS-J, Olsen EW. Steroid anesthetics and naturally occurring analogs modulate the γ-aminobutyric acid receptor complex at a site distinct from barbiturates. J Pharmacol Exp Ther 1989; 248:960–966.

52. Brot MD, Akwa Y, Purdy RH, Koob GF, Britton KT. The anxiolytic-like effects of the neurosteroid allopregnanolone: interactions with GABA$_A$ receptors. Eur J Pharmacol 1997; 325:1–7.

53. Vivian JA, Barros HMT, Manitiu A, Miczek KA. Ultrasonic vocalizations in rat pups: modulation at the γ-aminobutyric acid$_A$ receptor complex and the neurosteroid recognition site. J Pharmacol Exp Ther 1997; 282:318–325.

54. Reddy DS, Kulkarni SK. Sex and estrous cycle-dependent changes in neurosteroid and benzodiazepine effects on food consumption and plus-maze learning behaviors in rats. Pharmacol Biochem Behav 1999; 62:53–60.

55. Deutsch SI, Park CH, Hitri A. Allosteric effects of a GABA receptor–active steroid are altered by stress. Pharmacol Biochem Behav 1994; 47:913–917.

56. Xue BG, Whittemore ER, Park CH, Woodward RM, Lan NC, Gee KW. Partial agonism by 3α,21-dihydroxy-5β-pregnan-20-one at the γ-aminobutyric acid$_A$ receptor neurosteroid site. J Pharmacol Exp Ther 1997; 281:1095–1101.

57. Lambert JJ, Belelli D, Harney SC, Peters JA, Frenguelli BG. Modulation of native and recombinant GABA$_A$ receptors by endogenous and synthetic neuroactive steroids. Brain Res Rev 2001; 37:68–80.

58. Harrison NL, Majewska MD, Harrington JW, Barker JL. Structure-activity relationships for steroid interactions with the γ-aminobutyric acid$_A$ receptor complex. J Pharmacol Exp Ther 1987; 241:346–353.

59. Puia G, Santi M, Vicini S, Pritchett DB, Purdy RH, Paul SM, Seeburg PH, Costa E. Neurosteroids act on recombinant human GABA$_A$ receptors. Neuron 1990; 4:759–765.

60. Purdy RH, Morrow AL, Blinn JR, Paul SM. Synthesis, metabolism, and pharmacological activity of 3α-hydroxy steroids which potentiate GABA-receptor-mediated chloride ion uptake in rat cerebral cortical synaptoneurosomes. J Med Chem 1990; 33:1572–1581.

61. Kokate TG, Svensson BE, Rogawski MA. Anticonvulsant activity of neurosteroids: correlation with γ-aminobutyric acid–evoked chloride current potentiation. J Pharmacol Exp Ther 1994; 270:1223–1229.

62. Wetzel CH, Vedder H, Holsboer F, Zieglgansberger W, Deisz RA. Bidirectional effects of the neuroactive steroid tetrahydrodeoxycorticosterone on GABA-activated Cl$^-$ currents in cultured rat hypothalamic neurons. Br J Pharmacol 1999; 127: 863–868.

63. Bowers BJ, Wehner JM. Biochemical and behavioral effects of steroids on GABA$_A$ receptor function in long- and short-sleep mice. Brain Res Bull 1992; 29:57–68.

64. Teschemacher A, Zeise ML, Holsboer F, Zieglgansberger W. The neuroactive steroid 5α-tetrahydrodeoxycorticosterone increases GABAergic postsynaptic inhibition in rat neocortical neurons in vitro. J Neuroendocrinol 1995; 7:233–240.

65. Zhu WJ, Vicini S. Neurosteroid prolongs GABA$_A$ channel deactivation by altering kinetics of desensitized states. J Neurosci 1997; 17:4022–4031.

66. Devaud LL, Purdy RH, Finn DA, Morrow AL. Sensitization of γ-aminobutyric acid$_A$ receptors to neuroactive steroids in rats during ethanol withdrawal. J Pharmacol Exp Ther 1996; 278:510–517.

67. Grobin AC, Morrow AL. 3α-Hydroxy-5α-pregnan-20-one levels and GABA$_A$ receptor–mediated ^{36}Cl$^-$ flux across development in rat cerebral cortex. Dev Brain Res 2001; 31:31–39.

68. Challachan H, Cotrel GA, Hather NY, Nooney JM, Peters JA. Modulation of the GABA$_A$ receptor by progesterone metabolites. Proc R Soc Lond B 1987; 231:359–369.

69. Twyman RE, Macdonald RL. Neurosteroid regulation of GABA$_A$ receptor single-channel kinetic properties of mouse spinal cord neurons in culture. J Physiol (Lond) 1992; 456:215–245.

70. Lambert JJ, Belelli D, Shepherd SE, Pistis M, Peters JA. The selective interaction of neurosteroids with the GABA$_A$ receptors. In: Baulieu E-E, Robel P, Schumacher M, eds. Neurosteroids: A New Regulatory Function in the Nervous System. Totowa, NJ: Humana Press, 1999:125–142.

71. MacDonald RL, Olsen RW. GABA$_A$ receptor channels. Annu Rev Neurosci 1994; 17:569–602.

72. Cooper EJ, Johnston GA, Edwards FA. Effects of a naturally occurring neurosteroid on GABA$_A$ IPSCs during development in rat hippocampal or cerebellar slices. J Physiol 1999; 521:437–449.

73. Lambert JJ, Belelli D, Hill-Venning C, Peters JA. Neurosteroids and GABA$_A$ receptor function. Trends Pharmacol Sci 1995; 16:295–303.

74. Belelli D, Lambert JJ, Peters JA, Gee KW, Lan NC. Modulation of human recombinant GABA$_A$ receptors by pregnanediols. Neuropharmacology 1996; 35:1223–1231.

75. Wang M, Seippel L, Purdy RH, Bäckström T. Relationship between symptom severity and steroid variation in women with premenstrual syndrome: study on serum pregnenolone, pregnenolone sulfate, 5α-pregnane-3,20-dione and 3α-hydroxy-5α-pregnan-20-one. J Clin Endocrinol Metab 1996; 81:1076–1082.

76. Purdy RH, Morrow AL, Moore PH Jr, Paul SM. Stress-induced elevations of γ-aminobutyric acid type A receptor-active steroids in the rat brain. Proc Natl Acad Sci USA 1991; 88:4553–4557.

77. Rho JM, Donevan SD, Rogawski MA. Direct activation of GABA$_A$ receptors by barbiturates in cultured rat hippocampal neurons. J Physiol 1996; 497(Pt 2):509–522.

78. Barnard EA, Skolnick P, Olsen RW, Mohler H, Sieghart W, Biggio G, Braestrup C, Bateson AN, Langer SZ. International Union of Pharmacology. XV. Subtypes of γ-aminobutyric acid$_A$ receptors: classification on the basis of subunit structure and receptor function. Pharmacol Rev 1998; 50:291–313.

79. Sigel E, Baur R, Trube G, Möhler H, Malherbe P. The effect of subunit composition of rat brain GABA$_A$ receptors on channel function. Neuron 1990; 5:703–711.

80. Mathews GC, Bolos-Sy AM, Holland KD, Isenberg KE, Covey DF, Ferrendelli JA, Rothman SM. Developmental alteration in GABA$_A$ receptor structure and physiological properties in cultured cerebellar granule neurons. Neuron 1994; 13:149–158.

81. Whittemore ER, Yang W, Drewe JA, Woodward RM. Pharmacology of the human γ-aminobutyric acid$_A$ receptor α_4 subunit expressed in *Xenopus laevis* oocytes. Mol Pharmacol 1996; 50:1364–1375.

82. Davies PA, Hanna MC, Hales TG, Kirkness EF. Insensitivity to anesthetic agents conferred by a class of GABA$_A$ receptor subunit. Nature 1997; 385:820–823.

83. Shingai R, Sutherland ML, Barnard EA. Effects of subunit types of the cloned GABA$_A$ receptor on the response to a neurosteroid. Eur J Pharmacol 1991; 206:77–80.

84. Gee KW, Lan NC. γ-Aminobutyric acid$_A$ receptor complexes in rat cortex and spinal cord show differential responses to steroid modulation. Mol Pharmacol 1991; 40:995–999.

85. Lan NC, Gee KW, Bolger MB, Chen JS. Differential responses of expressed recombinant human γ-aminobutyric acid$_A$ receptors to neurosteroids. J Neurochem 1991; 57:1818–1821.

86. Sapp DW, Witte U, Turner DM, Longoni B, Kokka N, Olsen RW. Regional variation in steroid anesthetic modulation of [^{35}S]TBPS binding to γ-aminobutyric acid$_A$ receptors in rat brain. J Pharmacol Exp Ther 1992; 262:801–806.

87. Puia G, Ducic I, Vicini S, Costa E. Does neurosteroid modulatory efficacy depend on GABA$_A$ receptor subunit composition? Receptors Channels 1993; 1:135–142.

88. Hadingham KL, Wingrove PB, Wafford KA, Bain C, Kemp JA. Role of the β-subunit in determining the pharmacology of human γ-aminobutyric acid type A receptors. Mol Pharmacol 1993; 44:1211–1218.

89. Hauser CAE, Chesnoy-Marchais D, Robel P, Baulieu EE. Modulation of recombinant $\alpha_6\beta_2\gamma_2$ GABA$_A$ receptors by neuroactive steroids. Eur J Pharmacol 1995; 289:249–257.

90. Wohlfarth KM, Bianchi MT, Macdonald RL. Enhanced neurosteroid potentiation of ternary GABA$_A$ receptors containing the δ subunit. J Neurosci 2002; 22:1541–1549.

91. Zhu WJ, Wang JF, Krueger KE, Vicini S. δ-Subunit inhibits neurosteroid modulation of GABA$_A$ receptors. J Neurosci 1996; 16:6648–6656.

92. Morris KD, Moorefield CN, Amin J. Differential modulation of the γ-aminobutyric acid type C receptor by neuroactive steroids. Mol Pharmacol 1999; 56:752–759.

93. Zhang D, Pan Z, Awobuluyi M, Lipton SA. Structure and function of GABA$_C$ receptors: a comparison of native versus recombinant receptors. Trends Pharmacol Sci 2001; 22:121–132.

94. Rudolph U, Crestani F, Mohler H. GABA$_A$ receptor subtypes: dissecting their pharmacological functions. Trends Pharmacol Sci 2001; 22:188–194.

95. Mihalek RM, Banerjee PK, Korpi ER, Quinlan JJ, Firestone LL, Mi ZP, Lagenaur C, Tretter V, Sieghart W, Anagnostaras SG, Sage JR, Fanselow MS, Guidotti A, Spigelman I, Li Z, DeLorey TM, Olsen RW, Homanics GE. Attenuated sensitivity to neuroactive steroids in γ-aminobutyrate type A receptor delta subunit knockout mice. Proc Natl Acad Sci USA 1999; 96:12905–12910.

96. Spigelman I, Li Z, Banerjee PK, Mihalek RM, Homanics GE, Olsen RW. Behavior and physiology of mice lacking the GABA$_A$-receptor δ subunit. Epilepsia 2002; 43(Suppl 5):3–8.

97. Herbison AE. Physiological roles for the neurosteroid allopregnanolone in the modulation of brain function during pregnancy and partirution. Progr Brain Res 2001; 133:39–47.

98. Smith SS. Withdrawal properties of a neuroactive steroid: implications for GABA$_A$ receptor gene regulation in the brain and anxiety behavior. Steroids 2002; 67:519–528.

99. Leidenheimer NJ, Chapell R. Effects of PKC activation and receptor desensitization on neurosteroid modulation of GABA$_A$ receptors. Mol Brain Res 1997; 52:173–181.

100. Fancsik A, Linn DM, Tasker JG. Neurosteroid modulation of GABA IPSCs is phosphorylation dependent. J Neurosci 2000; 40:3067–3075.

101. Covey DF, Evers AS, Mennerick S, Zorumski CF, Purdy RH. Recent developments in structure-activity relationships for steroid modulators of GABA$_A$ receptors. Brain Res Rev 2001; 37:91–97.

102. Han M, Zorumski CF, Covey DF. Neurosteroid analogues. 4. The effect of methyl substitution at the C-5 and C-10 positions of neurosteroids on electrophysiological activity at GABA$_A$ receptors. J Med Chem 1996; 39:4218–4232.

103. Marrow AL, Pace JR, Purdy RH, Paul SM. Characterization of steroid interactions with γ-aminobutyric acid receptor-gated chloride ion channels: evidence for multiple steroid recognition sites. Mol Pharmacol 1990; 37:263–270.

104. Hogenkamp DJ, Hasan Tihar SH, Hawkinson JE, Upasani RB, Alauddin M, Kimbrough CL, Acosta-Burruel M, Whittemore ER, Woodward RM, Lan NC, Gee KW, Bolger MB. Synthesis and in vitro activity of 3β-substituted-3α-hydroxy-pregnan-20-ones: allosteric modulators of the GABA$_A$ receptor. J Med Chem 1997; 40:61–72.

105. McCauley LD, Liu V, Chen JS, Hawkinson JE, Lan NC, Gee KW. Selective actions of certain neuroactive pregnanediols at the γ-aminobutyric acid type A receptor complex in rat brain. Mol Pharmacol 1995; 47:354–362.

106. Follesa P, Concas A, Porcu P, Sanna E, Serra M, Mostallino MC, Purdy RH, Biggio G. Role of allopregnanolone in regulation of GABA$_A$ receptor plasticity during long-term exposure to and withdrawal from progesterone. Brain Res Rev 2001; 37:81–90.

107. Roca DJ, Schiller GD, Friedman L, Rozenberg I, Gibbs TT, Farb DH. γ-Aminobutyric acid$_A$ receptor regulation in culture: altered allosteric interactions following prolonged exposure to benzodiazepines, barbiturates, and methylxanthines. Mol Pharmacol 1990; 37:710–719.

108. Friedman L, Gibbs TT, Farb DH. γ-Aminobutyric acid$_A$ receptor regulation: chronic treatment with pregnanolone uncouples allosteric interactions between steroid and benzodiazepine recognition sites. Mol Pharmacol 1993; 44:191–197.

109. Yu R, Ticku MK. Chronic neurosteroid treatment produces functional heterologous uncoupling at the γ-aminobutyric acid type A/benzodiazepine receptor complex in mammalian cortical neurons. Mol Pharmacol 1995; 47:603–610.

110. Yu R, Ticku MK. Chronic neurosteroid treatment decreases the efficacy of benzodiazepine ligands and neurosteroids at the γ-aminobutyric acid$_A$ receptor complex in mammalian cortical neurons. J Pharmacol Exp Ther 1995; 275:784–789.

111. Smith SS, Gong QH, Hsu FC, Markowitz RS, ffrench-Mullen JMH, Li X. GABA$_A$ receptor α4-subunit suppression prevents withdrawal properties of an endogenous steroid. Nature 1998; 392:926–930.

112. Smith SS, Gong QH, Li X, Moran MH, Bitran D, Frye CA, Hsu F-C. Withdrawal from 3α-OH-5α-pregnan-20-one using a pseudopregnancy model alters the kinetics of hippocampal GABA$_A$-gated current and increases the GABA$_A$ receptor α4 subunit in association with increased anxiety. J Neurosci 1998; 18:5275–5284.

113. Follesa P, Cagetti E, Mancuso L, Biggio F, Manca A, Maciocco E, Massa F, Desole MS, Carta M, Busonero F, Sanna E, Biggio G. Increase in expression of the GABA$_A$ receptor α4 subunit gene induced by withdrawal of, but not by long-term treatment with, benzodiazepine full or partial agonists. Mol Brain Res 2001; 92:138–148.

114. Brussaard AB, Kits KS, Baker RE, Willems WP, Leyting-Vermeulen JW, Voorn P, Smit AB, Bicknell RJ, Herbison AE. Plasticity in fast synaptic inhibition of adult oxytocin neurons caused by switch in GABA$_A$ receptor subunit expression. Neuron 1997; 19:1103–1114.

115. Park-Chung M, Malayev A, Purdy RH, Gibbs TT, Farb DH. Sulfated and unsulfated steroids modulate γ-aminobutyric acid$_A$ receptor function through distinct sites. Brain Res 1999; 830:72–87.

116. Majewska MD. Neurosteroids: endogenous bimodal modulators of the GABA$_A$ receptor. Mechanism of action and physiological significance. Prog Neurobiol 1992; 38:379–395.

117. Sousa A, Ticku MK. Interactions of the neurosteroid dehydroepiandrosterone sulfate with the GABA$_A$ receptor complex reveals that it may act via the picrotoxin site. J Pharmacol Exp Ther 1997; 282:827–833.

118. Majewska MD, Schwartz RD. Pregnenolone sulfate: an endogenous antagonist of the γ-aminobutyric acid receptor complex in brain? Brain Res 1987; 404:355–360.

119. Majewska MD, Demirgoren S, Spivak CE, London ED. The neurosteroid dehydro-epiandrosterone sulfate is an allosteric antagonist of the GABA$_A$ receptor. Brain Res 1990; 526:143–146.

120. Mienville JM, Vicini S. Pregnenolone sulfate antagonizes GABA$_A$ receptor–mediated currents via a reduction of channel opening frequency. Brain Res 1989; 489:190–194.

121. Akk G, Bracamontes J, Steinbach JH. Pregnenolone sulfate block of GABA$_A$ receptors: mechanism and involvement of a residue in the M2 region of the α subunit. J Physiol (Lond) 2001; 532:673–684.

122. Wu FS, Gibbs TT, Farb DH. Pregnenonolone sulfate: a positive allosteric modulator at the N-methyl-D-aspartate receptor. Mol Pharmacol 1991; 40:333–336.

123. Bowlby MR. Pregnenolone sulfate potentiation of N-methyl-D-aspartate receptor channels in hippocampal neurons. Mol Pharmacol 1993; 43:813–819.

124. Irwin RP, Lin SZ, Rogawski MA, Purdy RH, Paul SM. Steroid potentiation and inhibition of N-methyl-D-aspartate receptor-mediated intracellular Ca^{2+} responses: structure-activity studies. J Pharmacol Exp Ther 1994; 271:677–682.

125. Yaghoubi N, Malayev A, Russek SJ, Gibbs TT, Farb DH. Neurosteroid modulation of recombinant ionotropic glutamate receptors. Brain Res 1998; 803:153–160.

126. Malayev A, Gibbs TT, Farb DH. Inhibition of the NMDA response by pregnenolone sulphate reveals subtype selective modulation of NMDA receptors by sulphated steroids. Br J Pharmacol 2002; 135:901–909.

127. Guazzo EP, Kirkpatrick PJ, Goodyer IM, Shiers HM, Herbert J. Cortisol, dehydroepiandrosterone (DHEA), and DHEA sulfate in the cerebrospinal fluid of man: relation to blood levels and the effects of age. J Clin Endocrinol Metab 1996; 81:3951–3960.

128. Vallée M, Mayo W, Darnaudéry M, Corpéchot C, Young J, Koehl M, Le Moal M, Baulieu EE, Robel P, Simon H. Neurosteroids: deficient cognitive performance in aged rats depends on low pregnenolone sulfate levels in the hippocampus. Proc Natl Acad Sci USA 1997; 94:14865–14870.

129. Friess E, Schiffelholz T, Steckler T, Steiger A. Dehydroepiandrosterone—a neurosteroid. Eur J Clin Invest 2000; 30(suppl 3):46–50.

130. Belelli D, Bolger MB, Gee KW. Anticonvulsant profile of the progesterone metabolite 5α-pregnan-3α-ol-20-one. Eur J Pharmacol 1989; 166:325–329.

131. Wieland S, Belluzzi JD, Stein L, Lan NC. Comparative behavioral characterization of the neuroactive steroids 3α-OH,5α-pregnan-20-one and 3α-OH,5β-pregnan-20-one in rodents. Psychopharmacology 1995; 118:65–71.

132. Gasior M, Carter RB, Goldberg SR, Witkin JM. Anticonvulsant and behavioral effects of neuroactive steroids alone and in conjunction with diazepam. J Pharmacol Exp Ther 1997; 282:543–553.

133. Frye CA, Scalise TJ. Anti-seizure effects of progesterone and 3α,5α-THP in kainic acid and perforant pathway models of epilepsy. Psychoneuroendocrinology 2000; 25:407–420.

134. Frye CA. The neurosteroid 3α,5α-THP has anti-seizure and possible neuroprotective effects in an animal model of epilepsy. Brain Res 1995; 696:113–120.

135. Kokate TG, Cohen AL, Karp E, Rogawski MA. Neuroactive steroids protect against pilocarpine- and kainic acid-induced limbic seizures and status epilepticus in mice. Neuropharmacology 1996; 35:1049–1056.

136. Holmes GL, Weber DA, Kloczko N, Zimmerman AW. Relationship of endocrine function to inhibition of kindling. Brain Res 1984; 318:55–59.

137. Carter RB, Wood PL, Wieland S, Hawkinson JE, Belelli D, Lambert JJ, White HS, Wolf HH, Mirsadeghi S, Tahir SH, Bolger MB, Lan NC, Gee KW. Characterization of the anticonvulsant properties of ganaxolone (CCD 1042; 3α-hydroxy-3β-methyl-5α-pregnan-20-one), a selective, high-affinity, steroid modulator of the γ-aminobutyric acid$_A$ receptor. J Pharmacol Exp Ther 1997; 280:1284–1295.

138. Edwards HE, Burnham WM, MacLusky NJ. Testosterone and its metabolites affect afterdischarge thresholds and the development of amygdala kindled seizures. Brain Res 1999; 838:151–157.

139. Gasior M, Ungard JT, Beekman M, Carter RB, Witkin JM. Acute and chronic effects of the synthetic neuroactive steroid, ganaxolone, against the convulsive and lethal effects of pentylenetrazol in seizure-kindled mice: comparison with diazepam and valproate. Neuropharmacology 2000; 39:1184–1196.

140. Członkowska AI, Krzążcik P, Sienkiewicz-Jarosz H, Siemiątkowski M, Szyndler J, Bidzinski A, Płaźnik A. The effects of neurosteroids on picrotoxin-, bicuculline- and NMDA-induced seizures, and a hypnotic effect of ethanol. Pharmacol Biochem Behav 2000; 67:345–353.

141. Tsuda M, Suzuki T, Misawa M. Modulation of the decrease in the seizure threshold of pentylenetetrazole in diazepam-withdrawn mice by the neurosteroid 5α-pregnan-3α,21-diol-20-one (alloTHDOC). Addict Biol 1997; 2:455–460.

142. Reddy DS, Kim H-Y, Rogawski MA. Neurosteroid withdrawal model of perimenstrual catamenial epilepsy. Epilepsia 2001; 42:328–336.

143. Reddy DS, Castaneda DC, O'Malley BW, Rogawski MA. Seizure resistance of progesterone receptor knockout mice. FASEB J 2001; 15:A223–223.

144. Rupprecht R, Reul JM, Trapp T, Van Steensel B, Wetzel C, Damm K, Zieglgansberger W, Holsboer F. Progesterone receptor-mediated effects of neuroactive steroids. Neuron 1993; 11:523–530.

145. Landgren S, Backstrom T, Kalistratov G. The effect of progesterone on the spontaneous interictal spike evoked by the application of penicillin to the cat's cerebral cortex. J Neurol Sci 1978; 36:119–133.

146. Bäckström T, Zetterlund B, Blom S, Romano M. Effect of intravenous progesterone infusions on the epileptic discharge frequency in women with partial epilepsy. Acta Neurol Scand 1984; 69:240–248.

147. Herzog AG. Progesterone therapy in women with complex partial and secondary generalized seizures. Neurology 1995; 45:1600–1662.

148. Kokate TG, Banks MK, Magee T, Yamaguchi S, Rogawski MA. Finasteride, a 5α-reductase inhibitor, blocks the anticonvulsant activity of progesterone in mice. J Pharmacol Exp Ther 1999; 288:679–684.

149. Lydon JP, DeMayo FJ, Funk CR, Mani SK, Hughes AR, Montgomery CA Jr, Shyamala G, Conneely OM, O'Malley BW. Mice lacking progesterone receptor exhibit pleiotropic reproductive abnormalities. Genes Dev 1995; 9:2266–2278.

150. Parsons B, Rainbow TC, MacLusky NJ, McEwen BS. Progestin receptor levels in rat hypothalamic and limbic nuclei. J Neurosci 1982; 2:1446–1452.

151. Edwards HE, Epps T, Carlen PL, MacLusky N. Progestin receptors mediate progesterone suppression of epileptiform activity in tetanized hippocampal slices in vitro. Neuroscience 2001; 101:895–906.

152. Reddy DS, Kulkarni SK. Proconvulsant effects of neurosteroid pregnenolone sulfate and dehydroepiandrosterone sulfate in mice. Eur J Pharmacol 1998; 345:55–59.

153. Kokate TG, Juhng KN, Kirkby RD, Llamas J, Yamaguchi S, Rogawski MA. Convulsant actions of the neurosteroid pregnenolone sulfate in mice. Brain Res 1999; 831:119–124.

154. Logothetis J, Harner R, Morrell F, Torres F. The role of estrogens in catamenial exacerbation of epilepsy. Neurology 1959; 9:352–360.

155. Woolley CS, Schwartzkroin PA. Hormonal effects on the brain. Epilepsia 1998; 39(suppl 8):S2–S8.

156. Logothetis J, Harner R. Electrocortical activation by estrogens. Arch Neurol 1960; 3:290–297.

157. Woolley DE, Timiras PS. Estrous and circadian periodicity and electroshock convulsions in rats. Am J Physiol 1962; 202:379–382.

158. Nicoletti F, Speciale C, Sortino MA, Summa G, Caruso G, Patti F, Canonico PL. Comparative effects of estradiol benzoate, the antiestrogen clomiphene citrate and the progestin medroxyprogesterone acetate on kainic acid–induced seizures in male and female rats. Epilepsia 1985; 26:252–257.

159. Buterbaugh GG, Hudson GM. Estradiol replacement to female rats facilitates dorsal hippocampal but not ventral hippocampal kindled seizure acquisition. Exp Neurol 1991; 11:55–64.

160. Woolley CS. Estradiol facilitates kainic acid-induced, but not flurothyl-induced, behavioral seizure activity in adult female rats. Epilepsia 2000; 41:510–515.

161. Frye CA, Reed TA. Androgenic neurosteroids: anti-seizure effects in an animal model of epilepsy. Psychoneuroendocrinology 1998; 23:385–399.

162. Uzunov DP, Cooper TB, Costa E, Guidotti A. Fluoxetine-elicited changes in brain neurosteroid content measured by negative ion mass fragmentography. Proc Natl Acad Sci USA 1996; 93:12599–12604.

163. Uzunov V, Sheline Y, Davis JM, Rasmusson A, Uzunov DP, Costa E, Guidotti A. Increase in the cerebrospinal fluid content of neurosteroids in patients with unipolar major depression who are receiving fluoxetine or fluvoxamine. Proc Natl Acad Sci USA 1998; 95:3239–3244.

164. Rapkin AJ, Morgan M, Goldman L, Brann DW, Simone D, Mahesh VB. Progesterone metabolite allopregnanolone in women with premenstrual syndrome. Obstet Gynecol 1997; 190:709–714.

165. Rupprecht R. Neuroactive steroids: mechanisms of action and neuropsychopharmacological properties. Psychoneuroendocrinology 2003; 28:139–168.

166. Reddy DS. Clinical potentials of endogenous neurosteroids. Drugs Today 2002; 38:465–485.

167. Newmark ME, Penry JK. Catamenial epilepsy: a review. Epilepsia 1980; 21:281–300.

168. Tauboll E, Lundervold A, Gjerstad L. Temporal distribution of seizures in epilepsy. Epilepsy Res 1991; 8:153–165.

169. Duncan S, Read CL, Brodie MJ. How common is catamenial epilepsy? Epilepsia 1993; 34:827–831.

170. Herzog AG, Klein P, Ransil BJ. Three patterns of catamenial epilepsy. Epilepsia 1997; 38:1082–1088.

171. Bäckström T. Epileptic seizures in women related to plasma estrogen and progesterone during the menstrual cycle. Acta Neurol Scand 1976; 54:321–347.

172. Jacono JJ, Robinson J. The effects of estrogen, progesterone, and ionized calcium on seizures during the menstrual cycle in epileptic women. Epilepsia 1997; 28:571–577.

173. Laidlaw J. Catamenial epilepsy. Lancet 1956; 271:1235–1237.

174. Concas A, Mostallino MC, Porcu P, Folesa P, Barbaccia ML, Trabucchi M, Purdy RH, Grisenti P, Biggio G. Role of brain allopregnanolone in the plasticity of γ-aminobutyric acid type A receptor in rat brain during pregnancy and after delivery. Proc Natl Acad Sci USA 1998; 95:13284–13289.

175. File SE. The history of benzodiazepine dependence: a review of animal studies. Neurosci Biobehav Rev 1990; 14:135–146.

176. Kokka N, Sapp DW, Taylor AM, Olsen RW. The kindling model of alcohol dependence: similar persistent reduction in seizure threshold to pentylenetetrazol in animals receiving chronic ethanol or chronic pentylenetetrazol. Alcoholism 1993; 17:525–531.

177. Bonuccelli U, Melis GB, Paoletti AM, Fioretti P, Murri L, Muratorio A. Unbalanced progesterone and estradiol secretion in catamenial epilepsy. Epilepsy Res 1989; 3:100–106.

178. Reddy DS, Rogawski MA. Enhanced anticonvulsant activity of neuroactive steroids in a rat model of catamenial epilepsy. Epilepsia 2001; 42:337–344.

179. Czlonkowska AI, Krzascik P, Sienkiewicz-Jarosz H, Siemiatkowski M, Szyndler J, Maciejak P, Bidzinski A, Plaznik A. Rapid down-regulation of GABA$_A$ receptors after pretreatment of mice with progesterone. Pol J Pharmacol 2001; 53:385–388.

180. Concas A, Follesa P, Barbaccia ML, Purdy RH, Biggio G. Physiological modulation of GABA$_A$ receptor plasticity by progesterone metabolites. Eur J Pharmacol 1999; 375:225–235.

181. Devaud LL, Fritschy JM, Morrow AL. Influence of gender on chronic ethanol-induced alterations in GABA$_A$ receptors in rats. Brain Res 1998; 796:222–230.

182. Moran MH, Goldberg M, Smith SS. Progesterone withdrawal. II. Insensitivity to the sedative effects of a benzodiazepine. Brain Res 1998; 807:91–100.

183. Sundstrom I, Nyberg S, Bäckström T. Patients with premenstrual syndrome have reduced sensitivity to midazolam compared to control subjects. Neuropsychopharmacology 1997; 17:370–381.

184. Wihlbäck A-C, Sundstrom-Poromaa I, Nyberg S, Bäckström T. Sensitivity to a neurosteroid is increased during addition of progestagen to postmenopausal hormone replacement therapy. Neuroendocrinology 2001; 73:397–407.

185. Reddy DS, Rogawski MA. Chronic treatment with the neuroactive steroid ganaxolone in the rat induces anticonvulsant tolerance to diazepam but not to itself. J Pharmacol Exp Ther 2000; 295:1241–1248.

186. Herzog AG. Intermittent progesterone therapy and frequency of complex partial seizures in women with menstrual disorders. Neurology 1986; 26:601–610.

187. Monaghan EP, Navalta LA, Shum L, Ashbrock DW, Lee DA. Initial human experience with ganaxolone, a neuroactive steroid with antiepileptic activity. Epilepsia 1997; 38:1026–1031.

188. Reddy DS, Rogawski MA. Enhanced anticonvulsant activity of ganaxolone after neurosteroid withdrawal in a rat model of catamenial epilepsy. J Pharmacol Exp Ther 2000; 294:909–915.

189. White HS, Woodhead JH, Franklin MR, Swinyard EA, Wolf HA. General principles. Experimental selection, quantification, and evaluation of antiepileptic drugs. In: Levy RH, Mattson RH, Meldrum BS, eds. Antiepileptic Drugs, 4th ed. New York: Raven Press, 1995:99–110.

190. Löscher W, Rundfeldt C, Honack D, Ebert U. Long-term studies on anticonvulsant tolerance and withdrawal characteristics of benzodiazepine receptor ligands in different seizure models in mice. I. Comparison of diazepam, clonazepam, clobazam and abecarnil. J Pharmacol Exp Ther 1996; 279:561–572.

191. Haigh JRM, Feely M. Tolerance to the anticonvulsant effect of benzodiazepines. Trends Pharmacol Sci 1988; 9:361–366.

192. Kokate TG, Yamaguchi S, Pannel LK, Rajamani U, Carroll DM, Grossman AB, Rogawski MA. Lack of anticonvulsant tolerance to the neuroactive steroid pregnanolone in mice. J Pharmacol Exp Ther 1998; 287:553–558.

193. Ramsay MAE, Savege TM, Simpson BRJ, Goodwin R. Controlled sedation with alphaxalone-alphadolone. Br Med J 1974; 2:656–659.

194. Wieland S, Belluzzi J, Hawkinson JE, Hogenkamp D, Upasani R, Stein L, Wood PL, Gee KW, Lan NC. Anxiolytic and anticonvulsant activity of a synthetic neuroactive steroid Co 3-0593. Psychopharmacology 1997; 134:46–54.

195. Marshall FH, Stratton SC, Mullings J, Ford E, Worton SP, Oakley NR, Hagan RM. Development of tolerance in mice to the sedative effects of the neuroactive steroid minaxolone following chronic exposure. Pharmacol Biochem Behav 1997; 58:1–8.

196. Czlonkowska AI, Krzascik P, Sienkiewicz-Jarosz H, Siemiatkowski M, Szyndler J, Maciejak P, Bidzinski A, Plaznik A. Tolerance to the anticonvulsant activity of midazolam and allopregnanolone in a model of picrotoxin seizures. Eur J Pharmacol 2001; 425:121–127.

197. Herzog AG. Psychoneuroendocrine aspects of temporolimbic epilepsy. Part II: Epilepsy and reproductive steroids. Psychosomatics 1999; 40:102–108.

198. Monteleone P, Luisi S, Tonetti A, Bernardi F, Genazzani AD, Luisi M, Petraglia F, Genazzani AR. Allopregnanolone concentrations and premenstrual syndrome. Eur J Endocrinol 2000; 142:269–273.

199. Costa AM, Spence KT, Smith SS, ffrench-Mullen JM. Withdrawal from the endogenous steroid progesterone results in GABA$_A$ currents insensitive to benzodiazepine modulation in rat CA1 hippocampus. J Neurophysiol 1995; 74:464–469.

200. Tan SY, Mulrow PJ. The contribution of the zona fasciculata and glomerulosa to plasma 11-deoxycorticosterone levels in man. J Clin Endocrinol Metab 1975; 41:126–130.

201. Kater CE, Biglieri EG, Brust N, Chang B, Hirai J, Irony I. Stimulation and suppression of the mineralocorticoid hormones in normal subjects and adrenocortical disorder. Endocr Rev 1989; 10:149–164.

202. Barbaccia ML, Roscetti G, Trabucchi M, Mostallino MC, Concas A, Purdy RH, Biggio G. Time-dependent changes in rat brain neuroactive steroid concentrations and GABA$_A$ receptor function after acute stress. Neuroendocrinology 1996; 63:166–172.

203. Barbaccia ML, Roscetti G, Trabucchi M, Purdy RH, Mostallino MC, Perra C, Concas A, Biggio G. Isoniazid-induced inhibition of GABAergic transmission enhances neurosteroid content in the rat brain. Neuropharmacology 1996; 35:1299–1305.

204. Barbaccia ML, Roscetti G, Trabucchi M, Purdy RH, Mostallino MC, Concas A, Biggio G. The effects of inhibitors of GABAergic transmission and stress on brain and plasma allopregnanolone concentrations. Br J Pharmacol 1997; 120:1582–1588.

205. Barbaccia ML, Concas A, Serra M, Biggio G. Stress and neurosteroids in adult and aged rats. Exp Gerontol 1998; 33:697–712.

206. Serra M, Pisu MG, Littera M, Papi G, Sanna E, Tuveri F, Usala L, Purdy RH, Biggio G. Social isolation–induced decreases in both the abundance of neuroactive steroids and GABA$_A$ receptor function in rat brain. J Neurochem 2000; 75:732–740.

207. Vallee M, Rivera JD, Koob GF, Purdy RH, Fitzgerald RL. Quantification of neurosteroids in rat plasma and brain following swim stress and allopregnanolone administration using negative chemical ionization gas chromatography/mass spectrometry. Anal Biochem 2000; 287:153–166.

208. Feldman RG, Paul NL. Identity of emotional triggers in epilepsy. J Nerv Ment Dis 1976; 162:345–353.

209. Minter RE. Can emotions precipitate seizures—a review of the question. J Fam Pract 1979; 8:55–59.

210. Temkin NR, Davis GR. Stress as a risk factor for seizures among adults with epilepsy. Epilepsia 1984; 25:450–456.

211. Soubrie P, Thiebot MH, Jobert A, Montastruc JL, Hery F, Hamon M. Decreased convulsant potency of picrotoxin and pentetrazol and enhanced [^{3}H]flunitrazepam cortical binding following stressful manipulations in rats. Brain Res 1980; 189:505–517.

212. Pericic D, Švob D, Jazvinšćak M, Mirković K. Anticonvulsive effect of swim stress in mice. Pharmacol Biochem Behav 2000; 66:879–886.

213. Abel EL, Berman RF. Effects of water immersion stress on convulsions induced by pentylenetetrazol. Pharmacol Biochem Behav 1993; 45:823–825.

214. Frucht MM, Quigg M, Schwaner C, Fountain NB. Distribution of seizure precipitants among epilepsy syndromes. Epilepsia 2000; 41:1534–1539.

215. Conforti N, Feldman S. Effect of cortisol on the excitability of limbic structures of the brain in freely moving rats. J Neurol Sci 1975; 26:29–38.

216. Roberts AJ, Keith LD. Corticosteroids enhance convulsion susceptibility via central mineralocorticoid receptors. Psychoneuroendocrinology 1995; 20:891–902.

217. Ehlers CL, Henriksen SJ, Wang M, Rivier J, Vale W, Bloom FE. Corticotropin releasing factor produces increases in brain excitability and convulsive seizures in rats. Brain Res 1983; 278:332–336.

218. Baram TZ, Schultz L. Corticotropin-releasing hormone is a rapid and potent convulsant in the infant rat. Dev Brain Res 1991; 61:97–101.

219. Wasserman MJ, Neville BS, Belton R, Millichamp JG. The effect of corticotropin (ACTH) on experimental seizures. Neurology 1965; 15:1136–1141.

220. Tartara A, Bo P, Maurelli M, Savoldi F. Centrally administered N-terminal fragments of ACTH (1-10, 4-10, 4-9) display convulsant properties in rabbits. Peptides 1983; 4:315–318.

221. Klein R, Livingston S. The effect of adrenocorticotrophic hormone in epilepsy. J Pediatr 1950; 37:733–742.

222. Sorel L, Dusaucy-Bauloye A. A propos de 21 cas d'hypsarrhythmia de Gibbs: son traitement spectaculaire par l'ACTH. Acta Neurol Belg 1958; 58:130–141.

223. Wong M, Trevathan E. Infantile spasms. Pediatr Neurol 2001; 24:89–98.

224. Rogawski MA, Reddy DS. Neurosteroids and infantile spasms: the deoxycorticosterone hypothesis. Int Rev Neurobiol 2002; 49:199–219.

225. Snead OC 3rd. How does ACTH work against infantile spasms? Bedside to bench. Ann Neurol 2001; 49:288–289.

226. Crosley CJ, Richman RA, Thorpy MJ. Evidence for cortisol-independent anticonvulsant activity of adrenocorticotropic hormone in infantile spasms. Ann Neurol 1980; 8:220.

227. Thompson J, Holmes GL. Failure of ACTH to alter transfer kindling in the immature brain. Epilepsia 1987; 28:17–19.

228. Baram TZ, Schultz L. ACTH does not control neonatal seizures induced by administration of exogenous corticotropin-releasing hormone. Epilepsia 1995; 36:174–178.

229. Monaghan EP, McAculey JW, Data JL. Ganaxolone: a novel positive allosteric modulator of the GABA$_A$ receptor complex for the treatment of epilepsy. Exp Opin Invest Drugs 1999; 8:1663–1671.

230. Kerrigan JF, Shields WD, Nelson TY, Bluestone DL, Dodson WE, Bourgeois BF, Pellock JM, Morton LD, Monaghan EP. Ganaxolone for treating intractable infantile spasms: a multicenter, open-label, add-on trial. Epilepsy Res 2000; 42:133–139.

231. Finn DA, Roberts AJ, Crabbe JC. Neuroactive steroid sensitivity in withdrawal seizure-prone and -resistant mice. Alcohol Clin Exp Res 1995; 19:410–415.

232. Morrow AL, Van Doren MJ, Penland SN, Matthews DB. The role of GABAergic neuroactive steroids in ethanol action, tolerance and dependence. Brain Res Rev 2001; 37:98–109.

233. Van Doren MJ, Matthews DB, Janis GC, Grobin AC, Devaud LL, Morrow AL. Neuroactive steroid 3α-hydroxy-5α-pregnan-20-one modulates electrophysiological and behavioral actions of ethanol. J Neurosci 2000; 20:1982–1989.

234. Devaud LL, Purdy RH, Morrow AL. The neurosteroid, 3α-hydroxy-5α-pregnan-20-one, protects against bicuculline-induced seizures during ethanol withdrawal in rats Alcohol Clin Exp Res 1995; 19:350–355.

235. Buck KJ, Harris RA. Benzodiazepine agonist and inverse agonist actions on GABA$_A$ receptor–operated chloride channels. II. Chronic effects of ethanol. J Pharmacol Exp Ther 1990; 253:713–719.

236. Romeo E, Brancati A, De Lorenzo A, Fucci P, Furnari C, Pompili E, Sasso GF, Spalletta G, Troisi A, Pasini A. Marked decrease of plasma neuroactive steroids during alcohol withdrawal. Clin Neuropharmcol 1996; 19:366–369.

237. Herzog AG. Reproductive endocrine considerations and hormonal therapy for men with epilepsy. Epilepsia 1991; 32(suppl 6):S34–S37.

238. Werboff LH, Havlena J. Audiogenic seizures in adult male rats treated with various hormones. Gen Comp Endocrinol 1963; 3:389–397.

239. Schwartz-Giblin S, Korotzer A, Pfaff DW. Steroid hormone effects on picrotoxin-induced seizures in female and male rats. Brain Res 1989; 476:240–247.

240. Thomas J, McLean JH. Castration alters susceptibility of male rats to specific seizures. Physiol Behav 1991; 49:1177–1179.

241. Pesce ME, Acevedo X, Bustamante D, Miranda HE, Pinardi G. Progesterone and testosterone modulate the convulsant actions of pentylenetetrazol and strychnine in mice. Pharmacol Toxicol 2000; 87:116–119.

242. Thomas J, Yang YC. Allylglycine-induced seizures in male and female rats. Physiol Behav 1991; 49:1181–1183.

243. Herzog AG, Seibel MM, Schomer DL, Vaitukaitis JL, Geschwind N. Reproductive endocrine disorders in men with partial seizures of temporal lobe origin. Arch Neurol 1986; 43:347–350.

244. Martini L. Androgen metabolism in the brain. Neuroendocrinol Lett 1992; 14:315–318.

245. Martini L, Melcangi RC, Maggi R. Androgen and progesterone metabolism in the central and peripheral nervous system. J Steroid Biochem Mol Biol 1993; 47:195–205.

246. Frye CA, Duncan JE, Basham M, Erskine MS. Behavioral effects of 3α-androstanediol. II: Hypothalamic and preoptic area actions via a GABAergic mechanism. Behav Brain Res 1996; 79:119–130.

247. Frye CA, Van Keuren KR, Erskine MS. Behavioral effects of 3α-androstanediol. I: Modulation of sexual receptivity and promotion of GABA-stimulated chloride flux. Behav Brain Res 1996; 79:109–118.

248. Frye CA, Park D, Tanaka M, Rosellini R, Svare B. The testosterone metabolite and neurosteroid 3α-androstanediol may mediate the effects of testosterone on conditioned place preference. Psychoneuroendocrinology 2001; 26:731–750.

249. Herzog AG, Klein P, Jacobs AR. Testosterone versus testosterone and testolactone in treating reproductive and sexual dysfunction in men with epilepsy and hypogonadism. Neurology 1998; 50:782–784.

250. Herzog AG. Seizure control with clomiphene therapy. A case report. Arch Neurol 1988; 45:209–210.

251. Herzog AG. Progesterone therapy in women with epilepsy: a 3-year follow-up. Neurology 1999; 52:1917–1918.

252. Laxer K, Blum D, Abou-Khalil BW, Morrell MJ, Lee DA, Data JL, Monaghan EP. Assessment of ganaxolone's anticonvulsant activity using a randomized, double-blind, presurgical trial design. Ganaxolone Presurgical Study Group. Epilepsia 2000; 41:1187–1194.

253. McAuley JW, Moore, JL, Reeves AL, Flyak J, Monaghan EP, Data J. A pilot study of the neurosteroid ganaxolone in catamenial epilepsy: clinical experience in two patients. Epilepsia 2001; 42(suppl 7, Abstract 1.267).

254. Liptakova S, Velisek L, Veliskova J, Moshe SL. Effect of ganaxolone on flurothyl seizures in developing rats. Epilepsia 2000; 41:788 793.

255. Belelli D, Herd MB. The contraceptive agent Provera enhances GABA$_A$ receptor-mediated inhibitory neurotransmission in the rat hippocampus: evidence for endogenous neurosteroids? J Neurosci 2003; 23:10013–10020.

256. Naum G, Cardozo J, Golombek DA. Diurnal variation in the proconvulsant effect of 3-mercaptopropionic acid and the anticonvulsant effect of androsterone in the Syrian hamster. Life Sci 2002; 71:91–98.

257. Snead OC 3rd. Ganaxolone, a selective, high-affinity steroid modulator of the γ-aminobutyric acid-A receptor, exacerbates seizures in animal models of absence. Ann Neurol 1998; 44:688–691.

18

Impact of Neuroendocrine Factors on Seizure Genesis and Treatment

Pavel Klein

Georgetown University Hospital
Washington, D.C., U.S.A.

INTRODUCTION

Hormones affect seizures. They modulate the expression of individual seizures in patients with epilepsy. They may also, in some situations, contribute to the development of an enduring state of spontaneous recurrent seizures—i.e., a process referred to as "epileptogenesis."

Modulation of seizure occurrence by hormonal changes in patients with epilepsy may be more common than is appreciated. Among the factors that precipitate seizures, stress is the most common, triggering seizures in 30–60% of patients with epilepsy. Among women, events related to the reproductive life cycle are also commonly associated with change in seizure manifestation and development. About 20% of women may develop epilepsy during the time around menarche ("perimenarche"); 15–30% of girls with preexisting seizures experience seizure exacerbation during perimenarche; about a third of women with refractory epilepsy have seizure exacerbation in relation to their menstrual cycle ("catamenial epilepsy"); and seizure occurrence changes during pregnancy and perimenopause in 20–50% of women. These clinical effects are likely due, in part or completely, to the associated hormonal changes. Thus, hormonal changes may be a common cause of disturbed—usually increased—seizure expression in patients with epilepsy. Understanding the hormonal changes involved may have important consequences for the treatment of patients with epilepsy and, possibly, for prevention of epilepsy in certain at risk patient populations.

In the present chapter, I will discuss the effect of sex hormones and stress hormones on seizure expression and on epileptogenesis, as well as the therapeutic potential of hormonal manipulation on treatment of seizures. I shall first discuss the basic scientific data concerning hormonal influence on neuronal excitability and seizures. I shall then outline the clinical settings where hormonal modulation of seizure expression or development may be important. Finally, I shall review hormonal treatments of epilepsy. Because more is known about the role of hormones in precipitating individual seizures in patients with established epilepsy than about their role in epileptogenesis, I will discuss the role of hormones in seizure provocation in more detail than their role in true epileptogenesis.

HORMONAL EFFECTS ON NEURONAL EXCITABILITY AND SEIZURES: ANIMAL DATA

Gonadal and adrenal steroid hormones have a wide-ranging influence upon neuronal activity in the central nervous system (CNS). Steroidal effects in the CNS occur by both receptor-mediated (genomic) and membrane (nongenomic) mechanisms, with long and short latencies of action, respectively (1,2). The effects of these hormones and related neuropeptides on neuronal excitability and in animal seizure models are discussed briefly below; a more detailed treatment can be found in the preceding chapter in this volume.

Estrogens increase neuronal excitability and facilitate seizure occurrence and epileptogenesis. Progesterone has the opposite effect: it inhibits neuronal excitability, seizures and epileptogenesis.

Estrogens

In adult female rats, seizure threshold fluctuates during the estrous cycle. Susceptibility to seizures is highest during proestrus, when serum estrogen levels are highest (3). Estrogens lower seizure threshold in different animal seizure models in both physiological and pharmacological doses and promote seizure kindling and epileptogenesis in animals in different brain regions, including the amygdala, the hippocampus, and the neocortex (4–12). Interestingly, physiological doses of estradiol (E2) facilitate seizure kindling in both female and male rats (6,8). Pharmacological doses of estrogens activate spike discharges and, in animals with preexisting cortical lesions, may induce seizures, including fatal status epilepticus (4,5). However, ovariectomy in adult rats does not alter seizure threshold (7). Thus, lack of estrogen may not protect against seizures, while excess of estrogen promotes them.

Estrogens affect neuronal excitability by genomically dependent mechanisms, by nongenomic, direct effects on neuronal membrane, and by affecting neuronal plasticity and the number of excitatory synapses. The genomic mechanisms are mediated by cytosolic neuronal estrogen receptors (ERs). Estrogen receptors (α, β) are present in neurons in different parts of the CNS. In addition to the anterior and mesiobasal parts of the hypothalamus, where they modulate the activity of neurons involved in the control of endocrine and behavioral functions associated with reproductions, they are found in great density in the cortical and medial amygdaloid nuclei, and in lesser numbers in the hippocampal pyramidal cell layer and the subiculum and the neocortex (13–15). ER-containing neurons colocalize with other neurotransmitters, including γ amino butyric acid (GABA) (1,16). By regulating the expression of genes affecting the activity, release, and postsynaptic action of different neurotransmitters and neuromodulators, estrogens may act to increase the excitability of neurons which concentrate estradiol. For instance, E2 reduces GABA synthesis in the corticomedial amygdala by decreasing the activity of glutamic acid decarboxylase (17).

Estrogens also exert a direct excitatory effect at the neuronal membrane, where E2 augments both the N-methyl-D-aspartate (NMDA) and non-NMDA glutamate receptor activity (18–20). This enhances the resting discharge rates of neurons in a number of brain areas (19). For instance, in the hippocampus, E2 increases excitability of the hippocampal CA1 pyramidal neurons and induces repetitive firing in response to Schaffer collateral stimulation (20,21). Finally, estrogens potentiate neuronal excitability by regulating neuronal plasticity and synaptogenesis. E2 increases the density of dendritic spines carrying excitatory, NMDA receptor–containing synapses on hippocampal CA1 pyramidal neurons (22,23). The density of the excitatory synapses fluctuates during the estrous cycle, being highest by about one-third during the proestrus, when estrogen levels are highest, compared to diestrus when they are low. It decreases markedly following oophorectomy (22). The estrogen-driven increase in excitatory synapses results in enhanced excitatory input to the CA1 neurons, in neuronal excitability, and in synchronization of neuronal outflow that is critical to formation of paroxysmal depolarization shifts, seizure genesis, and propagation (24).

Progestins

Progesterone depresses neuronal firing (18), lessens epileptiform discharges, and elevates seizure threshold in animal models of epilepsy (25,26), increasing seizure threshold in female, but not male, rats (6,7). Seizure threshold during the rat estrous cycle correlates with serum progesterone levels. It is highest during diestrus, when serum progesterone level is highest, suggesting a protective effect of progesterone against seizures. Progesterone inhibits seizure occurrence in animals with existing seizures in models of epilepsy that include both limbic and neocortical localization-related epilepsy (5,7,11,26). Progesterone inhibits epileptogenesis in different animal models of epilepsy, including amygdaloid and hippocampal electrical kindling and kainate models of limbic epilepsy (6,11,27,28). Inhibition of kindling is particularly prominent in immature animals in which progesterone is strongly protective against seizure development, particularly against limbic seizure kindling (7,27). The anticonvulsant effect of progesterone is largely mediated by its metabolite, 3-α-hydroxy-5-α-pregnan-20-one, allopregnanolone (29,30) (see below).

Like estrogens, progesterone affects neuronal excitability by genomic mechanisms, nongenomic membrane effects and by influencing synaptic plasticity. Progesterone receptors are found in most ER-containing brain regions, and in areas such as cerebral cortex that lack estrogen receptors (31). As with E2, progesterone may influence, via genomic mechanisms, the enzymatic activity controlling the synthesis and release of various neurotransmitters and neuromodulators produced by progesterone receptor containing neurons (1).

Progesterone's direct membrane effects are inhibitory (see below). Chronic progesterone exposure decreases the number of dendritic spines and synapses on hippocampal CA1 pyramidal neurons, counteracting the stimulatory effects of E2 (22).

Neuroactive Steroids

Most of the membrane effect of progesterone is due to the action of its 3α-hydroxylated metabolite, 3α-hydroxy-5α-pregnane-20-one or allopregnanolone (AP) (2,32). Allopregnanolone and the 3α,5α-hydroxylated natural metabolite of the mineralocorticoid deoxycorticosterone, allotetrahydrodeoxycorticosterone (allo-THDOC), are the two most potent of a number of endogenous neuroactive steroids with a direct membrane effect on neuronal excitability (2,32–34). Allopregnanolone (but not allo-THDOC) is devoid of hormonal effects and may, together with other related neuroactive steroids, be thought of as an endogenous regulator of brain excitability with anxiolytic, anticonvulsant and sedative-hypnotic properties (2,35).

Allopregnanolone and allo-THDOC hyperpolarize hippocampal and other neurons by potentiating GABA-mediated synaptic inhibition. They act as positive allosteric modulators of the GABA-A receptor, interacting with a steroid-specific site near the receptor to facilitate inward chloride flux through the channel, thereby prolonging the inhibitory action of GABA on neurons (2,32,33,35). At high micromolar concentrations, allopregnanolone also has a direct effect at the GABA-A receptor to induce chloride currents, but this is not likely to be of physiological significance (2,32). Allopregnanolone is one of the most potent ligands of GABA-A receptors in the CNS, with affinities similar to the potent benzodiazepines, and approximately a thousand times higher than pentobarbital (2,33). The parent steroid, progesterone, enhances GABA-induced chloride currents only weakly and only in high concentrations (2,34).

Plasma and brain levels of allopregnanolone parallel those of progesterone in rats, and in normal women plasma levels of AP correlate with progesterone levels during the menstrual cycle and pregnancy (2). However, brain activity of progesterone and AP is not dependent solely on ovarian and adrenal production, as they are both synthesized de novo in the brain (36). Their synthesis is region specific and includes the cortex and the hippocampus (36). In contrast, allo-THDOC is only synthesized by the adrenal gland and not in the brain (2).

Allopregnanolone, allo-THDOC, and a 3-α hydroxylated deoxycorticosterone metabolite, dihydrodeoxycorticosterone (DH-DOC), have potent anticonvulsant effects in animal seizure models, including bicuculine-, metrazol-, picrotoxin-, pentylenetetrazol-, pilocarpine, and kainic acid-induced seizures (30,37–39). Allopregnanolone is also effective against status epilepticus, but is ineffective against electroshock and strychnine-induced seizures (32,41).

Allopregnanolone's anticonvulsant properties resemble those of the benzodiazepine clonazepam (29,32,41); allopregnanolone is less potent than clonazepam but may have lower relative toxicity (29,41). However, an important difference in the anticonvulsant action of the benzodiazepines and allopregnanolone is that while the anticonvulsant effect of benzodiazepines habituates, that of allopregnanolone does not (39). Allopregnanolone's anticonvulsant effect is greater in female rats in diestrus (equivalent to human midluteal phase) than in estrus (equivalent to ovulation) or in the male. This may be due to increased functional sensitivity of the GABA-A receptor complex to allopregnanolone during diestrus. It correlates with higher seizure threshold during diestrus (42,43).

In contrast, some of the sulfated neuroactive steroids have excitatory neuronal effects. They include pregnenolone sulfate and dehydroepiandrosterone sulfate (DHEAS), the naturally occurring sulfated esters of the progesterone precursor pregnenolone and of the progesterone metabolite DHEA (2,44). These steroids increase neuronal firing when directly applied to neurons by negatively modulating the GABA-A receptor (2), and by facilitating glutamate-induced excitation at the NMDA receptor (45). In animals, pregnenolone sulfate and DHEAS have a proconvulsant effect (44). The proconvulsant effect is prevented by chronic pretreatment with progesterone (44).

Androgens

The effect of androgens on experimental seizures is uncertain (reviewed in 46).

Adrenal Steroids

Progesterone, allopregnanolone, TH-DOC, DH-DOC, pregnenolone sulfate and DHEAS are all adrenally produced steroids. Their neuroactive actions in relation to experimental epilepsy are discussed above.

Glucocorticoids (GCs) facilitate epileptiform discharges and seizures in animal models (5,47 50). Corticosterone and dexamethasone exacerbate kainic acid-, pentylenetetrazol-induced and other forms of seizures, while adrenalectomy attenuates them, as does administration of the steroid synthesis inhibitor, aminoglutethimide, of the mineralocorticoid antagonists spironolactone and RU-26752, and chronic downregulation of the hypothalamopituitary adrenal (HPA) axis with prolonged low-dose cortisone treatment (48–50). GCs also facilitate the development of cocaine and alcohol withdrawal-caused seizures (48,51).

Glucocorticoids increase neuronal excitability (52–54). The mechanism has not been elucidated (2). Two types of GC receptor are found in the brain. type I (mineralocorticoid receptor, MR), with high affinity for corticosterone and aldosterone, and type II (glucocorticoid receptor, GR), with low affinity for corticosterone—10 times lower than MR (55). Both receptor subtypes are present in the principal cells of the hippocampus (including the dentate gyrus), and thus modulate the excitability of these neurons (56). Normal basal levels of corticosterone occupy the majority of the MR receptors. Stimulation of these receptors reduces the activity of voltage-gated calcium channels and enhances long-term potentiation (LTP). Higher amounts of corticosterone activate glucocorticoid receptors. This facilitates voltage-gated calcium channels but inhibits LTP. During the diurnal surge of corticosterone and following stress, the mineralocorticoid and glucocorticoid receptors are both maximally occupied. Such high level of glucocorticoid receptor activation markedly increases calcium currents, induces expression of NMDA receptor subunit 1 (NR1) mRNA expression in hippocampal neurons (56). It is these higher levels of corticosterone that are associated with a decrease in the action potential threshold (54).

Glucocorticoids also affect neuronal survival and, like estrogens, plasticity (57–59). Chronic glucocorticoid excess results in hippocampal pyramidal neuronal loss and in loss of dendritic spines and branching (58,59). Glucocorticoid elevation exacerbates hypoxia-, stress-, and seizure-induced CA3 pyramidal neuronal loss by potentiating glutamate (i.e., NMDA) receptor-dependent excitotoxicity, and by limiting neuronal energy supply by inhibiting glucose uptake (58). Adrenalectomy has a protective effect in all these situations (58).

CRH

Corticotropin-releasing hormone (CRH) is a neuropeptide which controls the release of ACTH. It is important in the endocrine and behavioral regulation of the stress response (60). It is found in the hypothalamus, where it acts as adrenocorticotropin (ACTH) releasing hormone, but also in the amygdala, hippocampus, and the cortex (61).

CRH acts as an excitatory neurotransmitter or neuromodulator. It induces arousal and, in higher doses, epileptiform discharges and seizures. The seizures start in the amygdala and may spread to the hippocampus and the cortex (62–66). In adult animals, the seizures occur with a latency of a few hours (63), suggesting that the effect could be mediated by CRH-induced increase in glucocorticoid activity rather than by CRH itself. In fact, CRH-induced seizures are potentiated by chronic glucocorticoid administration (67). However, in neonatal rats the convulsant effect occurs within 2 min and at a 200-fold lower dose. Further, seizures manifest before any changes in serum corticosterone can be seen. It may therefore be due to a direct effect of CRH itself (65). Tolerance develops to the seizure-inducing effect of CRH after 2 days (64). This may be due to seizure-induced production of CRH-binding protein (CRF-BP) (68). However, the potentiating effect of CRH on non-CRH induced seizures is long-lasting (64). It could thus contribute toward kindling and development of seizures after an acute CNS insult such as febrile status epilepticus.

CRH has an excitatory effect on neurons. It increases neuronal firing in the hippocampus by decreasing afterhyperpolarization of CA1 and CA3 hippocampal pyramidal cells and of the dentate hilus granule cells (62,68). The mechanism of the excitatory effect is unknown.

CRH-induced epileptiform discharges and seizures are suppressed by carbamazepine, verapamil, clonidine (66), a number of CRH non-selective peptide antagonists, and the selective nonpeptide CRH receptor type 1 antagonist NBI 27914 (Neurocrine Biosciences) (69). The CRH-1 receptor mediates the excitatory actions of CRH in the developing rat brain (70). The selective CRH-1 antagonist α-helical-CRH elevates seizure threshold in an infant rat febrile seizure model in a manner similar to phenobarbital (71).

While CRH can induce limbic seizures, limbic seizures, in turn, activate hippocampal and amygdaloid CRH-producing neurons (68,72). A positive feedback loop may thus exist between limbic seizures and CRH.

CRH, like glucocorticoids, exacerbates seizure-induced hippocampal neuronal loss (73). Unlike other convulsants that do not cause neuronal loss in the neonatal age, CRH-induced status epilepticus in neonatal rats results in neuronal loss in the hippocampal CA3 region, the amygdala and the pyriform cortex (73). Possibly as a result of this, CRH lowers the animals' subsequent threshold to kainic acid-induced seizures (74). A CRH antagonist, astressin, protects against seizure-related hippocampal neuronal loss when injected intracerebroventricularly either before or after seizures (75).

HORMONAL EFFECTS ON SEIZURES AND EPILEPTOGENESIS: CLINICAL DATA

Changes in reproductive hormonal status associated with menarche, menstrual cycles, pregnancy, and menopause may all affect clinical manifestation of seizures.

Menarche

There is increased susceptibility to development of seizures around the time of menarche (76)—i.e., "perimenarche" (77-81). This is not reflected in epidemiological studies, the majority of which do not show an increased incidence of seizures during the age associated with menarche or puberty (82). This may be due to a number of reasons.

First, most epidemiological studies concentrate on age brackets, typically at 5-year intervals, rather than endocrine events such as puberty or menarche. Because the endocrine events may gradually evolve over many years and because their age may not be the same in different subjects, patient grouping by age may not detect these events. In one study where the age bracket was 1 year only, a rise in the incidence of seizures during the 15th year of life was seen (83).

Second, some seizures—for example, absence seizures and the primary idiopathic benign partial epilepsies of childhood—remit spontaneously during adolescence, while others, such as juvenile myoclonic epilepsy, begin during adolescence. These opposing effects might cancel each other out in studies of overall incidence and prevalence of epilepsy.

Third, puberty and sexual maturation are protracted, multifaceted endocrinological events with different hormonal changes occurring during different stages of the 7- to 10-year-long process. This makes correlation with possible seizure onset (or remission) difficult without specifically directed prospective studies, which do not exist.

However, several studies have shown that in women, seizures commonly start during perimenarche (79–81). In a recent questionnaire survey, 19% of 165 adult women with epilepsy reported seizure onset at menarche (80), including 33% of women with primary generalized epilepsy and 14% women with partial epilepsy. This was confirmed in another study, which compared seizure onset during menarche and perimenarche to seizure onset during other childhood periods. Of 76 consecutively evaluated women whose seizures began between the ages of 0.5 and 18 years, seizure onset occurred within 2 years of menarche in 35% of women. In 17%, seizures began during the year of menarche (81). Primary generalized and localization-related epilepsies were equally likely to start during perimenarche.

In addition, several studies have shown an increased risk of exacerbation of seizures during puberty. Rosciszewska showed in the 1970s that approximately one-third of girls with preexisting seizures experience seizure exacerbation during puberty (77). Another third of girls showed improvement in seizure control, while the remaining third was not affected by sexual maturation. Seizure exacerbation is more likely to occur in girls with focal epilepsies, with refractory seizures, with evidence of CNS damage, and with delayed menarche. In more recent studies, 13–38% of girls experienced seizure exacerbation during perimenarche/puberty (80,81).

Changes in reproductive hormones may be responsible for these observations. Sexual maturation begins with adrenarche, usually between the age of 8 and 10 years. It is initiated by a marked increase in the secretion of dehydroepiandrosterone sulfate (DHEAS) and DHEA (84). During perimenarche, which follows, ovarian secretion of estrogens precedes secretion of progesterone. Ovarian secretion of estrogens begins during thelarche (median age, 9.8 years) (85), and increases steadily through menarche (median age, 12.8 years) (86) until the onset of ovulation. In contrast, ovarian secretion of progesterone does not begin until menstrual cycles become ovulatory, 12–18 months after menarche in the majority of girls (85), with parallel increase in serum allopregnanolone levels in late puberty (87). Thus, the DHEAS and estrogen secretion precedes that of progesterone by 2–6 and 2–4 years, respectively.

Localization-related epilepsy is not uncommonly due to an underlying focal lesion. Patients with CNS insults such as severe head trauma, infections, complex febrile seizures, perinatal insults, and developmental disorders have an increased risk for developing seizures (88–91). Epilepsy may occur after a variable period which may last for years after the original insult (91). According to the "two-hit" hypothesis of epileptogenesis, reorganization of neuronal networks after the first insult may increase neuronal excitability, but not sufficiently to result in epilepsy (92). A second event ("hit") later in life may further lower seizure threshold and result in the appearance of epilepsy. Continued exposure of the brain during this time to the proconvulsant effects of estrogen and DHEAS, without the anticonvulsant effect of progesterone, may facilitate kindling of a preexisting CNS lesion into an epileptic focus and thus provide the "second hit" of epileptogenesis in susceptible females.

Animal studies support this hypothesis. Both DHEAS and estrogen promote epilepsy kindling, while progesterone retards it (3,7,27,44,93). Female rats ovariectomized before puberty have a higher seizure threshold in adulthood than to control animals (7,93). The difference in seizure threshold between ovariectomized and intact animals only starts at the time of sexual maturation. Rats castrated after puberty do not differ from control animals (3). This suggests that castration before puberty may be protective against later development of seizures. This is likely due to the estrogenic effect of maturing ovaries, for exposure of young female rats to even a single high dose of estrogen before maturation results in a permanent increase in neuronal excitability and a lowering of seizure threshold that persists well into adulthood (94). In contrast, administration of progesterone to rats shortly before sexual maturation is strongly protective against amygdaloid seizure kindling (27).

The hormonal effects on epileptogenesis during sexual maturation could be due to the effects of gonadal hormones on neuronal plasticity and synaptogenesis. As noted earlier, in the adult female rat, the density of excitatory synapses on the apical dendrites of CA1 pyramidal neurons is increased by estrogen and reduced by progesterone (22,23). Ovariectomized animals treated with estradiol without progesterone, a situation analogous to human perimenarche, show a 30% increase of the density of the dendritic spines associated with excitatory synapses. These new synaptic connections form especially between previously unconnected hippocampal neurons (24). They thus facilitate synchronization of neuronal discharge and generation and/or propagation of seizures. The increase in excitatory synapses formation is opposed by progesterone (22). It is possible that by promoting excitatory synaptogenesis and transmission, prolonged, continued exposure of the brain to DHEAS and estrogen without progesterone during adrenarche and perimenarche could facilitate "kindling" of a previously lesioned brain and provide the "second hit" of epileptogenesis in susceptible females.

The prolonged imbalance between the excitatory and inhibitory neuroactive steroids during perimenarche and the same pathophysiological mechanisms may also be responsible for the observed seizure exacerbation during perimenarhce in girls with partial epilepsy.

Catamenial Epilepsy

Catamenial (from Greek *katamenia*: *kata*, by; *men*, month) epilepsy refers to seizure exacerbation in relation to the menstrual cycle. Seizures do not occur randomly in the majority of men and women with epilepsy. They tend to cluster in > 50% of cases (95). In women, such clustering may relate to the menstrual cycle. This has been recognized since the 19th century (76). Based on the analysis of both seizure frequency (average daily seizure frequency during four phases of the menstrual cycle) and the nature of menstrual cycles, Herzog et al. described three patterns of catamenial seizure exacerbation (96). The first pattern (C1) involved seizure exacerbation during the perimenstrual phase (menstrual cycle days −3 to 3, with the first day of menstrual blood flow being the first day of the cycle). The second (C2) pattern involved seizure exacerbation during periovulatory phase (days 10–13). Both C1 and C2 occurred in women with normal ovulatory cycles. In the third pattern (C3), seizures were exacerbated during the entire second half (days 10 to 3) of anovulatory cycles.

Clinical determination of such exacerbation is made by daily seizure count averaged during the different phases of the menstrual cycle (perimenstrual, day −3 to 3; follicular, day 4–10; periovulatory, day 11–16; and luteal, day 17 to day 3) and the determination of midluteal (menstrual cycle day 20–22) serum progesterone level to distinguish between normal and anovulatory menstrual cycles (> 6 ng/mL in normal ovulatory cycles). Herzog et al. proposed a definition of catamenial epilepsy based on the severity of seizure exacerbation: a twofold increase in average daily seizure frequency during the phases of exacerbation relative to the baseline phases. Using this definition, approximately one-third of women with intractable partial epilepsy have catamenial seizure exacerbation (96).

Menstrually related hormonal fluctuations of estrogen and progesterone likely underlie catamenial seizure exacerbation. Estrogens activate epileptiform discharges and may induce seizures in women with epilepsy (97). In contrast, progesterone given in doses resulting in luteal phase plasma levels suppresses epileptiform discharges (98). Accordingly, changes in reproductive hormonal status associated with menstrual cycles may affect the clinical manifestation of seizures (96,99).

Both progesterone deficiency and estrogen excess relative to progesterone may contribute to the catamenial pattern of seizure exacerbation in both normal women and in women with menstrual irregularities (96,99). In rats, seizure propensity is greatest during proestrus, when the serum estrogen levels are highest, and lowest during diestrus, when the progesterone levels are highest (XXX) (62). In women with epilepsy, seizure frequency is similarly high during the periovulatory surge of serum estrogen levels, and is low when serum progesterone levels are high during the luteal phase in normally ovulating women. The periovulatory seizure exacerbation may be related to the periovulatory surge in estrogen secretion. Seizure exacerbation pre/perimenstrually may be related to the fall in serum progesterone levels (38,96). This may be due to the withdrawal of the progesterone metabolite, allopregnanolone. In an animal model of catamenial epilepsy, abrupt withdrawal of allopregnanolone can be achieved biochemically with finasteride, a 5-α reductase inhibitor which blocks the conversion of progesterone to allopregnanolone. Such withdrawal is associated with marked increased seizure susceptibility (38). Although the mechanism underlying this effect is not clear, it has been suggested that allopregnanolone's modulating effect on the GABA-A receptor may be responsible. Progesterone withdrawal is associated with a change in the expression of GABA-A receptor subunits and properties, a reduction in GABA inhibition and an increase in neuronal excitability. Specifically, an increased production of the α4 subunit of the GABA-A receptor has been observed, a subunit that confers resistance of the GABA-A receptor to GABA and to benzodiazepines (100). These findings have not been confirmed, however (101).

In women with anovulatory cycles, seizure exacerbation is seen during the whole second half of the cycle (98). During an anovulatory cycle, estrogen levels rise at the end of the follicular phase and stay elevated throughout the luteal phase until premenstrually, as in normally menstruating women; but there is little or no progesterone secretion. Thus, there is estrogen:progesterone (E/P) imbalance with relative excess of estrogen throughout the whole second half of the menstrual cycle, with associated seizure exacerbation (102).

Premenstrual exacerbation of seizures may also be related to a premenstrual decline in AED levels. This occurs in women treated with AEDs metabolized by hepatic microsomal enzymes of the CYP3A subfamily, which also metabolizes gonadal steroids. Competition between the hormones and AEDs (such as phenytoin) results in greater phenytoin metabolism when gonadal serum levels decline premenstrually, accounting for the decline in AED level (103,104).

Reproductive Endocrine Disorders and the Development and Exacerbation of Epilepsy

Reproductive endocrine disorders may favor the development of temporal lobe epilepsy (TLE) in women. As noted above, women with anovulatory cycles have continued ovarian secretion of estrogen with failure of progesterone secretion during the luteal phase of the cycle. The resulting continuous exposure of the amygdala and the hippocampus to estrogen without the normal cyclical progesterone effects may promote interictal epileptiform activity and the possibility of "kindling" (105).

Epilepsy itself is associated with an increased incidence of reproductive endocrine disorders. Approximately 20% of women with TLE suffer from polycystic ovarian syndrome, while another 5% each may suffer from hypothalamic hypogonadism and hyperprolactinemia (106). All these conditions are associated with anovulatory menstrual cycles. One-third of all menstrual cycles of women with epilepsy have been estimated to be anovulatory (107). The chronically increased E/P ratio may promote seizure occurrence. Anovulatory cycles are associated with more frequent seizures (102,108). Thus, a positive-feedback cycle may be envisaged, whereby TLE leads to endocrine reproductive disorders with failure of ovulation, which in turn further exacerbates the seizure disorder.

Menopause

The effect of menopause on epilepsy has not been studied extensively. The term menopause refers to a complex process that encompasses menopause, cessation of all menstruation, and perimenopause, the preceding decline in reproductive endocrine function. Perimenopause often extends for several years. The decline in progesterone secretion occurs early in perimenopause, as ovulatory cycles change to anovulatory, an early endocrine change of the perimenopause. In contrast, estrogen secretion remains normal through most of perimenopause and may even increase episodically during it when, as a result of erratic follicular development, multiple follicles develop during some menstrual cycles (109,110). Estrogen levels only drop consistently late in perimenopause, during the last few months before cessation of menses—as the follicle pool becomes exhausted (109,110). Thus, for a period of time lasting up to several years, there may be relative excess of serum estrogen levels compared to serum progesterone levels.

Based on the pattern of hormonal change, an evolving seizure pattern with seizure exacerbation during the perimenopause might be expected: initial seizure exacerbation when progesterone secretion declines, but estrogen secretion continues, followed by stabilization or improvement after menopause, as estrogen secretion ceases. This pattern was, in fact, shown to occur in a recent questionnaire study. Sixty-four percent of women experienced seizure exacerbation, and only 13% of women experienced seizure improvement during the perimenopause. In contrast, 43% of women had seizure improvement during the menopause, with only 31% experiencing seizure exacerbation (111). Hormone replacement therapy may further affect seizure expression during perimenopause/menopause. Sixty-three percent of the women with seizure exacerbation during menopause were taking estrogen hormone replacement therapy (HRT) (111). Interestingly, partial epilepsy may begin during the climacteric, sometime without an apparent cause. This occurred in 8/61 (13%) of menopausal women in one study (112). It is possible that the chronic exposure of the brain to estrogen without progesterone during the perimenopausal years could promote epileptogenesis in women with minor, occult CNS lesions in a way similar to the suggested epileptogenic effect of perimenarche. No studies have addressed this possibility.

Pregnancy

Pregnancy has variable effects on epilepsy. A small number of women experience seizures for the first time during pregnancy, and have seizures only during pregnancy (113). In about one-third of women, seizures worsen during pregnancy (113,114). In about one-sixth of women, seizures decrease in frequency. Nonhormonal factors affecting seizure occurrence during pregnancy include altered medication compliance, AED absorption, body space distribution, protein binding, liver metabolism, and renal clearance. Profound hormonal changes occur during pregnancy, including up to 10-fold increases in estrogens, progesterone, cortisol, DHEAS, and other neuroactive hormones. In the only study of the effects of hormones on seizures during pregnancy to date, no association was seen between serum progesterone and estrogen levels and E/P ratios and seizure frequency during pregnancy (115). Other hormones have not been examined.

Stress

Stress is probably the most common precipitant of seizures (116–118). Several surveys have shown that in 30–60% of epileptic patients, seizure occurrence is related to stress, stressful events, or subjectively perceived change in stress levels (116–122). In contrast, studies relating seizure diaries to life events or subjective distress have shown a more variable relationship of seizures to stress, with 14–58% of patients having an increase or, occasionally, decrease in seizure frequency with stress (119,120,123,124). Several reports have documented seizure triggering in a controlled setting by exposure to emotionally stressful stimuli during a clinical interview or videotape presentation (125–128). Approximately one-third of stress-related seizure facilitation may be due to seizure facilitation by concomitant sleep deprivation; the remainder of the effect is due to stress itself, unrelated to other stress-associated physiological and behavioral factors that might alter seizure threshold, such as medication compliance or alcohol or other substance abuse (118).

The effect of stress on seizures is likely a direct effect of stress-related physiological changes on neuronal excitability and seizure threshold. Stress affects neuronal excitability and epileptiform discharges in both animals and in patients with epilepsy. In the monkey, spike discharges and seizure frequency increase under social stress (129). In mice, brief restraint lowers seizure threshold to pentylenetetrazol- and electroshock-induced seizures, starting immediately after restraint. This effect is abrogated by adrenalectomy, suggesting that the increase in excitability is mediated by the adrenal gland (130). In contrast, more prolonged stress lasting 10 min may increase seizure threshold (52,131). In human studies, a stress interview structured to elicit maximal emotional response activated interictal epileptiform spike activity within 30 s to minutes in 12/44 (27%) patients with epilepsy, and in almost 50% among the patients with partial epilepsy (125,126). About 10% of patients developed a partial seizure during or following the interview (125,126). Reduction of epileptiform activity during stress was seen in 5% of patients. In one patient undergoing depth electrode recording, an emotional challenge triggered a seizure that started after 3 min in the left amygdala (128).

Stress response includes the activation of the amygdalohypothalamopituitary adrenal hormonal axis. Release of corticotropin-releasing hormone (CRH) leads to release of adrenocorticotropic hormone (ACTH) from the pituitary, which stimulates adrenal steroid secretion. As discussed earlier, CRH and a number of adrenal steroids affect neuronal excitability and seizures.

CRH acts as an excitatory neuromodulator. It increases neuronal firing in the hippocampus and induces epileptiform discharges and seizures in animals (62,64,65). CRH-containing neurons are concentrated in the central nucleus of the amygdala, where they mediate the autonomic and behavioral aspects of the stress response (132,133). CRH-induced seizures start in the amygdala and spread to the hippocampus and cortex (64,65). CRH neurons are activated under stress conditions (134,135). Thus, stress may activate CRH-containing neurons in the limbic system and CRH-mediated increase in neuronal excitability may result in seizure facilitation.

Glucocorticoids also increase neuronal excitability and facilitate epileptiform discharges and seizures in animal models, with a latency of hours (47,49,52,136). This effect is likely mediated by neuronal glucocorticoid receptors, as discussed previously. There is a high density of glucocorticoid receptors in the hippocampus, the amygdala, and the septum. Two types of glucocorticoid receptors are found in the brain. The glucocorticoid (type II) receptor has low affinity for glucocorticoids and is only activated during times of high glucocorticoid levels, such as that seen during stress (137). Activation of this receptor might be important in lowering the seizure threshold at the time of stress.

Other adrenal neuroactive steroids also affect the seizure threshold. Pregnenolone sulfate (PS) and DHEAS both lower seizure threshold in animals (44,138). This is thought to occur by antagonism of GABA-A-mediated neuronal hyperpolarization, and potentiation of NMDA receptor–mediated glutamatergic neuronal excitation (2). In contrast, allopregnanolone and the metabolites of the mineralocorticoid deoxycorticosterone, dihydroxycorticosterone (DH-DOC) and tetrahydroxydeoxycorticosterone (TH-DOC), exert a potent anticonvulsant effect in a number of animal seizure models by enhancing GABA-A receptor-mediated synaptic inhibition (2,29,33,131). Some of these neurosteroids (e.g., allopregnanolone) are synthesized in the brain acutely following stress, independently of their adrenal synthesis (2,36). Withdrawal of this anticonvulsant effect could promote seizure activity when stress is terminated.

Finally, noradrenergic activity which is increased as part of the stress response exerts an anticonvulsant effect The locus coeruleus is the principal source of ascending noradrenergic fibers. Activation of the locus coeruleus, which occurs in response to stress, elevates seizure threshold in animals and has been postulated as a possible important mechanism underlying the therapeutic anticonvulsant effect of vagus nerve stimulation (139).

Thus, stress induces both pro-convulsant and anticonvulsant neuroendocrine and neuronal changes. These observations may explain why stressful events can be associated with both increased and decreased seizure frequency (119,120). Stress-related seizure precipitation can occur with variable latency after change in stress level. The latency ranges from minutes through hours to days, and may even include seizure precipitation during relief from stress (118). This suggests that more than one pathophysiological mechanism may mediate stress-related seizure modulation. Seizure facilitation that occurs within minutes of a stressful event might result from activation of central CRH neurons, leading to augmentation of neuronal excitation, or from an acute increase in the CNS excitatory neurosteroids such as PS or DHEAS. Seizures occurring half an hour to hours after a stressful event could result from activation of the HPA axis and increased adrenal secretion of the proconvulsants cortisol, PS, and DHEAS. Increase in seizure frequency associated with chronic stress may be harder to explain, but could be mediated by chronically elevated release of cortisol from the adrenals. Finally, seizure occurrence at the end of a stressful event, i.e., with termination of stress, might result from withdrawal of GABA-potentiating neurosteroids such as allopregnanolone, DH-DOC, and TH-DOC, secreted acutely during the stressful event, or from reduction of noradrenergic activity. The protective effect of stress reported in some patients might similarly be mediated by increased secretion of TH-DOC, DH-DOC, or allopregnanolone (2,131).

If stress alters seizure threshold acutely, could sustained high levels stress permanently increase excitability of selected neuronal tissue—for instance, in the limbic system—and promote epileptogenesis? In neonatal animals, acute CRH-induced status epilepticus exposure results in neuronal loss in the hippocampal CA3 region, amygdala and the pyriform cortex (73) and in a long-lasting potentiation of subsequent non-CRH induction (e.g., kainic acid induced) (74), suggesting that this might be the case (64). Clinical data are sparse in this respect. Several cases have been reported in which seizures starting shortly after sexual abuse (without apparent head trauma) were followed by seizure exacerbation during heightened symptoms of the posttraumatic stress disorder (PTSD) (140). There is an increased prevalence of PTSD among patients with intractable epilepsy: 37% versus 5–10% in the general population (141).

HORMONAL TREATMENT IN EPILEPSY

Hormonal treatment of seizures may rationally be aimed at those endocrinologic aspects of seizures that act to cause, exacerbate, or ameliorate them. Endocrine intervention to prevent epileptogenesis has not been attempted to date. Progesterone may have an anticonvulsant effect, whereas estrogen, CRH, and cortisol may have pro-convulsant effects. Thus, treatment with progesterone, estrogen antagonists and medications that suppress the activity of the hypothalamopituitary adrenal axis may prove to be useful adjunct treatment in the appropriate epilepsy patients.

Gonadal Hormone-Based Treatment

Progesterone

As noted previously, low progesterone levels or progesterone withdrawal may be a factor in the increased seizure frequency seen perimenstrually in women with catamenial epilepsy and normal ovulatory cycles, and during the entire luteal phase of women with anovulatory cycles (96,99,102). Progesterone may be expected to benefit these women.

Synthetic progestin therapy may also be considered. Oral forms of synthetic progestins have yielded inconsistent results. Little or no benefits have been noted in a number of studies (142) with cyclically administered oral forms such as the testosterone-derived norethisterone (143), although occasional benefits have been described in single case reports with its continuous use, and of the hydroxyprogesterone derivative medroxyprogesterone acetate (142,144).

Intramuscularly (IM)-administered synthetic progestins may be more beneficial than these oral forms (116). In one open-label study of 13 women with refractory partial seizures and normal ovulatory cycles, a medroxyprogesterone dose large enough to induce amenorrhoea (i.e., 120–150 mg every 6–12 weeks) resulted in a 40% seizure reduction (116), from an average of eight seizures per month to five seizures per month. It was unclear whether the effect was due to direct anticonvulsant activity of MPA or to the hormonal consequences of the medroxyprogesterone-induced amenorrhea (i.e., loss of periovulatory estrogen surge).

One patient who had absence rather than partial seizures did not improve. Weekly doses of 400 mg of IM depomedroxyprogesterone may be more effective (145). Potential side effects include depression, sedation, breakthrough vaginal bleeding, and lengthy delay in the return of regular menstrual cycles, the last side effect following only the depo-, not oral medroxyprogesterone administration (116).

On the other hand, natural progesterone may be a more effective treatment than synthetic progestins (146–148). In one open-label trial, 25 women with catamenial exacerbation of complex partial seizures of temporal lobe origin with or without secondary generalization, 14 with inadequate luteal phase or anovulatory cycles, and 11 with normal cycles and perimenstrual seizure exacerbation received natural progesterone in doses sufficient to produce physiological luteal range progesterone serum levels of 5–25 ng/mL. Seventy-two percent of the women improved; there was a 55% decline in average seizure frequency, from 0.39 to 0.18 daily seizures (147). Progesterone was administered as lozenges, 200 mg TID on days 23–25 of each menstrual cycle for perimenstrual exacerbation, and on days 15–25 of each menstrual cycle, with taper over days 26–28, for exacerbations lasting throughout the entire luteal phase. Similar findings had previously been found in a smaller study using progesterone vaginal suppositories (106). Side effects included mild fatigue, depression, weight gain, fluid retention, and breakthrough bleeding. All side effects resolved promptly with dose reduction or medication withdrawal. The observations of the larger study were subsequently extended for 3 years, with continued improvement in seizure control at the same level and with no significant side effects during the 3 years of treatment (148). A multicenter, double-blind, randomized, placebo-controlled trial is currently in progress.

Natural progesterone is available as a soybean or yam extract in lozenge, micronized capsule, cream, and suppository form. The usual daily regimen to achieve physiological luteal range serum levels ranges from 100 to 200 mg TID (147). The synthetic progestins are not equivalent because the natural progesterone is metabolized to allopregnanolone (which possesses anticonvulsant activity), whereas the synthetic progestins are not (2,149). Potential side effects may include sedation, depression, weight gain, breast tenderness, and breakthrough vaginal bleeding, all readily reversible upon discontinuation of the hormone or lowering of the dose.

Neuroactive Steroids

The experimental data on the cellular effects of the GABA-mimetic neuroactive steroids such as allopregnanolone and TH-DOC would suggest that these compounds may have a potent anticonvulsant effect (2), a suggestion borne out in animal studies (29,40,41,131).

Two older studies have investigated the antiepileptic potential of some neuroactive steroids. In one study, the 21-acetate form of deoxycorticosterone was found to be effective in 6/10 patients with refractory seizures (150). Its effect may have been due to its neuroactive steroid metabolite, TH-DOC (32). In a second study, the synthetic neuroactive pregnane steroid anaesthetic, alphaxalone, was effective in treating status epilepticus (151).

The antiepileptic potential of allopregnanolone has received considerable attention. Allopregnanolone and other related, naturally occurring neuroactive steroids with anticonvulsant properties produce motor impairment with a low therapeutic:toxic ratio, and have very short half-lives (29). Allopregnanolone modified synthetically by the incorporation of a 3β-methyl group (ganaxolone) has a better therapeutic:toxic ratio in animal studies of pentylenetetrazol-, pilocarpine-, and bicuculline-induced seizures, and prolongs allopregnanolone's half-life (29,152). Tolerance to the anticonvulsant effect, such as that seen with benzodiazepines, does not occur with ganaxolone in animal studies (153). In an open-label study of children and adolescents with refractory partial or generalized seizures, 6/15 patients had a > 50% seizure reduction. Nine of 15 patients had mild to moderate side effects. There was no evidence of altered metabolism of other AEDs (154). In another open-label pediatric study of children aged 20–60 months with refractory seizures and a history of infantile spasms during the first year of life, approximately one-third of patients improved (155). A double-blind, randomized, placebo-controlled multi-center trial of 50 adult patients with refractory partial complex seizures withdrawn from all AEDs as part of presurgical evaluation showed a trend toward efficacy (155a). Fifty percent of ganaxolone-treated patients were withdrawn from the study because of seizures versus 75% of placebo-treated patients ($P = .0795$). Side effects were similar between the ganaxolone and the placebo-treated groups. Unfortunately, the patient number was smaller, the study duration shorter, and the response of the placebo group better than in similar presurgical studies, i.e., studies of felbamate, gabapentin, and oxcarbazepine, likely accounting for the lack of statistical significance. Owing to financial contraints of Cosensys, the company developing ganaxolone, no further developments of ganaxolone have occurred since that trial.

Clomiphene

Clomiphene citrate is an estrogen analogue with both estrogenic and antiestrogenic effects that are dose dependent. In clinical use, it acts primarily as an anti-estrogen at the hypothalamic and pituitary level to stimulate gonadotropin secretion, ovulation, and fertility. It exerts an anticonvulsant effect in rats in a dose-related fashion (6). Remarkable reductions in seizure frequency have been reported in isolated cases involving both men and women (156,157). In one series of 12 women who had complex partial seizures and menstrual disorders (polycystic ovarian syndrome or inadequate luteal phase cycles) and who were given clomiphene, 10 improved, often dramatically, with an average 87% drop in seizure frequency (158). Improvement in seizure frequency occurred in those women who had normalization of menstrual cycles and of luteal progesterone secretion. The only two women who did not improve continued to have menstrual abnormalities.

Thus, clomiphene may be a useful adjunct antiepileptic treatment in women with menstrual disorders. It is administered in dosages from 25 to 100 mg/d on days 5–9 of each menstrual cycle in women, and 25–50 mg/d or on alternate days in men. Unfortunately, side effects can be significant, and include unwanted pregnancy, ovarian overstimulation syndrome, transient breast tenderness, and pelvic cramps. Furthermore, seizure frequency may increase during the enhanced preovulatory rise in serum estradiol levels in some women. Clomiphene treatment, therefore, should be restricted to situations where irregular anovulatory cycles cannot be readily normalized with cyclic progesterone use.

Testosterone and Aromatase Inhibitors

We have reported improvement in seizures in a couple of patients treated for AED-related hyposexuality with testosterone and testolactone, an inhibitor of the enzyme aromatase, which inhibits conversion of estrogens and androgens (159). Treatment with testosterone alone was ineffective. The successful treatment was associated with normalization of previously elevated estradiol levels, suggesting that the anticonvulsant effect of testolactone may be due to reduction of the pro-convulsant effects of estrogen. A larger study with a newer aromatase inhibitor is currently under way.

LHRH Agonists

Lowering of estrogen levels by induction of menopause is expected to improve seizure control. Medical menopause can be achieved by chronic usage of one of the long-acting LHRH analogs. Long-term suppression of gonadotropin and ovarian secretion develops after an initial 3- to 4-week long phase of reproductive endocrine stimulation. One patient with severe refractory seizures with perimenstrual exacerbation has been reported to improve markedly after treatment with the LHRH agonist goserelin (160). One open-label study of 10 patients with catamenial seizures showed improvement in 8/10 patients, with adverse effects, including hot flashes and headache occurring in 8/10 patients (161). My own experience in a few cases suggests that seizure control may improve modestly, but seizure exacerbation during the first month stimulation phase may preclude their use in some cases. Moreover, the immediate and long-term effects of hypoestrogenism need to be considered.

Adrenal Steroid- and CRH-Based Treatments

Both ACTH and prednisone have been used extensively in the treatment of refractory infantile spasms and other primarily generalized seizures of childhood (reviewed in 162). They have been successfully used in another childhood epileptic syndrome, the Landau-Kleffner syndrome (aka acquired epileptic aphasia) (162), but not in other forms of partial epilepsy. In infantile spasms, low-dose ACTH and prednisone are equally efficacious, but a high dose of ACTH ($150\,IU/m^2/d$) is considerably more effective than prednisone during a 2-week-long course (162,163) Longer usage of high-dose ACTH may be limited by severe side effects (162). The mechanism of ACTH anticonvulsant activity is uncertain. It may include suppression of CRH and its epileptogenic activity (164). There are also some data to suggest that ACTH may stimulate the production of endogenous steroids with anticonvulsant activity (165).

One study reported three patients with refractory seizures and hypercortisolemia whose seizures became controlled upon normalization of the cortisol levels by ketoconazole (166). Wider anticonvulsant potential of ketoconazole or other potential suppressors of cortisol synthesis, including low-dose prednisone and aminoglutethimide, and antagonists of the corticosteroid receptors, such as spironolactone (49), has not been explored.

In animal studies, administration of a CRH receptor antagonist is protective against both seizures and seizure-related hippocampal neuronal loss (75). The possibility of treating seizures and ictus-related excitatory neuronal injury by antagonizing CRH activity has been examined in a Phase I clinical study. The competitive CRH antagonist α-helical-CRH failed to cross the blood-brain barrier and was ineffective in the treatment of infantile spasms in a small group of children (167).

Oral small-molecule nonpeptidal CRF receptor antagonists, for instance, the recently developed nonpeptidal CRF receptor 1 blocker (NBI 27914; Neurocrine Biosciences), are potential candidates for testing in epilepsy, including, given the great sensitivity to the excitatory effect of CRH of developing CNS (65), in childhood epilepsies. Reduction of CRH activity by means of stimulating the activity of CRH-binding peptide may be another possible, as yet untested therapeutic avenue.

REFERENCES

1. McEwen B. Nongenomic and genomic effects of steroids on neural activity. Trends Pharmacol Sci 1991; 12:141–147.
2. Paul SM, Purdy RH. Neuroactive steroids. FASEB J 1992; 6:2311–2322.
3. Teresawa E, Timiras P. Electrical activity during the estrous cycle of the rat: cyclic changes in limbic structures. Endocrinology 1968; 83:207.
4. Logothetis J, Harner R. Electrocortical activation by estrogens. Arch Neurol 1960; 3:290–297.
5. Marcus EM, Watson CW, Goodman PL. Effects of steroids on cerebral electrical activity. Arch Neurol 1966; 15:521–532.
6. Nicoletti F, Speciale C, Sortino MA, et al. Comparative effects of estradiol benzoate, the antiestrogen clomiphene citrate and the progestin medroxyprogesterone acetate on kainic acid-induced seizures in male and female rats. Epilepsia 1985; 26:252–257.
7. Woolley DE, Timiras PS. The gonad-brain relationship: effects of female sex hormones on electroshock convulsions in the rat. Endocrinology 1962; 70:196–209.
8. Hom AC, Buterbaugh GG. Estrogen alters the acquisition of seizures kindled by repeated amygdala stimulation or pentylenetetrazol administration in ovariectomized female rats. Epilepsia 1986; 27:103–108.
9. Buterbaugh GG, Estradiol replacement facilitates acquisition of seizures kindled from the anterior neocortex in female rats. Epilepsy Res 1989; 1989:207–215.
10. Buterbaugh GG, Hudson GM. Estradiol replacement to female rats facilitates dorsal hippocampal but not ventral hippocampal kindled seizure acquisition. Exp Neurol 1991; 111:54–64.
11. Edwards HE, Burnham WM, Mendonca A, et al. Steroid hormones affect limbic afterdischarge thresholds and kindling rates in adult female rats. Brain Res 1999; 838:136–150.
12. Woolley CS. Estradiol facilitates kainic acid-induced, but not fluorothyl-induced, behavioral seizure activity in adult female rat. Epilepsia 2000; 41:510–515.
13. Pfaff DW, Keiner M. Estradiol-concentrating cells in the rat amygdala as part of a limbic-hypothalamic hormone-sensitive system. In: The Neurobiology of the Amygdala. New York: Plenum Publishing, 1973:775–792.
14. Simerly RB, Chang M, Muramatsu M, Swanson LW. Distribution of androgen and estrogen receptor mRNA-containing cells in the rat brain: and in situ hybridization study. J Comp Neurol 1990; 294:76–95.
15. Shughrue PJ, Lane MV, Merchenthaler I. Comparative distribution of estrogen receptor and mRNA in the rat central nervous system. J Comp Neurol 1997; 388:507–525.
16. Flugge G, Oertel WH, Wuttke W. Evidence for estrogen-receptive GABAergic neurons in the preoptic/anterior hypothalamic area of the rat brain. Neuroendocrinology 1986; 43:1–5.

17. Wallis GJ, Luttge W. Influence of estrogen and progesterone on glutamic acid decarboxylase activity in discrete regions of rat brain. J Neurochem 1980; 34: 609–613.

18. Smith SS, Waterhouse BD, Woodward DJ. Sex steroid effects on extrahypothalamic CNS. II. Progesterone, alone and in combination with estrogen, modulates cerebellar responses to amino acid neurotransmitters. Brain Res 1987; 422:52–62.

19. Smith, SS. Estrogen administration increases neuronal responses to excitatory amino acids as a long term effect. Brain Res 1989; 503:354–357.

20. Wong M, Moss R. Long-term and short-term electrophysiological effects of estrogen on the synaptic properties of hippocampal CA1 neurons. J Neurosci 1992; 12: 3217–3225.

21. Kawakami M, Teresawa WAE, Ibuki T. Changes in multiple unit activity in the brain during the estrous cycle. Neuroendocrinology 1970; 6:30–48.

22. Woolley CS, McEwen BS. Role of estradiol and progesterone in regulation of hippocampal dendritic spine density during the estrous cycle in the rat. J Comp Neurol 1993; 336:293–306.

23. Wooley CS, Wenzel H, Schwartzkroin PA. Estradiol increases the frequency of multiple synapse boutons in the hippocampal CA1 region of the adult female rat. J Comp Neurol 1996; 373:108–117.

24. Yankova M, Hart JA, Woolley CS. Estrogen increases synaptic connectivity between single presynaptic inputs and multiple postsynaptic CA1 pyramidal cells: a serial electron-microscopic study. Proc Natl Acad Sci USA 2001; 98:3525–3530.

25. Landgren S, Backstrom T, Kalistratov G. The effect of progesterone on the spontaneous interictal spike evoked by the application of penicillin to the cat's cerebral cortex. J Neurol Sci 1978; 36:119–133.

26. Landgren S, Aasly J, Backstrom T, et al. The effect of progesterone and its metabolites on the interictal epileptiform discharge in the cat's cerebral cortex. Acta Physiol Scand 1987; 131:33–42.

27. Holmes GL, Weber DA. The effect of progesterone kindling: a developmental study. Dev Brain Res 1984; 16:45–53.

28. Frye CA, Scalise TJ, Anti seizure effects of progesterone and 3alpha, 5alpha-THP in kainic acid and perforant pathway models of epilepsy. Psychoneuroendocrinology 2000; 25:407–420.

29. Kokate TG, Svensson BE, Rogawski MA. Anticonvulsant activity of neurosteroids: correlation with g-aminobutyric acid–evoked chloride current potentiation. J Pharmacol Exp Ther 1994; 270:1223–1229.

30. Kokate TG, Banks MK, Magee T, et al. Finasteride, a 5a-reductase inhibitor, blocks the anticonvulsant activity of progesterone in mice. J Pharmacol Exp Ther 1999; 288:679–684.

31. McEwen BS, Davis P, Gerlach J. Progestin receptors in the brain and pituitary gland. In: Bardin M.-J.J, Milgrom CW. eds. Progesterone and Progestins. New York: Raven Press, 1983:59–76.

32. Gee KW, McCauley LD, Lan NC. A putative receptor for neurosteroids on the GABA receptor complex: the pharmacological properties and therapeutic potential of epalons. Crit Rev Neurobiol 1995; 9:207–227.

33. Majewska MD, Harrison NL, Schwartz RD, et al. Steroid hormone metabolites are barbiturate-like modulators of the GABA receptor. Science 1986; 232:1004–1007.

34. Wu FS, Gibbs TT, Farb DH. Inverse modulation of g-aminobutyric acid- and glycine-induced currents by progesterone. Mol Pharmacol 1990; 37:597–602.

35. Wilson MA. GABA physiology: modulation by benzodiazepines and hormones. Crit Rev Neurobiol 1996; 10:1–37.

36. Cheney DL, Uzunov D, Vosta E, et al. Gas chromatographic–mass fragmentographic quantitation of 3a-hydroxy-5a-pregnan-20-one (allopregnanolone) and its precursors in blood and brain of adrenalectomized and castrated rats. J Neurosci 1995; 15: 4641–4650.

37. Gasior M, Ungard JT, Beekman M, et al. Acute and chronic effects of synthetic neuroactive steroid, ganaxolone, against the convulsive and lethal effects of pentylenetetrazol in seizure-kindled mice: comparison with diazepam and valproate. Neuropharmacology 2000; 39:1184–1196.

38. Reddy DS, Kim HY, Rogawski MA. Neurosteroids withdrawal model of perimenstrual catamenial epilepsy. Epilepsia 2001; 42:328–337.

39. Reddy DS, Rogawski MA. Enhanced anticonvulsant activity of neuroactive steroids in a rat model of catamenial epilepsy. Epilepsia 2001; 42:337–344.

40. Belleli D, Bolger MB, Gee KW. Anticonvulsant profile of the progesterone metabolite 5a-pregnan-3a-ol-20-one. Eur J Pharmaol 1989; 166:325–329.

41. Kokate TG, Cohen AL, Karp E, Rogawski MA. Neuroactive steroids protect against pilocarpine- and kainic acid–induced limbic seizures and status epilepticus in mice. Neuropharmacology 1996; 35:1049–1056.

42. Finn DA, Gee KW. The estrus cycle, sensitivity to convulsants and the anticonvulsant effect of a neuroactive steroid. J Pharmacol Exp Ther 1994; 271:164–170.

43. Finn DA, Gee KW. The influence of estrus cycle phase on neurosteroid potency at the GABA-A receptor complex. J Pharmacol Exp Ther 1994; 265:1374–1379.

44. Reddy DS, Kulkami SK. Proconvulsant effects of neurosteroids pregnenolone sulfate and dehydroepiandrosterone sulfate in mice. Eur J Pharmacol 1998; 345:55–59.

45. Irwin RP, Maragakis NJ, Rogawski MA, et al. Pregnenolone sulfate augments NMDA receptor mediated increases in intracellular Ca^{2+} in cultured rat hippocampal neurons. Neusosci Lett 1992; 141:30–34.

46. Klein P, Herzog AG. Endocrine asepects of partial epilepsy. In: Knigge K, Pretel S, Wagner JE, eds. MCH and Seizures: Neuromolecular and Neuroendocrine Aspects. Trivandrum, India: Research Signpost, 1997.

47. Lee PH, Grimes L, Hong JS. Glucocorticoids potentiate kainic acid–induced seizures and wet dog shakes. Brain Res 1989; 480:322–325.

48. Roberts AJ, Crabbe JC, Keith LD. Type I corticosteroid receptors modulate PTZ-induced convulsions of withdrawal seizure prone mice. Brain Res 1993; 626:143–148.

49. Roberts AJ, Keith LD. Mineralocorticoid receptors mediate the enhancing effects of corticosterone on convulsion susceptibility in mice. J Pharmacol Exp Ther 1994; 270: 505–511.

50. Krugers HJ, Knollema S, Kemper RH, et al. Down-regulation of the hypothalamo-pituitary-adrenal axis reduces brain damage and number of seizures following hypoxia/ischaemia in rats. Brain Res 1995; 690:41–47.

51. Kling MA, Smith MA, Glowa JR, et al. Facilitation of cocaine kindling by glucocorticoids in rats. Brain Res 1993; 629:163–166.

52. Woodbury DM. Effect of adrenocortical steroids and adrenocorticotropic hormone on electroshock seizre threshold. J Pharmacol Exp Ther 1952; 105:27–36.

53. Dafny N, Phillips MI, Newman TA, Gilman S. Dose effect of cortisol on single unit activity in hypothalamus, reticular formation and hippocampus of freely behaving rats correlated with plasma steroid levels. Brain Res 1973; 59:257–272.

54. Birnstiel S, List TJ, Beck SG. Chronic corticosterone treatment maintains synaptic activity of CA1 hippocampal pyramidal cells: acute high corticosterone administration increases action potential number. Synapse 1995; 20:117–124.

55. Reoul J, DeKloet R. Two receptor systems for corticosterone in rat brain: microdictribution and differential occupation. Endocrinology 1985; 117:2505–2511.

56. McEwen BS. Neurobiology of interpreting and responding to stressful events: paradigmatic role of the hippocampus. In: McEwen B, ed. Handbook of Physiology. Section 7: The Endocrine System, Vol IV. New York: Oxford University Press, 2001:139–178.

57. Sapolsky RM, Krey LC, McEwen BS. Prolonged glucocorticoid exposure reduces hippocampal neuron number: implication for ageing. J Neurosci 1985; 1985: 1222–1227.

58. Sapolsky RM. The physiological relevance of glucocorticoid endangerment of the hippocampus. Ann NY Acad Sci 1994; 746:294–304.

59. Woolley CS, Gould E, McEwen BS. Exposure to excess glucocorticoids alters dendritic morphology of adult hippocampal pyramidal neurons. Brain Res 1990; 531:225–231.

60. De Souza EB, Pernin MH, Insel TR, et al. Corticotropin releasing factor receptors in rat forebrain: autoradiographic adentification. Science 1984; 224:1449–1451.

61. Dunn AJ, Berridge CW. Physiological and behavioral responses to corticotopin-releasing factor administration: is CRF a mediator of anxiety or stress responses? Brain Res Rev 1990; 15:71–100.

62. Aldenhoff GB, Gruol DL, Rivier J, et al. Corticotropin releasing factor decreases post-burst hyperpolarisation and excites hippocampal pyramidal neurons in vitro. Science 1983; 221:875–877.

63. Ehlers CL, Henriksen SJ, Wang M, et al. Corticotropoin releasing factor produces increases in brain excitability and convulsive seizures in rats. Brain Res 1983; 278:332–336.

64. Weiss SR, Post RM, Gold PW, et al. CRF-induced seizures and behavior: interaction with amygdala kindling. Brain Res 1986, 372:345–351.

65. Baram TZ, Hirsch E, Snead CO, et al. Corticotropin-releasing hormone–induced seizures in infant rats originate in the amygdala. Ann Neurol 1992; 31:488–494.

66. Marrosu F, Giagheddu M, Gessa GL, et al. Clonidine prevents corticotropin releasing factor-induced epileptogenic activity in rats. Epilepsia 1992; 33:435–438.

67. Rosen JB, Pishevar SK, Weiss SR, et al. Glucocorticoid treatment increases the ability of CRH to induce seizures. Neurosci Lett 1994; 174:113–116.

68. Smith MA, Weiss SR, Berry RL, et al. Amygdala-kindled seizures increase the expression of corticotropin-releasing factor (CRF) and CRF-binding protein in GABAergic interneurons of the dentate hilus. Brain Res 1997; 745:248–256.

69. Baram TZ, Koutsoukos Y, Schultz L, Rivier J. The effect of astressin, a novel antagonist of corticotropin releasing hormone (CRH) on CRH-induced seizures in the infant rat: comparison with two other antagonists. Mol Psychiatry 1996; 1:223–226.

70. Baram TZ, Chalmers DT, Chen C, et al. The CRF1 receptor mediates the excitatory actions of corticotropin releasing factor (CRF) in the developing rat brain: in vivo evidence using a novel, selective, non-peptide CRF receptor antagonist. Brain Res 1997; 770:89–95.

71. Baram TZ, Schultz L. Corticotropin-releasing hormone receptor antagonist is effective for febrile seizures in the infant rat. Ann Neurol 1994; 36:487.

72. Pickut D, Phipps B, Pretel S, Applegate C. Effects of generalized convulsive seizures on corticotropin releasing factor neuronal systems. Brain Res 1996; 743:63–69.

73. Ribak CE, Baram TZ. Selective death of hippocampal CA3 pyramidal cells with mossy fiber afferents after CRH-induced status epilepticus in infant rats. Brain Res 1996; 791:245–251.

74. Baram TZ, Vishai-Elliner S, Schultz L. Seizure threshold to kainic acid in infant rats is markedly increased by corticotropin releasing hormone. Epilepsia 1995; 36:245–251.

75. Maecker H, Desai A, Dash R, et al. Astressin, a novel potent CRF antagonist, is neuroprotective in the hippocampus when administered after a seizure. Brain Res 1997; 744:166–170.

76. Gowers. A Manual of Diseases of the Nervous System. Philadelphia: Blakinson, 1893: 732–753.

77. Rosciszewska D. The course of epilepsy in girls at the age of puberty. Neurol Neurochir Pol 1975; 9:597–602.

78. Niijima S, Wallace SJ. Effects of puberty on seizure frequency. Dev Med Child Neurol 1989; 31:174–180.

79. Silveira DC, Guerreiro AM. Inicio de crises epilepticas na menarca. Neuro-Psiquiat (Sao Paulo) 1991; 49:434–436. (In Portuguese.)

80. Morrell MJ, Hamdy SF, Seale CG, Springer A. Self-reported reproductive history in women with epilepsy: puberty onset and effects of menarche and menstrual cycle on seizures. Neurology 1998; 50(suppl 4):A448.

81. Klein P. Onset of epilepsy at the time of menarche. Neurology 2003; 60:495–497.

82. Hauser WA, Annegers JF, Kurland LT. The prevalence of epilepsy in Rochester, Minnesota 1940–1980. Epilepsia 1991; 32:429–445.

83. Shamansky SL, Glase GH. Annual incidence of epilepsy and first seizure by age. Epilepsia 1979; 20:457–474.

84. Apter D, Vikho R. Serum pregnenolone, progesterone, 17-hydroxyprogesterone, testosterone and 5α-dihydrotestosterone during female puberty. J Clin Endocrinol Metab 1977; 45:1039–1046.

85. Speroff L, Glass RH, Kase NG. Clinical Gynecologic Endocrinology and Infertility, 5th ed. Baltimore: Willliams & Wilkins, 1994:365–370.

86. Herman-Giddens ME, Slora EJ, Wasserman RC, et al. Secondary sexual characteristics and menses in young girls seen in office practice: a study from the Pediatric Research Office Settings network. Pediatrics 1997; 99:505–512.

87. Genazzani AR, Bernardi F, Monteleone P, et al. Neuropeptides, neurotransmitters, neurosteroids, and the onset of puberty. Ann NY Acad Sci 2000; 900:1–9.

88. Hauser WA. The prevalence and incidence of convulsive disorders in children. Epilepsia 1994; 35(suppl 2):S1–S6.

89. Annegers JF, Grabow JD, Groover RV, et al. The incidence, causes and secular trends of head trauma in Olmstead County, Minnesota 1935–1974. Neurology 1980; 30: 912–919.

90. Annegers JF, Hauser WA, Beghi E, et al. The risk of unprovoked seizures after encephalitis and meningitis. Neurology 1988;38:1407–1410.

91. Marks DA, Kim J, Spencer DD, Spencer SS. Characteristics of intractable seizures following meningitis and encephalitis. Neurology 1992; 42:1513–1518.

92. Dichter M. Basic mechanisms in epilepsy: targets for therapeutic intervention. Epilepsia 1997; 38(suppl 9):S2–S6.

93. Hom AC, Leppik IE, Rask CA. Effects of estradiol and progesterone on seizure sensitivity in oophorectomized DBA/2J mice and C57/EL hybrid mice. Neurology 1993; 43:198–204.

94. Heim L. Effect of estradiol in brain maturation: dose and time relationship. Endocrinology 1966; 78:1130–1134.

95. Tauboll E, Lundervold A, Gjerstad L. Temporal distribution of seizures in epilepsy. Epilepsy Res 1991; 8:153–65.

96. Herzog AG, Klein P, Ransil BJ. Three patterns of catamenial epilepsy. Epilepsia 1997; 38:1082–1088.

97. Logothetis J, Harner R, Morrell F, et al. The role of estrogens in catamenial exacerbation of epilepsy. Neurology 1959; 9:352–360.

98. Backstrom T, Zetterlund B, Blom S, et al. Effects of intravenous progesterone infusions on the epileptic discharge frequency in women with partial epilepsy. Acta Neurol Scand 1984; 69:240–248.

99. Laidlaw WJ. Catamenial epilepsy. Lancet 1956; 271:1235–1237.

100. Smith SS, Gong QH, Hsu FC, et al. GABA-A receptor α4-subunit suppression prevents withdrawal properties of an endogenous steroid. Nature 1998; 392:926–930.

101. Concas A, Mostallino MC, Porcu P, et al. Role of brain allopregnanolone in the plasticity of gamma-aminobutyric acid type A receptor in rat brain during pregnancy and after delivery. Proc Natl Acad Sci USA 1998; 95:13284–13289.

102. Backstrom T. Epileptic seizures in women related to plasma estrogen and progesterone during the menstrual cycle. Acta Neurol Scand 1976; 54:321–347.

103. Roscizewska D, Buntner B, Guz I, et al. Ovarian hormones, anticonvulsant drugs and seizures during the menstrual cycle in women with epilepsy. J Neurol Neurosurg Psychiatry 1986.

104. Shavit G, Lerman P, Korczyn AD. Phenytoin pharmacokinetics in catamenial epilepsy. Neurology 1984; 34:959–961.

105. Sharf M, Sharf B, Bental E, Kuzminsky T. The electroencephalogram in the investigation of anovulation and its treatment by clomiphene. Lancet 1969; 1:750–753.

106. Herzog AG, Seibel MM, Schomer DL, et al. Reproductive endocrine disorders in women with partial seizures of temporal lobe origin. Arch Neurol 1986; 43:341–346.

107. Cummings LN, Giudice L, Morrell MJ. Ovulatory function in epilepsy. Epilepsia 1995; 36:353–357.

108. Mattson RH, Kramer JA, Caldwell BV, Cramer JA. Seizure frequency and the menstrual cycle: a clinical study. Epilepsia 1981; 22:242. (Abstract.)

109. Santoro N, Brown JR, Adel T, et al. Characterization of reproductive hormonal dynamics in the perimenopause. J Clin Endocrinol Metab 1996; 81:1495–1501.

110. Burger HC, Dudley EC, Hopper JL, et al. The endocrinology of the menopausal transition: a cross-sectional study of a population-based sample. J Clin Endocrinol Metab 1995; 80:3537–3545.

111. Harden CL, Pulver MC, Ravdin L, Jacobs AR. The effect of menopause and perimenopause on the course of epilepsy. Epilepsia 1999; 40:1402–1407.

112. Abbasi F, Krumholz A, Kittner SJ, Langenberg P. Effects of menopause on seizures in women with epilepsy. Epilepsia 1999; 40:205–210.

113. Knight AH, Rhind EG. Epilepsy and pregnancy: a study of 153 pregnancies in 59 patients. Epilepsia 1975; 16:99–110.

114. Schmidt D, Canger R, Avanzini G. Change in seizure frequency in pregnant epileptic women. J Neurol Neurosurg Psychiatry 1985; 46:751–755.

115. Ramsay E. Effect of hormones on seizure activity during pregnancy. J Clin Neurophysiol 1987; 4:23–25.

116. Mattson RH. Emotional effects on seizure occurrence. Adv Neurol 1991; 55:453–460.

117. Frucht MM, Quig M, Schwaner C, Fountain NB. Distribution of seizure preicipitants among epilepsy syndromes. Epilepsia 2000; 41:1534–1539.

118. Klein P, Pezzullo JC. Effect of stresss on localization-related epilepsy. Epilepsia 2000; 41(suppl 7):112.

119. Neugebauer R, Paik M, Hauser WA, et al. Stressful life events and seizure frequency in patients with epilepsy. Epilepsia 1994; 35:336–343.

120. Swinkels WA, Engelsman M, Kasteleijn-Nolst Trenite DG, et al. Influence of an evacuation in February 1995 in the Netherlands on the seizure frequency in patients with epilepsy: a controlled study. Epilepsia 1998; 39:1203–1207.

121. Spatt J, Langbauer G, Mamoli B. Subjective perception of seizure precipitants: results of a questionnaire study. Seizure 1998; 7:391–395.

122. Spector S, Cull C, Goldstein LH. Seizure precipitants and perceived self-control of seizures in adults with poorly-controlled epilepsy. Epilepsy Res 2000; 38:207–216.

123. Temkin NR, Davis GR. Stress as a risk factor for seizures among adults with epilepsy. Epilepsia 1984; 25:450–456.

124. Webster A, Mawer GE. Seizure frequency and major life events in epilepsy. Epilepsia 1989; 30:162–167.

125. Small JG, Stevens JR, Milstein V. Electro-clinical correlates of emotional activation of the electroencephalogram. J Nerv Ment Dis 1964; 138:146–155.

126. Stevens JR. Emotional activation of the EEG in patients with convulsive disorders. J Nerv Ment Dis 1959; 128:339–351.

127. Feldman RG, Paul NL. Identity of emotional triggers in epilepsy. J Nerv Ment Dis 1976; 162:345–353.

128. Groethuysen UC, Robinson DB, Haylett CH, et al. Depth electrographic recording of a seizure during a structured interview. Psychosom Med 1957; 19:354–362.

129. Lockard JS, Ward A. Epilepy: A Window to the Brain Mechanisms. New York: Raven Press, 1980.

130. Swinyard EA, Radhakrishgnan N, Goodman LS. Effect of brief restraint on the convulsive threshold of mice. J Pharmacol Exp Ther 1962; 138:337–342.

131. Reddy DS, Tabatabai N, Rogawski MA. Stress-induced deoxycorticosterone-derived neurosteroids modulate GABAa receptor functin and seizure susceptibility. J Neurosci 2000:Abstracts.

132. Swanson LW, Sawchenko P, Rivier J, et al. Organization of ovine corticotrophin-releasing factor immunoreactive cells and foibeers in the rat brain. Neuroendocrinology 1983; 36:165.

133. De Souza EB. Corticotrophin-releasing factor receptors: physiology, pharmacology, biochemistry and role in central nervous system and immune disorders. Psycho-neuroendocrinology 1995; 20:789–819.

134. De Waal WJ, Torn M, De Muinck Keizer-Schrama SM, et al. Long term sequelae of sex steroid treatment in the management of constitutionally tall stature. Arch Dis Child, 1995; 73:311–315.

135. Kalin NH, Takashani L, Chen FL. Restraint stress increases corticotropin-releasing hormone mRNA content in the amygdala and paraventricular nucleus. Brain Res 1994; 656:182–186.

136. Klein P, Herzog AG. Emerging applications of hormonal therapy of paroxysmal central nervous system disorders. Exp Opin Invest Drugs 1997; 6:1337–1349.

137. Joels M, De Kloet E, Mineralocorticoid and glucocorticoid receptors in the brain. Implications for ion permeability and transmitter systems. Prog Neurobiol 1994; 43:1–36.

138. Heuser G, Ling GM, Buchwald NA. Sedation or seizures as dose-dependent effects of steroids. Arch Neurol 1965; 13:195–203.

139. Naritoku DK, Terry WJ, Helfert RH. Regional induction of fos immunoreactivity in the brain by anticonvulsant stimulation of the vagus nerve. Epilepsy Res 1995; 22:53–62.

140. Greig E, Betts T. Epileptic seizures induced by sexual abuse. Pathogenic and pathoplastic factors. Seizure 1992; 1:269–274.

141. Rosenberg HJ, Rosenberg SD, Williamson PD, et al. A comparative study of trauma and posttraumatic stress disorder prevalence in epilepsy patients and psychogenic nonepileptic seizure patients. Epilepsia 2000; 41:447–452.

142. Mattson RH, Cramer J, Caldwell BV, et al. Treatment of seizures with medroxypro-gesterone acetate: preliminary report. Neurology 1984; 1984:1255–1258.

143. Dana Haeri J, Richens A. Effect of norethisterone on seizures associated with menstruation. Epilepsia 1983; 24:377–381.

144. Hall SM. Treatment of menstrual epilepsy with a progesterone only oral contraceptive. Epilepsia 1977; 18:235–236.

145. Klein P, Herzog AG. Hormonal effects on epilepsy in women. Epilepsia 1998; 39(suppl 8):S9–S16.

146. Herzog AG. Intermittent progesterone therapy and frequency of complex partial seizures in women with menstrual disorders. Neurology 1986; 36:1607–1610.

147. Herzog AG. Progesterone therapy in women with complex partial and secondary generalized seizures. Neurology 1995; 45:1660–1662.

148. Herzog AG. Progesterone therapy in women with epilepsy: a 3-year follow-up. Neurology 1999; 52:1917–1918.

149. Monaghan E, McAuley JW, Data JL. Ganoxolone: a novel positive allosteric modulator of the GABA(A) receptor complex for the treatment of epilepsy. Expert Opin Invest Drugs 1999; 8:1663–1671.

150. Aird RB, Gordon GS. Anticonvulsant properties of deoxycorticosterone. JAMA 1951; 1951:715–719.

151. Casaroli G, Munari C, Matteuzzi G, et al. L'Athesin nel tratt amento dello stato di male epilettico. Minerva-Anesthesiol 1980; 46:129–140.

152. Carter RB, Wood PL, Wieland S, et al. Characterization of the anticonvulsant properties of ganaxolone (CCD 1042;3a-hydroxy-3b-methyl-5a-pregnan-20-one), a selective, high affinity, steroid modulator of the g-aminobutyric acid receptor. J Pharmacol Exp Ther 1997; 280:1284–1295.

153. Reddy DS, Rogawski MA. Chronic treatment with the neuroactive steroid ganaxolone in the rat induces anticonvulsant tolerance to diazepam but not to itself. J Pharm Exp Ther 2000; 295:1342–1350.

154. Lechtenberg R, Villeneuve N, Monaghan EP, et al. An open label dose-escalation study to evaluate the safety and tolerability of ganaxolone in the treatment of refractory epilepsy in pediatric patients. Epilepsia 1996; 37(suppl 5):205.

155. Dodson WE, Bourgeois B, Kerrigan J, et al. An open label evaluation of safety and efficacy of ganaxolone in children with refractory seizures and history of infantile spasms. Epilepsia 1997; 38(suppl):15.

155a. Laxer K, Blum D, Abou Khalil BW, et al. Assessment of ganaxolone's anticonvulsant activity using a randomized, double-blind, presurgical trial design. Ganaxolone Presurgical Study Group. Epilepsia 2000; 41:1187–1194.

156. Herzog AG. Seizure control with clomiphene therapy: a case report. Arch Neurol 1988; 45:209–210.

157. Login IS, Dreifuss FE. Anticonvulsant activity of clomiphene. Arch Neurol 1983; 40:525.

158. Herzog AG. Clomiphene therapy in epileptic women with menstrual disorders. Neurology 1988; 38:432–434.

159. Herzog AG, Klein P, Jacobs AR. Testosterone versus testostereone and testolactone in treating reproductive and sexual dysfunction in men with epilepsy and hypogonadism. Neurology 1998; 50:782–784.

160. Haider Y, Barnett D. Catamenial epilepsy and goserelin. Lancet 1991; 2:1530.

161. Bauer J, Wildt L, Flugel D, Stefan H. The effect of a syntheric GnRH analogue on catamenial epilepsy: a study in ten patients. J Neurol 1992; 239: 284–286.

162. Snead OC. ACTH and prednisone: use in seizure disorders other than infantile spasms. In: Levy RH, Meldrum BS, eds. Antiepileptic Drugs. New York: Raven Press, 1995:941–948.

163. Baram TZ, Mitchell WG, Tournay A, et al. High-dose corticotropin (ACTH) versus prednisone for infantile spasms: a prospective, randomized, blinded study. Pediatrics, 1996; 97:375–379.

164. Baram TZ. Pathophysiology of infantile spasms: perspective on the putative role of the brain adrenal axis. Ann Neuol 1993; 33:231–236.

165. Eneroth P, Gustafsson JA. Excretion and anticonvulsant activity of steroid hormones in an infant with infantile spasm and hypsarrhythmia treated with excessive doses of ACTH. J Steroid Biochem 1972; 3:877–887.

166. Herzog AG, Sotrel A, Ronthal M. Reversible proximal myopathy in epilepsy-related Cushing's syndrome. Ann Neurol 1995; 38:306–307.

167. Baram TZ, Mitchell WG, Brunson K, Haden E. Infantile spasms: hypothesis-driven therapy and pilot human infant experiments using corticotropin-releasing hormone receptor antagonists. Dev Neurosci 1999; 21:281–289.

168. McEwen BS. How do sex and stress hormones affect nerve cells? Ann NY Acad Sci 1994; 743:1–16.

19

Chronobiology and Sleep: Implications for Seizure Propensity

Mark Quigg

University of Virginia
Charlottesville, Virginia, U.S.A.

INTRODUCTION

Circadian rhythms have marked effects on expression of epilepsy, influencing the timing of occurrence of seizures and the characteristics of interictal epileptiform discharges (IEDs). Circadian rhythms are not a singular entity but involve many systems within and without the central nervous system. Therefore, a circadian influence is not likely a single, unified mechanism. Rather, circadian rhythms are better thought of as endogenously mediated, excitatory, and inhibitory influences that vary with time of day and dynamically compete with other seizure precipitants to elevate or depress seizure threshold. In this chapter, I review basic concepts of chronobiology, the organization of the circadian timing system, the effects of epilepsy and seizures on circadian rhythms, and the influences of circadian rhythms on the timing of seizures.

CIRCADIAN TIMING SYSTEM

A circadian (Latin: *circa*, about; *dies*, day) rhythm is any self-sustained, behavioral or physiologic activity that spontaneously oscillates with a period of ~24 h. The solar light-dark cycle is an important *zeitgeber* (German: time-giver), an external time cue that entrains circadian rhythms to the local environment. Synchronization to the solar cycle is a widespread and highly conserved adaptation that confers advantages in survival and performance (1–3).

A principal feature of circadian rhythms is that, once isolated from zeitgebers, endogenously maintained circadian rhythms persist and free-run with a period of

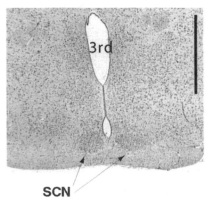

Figure 1. Photomicrograph of the SCN in the anterior hypothalamus in the rat. 3rd = 3rd ventricle. Bar = 100 μm.

~24 h, whereas exogenously maintained daily rhythms rapidly attenuate. Observation during constant environmental conditions, therefore, is the main test of whether a particular activity is truly circadian or is driven by external influences.

Many behaviors or physiologic activities fulfill the strict criteria of circadian rhythms. In animal experiments, the rest-activity cycle and core body temperature are predominant because of ease of use and accuracy in long-term measurements. Perhaps more relevant to epilepsy, however, are the circadian cycles of sleep-wake and neurohormones. Circadian rhythms are not the only endogenous biological rhythms. Ultradian rhythms such as the 90- to 100-min REM-NREM sleep cycle or the 1-min cyclic alternating pattern of arousal (4,5), and the infradian menstrual cycle (6) also may be important in precipitation of seizures or IEDs.

The paired suprachiasmatic nuclei (SCNs), located in the anterior hypothalamus, is the locus of the primary mammalian biological clock (Fig. 1). Ablation of the SCN attenuates circadian rhythms such as the cycles of rest-activity, body temperature, and corticosterone secretion (7–9). Transplantation of normal SCN cells into animals with genetically short circadian periods restores circadian rhythms with normal periods (10). Circadian oscillation is a property of individual neurons; for example, neuronal cultures of SCN maintain sustained rhythmic activity (11,12).

Knowledge of the basic genetic mechanism of the clock has advanced rapidly in the past 5 years. The clock consists of a set of genes that form an autoregulatory cycle of transcription and translation (for review see 13). The clock, as originally described in *Drosophila*, consists of four core genetic components. Two genes, *clock* and *bmal1*, comprise the positive components of a regulatory loop. These genes activate the transcription of two other genes that form a negative portion of the feedback loop, *timeless* and *period*. Through interactions with their own genes, proteins encoded by *timeless* and *period* inhibit their continued transcription. With time, the proteins degrade (the rate of degradation is but one determinant of the cycle's period), and their negative feedback effect weakens. *Clock* and *bmal1* are then free to activate transcription again, and the 24-h cycle resumes.

The primary neurotransmitter of SCN neurons is GABA. In the laboratory, circadian systems are susceptible to pharmacologic manipulation with agents active at the GABA receptor (14). Other peptides and transmitters important in clock function or its efferent signaling include somatostatin, acetylcholine, neuropeptide Y, and vasopressin (15,16).

The cyclic activity of the SCN and in turn the variety of circadian rhythms regulated by the SCN are synchronized to the solar light cycle. The SCNs exert their rhythmic influence through diffuse projections throughout the hypothalamus (17). Other efferents from the SCN, either directly or indirectly through hypothalamic connections, project to the thalamus and limbic system (17,18).

Some consider the pineal body a second component of the circadian timing system. In mammals, the pineal body synthesizes and secretes melatonin during the nocturnal portion of the light-dark cycle in a pattern dependent upon SCN activity and on the suppressive influence of light exposure (19). The primary function of melatonin in mammals is to transmit information concerning light-dark cycles and day length to organize behavior dependent on seasonal functions. It may act directly on SCN neurons in a feedback loop to induce phase shifts and entrainment (20).

The SCN is considered the primary circadian oscillator, but regions outside the SCN maintain rhythms that are either are subordinate to or may contribute to circadian regulation. Genes with direct roles in circadian regulation are expressed in other diverse systems such as the retina (21), liver, lung, and skeletal muscle (12), as well as in regions of the brain outside the SCN (Fig. 2). Recent gene chip experiments

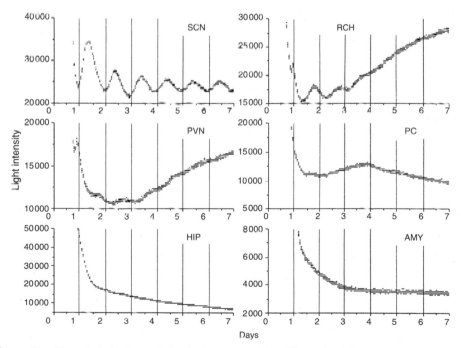

Figure 2. Circadian rhythms of the clock gene Per1 in different brain regions, as revealed by light emission from neuronal cultures in a transgenic rat in which luciferase is rhythmically expressed under control of the Per1 promoter (12). These data show persistent and self-sustained circadian rhythms of the SCN. Other brain regions are either arrhythmic or are rhythmic only for a short time (personal communication, Shin Yamazaki).

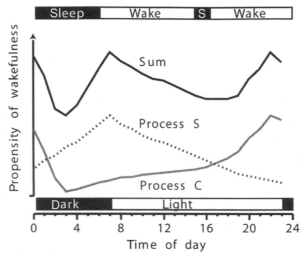

Figure 3. Interactions of sleep homeostasis and the circadian rhythm of arousal on sleep-wake state. Sleep debt, represented by Process S, gradually accumulates following the last episode of sleep, resulting in a gradually decreasing level of alertness until reset by a major sleep episode. The circadian rhythm of arousal, Processes C, counters sleep debt by gradually increasing its effect through the light phase of the cycle. The sum of Processes S and C is a biphasic rhythm of propensity of wakefulness, organizing sleep-wake states into a major nocturnal episode of sleep and a shorter "nap" during the late afternoon. (From Ref. 24.)

with *Drosophila* show that ~400 gene transcripts have significant circadian oscillations (22), but the functions of rhythmic expression of these diverse genes, within and without the traditional circadian timing system, remain unclear.

The sleep-wake cycle is arguably the most visible of circadian rhythms, and in fact is used synonymously with "circadian" in some reports of circadian effects in epilepsy. It is an oversimplification, since circadian timing and sleep-wake regulation comprise autonomous systems that mutually interact to regulate behavior (for review see 23). The temporal pattern of sleep-wakefulness can be represented by the following model (Fig. 3) (24): The homeostatic drive for sleep, Process S, gradually builds until reset by the next sleep episode. The 24-h cycle of arousal, Process C, gradually increases the propensity for alertness as the day continues and declines late in the dark phase of the solar cycle. Therefore, the patterns of sleep-wake states reflect the dual influences of sleep debt and circadian organization. Sleep states are "circadian" in that the overall effect of the circadian clock is to organize sleep-wake states into daily cycles (25). To date, experiments purporting to examine circadian mechanisms of seizure propensity have yet to adequately control for separate influences of sleep-wake state, circadian arousal, and sleep debt.

In addition to the above endogenous influences, sleep-wake cycles are uniquely susceptible to perturbation or interruption from exogenous influences, such as beepers and babies, as any medical resident or parent can attest. The self-sustained rhythm of arousal, however, continues without interruption, a property enabling *forced desynchronization protocols* in which sleep and wakefulness are assigned to different periods and phases from underlying circadian cycles (25).

Finally, a clear reason to differentiate sleep-wake state from circadian timing is the observation that, among mammalian species, secondary circadian rhythms maintain different phase relationships to rhythms of the primary circadian timing system. Nocturnal animals, those active during the dark phase of the solar cycle, maintain rhythms of body temperature and, cortisol secretion that peak at night. The opposite is true for diurnal animals (such as man) with daily rhythms of activity, body temperature, and cortisol secretion that are maximal during the light phase. In contrast, primary rhythms of the circadian timing system—SCN activity and melatonin—remain in phase across all mammalian species. The activity of SCN neurons oscillates daily with the metabolic or electrical activity maintained during the daytime, whether a species is diurnal or nocturnal (26,27). Similarly, light suppresses melatonin production so that the daily oscillation of melatonin peaks during the night in both diurnal and nocturnal animals (28).

In summary, studies of circadian phenomena in epilepsy have historically—and understandably—simplified the complex interactions among primary and secondary endogenous circadian rhythms and exogenous stimuli. These complexities delineate interactions among seizures, epilepsy, and circadian phenomena.

INTERACTIONS OF THE CIRCADIAN TIMING SYSTEM, EPILEPSY, AND SEIZURES

There are three areas important in the interactions among seizures, epilepsy, and circadian rhythms. The first is effects of seizures and epilepsy upon circadian regulation. The second is the effects on circadian rhythms on epileptogenesis, the specific process of brain injury leading to the recurrence of spontaneous epileptic seizures. The third is the effects of primary and secondary circadian rhythms on the occurrence of IEDs and seizures.

Effects of Seizures or Epilepsy on the Circadian Timing System

Possible perturbations of the circadian timing system and its subordinate rhythms include attenuation or loss of normal circadian rhythmicity as a result of the chronic epileptic lesion, transient attenuation or perturbation of rhythms as an acute symptom of epileptic seizures, or more fundamental alterations of circadian timing induced by epileptic events.

Attenuation of Circadian Rhythmicity in Chronic Epilepsy

The epileptic state represents a permanent alteration of neuronal excitability, which results in clinical seizures. The exact alteration varies with the pathogenesis of the specific epileptic syndrome. Because neuronal pathways connect the SCN to target regions that are responsible for individual rhythms, damage to those pathways or target regions could result in abnormalities manifested by changes in circadian amplitude or emergence of noncircadian rhythms.

One example of altered circadian rhythms in epilepsy is the nocturnal melatonin rhythm (29–31). Most studies in patients treated with anticonvulsant medications document an interictal decrease in nocturnal melatonin (29,31), but others in untreated patients show an increased nocturnal melatonin level (30). In a comparison of melatonin rhythms of photosensitive, epileptic children to those without photosensitivity, two out of three photosensitive children, compared to none of 11 epileptic children without photosensitivity, have attenuated nocturnal melatonin rhythms (32). Although the above data suggest that some alterations in rhythms can result from the actions of anticonvulsant medications, attenuation of melatonin rhythmicity could represent a nonspecific response to injury, as evidenced by attenuation or loss of the circadian rhythms of body temperature, cortisol, or melatonin in patients with epileptic encephalopathy (33) or in neuronal degenerative diseases (34).

Nevertheless, the basic machinery of the clock is robust; only complete destruction of the SCN renders animals arrhythmic. Circadian rhythms emerge in incomplete lesions of bilateral SCN (35,36). Similarly, in a study of hypothalamic pathology in a rat model of limbic epilepsy, all animals maintain circadian rhythms of temperature (37). Studies of patients with neurodegenerative diseases how that only those with the most severe and diffuse disease have clear circadian abnormalities (although most have disordered sleep) (34).

Along with the blunting of normal circadian rhythms, the epileptic lesion may also allow emergence of ultradian or infradian rhythms that may normally be suppressed by the primary circadian pacemaker. For example, circadian temperature rhythms of epileptic rats are more complex and polyphasic than normal rats, demonstrating ultradian rhythms with periods ranging from 2 to 16 h (37). Epileptic patients observed during a period of 72 h off anticonvulsant medications have circadian temperature and cardiac rhythms that are more variable in the timing of temperature peaks, nadirs, and periods (38), consistent with the either the effects of underlying ultradian rhythms or with instability of the circadian pacemaker. Ultradian rhythms can emerge in cases of specific brain lesions in experimental animals (39) and in nonspecific lesions attributable to brain injury in ICU patients (40). Immaturity in brain development is also associated with ultradian body temperature rhythms (41). Studies of long-term seizure diaries show that some patients develop infradian patterns of seizure recurrence with periods ranging from 18 to 20 days (42,43), implying that an occult, underlying nonlunar rhythm is present in these subjects. In summary, these studies show that epileptic lesion largely spares overall circadian function, but circadian rhythms may be attenuated or impaired to the extent that ultradian or infradian patterns emerge.

Seizures and Masking Effects

Many studies document postictal *masking* effects: transient, seizure-induced changes in normal function proportional to the physiologic severity of the seizure. Although the underlying rhythm is temporarily overcome, the masking stimulus has no long-lasting effect on period or phase of circadian rhythmicity. An illustration of masking is the transient disruption of the daily pattern of secretion of hormones following acute seizures (44,45). For example, severe, secondarily generalized partial seizures transiently elevate levels of noradrenaline, prolactin, vasopressin, and oxytocin (45). On the other hand, simple partial seizures that spare the limbic system may fail to cause detectable changes in prolactin (46). In this light, transient elevations in nocturnal melatonin seen immediately after partial-onset seizures can be interpreted as masking effects (31).

Seizures and Circadian Timing

Few studies have been designed to determine whether seizures affect clock function. A principal feature of circadian rhythms is that they can be entrained to the solar light-dark cycle. One specific alteration of circadian timing stems from shifts in phase necessary to synchronize organisms to the environmental light-dark cycle. For example, after transmeridian travel, humans reset their internal clocks by ∼1 h (47). Available studies disagree on the ability of seizures to perturb clock function.

Most show a null affect on circadian phase or period. Early studies on wild rats that measured locomotor activity before and after electrically induced convulsions show transient, postictal masking of the rest-activity cycle. The subsequent phase of locomotor activity after recovery remains unchanged (48).

Humans following electroconvulsive therapy (ECT) also demonstrate transient changes in amplitudes of daily temperature rhythms; shifts in phase are not observed (49). Similarly, in patients with spontaneous temporal lobe seizures captured during monitoring for epilepsy surgery, no clear effects on the phase of melatonin or temperature rhythms are seen (31). The sampling resolution in these studies (every 3 h in the last for example), however, is limited and might not be sensitive enough to detect small shifts in phase.

Other evidence suggests that seizures can shift the circadian phase. ACTH and cortisol levels were monitored in depressed patients before and after antidepressant or electroconvulsive therapy; the timing of the peak of ACTH and cortisol levels shifted from phase-advanced to normal values following both treatments (50). Phase shifts in this study, however, may reflect the treatment of depression rather than the specific effect of a provoked seizure.

The above studies, however, are designed to show predictable, group effects. Rather than a consistent and physiologic shift in phase (as in the physiologic response to light stimuli) (47), the circadian system may shift unpredictably in response to a pathologic stimulus. In a study of kindled rats, electrically provoked convulsions caused a variety of phase advances and delays in temperature rhythms (51). Other studies that document alterations in entrainment to light stimuli in epileptic rats (52), and variable and inconsistent maintenance of body temperature and cardiac rhythms in humans (38) suggest that epilepsy is associated with an altered capacity for entrainment and synchronization.

In summary, there are conflicting data on the effects of seizures on the circadian timing system. The focus on transient elevations or depressions of activity, rather than on its timing, has led to an inadequate evaluation of interactions between circadian timing and epilepsy. Studies suggest, however, that time cues may be important in keeping epileptic subjects properly synchronized to environmental cycles following epileptic seizures.

Circadian Effects on IEDs, Epileptogenic Lesions, and Seizures

The following discussion is summarized in Figure 4. This schematic lays out the preferential phase of occurrence of seizures or IEDs, or in some cases, phases of enhanced vulnerability to epileptogenic or ictogenic procedures, in a variety of human epileptic syndromes and in experimental models.

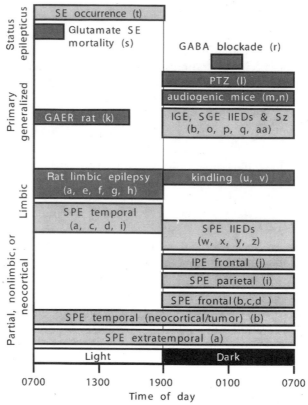

Figure 4. Summary of 27 studies of the preferential phase of occurrence of seizures or IEDs, or in some cases, phases of enhanced vulnerability to epileptogenic or ictogenic procedures, in a variety of human epileptic syndromes (light gray boxes) and in nocturnally active experimental models (dark gray boxes). In most studies, the time-of-day of phenomena are specified; in a few studies, as discussed in the text, sleep-wake state was made equivalent with the light-dark cycle by individual investigators. For comparison, studies performed at with point sampling (noon and midnight, for example) have been spread out to represent a whole photophase. Furthermore, slight variations in different light-dark schedules were ignored. Exceptions are those experiments with more frequent sampling across the clock that found effects confined to specific times of day. SPE, symptomatic partial epilepsy; IPE/IGE, idiopathic partial/generalized epilepsy; SGE, symptomatic generalized epilepsy; GAER, genetic absence epilepsy rat; SE, status epilepticus; Sz, seizure; IEDs, interictal epileptiform discharges; PTZ, pentylenetetrazole. References: a (87), b (88), c (124), d (91), e (78), f (125), g (86), h (85), i (42), j (90), k (83), l (81), m (57), n (77), o (68), p (126), q (62), r (82), s (127), t (54), u (58), v (59), w (67), x (65), y (61), z (66), aa (69).

Epileptogenic Lesions

The effects of time of day on the process of epileptogenesis (distinct from circadian influences on ictogenesis) have not been thoroughly studied. Human evidence indirectly suggests that epileptogenic events vary in occurrence by time of day. Status epilepticus, for example, can be considered an epileptogenic event attended by neuronal injury (53). Waterhouse et al. (54) report that a cohort of 1193 cases of status epilepticus in Richmond, VA, vary in occurrence by time of day in a unimodal distribution (54) with peak occurrence at 13:48 (personnel communication). Even though this preliminary report does not explore outcome, one may speculate that the clinical impact of status epilepticus can vary with etiology, treatment opportunities, or physiologic effects, all of which may vary by time of day. By analogy, epidemiological studies of the outcome of stroke by time day failed to demonstrate clear variables that distinguished strokes that occur in the morning (the peak time of stroke occurrence) versus those that occurred at other times of day (55).

Clinical sequelae of status epilepticus may not necessarily occur in phase with epileptic injury. For example, rats treated with monosodium L-glutamate at 07:00 (early in the light phase) have convulsions and convulsive status epilepticus that occurs more often and more severely than those treated at 15:00 (late in the light phase) or at 23:00 (middle of dark phase). Status epilepticus in the morning results in death in 70% of cases, compared to none at other times (56). Conversely, mice susceptible to audiogenic seizures experience a higher rate of fatal convulsions during the dark phase than during the light phase (57). The process of kindling brings more direct evidence that epileptogenic events vary by time of day. In nocturnal animals, the dark phase of the daily cycle is particularly vulnerable to epileptogenic injury. Rats undergoing electrical kindling of the amygdala require a smaller number of stimulations to achieve a fully kindled state, and develop after-discharges more quickly when stimuli are confined to dark phase of the daily cycle (58,59). Therefore, the differences in phases between the diurnally predominant occurrence and impact of status epilepticus and the nocturnally predominant effects of kindling suggests that these processes, in antiphase, are susceptible to different circadian influences.

Phasic Occurrence of Interictal Epileptiform Discharges

Interictal epileptiform discharges occur at a relatively high rate (in contrast to ictal discharges), thus facilitating their chronobiological study. Most studies concentrate on their occurrence at different sleep-wake states. Although examination of their occurrence is helpful in considering the specificity and sensitivity of EEG in diagnosis of epilepsy, the frequency of IEDs, notably in partial epilepsies, does not clearly predict the occurrence of ictal discharges (60). Generalized epilepsies, because distinctions between interictal and ictal discharges can be difficult, nevertheless share similarities with partial epilepsies in the modulation of IEDs by sleep-wake stages.

Most studies confirm that IEDs in both partial and generalized epilepsies occur in patterns tied to regulation of sleep-wake states (4,61–67). IEDs in symptomatic partial epilepsies appear most frequently during non-REM sleep and are suppressed during REM sleep (65–67). Generalized epilepsies share similar phasic distributions of IEDs. In the case of childhood absence epilepsy, a syndrome noted for frequent appearances of generalized 3-Hz discharges during routine, daytime EEG, spike-waves are further activated by non-REM sleep (68). Slow spike-waves discharges in epileptic encephalopathy also increase in persistence during non-REM sleep (69). Similarly, developmental disorders such as Landau-Kleffner syndrome or electrical status epilepticus during slow-wave sleep (ESES) exhibit IEDs that are either exacerbated by or are limited to appearance during slow-wave sleep, when they can become nearly continuous (70).

Long-term monitoring studies, performed in patients with a variety of epilepsy syndromes ranging from idiopathic partial (Rolandic epilepsy) to generalized polyspike wave epilepsy to temporal lobe epilepsy, show that IEDs occur in 90- to 110-min cycles, corresponding to the non-REM/REM ultradian cycles (4,62,63). The ultradian pattern of IED occurrence persists through the waking state (4,62).

Another similarity shared among the epilepsies is that IEDs are not only activated by non-REM sleep but undergo changes in distribution. During non-REM sleep focal spikes undergo generalization or appear bilaterally or contralaterally (61,66). Runs of 3-Hz discharges in absence epilepsy become disorganized and can appear as polyspike discharges (68). Conversely, the rare spikes during REM sleep are restricted in spatial distribution (66).

No studies have clearly examined whether IED occurrence is tied to a particular circadian phase independent from sleep-wake state. Kellaway and colleagues demonstrated that ultradian patterns of IED occurrence could be modeled by interactions of sleep-associated ultradian and circadian rhythms (63). Potential studies to examine circadian effects independent of sleep state are complicated by the finding that sleep deprivation activates IEDs in an independent fashion that supplements the activating effects of sleep state (71). Future studies on daily patterns of IEDs, therefore, may need to control for the duration from the last sleep episode. Available evidence, therefore, suggests that the nocturnal prevalence of IEDs is circadian only in that the timing system organizes and coalesces sleep-wake states into recognizable circadian and ultradian patterns of facilitation and inhibition (see Fig. 3).

Phasic Occurrence of Seizures

Studies of the chronobiology of epilepsy reveal several important findings. Epileptic seizures recur at preferred times of day. Seizures in specific animal models of epilepsy occur in true, endogenously mediated circadian patterns, implying that other epileptic conditions are susceptible to endogenous circadian modulation. Finally, the phasic patterns of seizure occurrence vary with the pathophysiology of the underlying epileptic syndrome.

The tendency of epileptic seizures to occur in temporal patterns was first described over 100 years ago. Gowers, in a study of 840 subjects, classifies patients into three groups based upon the daily distribution of "fits": "diurnal" (daytime onset, synonymous with wakefulness); "nocturnal" (nighttime onset—sleep); and "diffuse" (random onset) (72). Diurnal fits comprise 43% of the sample, nocturnal 20%, and diffuse 37%. The day- or nighttime occurrence of the first fit in a cluster fairly predicts that subsequent seizures would also occur within the preferred phase. Finally, transitions from sleep to wakefulness, especially in the morning, carries relatively high risk of seizure occurrence, at least 5% of the sample. Later studies based on observations of subjects in the asylums of the period expanded upon Gowers' findings by plotting seizure occurrence as a function of time of day (73–75). A "diffuse" distribution was associated with worse severity and duration of epilepsy (75).

These early studies established that seizures vary by time of day. Evidence that daily variations are in fact circadian are comes from case reports that demonstrate that seizures, like circadian rhythms, can shift in phase given changes in *zeitgebers*. Halberg reports that in a long-term seizure diary of an epileptic patient, seizures not only occur in a daily pattern, but the daily pattern shifts in response to a phasic change in the subject's daily work schedule (76).

The above studies share limitations. Studies were without benefit of EEG confirmation of seizure occurrence. Many seizures—especially nocturnal seizures—may have gone unobserved, and some seizures may have been mistaken for "hysteroid fits" (72). Furthermore, exposures to potential *zeitgebers* or other exogenous stimuli are difficult to limit in human subjects, so direct confirmation that epileptic seizures occur in an endogenous circadian pattern usually is precluded.

Rigorous environment controls, however, can be imposed on animal models of epilepsy. In mice with audiogenic convulsions, changes in phases of the light-dark cycle provoke comparable changes in phases of convulsions (77). Only one study thus far has conducted EEG monitoring under constant conditions to allow circadian rhythms to free-run (Fig. 5) (78). In this study, rats undergo electrical stimulation of the hippocampus, leading to self-sustained limbic status epilepticus (79). Animals develop spontaneously recurring limbic seizures, analogous to human complex partial seizures, and develop histological changes analogous to human mesial sclerosis (80). During continuous EEG monitoring in a 12–12 h light-dark cycle, nearly twice as many seizures occur during the light phase than during the dark phase. During constant darkness, seizures continue to occur in a strong pattern when referenced to the free-running circadian rhythm of body temperature. Limbic seizures, therefore, fulfill the explicit criteria of circadian phenomena. I infer

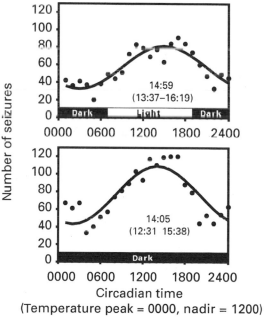

Figure 5. Distribution of spontaneous limbic seizures in an animal model of limbic epilepsy (78). Seizures recur preferentially during the daytime when animals are maintained in a regular light-dark cycle. The same circadian distribution is maintained when animals are monitored in constant darkness and isolated from other *zeitgebers*. The persistent pattern of seizure recurrence therefore fulfills the strict definition of circadian rhythmicity.

that the daily patterns of spontaneous seizures noted in other animal and human studies are also susceptible to the endogenous modulation of the circadian timing system.

Figure 5 compares the preferential phases of occurrence of a sample of animal models and human syndromes of partial and generalized epilepsies. The schematic highlights inconsistencies in phase within models of generalized epilepsies and models of limbic epilepsies. Animal models of generalized epilepsies, nocturnally active rats or mice, preferentially have greater susceptibility to seizures during the dark phase of the 24-h light-dark cycle (57,77,81,82). These animals have drug-induced or sensory-evoked seizures. In contrast, the spontaneous spike-wave discharges of genetic absence epilepsy rats (GAER) occur mainly during the light half of the cycle (83).

Similarly, models of limbic epilepsy also vary in phase depending on experimental protocol. Kindling experiments that involve triggered after-discharges or convulsions show greatest sensitivity during the dark (58,59), whereas spontaneous seizures in experimental models of limbic epilepsy occur predominantly during the light half of the cycle (78,84–87).

One explanation of the internal inconsistencies within groups of generalized and limbic models, therefore, is that provoked seizures occur out of phase with spontaneous seizures. Arousal, handling, and transient light exposure can occur during provocation of seizures and can thus confound comparisons.

Experiments that measure spontaneous epileptic events, however, show clear differences between generalized, partial neocortical, and partial limbic epilepsies. In diurnally active humans, IEDs of both generalized and partial epilepsies (discussed above), ictal discharges of generalized epilepsies (62,68,69,88,89), and ictal discharges of neocortical epilepsies (42,90,91) occur preponderantly during the dark half of the 24-h cycle. In nocturnally active models of generalized epilepsies in which epileptic events occur spontaneously, ictal discharges appear more frequently during the light portion of the cycle (83). Therefore, models of generalized epilepsies and human generalized and cortically based epilepsies manifest out of phase with each other. It follows, then, that circadian rhythms that occur antiphase between the two species can best modulate seizure occurrence in these syndromes. Sleep and other secondary circadian rhythms between diurnal and nocturnal species are out of phase. In summary, generalized epileptic events tend to occur during the circadian half-cycle in which sleep occurs.

A similar deduction leads to an opposite conclusion in the case of limbic epilepsies. In a comparison between experimental limbic epilepsy in rats and mesial temporal lobe epilepsy in humans, both species have peak incidences of limbic seizures during the light portion of the 24-h light-dark cycle (Fig. 5) (87). Rats, however, are nocturnal animals and have sleep-wake cycles 180° out of phase with those of diurnal humans. Rhythms of the primary circadian timing system occur in phase between diurnal and nocturnal animals. The finding that limbic seizures occur in phase among diurnal and nocturnal species implies a direct role of the circadian timing system on the modulation of seizure occurrence.

Primary Circadian Influences

To date there are only a few studies that examine direct involvement of the SCN or of the pineal body on seizure occurrence or seizure threshold. Indirect evidence, however, suggests that the circadian timing system may have effects on spontaneous seizure occurrence. There have been no studies addressing whether the circadian oscillation of the SCN directly affects epileptic seizures, although there may be direct connections from SCN to the limbic system (17,18). Hippocampal cells in culture produce daily oscillations in electrical activity that are not self-sustaining (11).

Several lines of evidence have suggested that melatonin possesses anticonvulsant properties. At a time when melatonin secretion is high, suppression of nocturnal seizure rate in limbic epilepsies can be demonstrated (78,84–87). Pinealectomy renders gerbils and parathyroidectomized rats susceptible to spontaneous convulsions, and melatonin administration confers partial protection against convulsions in pinealectomized gerbils (92). In kindled animals, melatonin decreases the duration of after-discharges (93) and increases the threshold current necessary to evoke after-discharges (94). Melatonin decreases epileptiform activity recorded from human hippocampal slices (95). Finally, adjunctive treatment with melatonin decreases seizures in humans (96,97).

However, in some situations, melatonin decreases (not increases) seizure thresholds (98). In addition, pinealectomy reduces seizure susceptibility in some species, opposite to its convulsion-inducing effect (92). Exogenous melatonin acts with much clearer efficacy in reducing seizures than does the endogenous cyclic increase in melatonin secretion (94,99).

Secondary Circadian Influences

Sleep-Wake State.   As discussed above, sleep, as organized by the circadian timing system, facilitates both the appearance and spread of IEDs in many epilepsy syndromes and promotes seizure occurrence in generalized epilepsy syndromes. State-dependent changes in cortical excitability and thalamocortical synchronization play important roles in the occurrence of epileptic seizures or related paroxysmal activity in generalized epilepsies (100). The work of Steriade and colleagues demonstrates that there is a progressive development from the hypersynchrony of non-REM sleep patterns to some forms of epilepticlike activities. Their work suggests that thalamocortical relay neurons are gradually recruited by cortical excitation into a hypersynchronous, epileptic state (101). However, thalamocortical interactions in the generation of seizures are not confined to the generalized epilepsies. Sleep spindles, mediated by GABA-ergic thalamocortical relay and reticular nucleus neurons (102), have been proposed to be present in the hippocampus as a finding associated with epilepsy (103). Growing experience in the functional anatomy of the limbic system suggest that interactions between the limbic system and thalamus comprise a network responsible for generation and maintenance of ictal discharges (104).

Hypothalamic Pituitary Adrenal Axis.   The three components of the hypothalamic pituitary adrenal (HPA) axis, corticotropin-releasing hormone (CRH), adrenocorticotropin hormone (ACTH), and corticosterone, all induce circadian rhythms that peak before and near the onset of locomotor activity (8,105,106). These rhythms depend on SCN input for their synchronization (8,107). Contrary to the traditional "top-down" regulatory model, activity of the SCN directly affects pituitary (ACTH) as well as hypothalamic (CRH) activity (107). All three components have been implicated in determining seizure threshold and the processes of epileptogenesis. Whereas CRH potentiates seizures (108,109), ACTH and corticosteroids are used as anticonvulsants in certain epileptic syndromes (110).

CRH is particularly interesting regarding the question of the circadian modulation of seizures. CRH neurons are not confined to the hypothalamus. Although the main population of CRH neurons resides in the PVN, CRH neurons are also present in the limbic system (111,112). These neurons are located mainly in the central nucleus of the amygdala (111,112) and also found in CA1, CA3, and granule cell and hilar layers of the dentate (111,113).

CRH secretion not only undergoes circadian changes but is a primary response to stress. Stressful stimuli immediately up-regulates transcription of CRH within neurons of the PVN (114). Because patients with epilepsy identify stress as an important precipitant of seizures (115), CRH is uniquely suited to promote epileptic seizures provoked by both exogenous stimuli and endogenous rhythms.

CRH is a potent pro-convulsant, especially in the immature brain (108,109). CRH is thought to amplify existing excitatory circuits to promote hyperexcitability (see review in 116). Therefore, CRH released during illness, stress, or in its daily cycle may facilitate epileptic seizures.

ACTH and corticosteroids are used in treatment of infantile spasms (110). Convulsions induced by CRH in infant rats do not cease with administration of ACTH independent of ACTH's effect on glucocorticoid production, suggesting that downregulation of CRH synthesis may be one route of ACTH and steroid anticonvulsant action (117). ACTH may have direct pharmacologic effects that vary with age. In infant rats, ACTH acts as a proconvulsant by reducing the threshold for electrically induced seizures. In adult rats, however, ACTH increases seizure threshold and slows down the rate of kindling (118).

Circadian aspects of neurosteroid regulation are just beginning to be elucidated. Estrogens potentiate IEDs and lower seizure thresholds. Progesterone, on the contrary, decreases IEDS and increases seizure thresholds. The anti-convulsant effects of progesterone are probably mediated by its metabolites containing 3α-hydroxy-5 substitutions. For example, 5α-pregnane-3α-ol-20-one (3α, 5α-THP or alloprogesterone) is active at the GABA-A receptor and possesses anticonvulsant, and possibly neuroprotective, properties (119). Androsterone acts differently on seizures provoked by inhibition of glutamate decarboxylase (thus depleting GABA), completely abolishing seizures at noon but incompletely effective at midnight (82). The GABA-ergic system itself undergoes diurnal changes with peak activity at night (120). By virtue of the interlinked metabolism of corticosteroids and sex steroids, neurosteroids may have a role in the circadian modulation of seizures.

Exogenous Rhythms

Daily and ultradian variations in anticonvulsant drugs can be important in patients with epilepsy because clusters of seizures may occur during troughs of anti-convulsant levels. Unfavorable drug timing in relationship to endogenous rhythms may complicate management of seizures. Carbamazepine, for example, has daily variations in autoinduction of its metabolism, showing more variability in total serum levels apparent during the day than during the night (121). In contrast, valproate is absorbed less completely at night because of nocturnal changes in gastrointestinal physiology that affect disintegration of tablets (122). Daily differences in effectiveness of anticonvulsants have been demonstrated in the electroshock rat model. Low-dose diazepam is less effective between 1800 and 2200 h, although the phasic effect attenuates with higher doses (123). In practice, however, most problems related to time-of-day effects of anticonvulsant medications stem from toxicities that are managed by adjustments in dose amounts or scheduling.

Finally, exogenous stress in the form of emotional stress (115) or physiologic arousal may exacerbate seizures, and daily recurring stress may contribute to an apparent schedule of seizure recurrence. For example, case studies show that changes in schedules (shift work) can cause a similar shift in the timing of seizures. Avoidance therapy, in these cases, may aid in management of regularly recurring seizures.

SUMMARY

In conclusion, this review has focused on the organization of the circadian timing system, its basic interactions with sleep-wake state, and its putative role in the modulation of epileptic seizures and IEDs. Future work is necessary to reveal dysfunction of circadian timing attributable to seizures and the mechanisms of circadian fluctuations in seizure propensity.

REFERENCES

1. Ouyang Y, Andersson CR, Kondo T, Golden SS, Johnson CA. Resonating circadian clocks enhance fitness in cyanobacteria. Proc Nat Acad Sci USA 1998; 95:8660–8664.
2. Recht L, Lew R, Schwartz W. Baseball teams beaten by jet lag. Nature 1995; 377:583.
3. DeCoursey PJ, Krulas JR, Mele G, Holley DC. Circadian performance of suprachiasmatic nuclei (SCN)-lesioned antelope ground squirrels in a desert enclosure. Physiol Behav 1997; 62:1099–1108.
4. Stevens JR, Kodoma H, Lonsbury B, Mills L. Ultradian characteristics of spontaneous seizure discharges recorded by radio telemetry in man. Electroencephalography Clin Neurophysiol 1971; 31:313–325.
5. Parrino L, Smerieri A, Spaggiari MC, Terzano MG. Cyclic alternating pattern (CAP) and epilepsy during sleep: how a physiological rhythm modulates a pathological event. Clin Neurophysiol 2000; 111:S39–S46.
6. Herzog AG, Klein P, Ransil BJ. Three patterns of catamenial epilepsy. Epilepsia 1997; 38:1082–1088.
7. Eastman C, Mistlberger R, Rechtschaffen A. Suprachiasmatic nuclei lesions eliminate circadian temperature and sleep rhythms in the rat. Physiol Behav 1984; 32:357–368.
8. Moore RY, Eicher VB. Loss of a circadian adrenal corticosterone rhythm following suprachiasmatic lesions in the rat. Brain Res 1972; 49:403.
9. Stephan F, Zucker I. Circadian rhythms in drinking behavior and locomotor activity of rats are eliminated by hypothalamic lesion. Proc Nat Acad Sci USA 1972; 69:1583–1586.
10. Ralph MR, Foster RG, Davis FC, Menaker M. Transplanted suprachiasmatic nucleus determines circadian period. Science 1990; 247:975–978.
11. Welsh DK, Logothetis DE, Meister M, Reppert SM. Individual neurons dissociated from the suprachiasmatic nucleus express independently phased circadian firing rhythms. Neuron 1995; 14:697–706.
12. Yamazaki S, Numano R, Michikazu A, Akiko H, Takahashi R, Ueda M, Block G, Yoshiyuki S, Menaker M, Tei H. Resetting central and peripheral circadian oscillators in transgenic rats. Science 2000; 288:682–685.

13. King D, Takahashi J. Molecular genetics of circadian rhythms in mammals. Annu Rev Neurosci 2000; 23:713–742.

14. Ralph M, Menaker M. Effects of diazepam on circadian phase advances and delays. Brain Res 1986; 372:405–408.

15. Rusak B, Bina KG. Neurotransmitters in the mammalian circadian system. Annu Rev Neurosci 1990; 13:387.

16. Kalsbeek A, Buijs RM. Rhythms of inhibitory and excitatory output from the circadian timing system as revealed by in vivo dialysis. In: Buijs RM, Kalsbeek A, Romijn HJ, Pennnartz CMA, Mirmiran M, eds. Progress in Brain Research. Vol. III. Amsterdam: Elsevier, 1996:273–293.

17. Buijs, RM. The anatomical basis for the expression of circadian rhythms: the efferent projections of the suprachiasmatic nucleus. In: Buijs RM, Kalsheek A, Romijn HJ, Pennartz CMA, Mirmiran M, eds. Progress in Brain Research. Vol. III. Amsterdam: Elsevier, 1996:229–240.

18. Peng Z, Grassi–Zucconi G, Bentivoglio M. Fos-related protein expression in the midline paraventricular nucleus of the rat hypothalamus: basal oscillation and relationship with limbic efferents. Exp Brain Res 1995; 104:21–29.

19. Kalsbeek A, Cutrera RA, Van Heerikhuize JJ. GABA release from suprachiasmatic nucleus terminals is necessary for the light-induced inhibition of nocturnal melatonin release in rats. Neuroscience 1999; 91:453–461.

20. Reppert SM, Weaver DR, Ebisawa T. Cloning and characterization of a mammalian melatonin receptor that mediates reproductive and circadian responses. Neuron 1994; 13:1177–1185.

21. Tosini G, Menaker M. Circadian rhythms in cultured mammalian retina. Science 1996; 272:419–421.

22. Claridge–Chang A, Wijnen H, Rajewski N, Young MW. Circadian regulation of gene expression systems in the *Drosophila* head. Neuron 2001; 32:657–671.

23. Aldrich MS, Neurobiology of sleep. In: Sleep Medicine. Vol. 53. Oxford: Oxford University Press, 1999:27–36.

24. Borbély AA. Sleep homeostasis and models of sleep regulation. In: Kryger M, Roth T, Dement W, eds. Principles and Practice of Sleep Medicine. 2nd ed. Philadelphia: W.B. Sanders, 1994:309–320.

25. Dijk D, Czeisler C. Contribution of the circadian pacemaker and the sleep homeostat to sleep propensity, sleep structure, electroencephalographic slow waves, and sleep spindle activity in humans. J Neurosci 1995; 15:3526–3538.

26. Schwartz WJ, Reppert SM, Eagan SM, Moore-Ede MC. In vivo metabolic activity of the SCN: a comparative study. Brain Res 1983; 274:184–187.

27. Inouye S-I. Circadian rhythms of neuropeptides in the suprachiasmatic nucleus. In: Buijs R, Kalsbeek H, Romijn H, Pennartz C, Mirmiriran M, eds. Progress in Brain Research: Hypothalamic Integration of Circadian Rhythms. Vol. III. Amsterdam: Elsevier, 1996:75–90.

28. Pang S, Lee P, Chan Y. Melatonin secretion and its rhythms in biological fluids. In: Reiter R, Yu H, eds. Melatonin: Biosynthesis Physiological Effects and Clinical Applications. Boca Raton: CRC Press, 1993:130–153.

29. Rao ML, Stefan H, Bauer J, Burr W. Hormonal changes in patients with partial epilepsy: attenuation of melatonin and prolactin circadian serum profiles. In: Dreifuss FE, ed. Chronopharmacology in Therapy of Epilepsies. New York: Raven Press, 1993:55–70.

30. Schapel GJ, Beran RG, Kennaway DL, McLoughney J, Matthews CD. Melatonin response in active epilepsy. Epilepsia 1995; 36:75–78.

31. Bazil CW, Short D, Crispin D, Zheng W. Patients with intractable epilepsy have low melatonin which increases following seizures. Neurology 2000; 55:1746–1748.

32. Miyamoto A, Itoh M, Hayashi K, Hara M, Fukuyama Y. Diurnal secretion of melatonin in epileptic children, photosensitivity, and an observation of altered circadian rhythm in a case of completely under dark living condition. No to Hattatsu. Brain Dev 1993; 25:405–411. (In Japanese.)

33. Laakso ML, Leinonen L, Hatonen T, Alila A, Heiskala H. Melatonin, cortisol and body temperature rhythms in Lennox-Gastaut patients with or without circadian rhythm sleep disorders. J Neurol 1993; 240:410–416.

34. Heikkila E, Hatonen T, Telakivi T, Laakso M, Heiskala H, Salmi T, Alila A, Santavuori P. Circadian rhythm studies in neuronal ceroid-lipofuscinosis (NCL). Am J Med Genet 1995; 5:229–234.

35. Satinoff E, Liran J, Clapman R. Aberrations of the circadian body temperature rhythms in rats with medial preoptic lesions. Am J Physiol 1982; 242:R352–R357.

36. Refinetti R, Kaufman C, Menaker M. Complete suprachiasmatic lesions eliminate circadian rhythmicity of body temperature and locomotor activity in golden hamsters. J Comp Physiol Sens Neural Behav Physiol 1994; 175:223–232.

37. Quigg M, Clayburn H, Straume M, Menaker M, Bertram EH. Hypothalamic neuronal loss and altered circadian rhythm of temperature in a rat model of mesial temporal lobe epilepsy. Epilepsia 1999; 40:1688–1696.

38. Baust W, Irmscher K, Jorg J, Sommer T. Studies on the circadian periodicity in patients with the awakening type of idiopathic epilepsy (author's transl). J Neurol 1976; 213:283–294.

39. Abrams R, Hammel H. Cyclic variations in hypothalamic temperature in unanesthetized rats. Am J Physiol 1965; 208:698–702.

40. Dauch W, Bauer S. Circadian rhythms in the body temperature of intensive care patients with brain lesions. J Neurol Neurosurg Psychiatry 1990; 53:245–247.

41. Thomas K. The emergence of body temperature rhythm in preterm infants. Nurs Res 1991; 40:98–102.

42. Quigg M, Straume M. Dual epileptic foci in a single patient express distinct temporal patterns dependent on limbic versus nonlimbic brain location. Ann Neurol 2000; 48: 117–120.

43. Binnie CD, Aarts JHP, Houtkooper MA, Laxminarayan R, Martins De Silva A, Meinardi H, Nagelkerke N, Overweg J. Temporal characteristics of seizures and epileptiform discharges. Electroencephalogr Clin Neurophysiol 1984; 58:498–505.

44. Meldrum B. Endocrine consequences of status epilepticus. Adv Neurol 1983; 34:399–403.

45. Meierkord H, Shorvon S, Lightman S. Plasma concentrations of prolactin noradrenaline, vasopressin and oxytocin during and after a prolonged epileptic seizure. Acta Neurol Scand 1994; 90:73–77.

46. Sperling MR, Pritchard PB, Engel JJ, Daniel C, Sagel J. Prolactin in partial epilepsy: an indicator of limbic seizures. Ann Neurol 1986; 20:716–722.

47. Czeisler C. The effect of light on the human circadian pacemaker. CIBA Found Symp 1995; 183:254–290.

48. Richter CP. Biological Clocks in Medicine and Psychiatry. Springfield, Il: Thomas, 1965.

49. Szuba M, Baxter LJ. Electroconvulsive therapy increases circadian amplitude and lowers core body temperature in depressed patients. Biol Psychiatry 1997; 42:1130–1137.

50. Linkowski P, Mendlewicz J, Kerhofs M, Leclerq R, Golstein J, Brasseur M, Copinschi G, Van Cauter E. 24-Hour profiles of adrenocorticotropin, cortisol and growth hormone in major depressive illness: effect of antidepressant treatment. J Clin Endocrinol Metab 1987; 65:141–152.

51. Quigg M, Straume M, Smith T, Menaker M, Bertram EH. Seizures induce phase shifts of rat circadian rhythm. Brain Res 2001; 913:165–169.

52. Sanabria ER, Scorza FA, Bortolotto ZA, Calderazzo-Filho LS, Cavalheiro EA. Disruption of light-induced c-Fos immunoreactivity in the suprachiasmatic nuclei of chronic epileptic rats. Neurosci Lett 1996; 216:105–108.

53. Meldrum B, Brierley J. Prolonged epileptic seizures in primates. Ischemic cell change and its relation to ictal physiological events. Arch Neurol 1973; 28:10–17.

54. Waterhouse E, Towne A, Boggs J, Garnett L, DeLorenzo R. Circadian distribution of status epilepticus. Epilepsia 1996; 37(suppl 5):137. (Abstract.)

55. Gur AY, Bornstein NM. Are there any unique epidemiological and vascular risk factors for ischaemic strokes that occur in the morning hours? Eur J Neurol 2000; 7:179–181.

56. Feria–Velasco A, Feria–Cuevas Y, Guitierrez–Padilla R. Chronobiological variations in the convulsive effect of monosodium L-glutamate when administered to adult rats. Arch Med Res 1995; 26:S127–S132.

57. Halberg F, Bittner JJ, Gully RJ. 24 Hour periodicity and audiogenic convulsions in I mice of various ages. Proc Soc Exp Biol Med 1955; 88:169.

58. Weiss G, Lucero K, Fernandez M, Karnaze D, Castillo N. The effect of adrenalectomy on the circadian variation in the rate of kindled seizure development. Brain Res 1993; 612:354–356.

59. Freeman FG. Development of kindled seizures and circadian rhythms. Behav Neural Biol 1980; 30:231–235.

60. Gotman J, Koffler D. Interictal spiking increases after seizures but does not after decreases in medication. Electroencephalography Clin Neurophysiol 1989; 72:7–15.

61. Montplaisir J, Laverdiere M, Saint-Hilaire JM. Sleep and focal epilepsy: contribution of depth recording. In: Sterman MB, Shouse MN, Passouant P, eds. Sleep and Epilepsy. New York: Academic Press, 1982:301–314.

62. Stevens JR, Lonsbury BL, Goel SL. Seizure occurrence and interspike interval. Telemetered Electroencephalogram Studies. Arch Neurol 1972; 26:409–419.

63. Kellaway P, Frost JJ, Crawley J. Time modulation of spike and wave activity in generalized epilepsy. Ann Neurol 1980; 8:491–500.

64. Kellaway P. Sleep and epilepsy. Epilepsia 1985; 26:S15–S30.

65. Malow BA, Lin X, Kushwaha R, Aldrich MS. Interictal spiking increases with sleep depth in temporal lobe epilepsy. Epilepsia 1998; 39:1309–1316.

66. Sammaritano M, Gigli GL, Gotman J. Interictal spiking during wakefulness and sleep and the localization of foci in temporal lobe epilepsy. Neurology 1991; 41:290–297.

67. Lieb J, Joseph JP, Engel J, Walker J, Crandall JP. Sleep state and seizure foci related to depth of spike activity in patients with temporal lobe epilepsy. Electroencephalogr Clin Neurophysiol 1980; 49:538–557.

68. Sato S, Dreifuss FE, Penry JK. The effect of sleep on spike-wave discharges in absence seizures. Neurology 1973; 23:1335–1345.

69. Degen R, Degen HE. Sleep and sleep deprivation in epileptology. In: Degen R, Rodin EA, eds. Epilepsy, Sleep and Sleep Deprivation. 2nd ed. Amsterdam: Elsevier, 1991:235–239.

70. Tassinari C, Michelucci R, Salvi F, Plasmati R, Rubboli G, Bureau M, Dalla BB, Roger J. The electrical status epilepticus syndrome [review]. Epilepsy Res Suppl 1992; 6: 111–115.

71. Fountain NB, Kim JS, Lee SI. Sleep deprivation activates epileptiform discharges independent of the activating effects of sleep. J Clin Neurophysiol 1998; 15:69–75.

72. Gowers W. Course of epilepsy. In: Gowers W, ed. Epilepsy and Other Chronic Convulsive Diseases: Their Causes, Symptoms and Treatment. New York: William Wood, 1885:157–164.

73. Griffiths GM, Fox JT. Rhythm in epilepsy. Lancet 1938; 2:409–416.

74. Patry F. The relationship of time of day, sleep, and other factors to the incidence of epileptic seizures. Am J Psychiatry 1931; 10:789–813.

75. Langdon-Down M, Brain WR. Time of day in relation to convulsions in epilepsy. Lancet 1929; 1:1029–1032.

76. Halberg F, Howard RB. 24 Hour periodicity and experimental medicine: examples and interpretation. Postgrad Med 1958; 24:349–358.

77. Poirel C. Circadian chronobiology of epilepsy: murine models of seizure susceptibility and theorectical perspectives for neurology. Chronobiologia 1990; 18:49–69.

78. Quigg M, Clayburn H, Straume M, Menaker M, Bertram EH. Effects of circadian regulation and rest-activity state on spontaneous seizures in a rat model of limbic epilepsy. Epilepsia 2000; 41:505–509.

79. Lothman EW, Bertram EH, Beckenstein JW, Perlin JB. Self-sustaining limbic status epilepticus induced by "continuous" hippocampal stimulation: electrographic and behavioral characteristics. Epilepsy Res 1989; 3:107–119.

80. Bertram EH, Lothman EW, Lenn NJ. The hippocampus in experimental chronic epilepsy: a morphometric analysis. Ann Neurol 1990; 27:43–48.

81. Eidman DS, Benedito MA, Leite JR. Daily changes in pentylenetetrazole-induced convulsions and open-field behavior in rats. Physiol Behav 1990; 47:853–860.

82. Naum G, Cardozo J, Golombek DA. Daily variation in the proconvulsant effect of 3-mercaptopropionic acid and the anticonvulsant effect of androsterone in the Syrian hamster. Life Sci. 2002; 71:91–98.

83. Faradji H, Rousset C, Debilly G, Vergnes M, Cespuglio R. Sleep and epilepsy: A key role for nitric oxide? [see comments]. Epilepsia 2000; 41:794–801.

84. Cavalhiero EA, Leite JP, Bortolotto ZA, Turski WA, Ikonomidou C, Turski L. Long-term effects of pilocarpine in rats: structural damage of the brain triggers kindling and spontaneous recurrent seizures. Epilepsia 1991; 32:778–782.

85. Hellier JL, Dudek FE. Spontaneous motor seizures of kainate-induced epileptic rats: effect of time of day and activity state. Epilepsy Res 1999; 35:47–57.

86. Bertram EH, Cornett JF. The evolution of a rat model of chronic spontaneous limbic seizures. Brain Res 1994; 661:157–162.

87. Quigg M, Straume M, Menaker M, Bertram EH. Temporal distribution of partial seizures: comparison of an animal model with human partial epilepsy. Ann Neurol 1998; 43:748–755.

88. Janz D. Epilepsy and the sleeping-waking cycle. In: Magnus O, Lorentz De Haas A, eds. The Epilepsies. Vol. 15. Amsterdam: North Holland, 1974:457–490.

89. Jovanivic UJ, Das Schlafverhalten de Epileptiker I. Schlafdauer, Schlaftiefe und Besonderheiten der Schlafperiodik. Deutch Z Nerven 1967; 190:159.

90. Hayman M, Scheffer I, Chinvarum R, Berlangieri S, Berkovic S. Autosomal dominant nocturnal frontal lobe epilepsy: demonstration of focal frontal onset and intrafamilial variation. Epilepsia 1997; 49:969–975.

91. Crespel A, Baldy-Moulinier M, Coubes P. The relationship between sleep and epilepsy in frontal and temporal lobe epilepsies: practical and physiopathologic considerations. Epilepsia 1998; 39:150–157.

92. Champney TH, Peterson SL. Circadian seasonal, pineal and melatonin influences on epilepsy. In: Reiter R, Yu H, eds. Melatonin: Physiological Effects Biosynthesis and Clinical Applications. Boca Raton: CRC Press, 1993:478–494.

93. Albertson TE, Peterson SL, Stark LG, Lakin ML, Winters WD. The anticonvulsant properties of melatonin on kindled seizures in rats. Neuropharmacology 1981; 20:61–66.

94. Mevissen M, Ebert U. Anticonvulsant effects of melatonin in amygdala-kindled rats. Neurosci Lett 1998; 257:13–16.

95. Fauteck JD, Bockmann J, Bockers TM, Wittkowski W, Kohling R, Lucke A, Straub H, Speckmann EJ, Tuxhorn I, Wolf P. Melatonin reduces low-Mg^{2+} epileptiform activity in human temporal slices. Exp Brain Res 1995; 107:321–325.

96. Molina-Carballo A, Munoz-Hoyos A, Reiter RJ, Sanchez-Forte M, Moreno-Madrid F, Rufo-Campos M, Molina-Font JA, Acuna-Castroviejo D. Utility of high doses of melatonin as adjunctive anticonvulsant therapy in a child with severe myoclonic epilepsy: two years experience. J Pineal Res 1997; 23:97–105.

97. Fauteck JD, Schmidt H, Lerchl A, Kurlemann G, Wittkowski W. Melatonin in epilepsy: first results of replacement therapy and first clinical results. Biol Signals Receptors 1999; 8:105–110.

98. Yehuda S, Mostofsky DI. Circadian effects of beta-endorphin, melatonin, DSIP, and amphetamine on pentylenetetrazol-induced seizures. Peptides 1993; 14:203–205.

99. Champney TH, Hanneman WH, Legare ME, Appel K. Acute and chronic effects of melatonin as an anticonvulsant in male gerbils. J Pineal Res 1996; 20:79–83.

100. Alovi M, Gloor P. Effects of transient functional depression of the thalamus on spindles and on bilateral synchronous epileptic discharges of feline generalized penicillin epilepsy. Epilepsia 1981; 22:443–452.

101. Steriade M, Contreras D. Relations between cortical and thalamic cellular events during transition from sleep patterns to paroxysmal activity. J Neurosci 1995; 15: 623–642.

102. Steriade M, Conteras D, Amzica F. Synchronized sleep oscillations and their paroxysmal developments. Trends Neurosci 1994; 17:199–208.

103. Malow BA, Carney PR, Kushwaha R, Bowes RJ. Hippocampal sleep spindles revisited: physiologic or epileptic activity? Clin Neurophysiol 1999; 110:687–693.

104. Bertram EH, Zhang DX, Mangan P, Fountain N, Rempe D. Functional anatomy of limbic epilepsy: a proposal for central synchronization of a diffusely hyperexcitable network. Epilepsy Res 1998; 32:194–205.

105. Atkinson HC, Waddell BJ. Circadian variation in basal plasma corticosterone and adrenocorticotropin in the rat: sexual dimorphism and changes across the estrous cycle. Endocrinology 1997; 138:3842–3848.

106. Kwak SP, Young EA, Morano I, Watson SJ, Akil H. Diurnal corticotropin-releasing hormone mRNA variation in the hypothalamus exhibits a rhythm distinct from that of plasma corticosterone. Neuroendocrinology 1992; 55:74–83.

107. Buijs RM, Wortel J, Van Heerikhuize JJ, Kalsbeek A. Novel environment induced inhibition of corticosterone secretion: physiological evidence for a suprachiasmatic nucleus mediated neuronal hypothalamo-adrenal cortex pathway. Brain Res 1997; 758:229–236.

108. Ehlers CL, Henriksen SJ, Wang M, Rivier J, Vale W, Bloom FE. Corticotropin releasing factor produces increases in brain excitability and convulsive seizures in rats. Brain Res 1983; 278:332–336.

109. Baram TZ, Schultz L. Corticotropin-releasing hormone is a rapid and potent convulsant in the infant rat. Brain Res 1991; 61:97–101.

110. Baram TZ, Mitchell WG, Tournay A, Snead OC, Hanson RA, Horton EJ. High-dose corticotropin (ACTH) versus prednisone for infantile spasms: a prospective, randomized, blinded study. Pediatrics 1996; 97:375–379.

111. Swanson LW, Sawchenko PE, Rivier J, Vale WW. Organization of ovine corticotropin-releasing factor immunoreactive cells and fibers in the rat brain: an immunohistochemical study. Neuroendocrinology 1983; 36:165–186.

112. Gray TS, Bingaman EW. The amygdala: corticotropin-releasing factor, steroids, and stress. Crit Revi Neurobiol 1996; 10:155–168.

113. Merchenthaler I. Corticotropin releasing factor (CRF)-like immunoreactivity in the rat central nervous system. Extrahypothalamic distribution. Peptides 1984; 5:53–69.

114. Kovacs K, Sawchenko P. Regulation of stress-induced transcriptional changes in the hypothalamic neurosecretory neurons. J Mol Neurosci 1996; 7:125–133.

115. Frucht MM, Quigg M, Schwaner C, Fountain NB. Seizure precipitants vary with epileptic syndrome. Epilepsia 2000; 41:1534–1539.

116. Baram TZ, Hatalski CG. Neuropeptide–meditated excitability: a key triggering mechanism for seizure generation in the developing brain. Trends Neurosci 1998; 21:471–476.

117. Baram TZ, Schultz L. ACTH does not control neonatal seizures induced by administration of exogenous corticotropin-releasing hormone. Epilepsia 1995; 36: 174–178.

118. Pranzatelli M. On the molecular mechanism of adrenocorticotropin hormone in the CNS: transmitters and receptors. Exp Neurol 1994; 125:142–161.

119. Frye C. The neurosteroid 3a,5a-THP has antiseizure and possible neuroprotective effects in an animal model of epilepsy. Brain Res 1995; 696:113–120.

120. Cardinali DP, Golombek DA. The rhythmic GABAergic system. Neurochem Res 1998; 23:611–618.

121. Macphee GJ, Butler E, Brodie MJ. Intradose and circadian variation in circulating carbamazepine and its epoxide in epileptic patients: a consequence of autoinduction of metabolism. Epilepsia 1987; 28:286–294.

122. Cloyd J. Pharmacokinetic pitfalls of present antiepileptic medications. Epilepsia 1991; 32:S53–S65.

123. Schmutz M, Baud J, Glatt A, Portet C, Baltzer V. Chronopharmacological investigations on tonic-clonic seizures on rats and their suppression by carbamazepine, oxcarbazepine, and diazepam. In: Dreifuss F, Meinardi H, Stefan H, eds. Chronopharmacology in Therapy of the Epilepsies. New York: Raven Press, 1990: 145–154.

124. Herman ST, Walczak TS, Bazil CW. Distribution of partial seizures during the sleep-wake cycle. Neurology 2001; 56:1453–1459.

125. Franceschi M, Perego L, Cavagnini F, Cattaneo AG, Invitti C, Caviezel F, Strambi LF, Smirne S. Effects of long-term antiepileptic therapy on the hypothalamic-pituitary axis in man. Epilepsia 1984; 25:46–52.

126. Jovanivic UJ. Forced normalization in the EEG (Landholt) and forced abnormalization of sleep electroencephalograms. Psychiatr Neurol 1966; 152:370–386. (In German.)

127. Velasco M, Diaz-de-Leon AE, Brito F, Velasco AL, Velasco F. Sleep-epilepsy interactions in patients with intractable generalized tonic seizures and depth electrodes in the centro median thalamic nucleus. Arc Med Res 1995; 26:S117–S125.

20

Psychopathology in Epilepsy: A Window to Brain Behavior Relationships

Rochelle Caplan
UCLA Neuropsychiatric Institute
Los Angeles, California, U.S.A.

INTRODUCTION

Our understanding of the behavioral aspects of epilepsy has evolved over time in parallel with changes in the scientific conceptualization of the biological basis of behavior. Seizures were considered a supernatural phenomenon in Babylon, in ancient Greece, and during the Middle Ages. Although epilepsy was first conceptualized as a brain disorder in the 18th and 19th centuries, patients with this disorder were demonized, branded as witches, treated as outcasts, and hospitalized in special colonies.

The scientific developments of the 20th century resulted in new diagnostic and treatment strategies for epilepsy and in studies of both "interictal" and "ictal" behaviors. Accelerated development of psychiatric methodologies, psychotropic medications, and neuroimaging techniques during the 1990s resulted in identification of high rates of psychopathology and poor quality of life in adults and in children with epilepsy.

The new millennium brings with it studies on the biological basis of the behavior disorders found in epilepsy, which is the focus of this chapter. As found in other chronic illnesses, coping with epilepsy involves a wide range of intrapersonal and interpersonal psychosocial factors that affect emotional and intellectual functioning (1). Owing space limitations, this chapter reviews studies on how brain involvement affects behavior, but will not address how psychosocial factors impact the complex behavioral constellations found in epilepsy.

To understand the biological basis of the psychopathology associated with epilepsy, the chapter identifies methodological difficulties involved in designing and conducting studies on this topic and presents kindling as a possible mechanism for these behavioral disorders. The chapter then reviews the findings of studies on the biological basis of depression, schizophrenialike psychosis, anxiety, aggression, attention deficit hyperactivity disorder (ADHD), and autism associated with epilepsy. It concludes with possible future research directions needed to delineate the biological underpinnings of psychopathology in epilepsy.

METHODOLOGICAL ISSUES

To understand the biological basis of the behavioral disturbances associated with epilepsy, it is important to determine how the underlying pathology and seizures lead to these behavioral problems. More specifically, we need to ascertain if epilepsy is associated with psychopathology because of focal and/or general effects of both the underlying pathology and seizures on brain structures and pathways involved in behavior.

Although early studies suggested specific behavioral disturbances associated with temporal lobe epilepsy in adults (2–4) and in children (5–8), these findings were not confirmed by later studies (9,10). Other than a schizophrenialike psychosis found only in adults (11) and children (6,12) with complex partial seizures, patients with both focal and generalized seizure disorders have similar psychopathology (3,12,13).

It has been difficult to design studies that examine how underlying pathology and seizures contribute to psychopathology for a variety of reasons. Prior to the development of magnetic resonance imaging (MRI) technology, there were no suitable methodologies for measuring subtle abnormalities of brain structure and function without unnecessary exposure of patients to radiation. Recent studies using MRI, magnetic resonance spectroscopy (MRS), and functional magnetic resonance imaging (fMRI) provide invaluable information on morphometry, neurochemical function, and cerebral blood flow and their relationship to behavior.

In addition, several methodological problems need to be addressed to adequately study the biological basis of psychopathology in epilepsy. In terms of study design, the effect of seizures (i.e., changes in seizure frequency, duration, and severity) on behavior should be studied prospectively, for adequate time periods, and using valid behavioral measures. Although cross-sectional and retrospective studies are cheaper and easier to conduct than prospective studies, they determine the association of underlying pathology and seizures with behavior rather than the effect of seizures on behavior. Moreover, the duration of longitudinal behavioral studies in children should reflect the amount of time needed to measure developmental changes in the target behaviors.

Furthermore, numerous biological and psychosocial confounding variables limit our ability to generalize the findings of behavioral studies in epilepsy patients. The confounding biological variables include associated neurological deficits, as well as seizure-related variables, such as type of seizure disorder, number (i.e., monotherapy vs. polytherapy), type and dose of antiepileptic drugs (AEDs), and localization and lateralization of EEG findings. Socioeconomic status, ethnicity, and family and social support systems are some of the confounding psychosocial variables. In addition, cognitive (i.e., normal intelligence vs. global or specific cognitive deficits), linguistic, and developmental variables (i.e., age of onset, duration of illness, chronological age) increase the heterogeneity of the patient groups studied.

To tease out the contribution of these confounding factors to the findings of behavioral studies in epilepsy patients, these studies need to be conducted on large representative samples of subjects. For example, children with epilepsy with early age of onset often have difficult-to-control seizures (necessitating high doses of AED polytherapy), low IQ scores, and impaired language development (see review in 12). Thus, in addition to the effects of the underlying pathology and ongoing seizures, these children are at high risk for behavioral disorders due to each of the confounding factors described above. The inclusion of a large number of subjects with adequate representation across ages of onset could obviate this problem.

In addition to sample size, the importance of adequate control groups for these studies cannot be overemphasized. For example, behavioral studies of epilepsy patients with siblings as "normal" control subjects might underestimate the relationship between seizure control and psychopathology because of familial transmission of psychopathology.

Moreover, the choice of behavioral instruments might underlie differences across studies in behavioral findings (see reviews in 14,15). More specifically, structured psychiatric interviews identify higher rates of psychopathology in both adults (15) and children with epilepsy (13) than self-report, teacher, and parent questionnaires, respectively.

Despite high rates of psychopathology in adults and children with epilepsy, the wide range of psychopathology suggests that the underlying pathology and/or seizures might have a nonspecific effect on behavior, as found in other brain disorders, such as head trauma (16). Prospective studies of large samples of patients, inclusion of adequate control groups, as well as use of suitable measures of underlying pathology, seizure-related variables (i.e., type of seizures, seizure frequency, AEDs, and EEG findings), and behavior are needed to determine the mechanisms of this non-specific effect.

MECHANISMS OF THE BIOLOGICAL BASIS OF PSYCHOPATHOLOGY IN EPILEPSY

Kindling might play a role in how underlying pathology contributes to seizures, makes them recur, and causes the associated behavioral impairments (see reviews in 17,18). Since Sevillano's original study demonstrating that low levels of electrical stimulation in the hippocampus caused spontaneous seizures (19), the findings of numerous animal studies underscore the possible role of kindling in adult and pediatric epilepsy (see reviews in 18,20). More specifically, these findings suggest that the underlying pathology might set off neuroplastic changes in limbic neural circuits and their associated neurotransmitters and maintain the cascade of events that lead to both recurrent seizures and psychopathology. Increased excitation, postictal depression, rearrangement of neural circuits, formation of abnormal neural circuits, and associated neurotransmitter changes might impact numerous neural circuits involved in the modulation of emotions, interface between emotions and cognition, and other higher level functions involved in behavior.

From the neuroanatomical perspective, the hippocampus, amygdala, parahippocampal, and entorhinal cortices are important structures involved in the kindling model of complex partial seizures (see review in 18). There are numerous pathways connecting these brain regions with each other and with the neocortex, particularly the frontal lobe. There is increasing evidence for involvement of these brain regions in animal behavior (21,22) and cognition (23,24), in normal human emotional, cognitive, and social functioning (see review in 25), and in psychopathology (21,26–28). Furthermore, neurotransmitter systems implicated indifferent psychiatric conditions appear to be affected by kindling (29,30), such as the NMDA receptor (see review in 17), dopamine (31,32), noradrenaline and 5-hydroxytryptophan (30), and γ-aminobutyric acid (GABA) (33).

From the developmental perspective, the effect of brief or prolonged seizures on the brain likely depend on age (34–36). Seizures impair ongoing developmental processes (37,38). In addition, early-life seizures, without causing overt cellular damage, might predispose the brain to the damaging effect of seizures later in life (39). Furthermore, some developmental processes might be more vulnerable to the effects of kindling than others. Thus, for example, kindled immature rats demonstrated altered emotionality and activity level, but no alteration in learning and memory (24).

In summary, kindling of the limbic system and the impact on neural circuits involving the limbic system might be one of the mechanisms through which the underlying pathology and ongoing seizures affect behavior in adults and children with epilepsy.

CLINICAL EVIDENCE FOR THE BIOLOGICAL BASIS OF PSYCHOPATHOLOGY IN EPILEPSY

Depression

Although depression is the most frequent psychiatric disturbance in adults with epilepsy, there has been only one epidemiological study addressing the rate of depression in a community sample (40). Some studies find depression in 25–80% (15,41–43) of adults with epilepsy and in 23–25% of children and adolescents with epilepsy (12,13,44,45). The variability of findings could reflect use of different instruments (i.e., self-report scales; structured psychiatric interviews; questionnaires filled out by family, caretakers) and sampling effects (i.e., hospital vs. community sample, chronicity of illness, poor vs. good seizure control, seizure type, age range of patients).

Neuroimaging studies of adults with depression unrelated to epilepsy demonstrate smaller volume (26) and hypometabolism of the hippocampus (27), particularly on the left. Several cross-sectional studies have found increased depression in epilepsy patients with left-sided compared to right-sided temporal lobe epilepsy (46–48). A recent cross-sectional study demonstrated an association between mesial temporal or hippocampal sclerosis and depression, assessed with Beck's Depression Inventory, a self-report scale in adults with temporal lobe epilepsy (49). The findings of this study, however, were unrelated to lateralization of the epilepsy focus. Other studies in adults with epilepsy have not confirmed the relationship between depression and hippocampal sclerosis or depression and hippocampal atrophy (50).

Van Elst et al. described enlarged left and right amygdala in adults with dysthymia and a relationship between increased amygdala volume on the left with a trend for volume increase on the right in adults with depression (51). Although these relationships have not been studied in patients with epilepsy and depression, intermittent explosive disorder was associated with depression, anxiety, and amygdala atrophy in a subgroup of temporal lobe epilepsy (TLE) adults with aggression and a history of encephalitis (51).

Using ^{18}F-2-deoxyglucose positron emission tomography (PET), Bromfield et al. (52) found bilateral inferior frontal hypometabolism in five TLE patients with depression compared to four TLE patients without depression and normal control subjects. From these PET findings, they concluded that depression associated with TLE was similar to primary affective disorder and to depression associated with Parkinson's disease. In a cross-sectional study of 53 patients with complex partial seizures, Victoroff et al. (48) found that left or right laterality of ictal onset and degree of interictal temporal lobe hypometabolism might be interdependent factors that contribute to the risk of depression assessed with a structured psychiatric interview.

Increased, rather than decreased, perfusion in the left hemisphere was found in another SPECT study comparing 10 TLE patients with and 10 without depression, but normal perfusion values compared to nondepressed control subjects (53). However, a cross-sectional SPECT study performed with ^{99m}Tc-HMPAO on a larger sample of 40 epilepsy patients did not confirm the notion of lateralization of cerebral blood flow in the patients with depression (47).

Regarding the effect of seizures on depression, several recent prospective studies that have used well established behavioral instruments demonstrated that fewer surgically treated patients with seizure control exhibit depression than those with poor seizure control. A 2-year prospective study conducted on 39 adults following temporal lobectomy demonstrated improvement in depression. This was ascertained in patients with post-surgical seizure control using the Center for Epidemiological Studies Depression Scale (54). Helmstaedter et al. (55) described freedom from seizures and absence of depression in 161 surgically treated adults with epilepsy who had improved quality of life when seen almost 5 years after surgery. Postsurgical seizure control also predicts the absence of depression, assessed with the Minnesota Multiphasic Personality Inventory (56).

In a community-based epidemiological study of 975 patients with relatively well-controlled epilepsy, Baker et al. (40) examined the relationship between outcome of epilepsy and psychosocial variables. After eliminating the effect of psychosocial factors, seizure control was the most robust variable associated with both depression, assessed with the Hospital Anxiety and Depression Scale. Regarding type of seizure disorder, based on a structured psychiatric interview, Perini et al. (42) found a significantly higher rate of depression in 55% of adults with TLE compared to 16% of patients with juvenile myoclonic epilepsy and 10% of diabetic patients. Thus, above and beyond the effects of chronic illness, seizure type appears to be related to the severity of depression in adults with epilepsy.

Based on structured psychiatric interviews (12,13) and a self-reporting instrument (44,45), 13–26% of children and adolescents with epilepsy have depression. To date, there have been no neuroimaging studies in children with epilepsy who have depression. Unlike adults, seizure frequency and type of seizure disorder are unrelated to the presence or absence of depression in children with complex partial seizure disorder and primary generalized epilepsy with absence (12,45).

Finally, both temporal lobe epilepsy and mesial temporal sclerosis appear to have a strong genetic component, irrespective of the seizure course, as demonstrated in a cross-sectional study of 22 unrelated families with 98 individuals with a history of seizures (58). Despite strong evidence for familial effects in depression (59), only one study has shown that children with epilepsy who are treated with phenobarbital and develop depression have a higher rate of maternal depression than those who do not develop depression (60). There have been no other studies that have examined whether adults and children with a family history of depression are more vulnerable to depression than those without a family history.

In summary, the depression of adults with epilepsy appears to be associated with morphometric and functional abnormalities in mesial temporal and inferior frontal regions, areas involved in the underlying seizure disorder and in depression unrelated to epilepsy. The severity of depression is also related to seizure control and type of seizure disorder. Thus, biological factors clearly contribute to the depression of adults with epilepsy.

Similar studies have not been conducted in children. Therefore, prospective studies on large samples of children with epilepsy are needed to determine if the morphometric and functional abnormalities found in adult epilepsy patients with depression reflect the underlying pathology and/or effects of ongoing seizures on brain development.

Psychosis

Interictal psychosis can present with mood-related or schizophrenialike symptoms. Among epilepsy patients with depression, only 2.3% develop psychosis (61), and there have been no studies to date on the biological underpinnings of affective psychosis associated with epilepsy.

The rate of nonaffective, schizophrenialike, interictal psychosis in adults with epilepsy is significantly higher than in the general population (11). This type of psychosis is thought to occur in TLE rather than in other types of seizure disorders in both adults (11) and children (6,12). However, based on a large sample of 196 adults with epilepsy who had interictal psychosis and 496 epilepsy patients without psychosis, Adachi et al. (62) found similar rates in those with temporal lobe epilepsy and other types of seizure disorder. Patients with temporal lobe epilepsy present more paranoid features and those with frontal lobe epilepsy hebephrenic or disorganized features (63).

Regarding nonsurgically induced schizophrenialike psychosis, early adult studies demonstrated more extensive brain involvement based on EEG evidence of bilateral foci and associated neurological deficits in adults with epilepsy who developed psychosis than in those who did not (64,65). Recent neuroimaging studies also confirm extensive brain involvement in patients who develop a schizophrenialike psychosis.

For example, Marsh et al. (66) described ventricular enlargement and smaller temporal lobe, frontoparietal, and superior temporal gyrus gray matter volumes among nine epilepsy patients with psychosis, 18 TLE patients without psychosis, and

46 schizophrenic patients, compared to 57 healthy control subjects. The extent of these abnormalities was greatest in the patients with epilepsy and psychosis. Unlike the nonpsychotic TLE patients, the psychotic patients with epilepsy and the schizophrenic patients did not have white matter deficits in the temporal lobe or smaller hippocampi compared to the normal subjects. Among 12 adults with a schizophrenialike psychosis associated with epilepsy, those with hallucinations had significantly greater T1-weighted abnormalities in the left temporal lobe than 38 adults with epilepsy and no psychiatric disorder (67). In a retrospective study of 1008 adults with temporal lobe epilepsy, Van Elst et al. (68) described a 16–18% increase in amygdala volume bilaterally in 26 adults with a schizophrenialike psychosis compared to 24 with temporal lobe epilepsy and no psychosis and 20 normal adults.

In an MRS study Maier et al. (69) reported that 12 TLE patients with psychosis had significant reduction in N-acetyl aspartate (NAA), particularly on the left, compared to 12 TLE patients without psychosis, 26 schizophrenic, and 38 normal control subjects. The epileptic patients with psychosis also had bilateral volume reduction in the hippocampus/amygdaloid complex compared to left hippocampus/amygdala volume reduction in the nonepileptic schizophrenic patients.

Using SPECT, Mellers et al. (70) found low blood flow in the left superior temporal gyrus during performance on a verbal fluency and word repetition task in 12 epilepsy patients with a schizophrenialike psychosis, compared to a greater increase in anterior cingulate blood flow in 11 schizophrenic patients. These authors concluded that, in these two patient groups, different pathophysiological mechanisms underlie impaired performance on the same task.

In terms of the underlying pathology, several studies suggest that epilepsy surgery with seizure control might aggravate or precipitate a schizophrenialike psychosis de novo when due to a developmental lesion, such as a ganlioglioma or dysmbryoplastic neuropithelioma (71,72). Several investigators maintain that there is an antagonism between ongoing seizures and psychotic manifestations or between ictal EEG evidence and psychosis or forced normalization (73,74). This might involve changes in GABA and dopamine levels secondary to seizure control (75). Suckling et al. (76) reported that six TLE patients with psychosis had more focal lesions outside the hippocampus, less severe CA1 loss, and a trend for a higher density of calbindin-immunoreactive neurons in CA1 than 26 TLE patients without psychosis.

Several studies provide evidence for an association between psychosis associated with epilepsy and age of onset and severity of seizure disorder (77–79). A retrospective study of 25 patients with epilepsy and psychosis, 25 patients with epilepsy and major depression, and 50 nonpsychiatric epilepsy patients demonstrated earlier age of onset of epilepsy and more severe epilepsy (78). These epilepsies were characterized by a history of status epilepticus, multiple seizure types, and greater severity of seizures in the patients with psychosis compared to nonpsychiatric controls (78).

In addition, early onset and a history of prolonged febrile convulsions were two factors associated with psychosis in 12/27,773 epilepsy patients (77). Adachi et al. (63) compared 246 patients with epilepsy and psychosis to 628 without psychosis and found the following correlates of psychosis: early age of onset, family history of psychosis, and borderline intellectual functioning (63). Finally, bitemporal seizure foci, clustering of seizures, absence of febrile convulsions, younger age at onset of epilepsy, and lower verbal and full-scale IQs were found in seven adults with chronic interictal psychosis compared to 29 adults with intractable TLE with no evidence of a psychiatric disorder (79).

A schizophrenialike psychosis is also found in ~10% of children with temporal lobe epilepsy (6,12). There have been no studies to date, however, on brain morphometry in these children. Unlike adults, children with a schizophrenialike psychosis do not have forced normalization (80). In fact, seizure control was associated with improvement in the psychotic manifestations in these children (80).

Caplan et al. (81) have shown that children with complex partial seizures who have a schizophrenialike psychosis have a significantly higher incidence of thought disorders, lower IQ scores, and greater EEG evidence for left, right, or bilateral epileptic activity than those without psychosis. A pilot morphometric study in 10 medically treated children with complex partial seizure disorder compared to age- and gender-matched normal children demonstrated that asymmetry of the hippocampi, amygdalae, and thalami was associated with different aspects of thought disorder also found in schizophrenic children (82). These findings suggest that, like adults, children with a schizophrenialike psychosis associated with complex partial seizures have more extensive brain involvement.

Some of the AEDs, particularly vigabatrin, zonisamide, levetiracetam, topiramate, and tiagibine can cause psychosis (see review in 83). The mechanisms for the development of psychosis induced by AEDs and which patients are vulnerable to this side effect are unclear.

In summary, interictal schizophrenialike psychosis in adults seems to involve decreased volume, impaired neurochemical function, and reduced blood flow, particularly in temporofrontal brain regions. There is extensive evidence for structural and functional abnormalities in these regions in schizophrenia (28,84). Moreover, excitatory neurotransmitters, such as glutamate, are increased during both seizures and psychosic episode (17). Involvement of common brain structures and networks in TLE and in schizophrenia might underlie the development of a schizophrenialike psychosis in this disorder.

An interictal schizophrenialike psychosis in children occurs in children with difficult-to-control complex partial seizure disorder. What makes some children vulnerable to this disorder and the underlying biological substrates, however, has not yet been adequately studied. Factors that might impact brain development, such as poor seizure control, early age of onset, and multiple foci, as well as a family history of psychosis, underscore the importance of determining the neurobiological underpinnings of a schizophrenialike psychosis associated with TLE in both adults and children.

Anxiety

An epidemiologic study in adult epileptic patients indicated that, like depression, self-reported anxiety occurs in ~39% of a community sample (40). Manchanda et al. (85) found anxiety to be the most frequent psychiatric disorder in a large sample of 300 patients with intractable epilepsy, most of whom (77%) had TLE. Blumer et al. (61) also reported frequent anxiety, albeit less frequently than atypical mood disorder in 97 patients undergoing inpatient video-EEG telemetry.

Despite evidence that kindling of the amygdala is involved in anxiety and in epilepsy (21), there have been no neuroimaging studies to date on the amygdala in patients with epilepsy associated with anxiety symptoms. However, anxiety persists after epilepsy surgery in temporal lobe epilepsy patients who continue to have fear auras, compared to other auras (86), and in those having undergone left-sided surgery (53). These findings imply that, in addition to the stress involved in adaptation to a chronic illness, anxiety associated with TLE might reflect limbic dysfunction involving the amygdala (42,86).

With regard to seizure type, 40% of patients with TLE had anxiety based on state and trait anxiety scales, but there was no evidence of anxiety in 18 juvenile myoclonic epilepsy and 20 diabetic patients (42). In terms of seizure control, as described for self-report of depression, Baker et al. (40) have shown that, after removing the robust effect of psychosocial variables, poor seizure control is associated with self-report of anxiety. There have been no studies on the association of age of onset and anxiety in adults with epilepsy.

Unlike adults with epilepsy, in children with complex partial seizures and children with primary generalized epilepsy with absence, there is no difference in the rate of anxiety disorder (12,13). The presence of anxiety disorder in children with these types of seizure disorder is unrelated to seizure control, AEDs, and age of onset. As described for adults with epilepsy, there have been no neuroimaging studies on the amygdala in these children.

Aggression

The exact frequency of aggression in patients with epilepsy is unknown, as there are no published epidemiological studies. However, aggression is one of the most common reasons for referring patients with epilepsy to a mental health clinician. In terms of the biological basis for aggression in epilepsy, Woermann et al. (87) found a relationship between reduction in gray matter in the left frontal lobe and aggression in adults with temporal lobe epilepsy who have intermittent explosive disorder. As previously mentioned, Van Elst et al. (51) reported that 20% of TLE patients with aggression have atrophy of the amygdala, a history of encephalitis, left-sided or bilateral EEG abnormalities. Furthermore, AEDs, such as barbiturates (88), benzodiazepines (89), and some of the newer AEDs, such as gabapentin (90), topiramate (91), and vigabatrin (92), also cause irritability and aggression, particularly when high doses of polytherapy are used.

In summary, the high clinical morbidity associated with aggression together and the relative dearth of information on the biological basis of aggression in patients with epilepsy underscore the importance of performing studies on this topic.

Attention Deficit Hyperactivity Disorder (ADHD)

In epileptic children, ADHD is found in ~25% of patients with normal cognition (12), and in ~5–7% with mental retardation (7,93). Despite early descriptions suggesting that hyperactivity was prominent in children with temporal lobe epilepsy (7,8), and attentional problems occurred in children with petit mal (94,95), the presence of ADHD does not appear to be related to the type of seizure disorder or to the degree of seizure control (12). Thus, 23% of children with complex partial seizure disorder and 25% of children with petit mal meet criteria for ADHD using a structured psychiatric interview (12). Several case studies suggest that certain AEDs, such as gabapentin (90,96), vigabatrin (92), phenobarbital (88,97), and topiramate (91), can also induce ADHD symptoms in children.

There are no published reports on the biological mechanisms underlying ADHD symptoms associated with epilepsy in children. However, greater deficits in attention in children with ADHD and complex partial seizure disorder, compared to those with ADHD without seizure disorder during the continuous performance task (98), suggest that the psychopathology underlying epilepsy and/or ongoing seizures might contribute to attentional impairments.

Autism

Young children with a history of infantile spasms exhibit a high rate of autism (11%), particularly those with EEG and CT evidence for temporal lobe abnormalities (99) and bilateral temporal hypometabolism on PET (100). Children with infantile spasms and tuberous sclerosis have a higher rate of autism (101), particularly those with tubers localized to the temporal lobe (102). About two-thirds of children with infantile spasms who also have autism meet criteria for hyperkinetic disorder (101), and ~15% of children with infantile spasms have severe "nonautistic" overactivity (57). Involvement of frontotemporal structures and pathways in infantile spasms might underlie the deficits in social communication and language (103), as well as the impaired visual attention (104) found in the autism associated with this seizure disorder.

CONCLUSIONS AND FUTURE DIRECTIONS

Austin et al. (105) have recently shown that behavioral disturbances predate the onset of epilepsy in some children, particularly if they have uncontrolled seizures. These findings suggest that behavioral disturbances might be integrally related to the pathogenesis and evolution of the underlying seizure disorder.

Therefore, prospective studies of large samples of children, adolescents, and adults with both new-onset and chronic epilepsy that use well-established behavioral measures, biological measures (e.g., EEG, evoked responses, neuroimaging), as well as appropriate control groups are needed to delineate the mechanisms underlying the behavioral disorders associated with epilepsy. The findings of these studies would be an important first step in designing future interventional studies.

The previously reviewed associations among the severity of the seizure disorder, the extent of brain involvement, and the morbidity of the psychopathology underscore the significance of conducting studies that would focus on mitigating both seizures and associated psychopathology. For example, extensive evidence for the psychotropic effects of AEDs highlights the need for drug studies on both seizures and psychopathology in patients with epilepsy. Use of functional and structural neuroimaging measures in these studies would advance our knowledge and provide a window of the biological mechanisms of the brain/behavior relationships in epilepsy.

REFERENCES

1. Caplan R. Epilepsy syndromes in childhood. In: Coffey CE, Brumback RA, eds. Textbook of Pediatric Neuropsychiatry. American Psychiatric Association Press. 1998: 977–1010.

2. Bear DM, Fedio P. Quantitative analysis of interictal behavior in temporal lobe epilepsy. Arch Neurol 1977; 34:454–467.

3. Hermann BP, Riel P. Interictal personality and behavioral traits in temporal lobe and generalized epilepsy. Cortex 1981; 17:125–128.

4. Geschwind N. Behavioural changes in temporal lobe epilepsy. Psychol Med. 1979; 9: 217–219.

5. Hoare P, Kerley S. Psychosocial adjustment of children with chronic epilepsy and their families. Dev Med Child Neurol 1991; 33:201–215.

6. Lindsay JJ, Ounsted C, Richards P. Long-term outcome in children with temporal lobe seizures. III. Psychiatric aspects in childhood and adult life. Dev Med Child Neurol 1979; 21:630–636.

7. Rutter M, Graham P, Yule W. A Neuropsychiatric Study in Childhood. London: S.I.M.P./William Heinemann, 1970.

8. Stores G. School-children with epilepsy at risk for learning and behavioral problems. Dev Med Child Neurol 1978; 20:502–508.

9. Apter A, Aviv A, Kaminer Y, Weizman A, Lerman P, Tyano S. Behavioral profile and social competence in temporal lobe epilepsy of adolescence. J Am Acad Child Adolesc Psychiatry 1991; 30:887–892.

10. Garyfallos G, Manos N, Adamopoulou A. Psychopathology and personality characteristics of epileptic patients: epilepsy, psychopathology and personality. Acta Psychiatr Scand 1988; 78:87–95.

11. Bredkjaer SR, Mortensen PB, Parnas J. Epilepsy and non-organic non-affective psychosis. National epidemiologic study. Br J Psychiatry 1998; 72:235–238.

12. Caplan R, Arbelle S, Magharious W, Guthrie D, Komo S, Shields WD, Chayasirisobhon S, Hansen R. Psychopathology in pediatric complex partial and primary generalized epilepsy. Dev Med Child Neurol 1998; 40:805–811.

13. Ott D, Caplan R, Guthrie D, Komo S, Chayasirisobhon S, Hansen R, Shields WD. Measures of psychopathology in children with complex partial seizures and primary generalized epilepsy with absence. J Am Acad Child Adolesc Psychiatry 2000; 40: 907–914.

14. Salzberg MR, Vajda FJ. Epilepsy, depression and antidepressant drugs J Clin Neurosci 2001; 8:209–215.

15. Glosser G, Zwil AS, Glosser DS, O'Connor MJ, Sperling MR. Psychiatric aspects of temporal lobe epilepsy before and after anterior temporal lobectomy. J Neurol Neurosurg Psychiatry 2000; 68:53–58.

16. Max JE, Roberts MA, Koele SL, Lindgren SD, Robin DA, Arndt S, Smith WL Jr, Sato Y. Cognitive outcome in children and adolescents following severe traumatic brain injury: influence of psychosocial, psychiatric, and injury-related variables. J Int Neuropsychol Soc 1999; 5:58–68.

17. Kraus JE. Sensitization phenomena in psychiatric illness: lessons from the kindling model. J Neuropsychiatry Clin Neurosci 2000; 12:328–343.

18. Leung LS, Ma J, McLachlan RS. Behaviors induced or disrupted by complex partial seizures. Neurosci Biobehav Rev 2000; 24:763–775.

19. McNamara JO. Kindling model of epilepsy. Adv Neurol 1986; 44:303–318.

20. Bragin A, Wilson CL, Engel J Jr. Chronic epileptogenesis requires development of a network of pathologically interconnected neuron clusters: a hypothesis. Epilepsia 2000; 41(suppl 6):S144–S152.

21. Adamec R, Young B. Neuroplasticity in specific limbic system circuits may mediate specific kindling induced changes in animal affect—implications for understanding anxiety associated with epilepsy. Neurosci Biobehav Rev 2001; 24:705–723.

22. Kalynchuk LE, Pinel JP, Treit D. Long-term kindling and interictal emotionality in rats: effect of stimulation site. Brain Res 1998; 779:149–157.

23. Hannesson DK, Howland J, Pollock M, Mohapel P, Wallace AE, Corcoran ME. Dorsal hippocampal kindling produces a selective and enduring disruption of hippocampally mediated behavior. J Neurosci 2001; 15(21):4443–4450.

24. Holmes GL, Chronopoulos A, Stafstrom CE, Mikati MA, Thurber SJ, Hyde PA, Thompson JL. Effects of kindling on subsequent learning, memory, behavior, and seizure susceptibility. Brain Res Dev Brain Res 1993; 21(73):71–77.

25. Adolphs R. The neurobiology of social cognition. Curr Opin Neurobiol 2001; 11:231–239.

26. Mervaala E, Fohr J, Kononen M, Valkonen-Korhonen M, Vainio P, Partanen K, Partanen J, Tiihonen J, Viinamaki H, Karjalainen AK, Lehtonen J. Quantitative MRI of the hippocampus and amygdala in severe depression. Psychol Med 2000; 30:117–1125.

27. Saxena S, Brody AL, Ho ML, Alborzian S, Ho MK, Maidment KM, Huang SC, Wu HM, Au SC, Baxter LR Jr. Cerebral metabolism in major depression and obsessive-compulsive disorder occurring separately and concurrently. Biol Psychiatry 2001; 50:159–170.

28. Sigmundsson T, Suckling J, Maier M, Williams S, Bullmore E, Greenwood K, Fukuda R, Ron M, Toone B. Structural abnormalities in frontal, temporal, and limbic regions and interconnecting white matter tracts in schizophrenic patients with prominent negative symptoms. Am J Psychiatry 2001; 158:234–243.

29. Ferencz I, Leanza G, Nanobashvili A, Kokaia Z, Kokaia M, Lindvall O. Septal cholinergic neurons suppress seizure development in hippocampal kindling in rats: comparison with noradrenergic neurons. Neuroscience 2001; 102:819–832.

30. Shouse MN, Staba RJ, Ko PY, Saquib SF, Farber PR. Monoamines and seizures: microdialysis findings in locus ceruleus and amygdale before and during amygdala kindling. Brain Res 2001; 892:176–192.

31. Gelbard HA, Applegate CD. Persistent increases in dopamine D2 receptor mRNA expression in basal ganglia following kindling. Epilepsy Res 1994; 17:23–29.

32. Kraus JE, Sensitization phenomena in psychiatric illness: lessons from the kindling model. J Neuropsychiatry Clin Neurosci 2000; 12:328–343.

33. Rossler AS, Schroder H, Dodd RH, Chapouthier G, Grecksch G. Benzodiazepine receptor inverse agonist-induced kindling of rats alters learning and glutamate binding. Pharmacol Biochem Behav 2000; 67(1):169–175.

34. Sankar R, Shin D, Mazarati AM, Liu H, Katsumori H, Lezama R, Wasterlain CG. Epileptogenesis after status epilepticus reflects age- and model-dependent plasticity. Ann Neurol 2000; 48:580–589.

35. Sperber EF, Veliskova J, Germano IM, Friedman LK, Moshe SL. Age-dependent vulnerability to seizures. Adv Neurol 1999; 79:161–169.

36. Sutula TP, Pitkanen A. More evidence for seizure-induced neuron loss: is hippocampal sclerosis both cause and effect of epilepsy? Neurology 2001; 57:169–170.

37. Wasterlain CC, Sankar R. Excitotoxicity and the developing brain. In: Avanzinin G, Fariello R, Heinemann U, Mutani R, eds. Epileptogenic and Excitotoxic Mechanisms. London: Libbey and Company, 1993:135–151.

38. Wasterlain CC, Thompson KW, Kornblum H, Mazarati AM, Shirasaka Y, Katsumori H. Long-term effects of recurrent seizures on the developing brain. In: Nehlig A, Motte J, Moshe SL, Plouin P, eds. Childhood Epilepsies and Brain Development. London: Libbey and Company, 1999:237–254.

39. Koh S, Storey TW, Santos TC, Mian AY, Cole AJ. Early-life seizures in rats increase susceptibility to seizure-induced brain injury in adulthood. Neurology 1999; 53:915–921.
40. Baker GA, Jacoby A, Chadwick DW. The associations of psychopathology in epilepsy: a community study. Epilepsy Res 1996 25:29–39.
41. Paradiso S, Hermann BP, Blumer D, Davies K, Robinson RG. Impact of depressed mood on neuropsychological status in temporal lobe epilepsy. J Neurol Neurosurg Psychiatry 2001; 70:180–185.
42. Perini GI, Tosin C, Carraro C, Bernasconi G, Canevini MP, Canger R, Pellegrini A, Testa G. Interictal mood and personality disorders in temporal lobe pilepsy and juvenile myoclonic epilepsy. J Neurol Neurosurg Psychiatry 1996; 61:601–615.
43. Mendez MF, Cummings JL, Benson DF. Depression in epilepsy. Significance and phenomenology. Arch Neurol 1986; 43:766–770.
44. Dunn DW, Austin JK, Huster GA. Symptoms of depression in adolescents with epilepsy. J Am Acad Child Adolesc Psychiatry 1999; 38:1132–1138.
45. Ettinger AB, Weisbrot DM, Nolan EE, Gadow KD, Vitale SA, Andriola MR, Lenn NJ, Novak GP, Hermann BP. Symptoms of depression and anxiety in pediatric epilepsy patients. Epilepsia 1998; 39:595–599.
46. Altshuler LL, Devinsky O, Post RM, Theodore W. Depression, anxiety, and temporal lobe epilepsy. Arch Neurol 1990; 47:284–288.
47. Schmitz EB, Moriarty J, Costa DC, Ring HA, Ell PJ, Trimble MR. Psychiatric profiles and patterns of cerebral blood flow in focal epilepsy: interactions between depression, obsessionality, and perfusion related to the laterality of the epilepsy. J Neurol Neurosurg Psychiatry 1997; 62:458 463
48. Victoroff J, Benson DF, Grafton ST. Depression in complex partial seizures. Arch Neurol 1994; 511:155–163.
49. Quiske A, Helmstaedter C, Lux S, Elger CE. Depression in patients with temporal lobe epilepsy is related to mesial temporal sclerosis. Epilepsy Res 2000; 39:121–125.
50. Lehrner J, Kalchmayr R, Serles W, Olbrich A, Pataraia E, Aull S, Bacher J, Leutmezer F, Groppel G, Deecke L, Baumgartner C. Health-related quality of life (HRQOL), activity of daily living (ADL) and depressive mood disorder in temporal lobe epilepsy patients. Seizure 1999; 8:88 92
51. Van Elst LT, Woermann F, Lemieux L, Trimble MR. Increased amygdala volumes in female and depressed humans. A quantitative magnetic resonance imaging study. Neurosci Lett 2000; 281(2 3):103.
52. Bromfield EB, Altshuler L, Leiderman DB, Balish M, Ketter TA, Devinsky O, Post RM, Theodore WH. Cerebral metabolism and depression in patients with complex partial seizures. Arch Neurol 1992; 49:617–623.
53. Ring HA, Acton PD, Scull D, Costa DC, Gacinovik S, Trimble MR. Patterns of brain activity in patients with epilepsy and depression. Seizure 1999; 8:390–397.
54. Derry PA, Rose KJ, McLachlan RS. Moderators of the effect of preoperative emotional adjustment on postoperative depression after surgery for temporal lobe epilepsy. Epilepsia 2000; 41:177–185.
55. Helmstaedter C, Kurthen M, Lux S, Johanson K, Quiske A, Schramm J, Elger CE. Temporal lobe epilepsy: longitudinal clinical, neuropsychological and psychosocial follow-up of surgically and conservatively managed patients. Nervenarzt 2000; 71: 629–642.
56. Hermann BP, Wyler A, Somes G. Preoperative psychological adjustment and surgical outcome are determinants of psychosocial status after anterior temporal lobectomy. J Neurol Neurosurg Psychiatry 1992; 55:491–496.
57. Caplan R, Gillberg C. Child psychiatric disorders. In: Engel J Jr, Pedley T, eds. Epilepsy: A Comprehensive Textbook. Vol. 2. New York: Raven Press, 1998:2125–2139.

58. Kobayashi E, Lopes-Cendes I, Guerreiro CAM, Sousa SC, Guerreiro MM, Cendes F. Seizure outcome and hippocampal atrophy in familial mesial temporal lobe epilepsy. Neurology 2001; 56:166–172.

59. Zubenko GS, Zubenko WN, Spiker DG, Giles DE, Kaplan BB. Malignancy of recurrent, early-onset major depression: a family study. Am J Med Genet 2001; 105: 690–699.

60. Brent DA, Crumrine PK, Varma R, Brown RV, Allan MJ. Phenobarbital treatment and major depressive disorder in children with epilepsy: a naturalistic follow-up. Pediatrics 1990; 85:1086–1091.

61. Blumer D, Montouris G, Hermann BP. Psychiatric morbidity in seizure. patients on a neurodiagnostic monitoring unit. J Neuropsychiatry Clin Neurosci 1995; 7:445–456.

62. Adachi N, Onuma T, Hara T, Matsuura M, Okubo Y, Kato M, Oana Y. Frequency and age-related variables in interictal psychoses in localization-related epilepsies. Epilepsy Res 2002; 48:25–31.

63. Adachi N, Onuma T, Nishiwaki S, Murauchi S, Akanuma N, Ishida S, Takei N. Interictal and post-ictal psychoses in frontal lobe epilepsy: a retrospective comparison with psychoses in temporal lobe epilepsy. Seizure 2000; 9:328–335.

64. Hermann BP, Whitman S. Neurobiological, psychosocial, and pharmacological factors underlying interictal psychopathology in epilepsy. Adv Neurol 1991; 55:439–452.

65. Stevens JR. Psychosis and epilepsy. Ann Neurol 1983; 14:347–348.

66. Marsh L, Sullivan EV, Morrell M, Lim KO, Pfefferbaum A. Structural brain abnormalities in patients with schizophrenia, epilepsy, and epilepsy with chronic interictal psychosis. Psychiatry Res 2001; 108:1–15.

67. Conlon P, Trimble MR, Rogers D. A study of epileptic psychosis using magnetic resonance imaging. Br J Psychiatry 1990; 156:231–235.

68. Van Elst LT, Baeumer D, Lemieux L, Woermann FG, Koepp M, Krishnamoorthy S, Thompson PJ, Ebert D, Trimble MR. Amygdala pathology in psychosis of epilepsy: a magnetic resonance imaging study in patients with temporal lobe epilepsy. Brain 2002; 125:140–149.

69. Maier M, Mellers J, Toone B, Trimble M, Ron MA. Schizophrenia, temporal lobe epilepsy and psychosis: an in vivo magnetic resonance spectroscopy and imaging study of the hippocampus/amygdala complex. Psychol Med 2000; 30:571–581.

70. Mellers JD, Toone BK, Lishman WA. A neuropsychological comparison of schizophrenia and schizophrenia-like psychosis of epilepsy. Psychol Med 2000; 30: 325–335.

71. Andermann LF, Savard G, Meencke HJ, McLachlan R, Moshe S, Andermann F. Psychosis after resection of ganglioglioma or DNET: evidence for an association. Epilepsia 1999; 40:83–87.

72. Roberts GW, Done DJ, Bruton C, Crow TJ. A "mock up" of schizophrenia: temporal lobe epilepsy and schizophrenia-like psychosis. Biol Psychiatry 1990; 28:127–143.

73. Wolf P. Acute behavioral symptomatology at disappearance of epileptiform EEG abnormality. Paradoxical or "forced" normalization. Adv Neurol 1991; 55:127–142.

74. Krishnamoorthy ES, Trimble MR. Forced normalization: clinical and therapeutic relevance. Epilepsia 1999; 40(suppl 10):S57–S64.

75. Ring HA, Trimble MR, Costa DC, George MS, Verhoeff P, Ell PJ. Effect of vigabatrin on striatal dopamine receptors: evidence in humans for interactions of GABA and dopamine systems. J Neurol Neurosurg Psychiatry 1992; 55:758–761.

76. Suckling J, Roberts H, Walker M, Highley JR, Fenwick P, Oxbury J, Esiri MM. Temporal lobe epilepsy with and without psychosis: exploration of hippocampal pathology including that in subpopulations of neurons defined by their content of immunoreactive calcium-binding proteins. Acta Neuropathol 2000; 99:547–554.

77. Kanemoto K, Kim Y, Miyamoto T, Kawasaki J. Presurgical postictal and acute interictal psychoses are differentially associated with postoperative mood and psychotic disorders. J Neuropsychiatry Clin Neurosci 2001; 13:243–247.

78. Schmitz EB, Robertson MM, Trimble MR. Depression and schizophrenia in epilepsy: social and biological risk factors. Epilepsy Res 1999; 35:59–68.

79. Umbricht D, Degreef G, Barr WB, Lieberman JA, Pollack S, Schaul N. Postictal and chronic psychoses in patients with temporal lobe epilepsy. Am J Psychiatry 1995; 152:224–231.

80. Caplan R. Shields WD, Mori L, Yudovin S. Middle childhood onset of interictal psychoses: case studies. J Child Adolesc Psychiatry 1991; 30:893–896.

81. Caplan R, Guthrie D, Komo S, Siddarth P, Chayasirisobhon S, Kornblum H, Sankar R. Social communication deficits in pediatric epilepsy. J Child Psychol Psychiatry Allied Disciplines 2002; 43:245–253.

82. Levitt J, Caplan R, Blanton R, Magharious W, Guthrie D, Komo S. Hippocampal morphology and communication deficits in pediatric complex partial seizure disorder. Annual Meeting of the American Academy of Child and Adolescent Psychiatry, Toronto, Canada, October 1997.

83. Besag FM. Behavioural effects of the new anticonvulsants. Drug Saf 2001; 24:513–536.

84. Hirayasu Y, Tanaka S, Shenton ME, Salisbury DF, DeSantis MA, Levitt JJ, Wible C, Yurgelun-Todd D, Kikinis R, Jolesz FA, McCarley RW. Prefrontal gray matter volume reduction in first episode schizophrenia. Cereb Cortex 2000; 11:374–381.

85. Manchanda R, Schaefer B, McLachlan RS, Blume WT, Wiebe S, Girvin JP, Parrent A, Derry PA. Psychiatric disorders in candidates for surgery for epilepsy. J Neurol Neurosurg Psychiatry 1996; 61:82–89.

86. Kohler CG, Carran MA, Bilker W, O'Connor MJ, Sperling MR. Association of fear auras with mood and anxiety disorders after temporal lobectomy. Epilepsia 2001; 42:674–681.

87. Woermann FG, Van Elst LT, Koepp MJ, Free SL, Thompson PJ, Trimble MR, Duncan JS. Reduction of frontal neocortical grey matter associated with affective aggression in patients with temporal lobe epilepsy: an objective voxel by voxel analysis of automatically segmented MRI. J Neurol Neurosurg Psychiatry 2000; 68:162–169.

88. Chen Y, Chi Chow J, Lee I. Comparison the cognitive effect of anti-epileptic drugs in seizure-free children with epilepsy before and after drug withdrawal. Epilepsy Res 2001; 44:65–70.

89. Sheth RD, Goulden KJ, Ronen GM. Aggression in children treated with clobazam for epilepsy. Clin Neuropharmacol 1994; 17:332–337.

90. Khurana DS, Riviello J, Helmers S, Holmes G, Anderson J, Mikati MA. Efficacy of gabapentin therapy in children with refractory partial seizures. J Pediatr 1996; 128: 829–833.

91. Elterman RD, Glauser TA, Wyllie E, Reife R, Wu SC, Pledger G. A double-blind, randomized trial of topiramate as adjunctive therapy for partial-onset seizures in children. Topiramate YP Study Group. Neurology 1999; 52:1338–1344.

92. Gobbi G, Pini A, Bertani G, Menegati E, Tiberti A, Valseriati D, Besana D, Rasmini P, Guerrini R, Belmonte A, Veggiotti P, Resi C, Lanzi G, Capovilla G, Galeone D, Milani S. Prospective study of first-line vigabatrin monotherapy in childhood partial epilepsies. Epilepsy Res 1999; 35:29–37.

93. Steffenburg U, Hagberg G, Viggedal G, Kyllerman M. Active epilepsy in mentally retarded children. I. Prevalence and additional neuroimpairments. Acta Paediatr 1995; 84:1147–1152.

94. Duncan CC. Application of event-related brain potentials to the analysis of interictal attention in absence epilepsy. In: Myslobodsky MS, Mirsky AF, eds. Elements of Petit Mal Epilepsy. New York: Peter Lang, 1988:341–364.

95. Mirsky AF. Information processing in petit mal epilepsy. In: Hermann BP, Seidenberg M, eds. Childhood Epilepsies: Neuropsychological, Psychosocial, and Intervention Aspects. New York: John Wiley & Sons, 1989:51–80.

96. Lee DO, Steingard RJ, Cesena M, Helmers SL, Riviello JJ, Mikati MA. Behavioral side effects of gabapentin in children. Epilepsia 1996; 37:87–90.

97. Domizio S, Verrotti A, Ramenghi LA, Sabatino G, Morgese G. Anti-epileptic therapy and behaviour disturbances in children. Childs Nerv Syst 1993; 9:272–274.

98. Semrud-Clikeman M, Wical B. Components of attention in children with complex partial seizures with and without ADHD. Epilepsia 1999; 40:211–215.

99. Riikonen R. A long-term follow-up study of 214 children with the syndrome of infantile spasms. Neuropediatrics 1982; 13:14–23.

100. Chugani HT, Da Silva E, Chugani DC. Infantile spasms. III. Prognostic implications of bitemporal hypometalbolism on positron emission tomography. Ann Neurol 1996; 3:643–649.

101. Riikonen R, Amnell G. Psychiatric disorders in children with earlier infantile spasms. Dev Med Child Neurol 1981; 23:747–760.

102. Bolton PF, Griffiths PD. Association of tuberous sclerosis of temporal lobes with autism and atypical autism. Lancet 1999; 349:392–395.

103. Caplan R, Siddarth P, Mathern G, Vinters H, Curtiss S, Levitt J, Asarnow R, Shields WD. Developmental outcome with and without successful intervention. In: Schwartzkroin PA, Rho J, eds. Epilepsy, Infantile Spasms, and Developmental Encephalopathy. Int Rev Neurobiol 2002: 49:269–284.

104. Jambaque I, Chiron C, Dulac O, Raynaud C, Sirota P. Visual inattention in West syndrome: a neuropsychological and neurofunctional imaging study. Epilepsia 1993; 34:692–700.

105. Austin JK, Harezlak J, Dunn DW, Huster GA, Rose DF, Ambrosius WT. Behavior problems in children before first recognized seizures. Pediatrics 2001; 107:115–122.

21
Novel Mechanisms of Drug Delivery

Jacquelyn L. Bainbridge, Janina Z.P. Janes, and D. Scott Pollock
Univeristy of Colorado Health Sciences Center
Denver, Colorado, U.S.A.

INTRODUCTION

A major focus of drug development is the formulation of novel drug delivery systems. Novel or new mechanisms of drug delivery offer patients the potential to enhance their quality of life by providing more convenient dosing intervals, fewer side effects, less drug-related toxicity, and better therapeutic control. New delivery systems are developed with certain patient populations in mind—for example, rectal diazepam gel (Diastat) in the pediatric population to abort acute repetitive seizures (ARS).

This chapter will focus on the novel mechanisms of drug formulation and delivery that enhance antiepileptic drug (AED) therapy. We will comment on the following novel AED preparations: (1) oxcarbazepine (Trileptal); (2) fosphenytoin (Cerebyx); (3) valproate sodium injection (Depacon); (4) carbamazepine extended release (Tegretol XR); (5) carbamazepine extended release (Carbatrol); (6) divalproex sodium extended release (Depakote ER); (7) extended phenytoin sodium (Phenytek); (8) lamotrigine (Lamictal) chewable dispersible tablets; (9) carbamazepine (Tegretol) chewable tablets; (10) topiramate (Topamax) sprinkle capsules; and (11) diazepam (Diastat) rectal gel. In addition, we will discuss future novel drug delivery systems for AEDs.

PRODRUGS

A prodrug is the inactive parent compound that is converted or metabolized to a drug with therapeutic activity (1). This approach to drug formulation is used to achieve sustained or rate- and time-controlled drug delivery, and is an alternative to sustained release formulations.

Oxcarbazepine (Trileptal)

Oxcarbazepine (OXC), an active 10-keto analog of carbamazepine (CBZ), is considered by some a prodrug (2–5). OXC was designed to be better tolerated than carbamazepine while maintaining equal efficacy (4). OXC is extensively and rapidly metabolized to the biologically active 10-monohydroxy metabolite (MHD). When patients need to be converted from carbamazepine to oxcarbazepine, a CBZ:OXC ratio of 1:1.5 is usually used for the conversion that can be made abruptly without need to titrate one drug or the other. Thus, a patient on 600 mg/d of carbamazepine is converted to 900 mg/day of OXC (6). Based on experience, some clinicians prefer a ratio of 1:1.2 of carbamazepine to OXC.

Fosphenytoin (Cerebyx)

Prodrugs can be developed to overcome insolubility of the parent compound. An example of this is fosphenytoin, designed to decrease the risk of cardiac arrhythmias and thrombophlebitis, which have been reported with IV phenytoin administration (7). It is a water-soluble phosphate ester of phenytoin that can be given through IV or IM routes, and is rapidly hydrolyzed within 15 min (8,9). Fosphenytoin is highly protein bound and competes with phenytoin for its binding site. Initially, this leads to a higher fraction of unbound phenytoin because fosphenytoin displaces phenytoin from the binding site. Equilibrium is achieved rapidly as more fosphenytoin is converted to phenytoin (10). Investigators have characterized the extent and the tolerability of IM loading doses of fosphenytoin. In an open-label, double-blind study, fosphenytoin produced therapeutic serum phenytoin concentrations within 5–20 min and was well tolerated (11).

Fosphenytoin dosage is expressed in phenytoin equivalents (PEs). Thus, 100 mg of phenytoin is equivalent to 100 mg fosphenytoin PE. There is no need to convert or recalculate dosing. Fosphenytoin can be infused up to 150 mg PE/min. In status epilepticus, an emergency situation defined operationally as a seizure (or seizures of seizures without full recovery) lasting >30 min, fosphenytoin should be given at 150 mg/min to mimic phenytoin given at its maximum infusion rate of 50 mg/min (12). Figure 1 is an example of phenytoin plasma concentrations following administration of 1200 mg PE fosphenytoin infused at 100 mg or 150 mg PE/min, and 1200 mg phenytoin infused at 50 mg/min to healthy volunteers (13). Consideration should be given to patients with severe renal impairment when choosing fosphenytoin over phenytoin due to the amount of phosphate delivered with fosphenytoin administration (0.0037 mmol phosphate/mg PE fosphenytoin) that is not eliminated by the kidney (13).

INJECTABLE PREPARATIONS

Immediate therapeutic blood levels are necessary in emergent situations, like status epilepticus. By avoiding the stomach, duodenum, and liver, some pharmacokinetic principles such as absorption and potential first-pass effect are circumvented (14). The IV or IM routes of administration can be useful when oral therapy is interrupted or when serum levels need to be elevated immediately to prevent seizures.

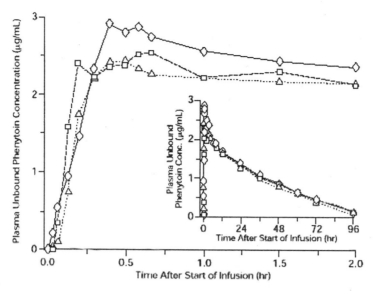

Figure 1. Phenytoin plasma concentration. (Courtesy of Pfizer Pharmaceuticals.)

Fosphenytoin (Cerebyx)

Fosphenytoin preparation does not require propylene glycol or ethanol for increased solubility, permitting faster and safer administration (15). Phenytoin preparation with propylene glycol and ethanol can cause thrombophlebitis, pain, burning, and irritation at the injection site (16). Tissue necrosis, phlebitis, and muscle damage can also be seen with phenytoin administration (17). Fosphenytoin is formulated for safe administration intramuscularly when nonemergent serum concentrations of phenytoin are required. Serum levels should be obtained two hours after an IV dose, and 4 h after an IM dose (18).

Purple glove syndrome has not been reported with fosphenytoin, as it has with phenytoin (11,19). Hypotension is documented less frequently with fosphenytoin than phenytoin when given by the IV route of administration (11,20,21). In status epilepticus, Lowenstein and Alldredge have illustrated a treatment algorithm utilizing fosphenytoin (22). Fosphenytoin produces fewer episodes of cardiac arrhythmias due to the reformulation of phenytoin. A unique side effect of fosphenytoin not encountered with phenytoin is parasthesias of the groin, head, neck, and abdomen, a phenomenon seen with other phosphate ester prodrugs (11).

Valproate Sodium Injection (Depacon)

Valproate sodium is a broad-spectrum antiepileptic drug (AED). The injectable formulation was designed initially as a temporary replacement (to be administered no more than 14 days) to the oral divalproex sodium (Depakote). Depacon is formulated to be only administered by the IV and not the IM route. When patients' drug therapy with Depakote is interrupted due to surgery or other conditions making oral therapy impractical or impossible, the IV formulation is given at similar doses on a milligram-to-milligram basis; e.g., Depacon 500 mg is equivalent to Depakote 500 mg. Current Food and Drug Administration (FDA) guidelines recommend that Depacon (diluted in at least 50 mL of dextrose 5%, sodium chloride 0.9%, or lactated Ringer's) be administered over 60 min, but at a rate no faster than 20 mg/min. If necessary, Depacon can be administered safely rapid infusion rates of (i.e., 1.5–3 mg/kg/min). In one clinical study, patients received up to 15 mg/ kg with a mean dose 1184 mg over 5–10 min, infusion rate of 1.5–3 mg/kg (23). Venkataraman and Wheless (24) studied rapid infusion at higher doses in 21 patients with epilepsy. These authors reported that Depacon was well tolerated at rates up to 6 mg/kg/min and at mean doses of 24 mg/kg (24). In order to maintain the patient's serum levels above 50 μg/mL when switching from IV to PO route, the oral dose must be administered within 1–2 h after the last IV dose for the patients who receive concomitant enzyme-inducing medications. For patients not on an enzyme-inducing medication, Depakote should be given within 2–4 h of the last IV dose of Depacon (25). If the patient is being converted to divalproex ER, the extended-release formulation should be given either concomitantly or at least 1 h after the last infusion of Depacon (26,27).

NEW EXTENDED-RELEASE FORMULATIONS

Carbamazepine (Tegretol XR)

Tegretol XR is widely used in the treatment of neuropathic pain, mood disorders, and partial seizures with or without secondary generalization. Traditional carbamazepine formulations were designed to be dosed at least three times a day. It is well known that compliance decreases as multiple daily doses increase (28). Noncompliance is the most common cause of breakthrough seizures in the patient with epilepsy (29). Tegretol XR was designed to provide more stable serum concentrations while allowing for potentially twice-daily dosing. The OROS drug delivery system was designed by Alza Corporation and used by Novartis Pharmaceuticals to manufacture Tegretol XR (Fig. 2). The principal mechanism of drug delivery involves osmotic release.

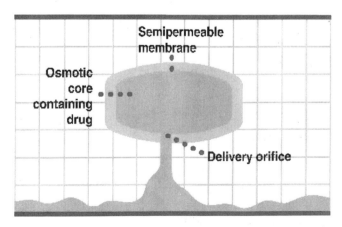

Figure 2. OROS XR. Tegretol XR. (From Novartis Pharmaceuticals Corp.)

Carbamazepine Extended Release (Carbatrol)

Carbamazepine extended-release capsules utilize the Microtrol formulation, a novel drug delivery system developed by Shire-Richwood. This new formulation was developed to be taken twice daily and to allow for greater dosing flexibility in different patient populations. Carbatrol can be swallowed whole or the capsule can be opened and the contents sprinkled on food. This is in contrast to valproate sodium delayed release (DR), which is designed for enteric protection, therefore diminishing its breakdown in the low pH milieu of the stomach (30). The Carbatrol formulation is ideal for children and for many elderly patients who have trouble swallowing whole tablets or capsules.

The Microtrol formulation utilizes immediate-release, extended-release, and enteric-release beads in a fixed ratio, which provides smoother, more predictable serum drug levels (Fig. 3). The uncoated, immediate-release beads constitute 25% of the capsule and dissolve immediately upon swallowing. The extended-release beads comprise 40% of capsule contents, and dissolution takes place over 8–12 h. This is accomplished via a polymer coat that allows slow diffusion of carbamazepine through tiny micropores. The final 35% represents enteric-release beads that are pH sensitive and thus allows for the slowest release of carbamazepine in the

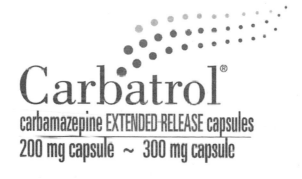

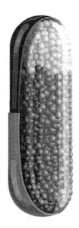

25%
Immediate-release beads
release carbamazepine almost as soon as swallowed for rapid absorption.[2]

40%
Extended-release beads
dissolve gradually over 8 to 12 hours to achieve steady state.[2]

35%
Enteric-release beads
with pH-sensitive coating release carbamazepine slowly in gut to maintain optimal levels.[2]

Figure 3. Microtrol formulation, Carbatrol. (From Shire-Richwood.)

small bowel (31). When switching patients from immediate-release formulation carbamazepine to Carbatrol, one should divide the total daily dose of carbamazepine in half. This is the dose of Carbatrol that the patient will take twice a day (31). No significant changes in seizure intensity or frequency have been observed with such mg-to-mg conversions (32). When taken every 12 h, Carbatrol is bioequivalent to carbamazepine immediate-release taken every 6 h (33). Carbatrol comes as 200- and 300-mg capsules, is not affected by GI transit time, and can be taken with food or on an empty stomach.

Divalproex Sodium Extended-Release (Depakote ER)

Depakote ER is not currently approved by the FDA for the treatment of epilepsy; rather, it is approved for migraine prevention. This formulation is intended for once-daily dosing. Depakote ER allows for smoother serum concentrations with a peak occurring ~4 h after ingestion. Depakote ER has an extended action lasting ~24 h. Fluctuations in the serum concentration of Depakote ER fluctuation are ~10–20% less then Depakote. However, Depakote ER and Depakote DR tablets are not bioequivalent. The bioavailability of Depakote ER on average when given once a day is 81–89% as compared to Depakote DR tablets given twice a day (34). Additionally, for Depakote ER, the maximum serum concentration (C_{max}) was lower and the minimum serum concentration was higher. This reinforces the need for higher daily doses of Depakote ER by ~14% as compared to Depakote DR (35).

Extended Phenytoin Sodium (Phenytek)

Extended phenytoin sodium was introduced to enhance patient's adherence when prescribed traditional phenytoin 300 mg/d. Under a traditional formulation, a patient would need to take three Dilantin Kapseals, 100 mg each per dose. This new formulation allows for convenient dosing when patients may or may not be on multiple medications. It is estimated that ~50% of patients who have epilepsy are noncompliant with their AEDs (36).

The Phenytek design uses an erodible matrix system for drug delivery. This system controls the rate at which phenytoin is released. The technology allows for reproducible dissolution and uniform profile (37). Each capsule of Phenytek, which is available in 200-mg and 300-mg units, contains two or three cylindrical erodible matrix tablets (200 mg, 300 mg) within each capsule. This allows the patient to take fewer capsules than the traditional formulation.

As the capsule shell dissolves and exposes the inside tablets, the outer surfaces of those tablets hydrate, form a gel layer, and begin to release phenytoin sodium. When the tablets move further along the gastrointestinal system, with continued fluid exposure, the gel layer still expands and the tablets continue to erode. This process continues until only small individual particles remain. The drug will continue to be released providing the conditions still exist for erosion (37) (Fig. 4). Fasting and fed studies indicate that the bioequivalence of Phenytek 300-mg capsules is equal to that of Dilantin Kapseals 300 mg (3 × 100 mg) (37). The half-life of Phenytek capsules is similar to that of Dilantin Kapseals.

Erodible-Matrix Delivery System‡

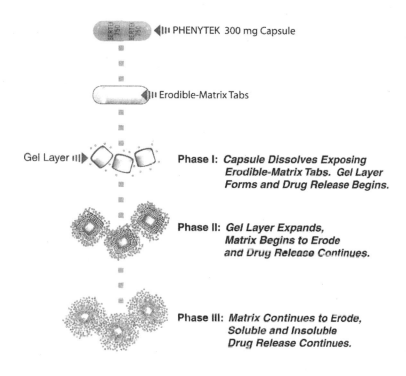

Gel Layer ॥▶

Phase I: *Capsule Dissolves Exposing Erodible-Matrix Tabs. Gel Layer Forms and Drug Release Begins.*

Phase II: *Gel Layer Expands, Matrix Begins to Erode and Drug Release Continues.*

Phase III: *Matrix Continues to Erode, Soluble and Insoluble Drug Release Continues.*

‡Artist's Interpretation.

Figure 4. Erodible matrix delivery system, Phenytek. (From Bertek Pharmaceuticals.)

CHEWABLE TABLETS

Lamotrigine (Lamictal) Chewable Dispersible Tablets

Lamotrigine is a broad-spectrum AED and is used commonly in the pediatric population, especially those with Lennox-Gastaut syndrome (LGS) (38–41). Lamotrigine has efficacy in the elderly as well: however, the traditional tablet strength limits its use in these two patient populations. The chewable dispersible tablet is berry flavored and available as 2-, 5-, and 25-mg tablets. Once the patient reaches his therapeutic dose after a dose escalation phase, the traditional tablet strength can then be used. The chewable tablets can be chewed, swallowed whole, or dispersed in at least 5 mL or 1 tsp water or diluted fruit juice. Approximately 1 min later, when the tablets are completely dispersed, the solution should be mixed and the entire amount taken immediately (42). This dosage form is considered therapeutically bioequivalent to the standard formulation, and the two forms are interchangable (43).

Carbamazepine (Tegretol) Chewable Tablets

The berry-flavored chewable carbamazepine tablets are available in 100-mg strength. The chewable formulation is beneficial in at least two populations—in pediatric patients, and in the elderly. It is a good alternative for adults who have difficulty swallowing and where precise dose escalation is required. The bioavailability of the chewable tablet is similar to other carbamazepine formulations, such as suspensions and slow-release tablets (44,45).

Topiramate (Topamax) Sprinkle Capsules

Topiramate is another broad-spectrum AED. Topiramate is used in the treatment of children and adults with primary generalized tonic-clonic seizures or with partial-onset seizures (46–49). Topiramate also has efficacy in Lennox-Gastaut syndrome (50). The new sprinkle capsule formulation is especially beneficial when a smaller dose is needed either for the pediatric population, in dose-escalation for adults, or in those adults who are unable to swallow whole tablets or capsules. It is available in 15- and 25-mg capsules that may be opened and sprinkled on food without affecting absorption. The capsule may also be swallowed whole.

Topiramate sprinkles may not be given through a nasogastric tube (NGT) because aggregation and clogging have been observed with this method of delivery. If topiramate is to be given through a NGT, the traditional formulation tablets must be crushed, suspended in water, and used immediately and not stored (51).

The unique sprinkle formulation of topiramate contains topiramate-coated beads in a hard gelatin capsule. Topiramate sprinkle capsules are bioequivalent to the traditional tablet formulation, and thus may be considered a therapeutic substitution. The contents of the sprinkle capsules may be emptied on top of a small amount (e.g., teaspoonful) of soft food, such as applesauce, custard, ice cream, oatmeal, pudding, or yogurt. All of the capsule's contents may be sprinkled out of the gelatin capsule onto a spoonful of soft food. The entire mixture of the topiramate sprinkles and food should be swallowed by the patient immediately after mixing to avoid loss of stability (52).

LIQUID PREPARATIONS

Many AEDs are manufactured in a liquid form for a variety of reasons. Patients in need of a liquid formulation are children, the elderly, the developmentally disabled, and adults who are unable to swallow oral preparations (53). Liquids can be used to precisely escalate the dose of AEDs with a known therapeutic index or dose-related toxicity. AEDs that are water soluble are formulated as solution, and those that are not water soluble are prepared as suspensions (54). Examples of AEDs that are commercially available as a solution in the United States are sodium valproate, gabapentin, and phenobarbital (an elixir). Vigabatrin is available in other countries as a solution. Examples of AEDs that are manufactured as a suspension are carbamazepine, phenytoin, primidone, felbamate, and oxcarbazepine. Suspension formulations should always be shaken before administration to ensure proper drug distribution throughout the liquid, thus providing for consistent dosage.

RECTAL FORMULATION

Rectal administration offers a beneficial route of administration where drugs are absorbed through passive diffusion. The surface area for drug absorption of the rectum is 1/10,000 as compared to the upper gastrointestinal (GI) tract. There is little intraluminal fluid in the rectum that may decrease drug absorption (55). Lipid-soluble drugs are better absorbed in the rectum than those that are not or less lipid soluble. In comparison to oral medications, first-pass metabolism is greatly reduced with rectal administration (15).

Diazepam (Diastat) Rectal Gel

Benzodiazepines are the drugs of choice for the management of status epilepticus and acute seizures (56). Rectal administration may be preferred when IV access is delayed or difficult. Additionally, rectal administration empowers the caregiver to treat acute repetitive seizures in the home or outpatient environment (such as schools). This delivery system is much more convenient than using diazepam solution rectally because it is prefilled with the appropriate dose. This product was designed to offer an easy, safe, and bioavailable alternative to administering diazepam IV (57).

An alternative to diazepam rectal gel is diazepam IV solution given rectally, but there are problems with this approach. This administration requires that the caregiver store the medication as specified by the company, measure the appropriate dose of diazepam with a syringe, administer it correctly, and dispose of needles appropriately, leaving much room for error (58). The novel formulation of diazepam rectal gel allows the patient to be treated at home instead of in the emergency department (ED).

This diazepam rectal delivery system is a nonsterile rectal gel provided in a prefilled, unit-dose syringe. Diazepam rectal gel is available in 2.5-, 5-, or 10-mg pediatric syringes with a 4.4-cm tip. It is available in adult syringes in 10, 15, and 20 mg with a 6-cm tip. In contrast to rectal lorazepam solution that has slower absorption, the high lipid solubility of diazepam rectal gel permits rapid absorption and penetration into the CNS (59). Diazepam rectal gel absorption proceeds more rapidly than oral or IM administration (60).

One study that compared IV diazepam to diazepam rectal gel demonstrated that mild cognitive effects could completely resolve within 4 h of administration of the rectal gel (57). Diazepam is well absorbed in the rectum, providing peak plasma concentrations in 1.5 h (61). The absolute bioavailability of diazepam rectal gel relative to diazepam injectable is 90.4% (57). Diazepam rectal gel contains diazepam, propylene glycol, ethyl alcohol (10%), hydroxypropyl methylcellulose, sodium benzoate, benzyl alcohol (1.5%), benzoic acid, and water.

FUTURE DEVELOPMENTS

The need for new and improved mechanisms of drug delivery still exists and is continually being investigated. There are many limitations of the current technology for AED delivery. A few limitations include CNS and systemic side effects, permeability of the AED across the blood-brain barrier (BBB) to the site of action, lack of uniform medication efficacy, and AED nonadherence. Novel mechanisms of drug delivery should then include medications that are delivered to the site of seizure generation and prior to onset of the event. Several examples of emerging approaches deserve mention.

Levetiracetam is approved as adjunctive treatment in the United States for the treatment of partial seizures in adults over 16 years of age. It is, however, being used in pediatrics, and the company is exploring use of a 10% solution (53).

A unique and important class of conotoxins, the ω-conotoxins isolated from the piscivorous species of cone snail, selectively inhibit neuronal voltage-sensitive calcium channels (VSCCs) found in mammals. ω-Conotoxins have varying affinity and selectivity for neuronal VSCC subtypes found in mammals, making them widely used research tools for defining the distribution and role of neuronal VSCC subtypes. Recently, one such conotoxin, CGX-1007 (Cognetix), has been identified as useful for the treatment of seizures (62).

CGX-1007 has high NMDA receptor subtype selectivity (63). This compound also has a high picomole potency. Plans for human delivery of this compound are through the Medtronic Synchromed Infusion Pump. Phase I human trials are complete and were performed with IV exposure to assess the human risk if the reservoir on the pump was missed by the needle used to refill. The compound is 17 amino acids in length, and to date there have not been any immunologic consequences. The proposed Phase IIA trial includes six patients with intrathecal infusion with the Medtronic pump. Three patients will be hospitalized to closely examine safety endpoints. Doses of CGX-1007 will be increased every 3 days to the maximum tolerated dose.

SP0294, also known as SPD 421, DP16, or DP-VPA, is valproate in a phospholipid carrier, currently in Phase I clinical trials. When this product is available, it will offer another AED with a novel mechanism of delivery (64). The agent is a prodrug that will allow delivery of the active drug to the site of seizure activity. This will limit many systemic side effects. The technology used with the phospholipid valproate is known as regulated activation of prodrugs (D-RAP) (65). The combination of valproic acid in the phospholipid complex is inert until seizure activity is sensed in the brain. At that moment valproic acid is cleaved from the complex after exposure to phospholipase A2 (PIA2) released at the site of epileptic activity (66). SPD 421 has been evaluated in one Phase I healthy-subject clinical trial and found to be well tolerated (67).

Omental tissue transplantation to the anterior perforated space and left temporal lobe has been evaluated in two patients (68). Transplanting fetal pig neurons into the epileptogenic zone of persons with epilepsy is currently being investigated along with stem cell transplantation. These cell and neuronal transplants and a device that could predict seizures up to 3 min before they occur are being researched (69).

Another investigational protocol underway is a direct brain infusion of muscimol (chemical similar to γ-aminobutyric acid, the major inhibitory neurotransmitter in the mammalian CNS) in patients undergoing standard epilepsy surgery. The objective of this protocol is to localize the epileptogenic focus, and may help in the treatment of patients with medically intractable epilepsy (70). This may be beneficial in aborting seizure activity since a higher drug concentration can be delivered to the site of action and less to other organs, thereby reducing the risk of systemic side effects.

Adenosine, an endogenous neuromodulator, reduces excitatory neuronal transmission and postsynaptic excitability. These effects are mediated by adenosine A_1 receptors (71). Under normal conditions, adenosine is found in low concentrations within the extracellular space. Researchers are investigating several mechanisms of adenosine delivery to block seizure activity. A group of researchers have engineered fibroblasts to release adenosine by inactivating the adenosine-metabolizing enzymes adenosine kinase and deaminase. Kindled rats were implanted with encapsulated semipermeable polymers of the engineered adenosine to study its effects on seizure activity. The local release of adenosine, resulting in concentrations < 25 nM at the site of action, was significant to suppress many seizures. This novel mechanism of therapy provides a potential therapeutic strategy for pharmacoresistant partial epilepsies (72).

Intravenous midazolam for febrile and prolonged seizures in children has been studied in the buccal (73,74), oral, rectal, and intranasal (75,76) routes of administration. For practical purposes, we will only discuss the buccal and intranasal routes of administration. Of note, other benzodiazepines have been examined in the sublingual and rectal routes of administration (77). Scott and colleagues reported rapid absorption and block of seizure activity after administration of buccal midazolam (73). The efficacy of buccal midazolam in comparison to rectal diazepam supports the use of the buccal route of administration (74). Buccal midazolam is preferred by some over intranasal midazolam due to fewer side effects and easier administration (78).

The implantable Vagus Nerve Stimulator (VNS, manufactured by Cyberonics) is currently available on the market (79). This device is placed in the upper chest area and wrapped around the left vagus nerve; it delivers periodic electrical pulses to abort seizure activity. Transcranial magnetic stimulation (TMS) is currently being studied in subjects with partial-onset seizures. The outcome of one such study has been mixed; the effect was short-lived and had only a mild impact on seizures (80).

There are several medications in clinical trials to date that are being evaluated for efficacy in patients with epilepsy. Although not representing novel mechanisms of delivery, these are future therapies that may become available for patients within the next few years (see Table 1).

It is now well accepted that certain forms of familial epilepsies are due to mutations in genes encoding proteins comprising voltage- or ligand-gated channels. These monogenetic epilepsies are currently being intensely investigated, and may lead to a better understanding of idiopathic epilepsies (79,80).

A new understanding of the mechanisms of AED failure is emerging. Most prominent is the role of the P-glycoprotein transporter system found throughout the body. This transporter system is found in the blood-brain barrier, liver, intestinal wall, biliary system, kidney, and placenta. Its role has been best characterized in cancer chemotherapy as a major cause of multidrug resistance (81,82). The P-glycoprotein system is a transporter system that pumps medications through the BBB (83,84). Much research is focused on ways to bypass the P-glycoprotein system by delivering AEDs directly to the site of action. Implantable microsystems would allow local delivery of minute doses of medication directly into the epileptogenic area, thus over coming the P-glycoprotein system (85,86). This can be accomplished

Table 1. Antiepileptic Drugs in Clinical Trials

Drug	Phase of study
Pregabalin	Phase III
Rufinamide	Phase III
Retigabine	Phase III
Carabersat	Phase II
Talamparel	Phase II
Valrocemide	Phase II
Harkoseride	Phase II
AWD131-138	Phase I
NPS 1776	Phase I
NW1015	Phase I
SP0294 (DP-VPA)	Phase I

by using an implantable pump with a catheter that delivers the drug to the epileptogenic area prior to a seizure, and minimizes the peripheral exposure of the medication (87,88). Drugs can also be used in this system even if they do not cross the BBB. The major risk of these systems involves surgery and its complications.

SUMMARY

Many novel delivery systems based on modifications of pharmacokinetic and pharmacodynamic variables have been reviewed in this chapter. All antiepileptic agents discussed represent the application of science and technology to minimize the side-effects profile, enhance convenience of the dosing interval, or obtain better therapeutic control. Through clinical trial validation the discussed medications have been much improved over their first-generation ancestors.

Currently available medications or formulations can still place some patients in the position of enduring recurrent and unpredictable seizures and adverse effects, thereby diminishing the patients' quality of life. The development of a pharmacokinetically enhanced AED that is peripherally administered may no longer be a rational approach, particularly as there is a greater appreciation of transport systems that can remove compounds outside of the BBB. The future treatment of epilepsy will likely depend on the development of drugs and delivery systems designed to provide precise local delivery of effective medications. To this end, the technological challenge will be to develop implantable microsystems that are cosmetically favorable to the patient, and that can be placed with minimal risk.

REFERENCES

1. Ansel HC, Allen LV, Popovich NG. Pharmaceutical Dosage Forms and Drug Delivery Systems, 7th ed. Philadelphia: Lippincott Williams & Wilkins, 1999:130.
2. Bialer M. Oxcarbazepine. Chemistry, biotransformation, and pharmacokinetics. In: Levy RH, Mattson RH, Medrum BS, Perucca E, eds. Antiepileptic Drugs, 5th ed. New York: Raven Press, 2002:458.

3. Shorvon S. Emergency treatment of epilepsy: acute seizures, serial seizures, seizure clusters and status epilepticus. In: Shorvon S, ed. Handbook of Epilepsy Treatment. Oxford, UK: Blackwell Science, 2000:118.

4. Sillanpaa ML. Carbamazepine and oxcarbazepine. In: Wyllie E, ed. The Treatment of Epilepsy. Philadelphia: Lippincott Williams & Wilkins, 2001:821–842.

5. Keltner NL, Folks DG. Psychotropic Drugs, 3rd ed. St. Louis: Mosby 2001:273.

6. Beydoun A. Safety and efficacy of oxcarbazepine results of randomized, double-blind trials. Pharmacotherapy 2000; 20(8 pt 2):S152–158.

7. Glauser TA, Graves NM. Phenytoin and fosphenytoin. In: Wyllie E, ed. The Treatment of Epilepsy, 3rd ed. Philadelphia: Lippincott Williams & Wilkins, 2001.

8. Shorvon S. Emergency treatment of epilepsy: acute seizures, serial seizures, seizure clusters and status epilepticus. In: Shorvon S, ed. Handbook of Epilepsy Treatment. Oxford, UK: Blackwell Science, 2000:189.

9. Leppik IE, Boucher BA, Wilder BJ. Pharmacokinetics in safety of phenytoin prodrug given IV in patients. Neurology 1990; 40:456–460.

10. Lai CM, Moore P, Quon CY. Binding of fosphenytoin, phosphate ester prodrug of phenytoin, to human serum proteins and competitive binding with carbamazepine, diazepam, phenobarbital, phenylbutazone, phenytoin, valproic acid or warfarin. Res Commun Mol Pathol Pharmacol 1995; 88:51–62.

11. Pryor FM, Ramsay RE, Gidal BE. Fosphenytoin: pharmacokinetics and tolerance of intramuscular loading doses. Epilepsia 2001, 42:245–250.

12. Eldon MA, Loewen GR, Voigtman RE. Pharmacokinetics and tolerance of fosphenytoin and phenytoin administration intravenously to healthy subjects. Can J Neurol Sci 1993; 20:S180.

13. Boucher BA. Fosphenytoin: a novel phenytoin prodrug. Pharmacotherapy 1996; 16:777–791.

14. Ansel HC, Allen LV, Popovich NG. Pharmaceutical Dosage Forms and Drug Delivery Systems, 7th ed. Philadelphia: Lippincott Williams & Wilkins, 1999:127.

15. Garnett WR, Cloyd JC. Dosage form considerations in the treatment of pediatric epilepsy. In: Pellock JM, Dodson WE, Bourgeois BFD, eds. Pediatric Epilepsy: Diagnosis and Therapy, 2nd ed. New York: Demos, 2001; 329–341.

16. Jameison BD, Dukes GF, Grouwer KLR. Venous irritation related to intravenous administration of phenytoin versus fosphenytoin. Pharmacotherapy 1994; 14:47–52.

17. Spengler RF, Arrowsmith JB, Kilarski DJ. Severe soft-tissue injury following intravenous infusion of phenytoin: patient and drug administration risk factors. Arch Intern Med 1988; 148:1329–1333.

18. Browne TR, Kugler AR, Eldon MA. Pharmacology and pharmakokinetics of fosphenytoin. Neurology 1996; 46(suppl 1):S3–S7.

19. O'Brien TJ, Cascino GD, So EL, Hanna DR. Incidence and clinical consequence of the purple glove syndrome in patients receiving intravenous phenytoin. Neurology 1998; 51:1034–1039.

20. Browne TR. Fosphenytoin (Cerebryx). Clin Neuropharmacol 1997; 20:1–12.

21. Luer MS. Fosphenytoin. Neurol Res 1998; 20:178–182.

22. Lowenstein DH, Alldredge BK. Status epilepticus. N Engl J Med 1998; 338:970–976.

23. Depacon. Package insert. Abbott Laboratories.

24. Venkataraman V, Wheless JW. Safety of rapid intravenous infusion of valproate loading doses in epilepsy patients. Epilepsy Res 1999; 35:147–153.

25. Cavanaugh JH, Hussein Z, Lamm J, Granneman GR. Pharmcokinetics of multiple oral dose divalproex sodium after intravenous loading dose administration in healthy volunteers. Drug Invest 1994; 7(1):1–7.

26. Dutta S, Cloyd JC, Granneman RG, Sommerville KW. Oral/intravenous maintanence dosing of valproate following intravenous loading: a simulation. Poster presented at American Epilepsy Society Annual Meeting, Nov 30 to Dec 5, 2001, Philadelphia.

27. Boggs JG, Nowack WJ, Maertens PM, Drinkard R. Successful initiation of antiepileptic therapy with a combination of Depacon and Depakote ER in the epilepsy monitoring unit. Poster presented at American Epilepsy Society Annual Meeting, Nov 30 to Dec 5, 2001, Philadelphia.

28. Cramer JA, Mattson RH, Prevey ML, Scheyer RD, Ouellette VL. How often is medication taken as prescribed. JAMA 1989; 261(22):3273.

29. Ciba-Geigy. Data on file.

30. Cloyd JC, Kriel RL, Jones-Saete CM. Comparison of sprinkle vs syrup formulations of valproate for bioavailability, tolerance, and preference. J Pediatr 1992; 120:634–638.

31. Shire-Richwood. Data on file.

32. Mirza WU, Rak IW, Thadani VM. Six month evaluation of Carbatrol (extended-release carbamazepine) in complex partial seizures. Neurology 1998; 51:1727–1729.

33. Garnett WR, Levy B, McLean AM. Pharmacokinetic evaluation of twice-daily extended-release carbamazepine (CBZ) and four-times-daily immediate-release CBZ in patients in epilepsy. Epilepsia 1998; 39(3):274–279.

34. Abbott Laboratories. Data on file.

35. Dutta S, Zhang Y, Selness DS, Lee LL, Williams LA, Sommerville KW. Comparsion of the bioavailability of unequal doses of divalproex sodium extended-release formulation relative to the delayed-release formulation in healthy volunteers. Epilepsy Res 2002; 49:1–10.

36. Leppik IE. How to get patients with epilepsy to take their medication: the problem with nonadherence. Postgrad Med 1990; 88(1):253–256.

37. Bertek Pharmaceuticals. Data on file.

38. Eriksson AS, Nergardh A, Hoppu K. The efficacy of lamotrigine in children and adolescents with refractory generalized epilepsy: a randomized, double-blind, crossover study. Epilepsia 1998; 39(5):495–501.

39. Motte J, Trevathan E, Arvidsson JF. Lamotrigine for generalized seizures associated with the Lennox-Gastaut syndrome. Lamictal Lennox-Gastaut Study Group. N Engl J Med 1997; 337(25):1807–1812.

40. Farrell K, Connolly MB, Munn R. Prospective, open-label, add-on study of lamotrigine in 56 children with intractable generalized epilepsy. Pediatr Neurol 1997; 16(3):201–205.

41. Motte J, Trevathan E, Arvidsson JVF. Lamotrigine for generalized seizures associated with the Lennox-Gastaut syndrome. N Engl J Med 1997; 337:1807–1812.

42. GlaxoSmithKline. Package insert, Lamictal Chewable.

43. Wheless J, Venkataraman V. New formulations of drugs in epilepsy. Exp Opin Pharmacother 1999; 1(1):49–60.

44. Patsalos PN. A comparitive pharmacokinetic study of conventional and chewable carbamazepine in epileptic patients. Br J Clin Pharmacol 1990; 29:574–577.

45. Wolf P, May T, Tiska G, Schreiber G. Steady state concentrations and diurnal fluctuations of carbamazepine in patients after different slow release formulations. Drug Res 1992; 42(1):284–288.

46. Privitera M, Fincham R, Penry J. Topiramate placebo-controlled dose-ranging trial in refractory partial epilepsy using 600-, 800-, and 1000-mg daily dosages. Neurology 1996; 46(6):1678–1683.

47. Faught E, Wilder BJ, Ramsay RE. Topiramate placebo-controlled dose-ranging trial in refractory partial epilepsy using 200-, 400-, and 600-mg daily dosages. Neurology 1996; 46(6):1684–1690.

48. Biton V, Montouris GD, Ritter F. A randomized, placebo-controlled study of topiramate in primary generalized tonic-clonic seizures. Neurology 1999; 52:1330–1337.

49. Elterman RD, Glauser TA, Wyllie E. A double-blind, randomized trial of topiramate as adjunctive therapy for partial-onset seizures in children. Neurology 1999; 52(7): 1338–1344.

50. Sachdeo RC, Glauser TA, Ritter F. A double-blind, randomized trial of topiramate in Lennox-Gastaut syndrome. Topiramate YL Study Group. Neurology 1999; 52(9): 1882–1887.

51. Ortho-McNeil. Data on file.

52. Ortho-McNeil. Package insert.

53. Bourgeois B. New dosages and formulations of AEDs for use in pediatric epilepsy. Neurology 2002; 58(suppl 7):S2–S5.

54. Bialer M, Cloyd JC. General principles: drug formulations and routes of administration. In: Levy RH, Mattson RH, Meldrum BS, eds. Antiepileptic Drugs, 4th ed. New York: Raven Press, 1995.

55. De Boer AG, Moolenaar F, De Leed LGJ. Rectal drug administration: clinical pharmacokinetic considerations. Clin Pharmacokinet 1982; 7:285–311.

56. Working Group on Status Epilepticus. Treatment of convulsive status epilepticus: recommendations of the Epilepsy Foundation of America's Working Group on Status Epilepticus. JAMA 1993; 270:854–859.

57. Cloyd JC, Lalonde RL, Beniak TE, Novack GD. A single-blind, crossover comparison of the pharmacokinetics and cognitive effects of a new diazepam rectal gel with intravenous diazepam. Epilepsia 1998; 39:520–526.

58. Cereghino RR, Mitchell WG, Murphy J, Kriel RL, Rosenfeld WE, Trevathan E. The North American Diastat Study Group. Neurology 1998; 51:1274–1282.

59. Schmidt D. Benzodiazepines: diazepam. In: Levy RH, Mattson RH, Meldrum BS, eds. Antiepileptic Drugs, 4th ed. New York: Raven Press, 1995:705–724.

60. Moolenaar F, Bakker S, Visser J, Huizinga T. Biopharmaceutics of rectal administration of drugs in man. IX. Comparative biopharmaceutics of diazepam after single rectal, oral, intramuscular and intravenous administration in man. Int J Pharmacol 1980; 5:127–137.

61. Xcel Pharmaceuticals, Inc. Data on file.

62. Lewis RJ. Ion channel toxins and therapeutics: from cone snail 10—venoms to ciguatera. Therapeutic Drug Monitoring 2000; 22:61–64.

63. McCabe RT. CGX-1007. Antiepileptic Drug Trials VI meeting. Oct 2001, Sonesta Beach Resort, FL.

64. Duncan JS. The promise of new antiepileptic drugs. Br J Clin Pharmacol 2002; 53:123–131.

65. Regulated Activation of Prodrugs (D-RAP) D-Pharm, Rehovot, Israel.

66. Perucca E, Kupferberg HJ. Drugs in development. Drugs in early clinical development. In: Levy RH, Mattson RH, Medrum BS, Perucca E, eds. Antiepileptic Drugs, 5th ed. New York: Raven Press, 2002:921–922.

67. Bialer M, Johannessen SI, Kupferberg HJ. Progress report on new antiepileptic drugs: a summary of the fifth Eilat conference (EILAT IV). Epilepsy Res 2001; 43:11–58.

68. Rafael H, Mego R, Moromizato P, Garcia W. Omental transplantation for temporal lobe epilepsy: report of two cases. Neurol India 2002; 50:71–74.

69. NINDS webpage reviewed 7-01-2001. www.ninds.nih.gov.

70. NINDS webpage. www.clinicaltrials.gov.

71. Dunwiddie TV. Adenosine and suppression of seizures. In: Delgado-Escueta AV, Wilson WA, Olsen RW, Porter RJ, eds. Jasper's Basic Mechanisms of the Epilepsies, 3rd ed. Advances in Neurology, Vol 79. Philadelphia: Lippincott Williams & Wilkins, 1999: 1001–1010.

72. Huber A, Padrun V, Deglon N, Aebischer P, Mohler H, Boison D. Grafts of adenosine-releasing cells suppress seizures in kindling epilepsy. Proc Natl Acad Sci USA 2001; 98:7611–7616.

73. Scott RC, Nesag FM, Boyd SG, Berry D, Neville BG. Buccal absorption of midazolam: pharmacokinetics and EEG pharmacodynamics. Epilepsia 1998; 39:290–294.

74. Scott RC, Besag FM, Neville BG. Buccal midazolam and rectal diazepam for the treatment of prolonged seizures in childhood and adolescence: a randomized trial. Lancet 1999; 353:623–626.

75. Koren G. Intranasal midazolam for febrile seizures: a step forward in treating a common and distressing condition. BMJ 2000; 321:64–65.

76. Lahat E, Goldran M, Barr J. Intranasal midazolam for childhood seizures. Lancet 1998; 352:620.

77. Anderson GD, Miller JW. Benzodiazepines. Chemistry, biotransformation, and pharmacokinetics. In: Levy RH, Mattson RH, Medrum BS, Perucca E, eds. Antiepileptic Drugs, 5th ed. New York: Raven Press, 2002:187–205.

78. Karl HW, Rosenberger JL, Larach MG, Ruffle JM. Transmucosal administration of midazolam for pre medication of pediatric patients. Comparison of the nasal and sublingual routes. Anesthesiology 1993; 78:885–891.

79. Vagus Nerve Stimulation Study Group. A randomized controlled trial of chronic vagus nerve stimulation for treatment of medically intractable seizures. Neurology 1995; 45:224–230.

80. Theodore WH, Hunter K, Chen R, Vega-Bermudez F, Boroojerdi B, Reeves-Tyer P, Werhahn K, Kelley KR, Cohen L. Transcranial magnetic stimulation for the treatment of seizures. A controlled study. Neurology 2002; 59:560–562.

81. Steinlein OK. Channelopathies can cause epilepsy in man. Eur J Pain 2002: 6(suppl A):27–34.

82. Kullmann DM. The neuronal channelopathies. Brain 2002; 125:1177–1195.

83. Silvermann JA. P-glycoprotein. In: Levy RH, Thummerl KE, Trager WE, eds. Metabolic Drug Interactions. Philadelphia: Lippincott Williams & Wilkins, 2000: 135–144.

84. Perucca E, Levy RH. General principles. Combination therapy and drug interactions. In: Levy RH, Mattson RH, Medrum BS, Perucca E, eds. Antiepileptic Drugs, 5th ed. New York: Raven Press, 2002:96–102.

85. Potschka H, Fedrowitz M, Loscher W. P-glycoprotein-mediated efflux of phenobarbital, lamotrigine, and felbamate at the blood-brain barrier: evidence from microdialysis experiments in rats. Neurosci Lett 2002; 327(3):173–176.

86. Potschka H, Loscher W. In vivo evidence for P-glycoprotein-mediated transport of phenytoin at the blood-brain barrier of rats. Epilepsia 2001; 42(10):1231–1240.

87. Eder HG, Stein A, Fisher RS. Interictal and ictal activity in the rat cobalt/pilocarpine model of epilepsy decreased by local perfusion of diazepam. Epilepsy Res 1997; 29:17–24.

88. Eder HG, Stein A, Fisher RS. Local perfusion of diazepam attenuates interictal and ictal events in the bicuculline model of epilepsy in rats. Epilepsia 1997; 38(5):516–521.

22
Deep Brain Stimulation: Why Should This Work?

Richard B. Kim

The Epilepsy Center of Hoag and Children's Hospitals
Newport Beach, California, U.S.A.

INTRODUCTION

Despite impressive advances in the surgical treatments of medically refractory epilepsy, many patients are not candidates for resective procedures or respond poorly to them. In the area of movement disorders, the recent revival of interest in ablative techniques has in turn sparked interest in chronic stimulation of deep brain structures. Stimulation has several advantages over ablation, chiefly reversibility and modifiability. The success and safety of deep brain stimulation (DBS) for movement disorders, as well as the efficacy of vagus nerve stimulation, provide the impetus for investigating the application of deep brain stimulation to epilepsy. In this chapter, the scientific bases and clinical results of stimulation of the thalamus, hippocampus, and subthalamic nucleus are discussed. Other brain targets have been explored, such as the cerebellum, locus coeruleus, caudate, and others, but there is insufficient experience to analyze outcomes; the reader is directed to previous reviews (1).

THALAMUS STIMULATION

Experimental Background

The widespread cortical afferents from the thalamus and its potent effects on cortical functioning have been studied in detail (2,3). The so-called specific nuclei demonstrate direct cortical connections, such as the ventralis lateralis (motor cortex), ventralis posterolatalis (sensory cortex), and the lateral geniculate (visual cortex). The nonspecific nuclei, such as the reticular nucleus, anterior nucleus, and intralaminar nuclei (of which one member is the centromedian nucleus [CM]), project more diffusely to broad areas of cortex.

The coupling of thalamic and cortical electrophysiologic activity has been demonstrated in a number of models. The augmenting rhythm is a biphasic cortical response to stimulation of specific thalamic nuclei (4). The recruiting rhythm results from stimulation of the nonspecific nuclei, and is a monophasic surface-negative potential that waxes and wanes over broad areas of cortex (4,5). The reticular nucleus is a key pacemaker for absence seizures which may be mediated by calcium currents (6). Epileptiform patterns are observed in several thalamic nuclei in generalized absence models, but they develop after cortical discharges (7,8). The nonspecific thalamus is therefore thought to play a role in the modulation or propagation of generalized seizures, but probably not in their generation (8,9). Kudo et al. found, for example, that the medial thalamic nuclei are important in the secondary generalization of penicillin-induced amygdala seizures in rats (10). Bertram and colleagues have also demonstrated a role of the medial thalamus, specifically the dorsomedial nucleus, in the propagation of limbic seizures (11,12). Stimulation of the medial thalamus produces excitatory responses in the amygdala and entorhinal cortex, suggesting that the medial thalamus may play a role in synchronization of limbic activity (13).

Monnier and associates (14,15) found that electrical stimulation of the medial thalamus produced desynchronization of the EEG. This would presumably have an anticonvulsant effect, leading these investigators to advocate this as a therapeutic option. The stimulation that produces EEG desynchronization is high frequency, in contrast to the low-frequency stimulation that produces recruiting rhythms. Stimulation of the CM has been shown to produce recruiting responses in the pyramidal tract (16,17), and this augments corticospinal responses to cortical stimulation (5). The CM therefore may be involved in corticospinal propagation of seizures. In monkeys with cortical alumina foci, Wilder and Schmidt (18) found that seizure termination often coincided with discharges appearing in the medial thalamus. They were able to terminate seizures by electrical stimulation of the medial thalamus.

The neuroanatomic substrates of seizures produced by pentylentetrazol (PTZ) infusion in rats has been extensively studied by Mirski and Ferrendelli (19–22). Electrical stimulation of the mammillary bodies was found to elevate the seizure threshold (23). Stimulation of AN, which in humans is a more favorable target than the mammillary bodies, was found to exert an anticonvulsant effect (24). In this study, as in those using mammillary body stimulation, high-frequency (100-Hz) bilateral AN stimulation did not affect the development of sharp wave bursts on EEG with PTZ infusion, but did result in a twofold higher dose requirement for the expression of clonic motor seizures (Fig. 1). Stimulation at low frequencies (<10 Hz) produced seizures (23). These investigators used autoradiographic, coagulative lesioning and pharmacological microinjections to study the anatomic and neurochemical basis of seizure expression. They described a synaptic pathway linking the anterior nucleus (AN) of the thalamus, mammillary complex of the posterior hypothalamus, and the dorsal and ventral segmental nuclei of the midbrain tegmentum (19–22). Efficacy of antiseizure effects depends on low to moderate current, high stimulation frequencies, and proper electrode placement.

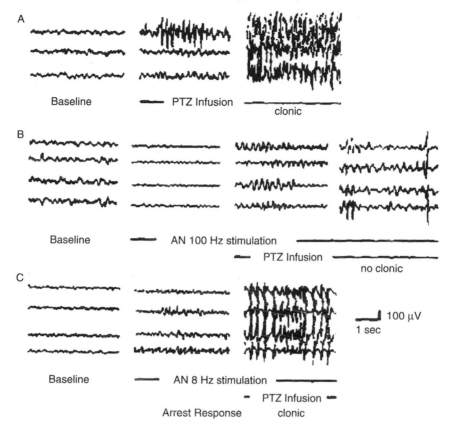

Figure 1. Cortical EEG before and during PTZ infusion. (A) Cortical (top), posterior thalamic (middle), and anterior thalamic (bottom) EEG tracings in a control animal. Note the early medium voltage burst activity in the cortical tracing. This is not associated with behavioral phenomena or subcortical activity. (B) Cortical EEG of an animal undergoing AN stimulation at 100 Hz. With stimulation, there is a decrease in baseline amplitude and a lack of both high-voltage synchronous activity and clonic activity during PTZ infusion. (C) Cortical EEG of an animal undergoing AN stimulation at 8 Hz. The animal displays behavioral arrest response during stimulation and has a major clonic seizure following a low dose of PTZ. (From Ref. 24.)

Clinical Data

Thalamocortical coupling of activity in epilepsy has been demonstrated in a number of studies in humans. Williams used depth electrode recording in a limited number of patients with absence epilepsy (25). Positron emission tomography ($H_2^{18}O$ PET) has been used recently to demonstrate thalamic hyperperfusion in absence epilepsy (26). Hajek et al. studied a patient with epilepsia partialis continua and found hypermetabolism of the ipsilateral thalamus on fluorodeoxyglucose PET (27). Detre et al. utilized the relatively superior spatial and temporal resolution of functional MRI (fMRI) compared to PET, and demonstrated concurrent activation of the ventrolateral thalamus ipsilateral to a frontal cortical epileptogenic lesion (28). Velasco and colleagues observed 3-Hz spike and wave complexes with 3-Hz stimulation of CM, while 8-Hz stimulation produced recruitinglike responses (29).

Cooper pioneered deep brain stimulation for epilepsy (30,31), and since that time several clinical series involving thalamic stimulation for epilepsy have been published (32–36). Cooper's group reported that many patients with epilepsy had favorable outcomes, but reporting of the data with respect to seizure types and quantification of benefit was limited. Velasco et al. (33) in Mexico City reported in 1987 on a group of five patients in whom they performed stimulation of the centromedian nucleus for medically intractable multifocal epilepsy. Stimulation was performed bilaterally through externalized electrode wires in daily sessions of 2 h each. Patients demonstrated a 60–100% reduction in frequency of generalized and partial-onset seizures. Much of this benefit occurred during times when stimulation was not taking place. The authors attribute this to the chronic theta rhythm observed after several weeks of CM stimulation, which they described subsequently (35).

The Velascos' initial experience has been extended over several studies. Predictors of good outcome were age 10–25 years, generalized tonic-clonic seizures, absence seizures, Lennox-Gastaut syndrome, and longer periods of stimulation. CM stimulation has no effect on complex partial seizures or on temporal epileptiform discharges (37).

Fisher et al. performed the first controlled study of thalamic stimulation (34). Seven patients received bilateral CM electrodes and implanted generators. Stimulation was delivered in double-blinded fashion, on in four patients for the first 3 months and off in the remaining three patients, then off for 3 months in all patients. In the final phase, patients received the opposite treatment from the initial phase. At the end of the 9-month study period, stimulation was unblinded. Stimulation parameters were as follows: 65 Hz, 0.1-msec pulse width, amplitude 0.5–10 V, on for 1 min and off for 4 min. Amplitude was set for half the sensory threshold so as to maintain the patients' blinding to stimulation. One patient experienced a reduction in generalized seizures from 12 to one per month. The remaining six patients did not demonstrate a significant effect, however. No patient experienced worsening of seizures, the onset of new seizure types, or cognitive sequelae to stimulation.

A comparison of these two clinical trials highlights some of the methodological difficulties that must be overcome when attempting to determine the effect of DBS on seizures. As is true for any stereotactic implantation procedure, physiologic verification of electrode position is the gold standard for target verification. Velasco et al. used stimulation at 8 Hz and observed a recruiting response to verify their correct location. Fisher et al. used purely anatomic localization methods from CT and MRI. This may account for some of the differences in effect between the two studies. Second is the issue of stimulation parameters. Velasco et al. used higher voltages and currents than Fisher et al. Finally, the patients in the Velasco study were not blinded, raising the very real possibility of a placebo effect.

The AN of the thalamus might be a good candidate to modulate seizures because of its involvement in the circuit of Papez, and in light of its connections with the mammillary bodies described in the previous section. Recently, Hodaie and colleagues (36) reported on the experience at the University of Toronto on five patients who underwent bilateral AN stimulation. Targeting was verified with microelectrode recording. After 3 days of monitoring through externalized leads, the leads were internalized, and all patients underwent a ramping up of their stimulation 4 weeks after implantation. Stimulation was delivered intermittently, 1 min on and 5 min off, at 100 Hz. Changes to the various parameters were performed during the treatment period. After at least 7 months of stimulation, the stimulators were turned off to assess the effect on seizure frequency. The mean reduction in seizure frequency was 54%, with a range of 24–89% (Fig. 2). Interestingly, the three patients with the greatest effect were those in whom low-frequency stimulation elicited a recruiting rhythm. Several other findings in this study are noteworthy. The reduction in seizures occurred immediately after electrode implantation, and was not significantly affected after stimulation was turned on 4 weeks later. A "microthalamotomy" effect has been described in the surgery for movement disorders, in which the insertion of the electrode produces the desired decrease in tremor and is thought to result from a microlesion (38). Another explanation is of course placebo effect since there was no sham operation group. The effect on seizures in this study was also not affected after the stimulation was turned off, after at least 7 months on. This may be a persistent microthalamotomy effect, or a long-lasting effect of stimulation.

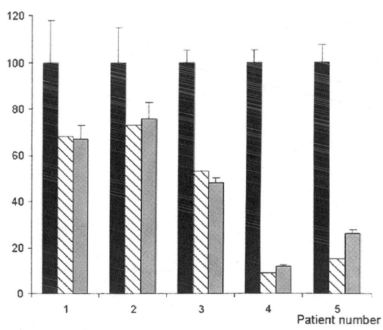

Figure 2. Reduction in seizure frequency in the five patients reported by Hodaie et al. (36), expressed as a percentage of baseline. Black bars: baseline seizure frequency. Hatched bars: change in seizure frequency after DBS electrode insertion, before stimulation. Gray bars: change in seizure frequency after DBS electrode stimulation. Note that the efficacy was realized with electrode insertion and that stimulation did not produce additional benefit. (From Ref. 36.)

SUBTHALAMIC NUCLEUS STIMULATION

Experimental Background

Iadarola and Gale have proposed and subsequently elucidated an endogenous epilepsy control system, referred to as the nigral control of epilepsy system (NCES) (39,40). The substantia nigra pars reticulata (SNr) is thought to exert a GABA-ergic inhibitory control over the superior colliculus, and in particular an area called the dorsal midbrain anticonvulsant zone (DMAZ). Blockade of this tonic inhibition by microinjection of GABA into the SNr causes potent excitation of collicular neurons (41). DMAZ neurons are the most sensitive to this modulation (42). A similar effect has also been produced by direct lesioning of the SNr (43,44). Blockade of the inhibition of the DMAZ in turn produces anticonvulsant effects in cortex (43–45). The SNr receives tonic excitatory glutamatergic input from STN (46–48), as well as phasic inhibitory GABA-ergic input from the striatum (45,47). Therefore, during normal resting conditions the STN acts to stimulate SNr and keep the NCES inactive. A summary of the proposed interactions in the NCES is depicted in Figure 3.

The NCES model has been fairly extensively studied using a variety of strategies. SNr has been inactivated by muscimol, a GABA agonist (45,48); gamma-vinyl-GABA, a GABA transaminase inhibitor (49,50); NMDA antagonists (51); substance P (52); opiates (53); and direct lesioning of SNpr (43,44). Activation of the striatum would be expected in this model to suppress the SNr's inhibitory

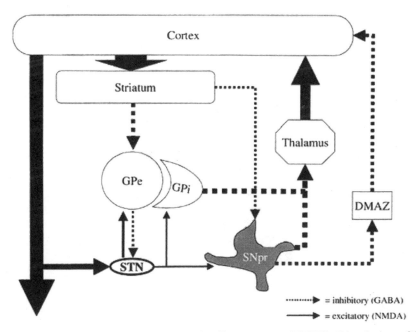

Figure 3.   Summary of the nigral control of epilepsy system (NCES). Stimulation of STN is thought to inhibit its excitatory influence on SNr, thereby releasing the inhibition of DMAZ and producing an anticonvulsant effect. GPe, globus pallidus pars externa; Gpi, globus pallidus pars interna. (From Ref. 63.)

modulation of the DMAZ and exert an anticonvulsant effect. This has been accomplished using NMDA analogs (54) and GABA antagonists (55). Lesioning of the striatum or GABA blockade with bicuculline injection into SNr attenuates the anticonvulsant effect. STN has been inhibited by microinjection of muscimol and by lesioning, both methods producing anticonvulsant effects (56).

A variety of rat epilepsy models have been used to validate this model. These include generalized electroshock (39,46), fluorothyl-induced clonic seizures (48), systemic bicuculline (58), and genetically determined petit mal epilepsy (45,59). Additional epilepsy models in which the NCES has been demonstrated to exert effects include intraperitoneal pilocarpine (51,56), bicuculline administration to area tempestas (58), and amygdala-kindled seizures (44,49,50,54,55). Activation of NCES does not appear to influence seizures in genetically epilepsy-prone rats with audiogenic seizures (45) or generalized nonconvulsive PTZ-induced seizures (13,24). In PTZ-induced seizures, the mammillary bodies and anterior nucleus of the thalamus are key modulators, as discussed earlier.

Some preliminary work on STN stimulation in animals has been reported. Vercueil and colleagues (60) studied a rat model that exhibited spontaneous absence seizures associated with generalized synchronous spike-and-wave discharges (genetic absence epilepsy in rats from Strasbourg; GAERS). High-frequency (130-Hz) bilateral stimulation was delivered to STN, resulting in interruption of ongoing spike-and-wave discharges following a 5-sec interval of stimulation. When stimulation was delivered continuously for 10 min, the effect was seen only within the first 2 min of stimulation, after which time there was no effect. When excitotoxic lesions were created bilaterally in STN, there was a 60% reduction in the mean duration of discharges but no complete elimination in any subject. Unilateral stimulation or lesioning produced no effect. The effect of STN stimulation is therefore transient, and thus the modulation effect of STN on the nigrotectal pathway appears subject to dynamic regulation.

Long-lasting seizure suppression was seen in the rat kainate model of limbic epilepsy (61). Bilateral STN stimulation reduced the number of seizures, while both bilateral and unilateral stimulation reduced seizure duration. The effect continued well after the period of stimulation.

Human Studies

The first patient with epilepsy to be treated with STN stimulation was reported by Benabid and colleagues in Grenoble after 30 months of follow-up (62). This was a 5-year-old girl with cortical dysplasia in motor cortex not amenable to resection. Bilateral stimulator leads were placed stereotactically. Stimulation was delivered at 130 Hz, pulse width at 90 μsec, and voltage increased from 0.8 to 5.2 V.

The investigators observed that seizures were reduced by a total of 80%. After 6 months, however, seizure frequency began to increase. Increasing the voltage caused a decrease in seizure frequency from 101 per month to 51 per month. This differs from observations in thalamic stimulation described earlier in this chapter, and suggests a voltage-dependent effect. However, the reason for the increasing seizure frequency despite constant voltage is unclear; the possibility of tolerance is certainly a troubling consideration. When stimulation was accidentally stopped, seizure frequency immediately increased, again in contrast to the results in the thalamus. The investigators also switched the stimulation protocol from continuous to intermittent, initiating stimulation holidays for 2 h/d. This was based on findings in the rat absence model from work in the same laboratory (60). The effect on seizures was more pronounced than with continuous stimulation, with a total 96% reduction in frequency. However, the period of observation with intermittent stimulation was too short to allow definitive conclusions.

Several more patients have undergone STN stimulation by the Grenoble group. In addition, the results of five patients who have been implanted in a collaboration between the Grenoble and Cleveland Clinic groups is available (63). Seizures were reduced by 80% in two patients, by 60% in one patient, and there was no effect in two patients. The Cleveland Clinic group has also reported on a patient with status epilepticus refractory to medications, who did not respond to STN stimulation (64). This patient required resection of primary motor cortex.

Alaraj and colleagues (65) have reported the results of a 14 year-old patient with Lennox-Gastaut syndrome, with myoclonic seizures, epileptic spasms, and generalized tonic-clonic seizures. The patient had >100 seizures per week. Bilateral STN stimulation resulted in a 75% reduction in myoclonic and absence seizures, with complete abolishment of generalized tonic-clonic seizures. The effect was sustained after 1 year of follow-up. Interestingly, the effect did not appear to be dependent on voltage or other stimulation parameters.

The studies of human subjects have provided valuable opportunities to study the interactions between STN and cortex. Both the Grenoble and the Cleveland Clinic groups have reported the findings of simultaneous recordings from scalp EEG and STN (63,66). These investigators found simultaneous epileptiform spike-wave discharges in both recordings, with the STN discharges reversed in polarity with respect to the scalp. Independent spikes were recorded from STN, however, without concomitant discharges from scalp (64). Ictal recordings have shown simultaneous discharges from scalp and the ipsilateral STN (64).

MECHANISMS OF DBS ACTION

The most commonly held view of the mechanism of DBS action is that high-frequency electrical stimulation in deep structures such as thalamic nuclei and subthalamic nucleus exerts an inhibitory effect. In STN, for example, the assumption of most studies has been that inhibition of this structure causes activation of the NCES, thereby suppressing seizures. More recent evidence, however, suggests that direct excitatory mechanisms may also play a role.

Parallels may be drawn from studies of DBS in patients with Parkinson's disease and other movement disorders. High-frequency stimulation of the VIM thalamus and globus pallidus produced similar clinical effects to the ablative lesions that DBS is quickly replacing (67). This has been shown to be frequency dependent; clinical improvement in movement disorders is achieved only at frequencies >100 Hz (68). This has also been seen in STN stimulation in the rat (69).

A recent study using patch-clamp recording in STN slices (70) reported that 1-min stimulation of the STN caused cessation of all spontaneous firing for up to

6 min. This effect was not prevented by blockers of ionophoric GABA and glutamate transmission, so it is probably not synaptically mediated. Instead, the effect is mediated by large reductions in voltage-gated Na^+ and Ca^{2+} currents. Therefore STN stimulation may exert a direct cellular inhibitory effect.

The studies discussed earlier in this chapter in which stimulation was applied to the mammillary bodies and to the anterior nucleus of the thalamus in a rat model of epilepsy showed that the antiseizure effects depended on high frequencies, in the range of 100 Hz (23). This is higher than would be expected to drive a polysynaptic pathway of inhibition. Moreover, low-frequency (10-Hz) stimulation drives seizures or produced recruiting rhythms, suggesting that direct activation of these areas is pro-convulsant. Excitotoxic lesioning produces effects similar to high-frequency stimulation, both in thalamus (22) and STN (60).

There is growing evidence that excitatory effects involving high-frequency (~100-Hz) stimulation may play a role in the clinical effects of DBS. Several clinical observations have raised this possibility. Stimulation of pyramidal tract fibers during surgical targeting of STN causes muscular contraction, while stimulation of the medial lemniscus evokes paresthesias (66). The high frequencies used for clinical application were employed. Functional MRI studies on patients with thalamic stimulation demonstrated activation in the thalamus, basal ganglia, and the primary cortical somatosensory and somatomotor areas (71).

Connections between STN and cortex would be expected to play a key role in modulating seizures. Direct corticosubthalamic pathways have been described from frontal motor (72), somatosensory (73), and insular cortex (74) in animals. Stimulation of STN at frequencies as high as 250 Hz produces cortical potentials in animal models (75), presumably via antidromic activation of a corticosubthalamic pathway. Preliminary data are available on cortical potentials evoked by STN stimulation in patients with epilepsy and Parkinson's disease (76). The investigators observed cortical evoked potentials with latencies in the range of 400 msec. When paired pulses were delivered with a 1-msec interpulse interval, the amplitude of the evoked potential was augmented by 50%. Such a short refractory period has been suggested to be more consistent with stimulation of axons rather than of cell bodies (76).

The immediate consequences of stimulation are probably more complex, however, than direct inhibition or stimulation. The results of Vercueil and colleagues (60) described above in the GAERS model of absence epilepsy in the rat showed that excitotoxic lesioning of STN yielded only part of the efficacy that stimulation did. The many elements within the field of stimulation, e.g., transmembrane channels, synapses, axon hillocks, axons of passage, etc., may each be expect to react to stimulation, with each individual reaction being excitatory or inhibitory. For example, STN stimulation produces both excitatory and inhibitory postsynaptic potentials in dopaminergic neurons of the SNr, with the EPSPs being monosynaptic and glutamatergic and the IPSPs being polysynaptic and GABA-ergic (77). The net effect of DBS, both locally and in more distant regions, will depend on the interplay of the individual responses. The individual component responses are likely to vary with stimulation parameters such as frequency and current, with differing net effects.

HIPPOCAMPAL STIMULATION

The role of the hippocampus and other medial temporal structures in the pathophysiology of medial temporal lobe epilepsy (MTLE) has been studied in great detail (for review, see 78). The pathologic hallmark of MTLE is mesial temporal sclerosis (MTS), characterized by severe neuronal loss, recurrent sprouting of mossy fibers, and hyperexcitability. Surgical resection of the medial structures has been demonstrated to produce seizure freedom in 70–90% of medically intractable patients. Despite its successes, surgical resection has significant limitations: Deficits in short-term memory and learning, especially for verbal material, may be seen in a significant percentage of patients with dominant-side surgery; bilateral disease cannot be treated with resection; the precise mechanisms of persistent seizures in patients who fail surgery are not understood. Stimulation of the hippocampus has thus received attention, albeit limited, for the possibility of overcoming these shortfalls.

The experimental basis for such therapy is even sparser than for thalamus or STN stimulation. Weiss and colleagues have shown that electrical stimulation of the amygdala after a kindling stimulus suppresses kindling, an effect termed quenching (79). A similar effect from hippocampus stimulation remains to be demonstrated.

The model of TLE in rats created by kainic acid injection into the amygdala (80) has been useful for studying hippocampal stimulation. Bragin and colleagues (81) used this model to perform subthreshold stimulation of the hippocampus and found that the rate of interictal epileptiform activity was decreased during 1-Hz and 50-Hz stimulation transiently, but returned to baseline within 30–60 min. There was no effect on the spontaneous seizure rate.

The investigators from Mexico City who helped pioneer clinical studies of thalamic stimulation for epilepsy have also published data on hippocampal stimulation for MTLE (82). Twelve patients were included in their study, but only two had bilateral depth electrodes within the hippocampi; the remaining 10 had basal temporal surface electrodes placed via craniotomy. Stimulation was delivered at 130 Hz, 450 μsec duration, and 200–400 μamp of current. In seven patients, the frequency of both complex partial and generalized tonic-clonic seizures diminished progressively until all seizures were abolished by day 6. The other patients did not have a significant response. An obvious flaw in this study is the inclusion of patients with basal temporal surface electrodes and no depth electrodes in the hippocampi. The report does not specify the response of the patients with hippocampal depth electrode stimulation. Neuropsychometric performance during stimulation was also not reported.

The major theoretical advantage of hippocampal stimulation over surgical resection would be the avoidance of memory deficits; that is, the preservation of normal hippocampal function while abolishing seizures. The preponderance of evidence shows that this does not occur, however. Early animal studies (83) have demonstrated amnestic effects of hippocampus stimulation. Lee and colleagues (84) found significantly impaired verbal learning with left hippocampus stimulation in patients with right MTLE, and impaired visuospatial learning with right hippocampus stimulation regardless of the laterality of MTLE. The same group of investigators observed verbal intrusion errors when hippocampus stimulation was applied to the side contralateral to the side of epileptogenicity (85).

SUMMARY AND FUTURE DIRECTIONS

A relative paucity of data exists from which a strong foundation for deep brain stimulation for epilepsy may be constructed. In the case of thalamic stimulation, there is much evidence for thalamocortical coupling of activity, particularly in the recruiting rhythm elicited by stimulation of nonspecific thalamic nuclei. Anticonvulsant effects have been demonstrated by stimulation of the medial thalamus, mammillary bodies, and anterior nucleus, among other sites. The precise cause-and-effect relationships in human epilepsies remain unclear. Clinical experience with thalamus stimulation has been limited thus far to small series, with widely varying results both between series and between patients within series. Taken together, the results on seizure control are interesting, but not yet of the magnitude to warrant widespread clinical use.

The experimental basis for the nigral control of epilepsy has been studied in detail. In this model, the SNr exerts tonic inhibitory control over the DMAZ region of the superior colliculus, which in turn activates widespread cortical regions. The STN has excitatory input to the SNr, thus acting to keep the NCES inactive. STN stimulation in this animal model is not as well worked out, and study in humans is in its infancy. As with thalamic stimulation, the clinical results have been varied but encouraging.

The dual goals of improved seizure control and minimizing the cognitive side effects of surgery for MTLE make hippocampal stimulation a seemingly attractive alternative. Animal experiments do not convincingly make the case for an antiepileptic effect, however, and if such an effect is present, it would appear to be extremely transient. Moreover, hippocampal stimulation has been shown convincingly to impair learning and verbal functioning. Nonetheless, the single published report on this therapy in humans suggests an anticonvulsant effect. This study had some limitations, and further studies are warranted.

As clinical studies move forward beyond the initial efforts described in this chapter, several key issues must be addressed. Among the most important of these is the selection of the targets of stimulation. In the thalamus, a number of nuclei have been studied in animal models of epilepsy. Human trials have been reported for centromedian and anterior nucleus stimulation. Targeting the anterior nucleus has a strong rationale based on the studies involving PTZ-induced seizures in rats, and the known anatomic connections of the anterior nucleus with the limbic system. Targeting the STN has a strong rationale based on the NCES model, although animal data on this treatment are scant.

As more experience is gained, different seizure types or clinical epilepsy syndromes may be found to respond better than others to different targets of stimulation. This relates to a second key issue of DBS trials: patient selection. Treating a homogeneous population may give consistent results, but the results cannot be generalized. As yet there is no a priori reason to select any seizure type for any target of DBS. Many other questions must be addressed in designing a clinical trial of DBS, such as the frequency of seizures, how many concurrent medications are allowed, whether patients with vagus nerve stimulators should be included, and many others.

The generators used for DBS allow a great deal of flexibility to the clinician in setting the parameters for stimulation; however, this creates many potential variables

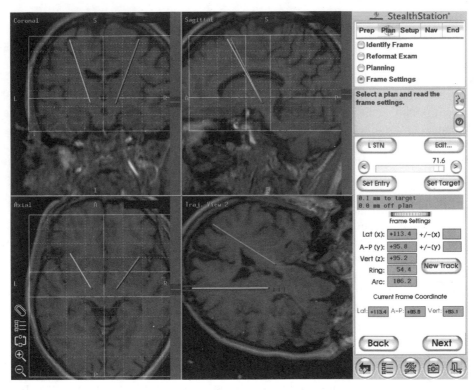

Figure 4. Example of stereotactic targeting of STN. Standard anatomic coordinates with reference to the AC-PC line are used in combination with direct imaging and an overlay of an anatomic atlas. Final positioning in the operating room is accomplished with microelectrode recording.

in a research trial. Few data exist to guide the investigator on the optimal parameters. Stimulus frequency should probably be in the high range, $\geq 100\,\mathrm{Hz}$, since low frequencies produce recruiting rhythms and may drive seizures, while high frequencies are effective in movement disorders in humans and epilepsy models in animals. Other stimulation parameters include bipolar versus monopolar stimulation, current, voltage, pulse width, and intermittent versus continuous stimulation.

Finally, the surgical technique should incorporate reliable targeting methods (Fig. 4). In most cases this means using not only anatomic (imaging) targeting but also microelectrode recording. The exception is in the hippocampus, which is a large enough structure that anatomic targeting routinely allows accurate electrode placement. Regardless of the target, postimplant MRI should be obtained to confirm accurate placement.

Since the pioneering efforts of Cooper and others in DBS for epilepsy, little progress has been made. The role, if any, for DBS in epilepsy remains to be defined. The next generation of clinical studies must be rigorously designed and carried out, and include sufficient numbers of patients to allow useful information to be gleaned.

REFERENCES

1. Krauss GL, Fisher RS. Cerebellar and thalamic stimulation for epilepsy. In: Devinsky O, Beric A, Dogali M, eds. Electrical and Magnetic Stimulation of the Brain and Spinal Cord. New York: Raven Press, 1994:231–245.
2. Jones EG. The Thalamus. New York: Plenum, 1985.
3. Steriade M. The Thalamus. Amsterdam: Elsevier Science Publishing, 1997.
4. Dempsey EW, Morison RS. The production of rhythmically recurrent cortical potentials after localized thalamic stimulation. Am J Physiol, 1942; 135:293–300.
5. Jasper H, Naquet R, King EE. Thalamocortical recruiting responses in sensory receiving areas in the cat. Electroencephalogr Clin Neurophysiol 1955; 7:99–114.
6. Coulter DA, Huguenard JR, Prince DA. Specific petit mal anticonvulsants reduce calcium currents in thalamic neurons. Neurosci Lett 1989; 98:74–78.
7. Fisher RS, Prince DA. Spike-wave rhythms in cat cortex induced by parenteral penicillin. Electroencephalographic features. Electroencephalogr Clin Neurophysiol 1977; 42:608–624.
8. Quesney LF, Gloor P, Kratzenberg E, Zumstein H. Pathophysiology of generalized penicillin epilepsy in the cat: role of cortical and subcortical structures. I. Systematic application of penicillin. Electroencephalogr Clin Neurophysiol 1977; 42:640–655.
9. Avoli M, Gloor P, Kostopoulos G, Gotman J. An analysis of penicillin-induced generalized spike and wave discharges using simultaneous recordings of cortical and thalamic single neurons. J Neurophysiol 1983; 50:819–837.
10. Kudo T, Yamauchi T. An ontogenic study of amygdala seizures induced by penicillin in rats. Exp Neurol 1988; 99:531–543.
11. Bertram EH, Zhang DX, Mangan P, Fountain N, Rempe D. Functional anatomy of limbic epilepsy: a proposal for central synchronization of a diffusely hyperexcitable network. Epilepsy Res 1998; 32:194–205.
12. Bertram EH, Mangan PS, Zhang D, Scott CA, Williamson JM. The midline thalamus: alterations and a potential role in limbic epilepsy. Epilepsia 2001; 42:967–978.
13. Zhang DX, Bertram EH. Midline thalamic region: widespread excitatory input to the entorhinal cortex and amygdala. J Neurosci 2002; 22:3277–3284.
14. Monnier M, Kalberer M, Krupp P. Functional antagonism between diffuse reticular and intralaminary recruiting projections in the medial thalamus. Exp Neurol 1960; 2:271–289.
15. Monnier M, Hoshi L, Krupp P. Moderating and activating systems in medio-central thalamus and reticular formation. Electroencephalogr Clin Neurophysiol Suppl 1963; 24:97.
16. Arduini A, Whitlock DG. Spike discharges in pyramidal system during recruitment waves. J Neurophysiol 1953; 16:430–436.
17. Purpura DP, Housepian EM. Alterations in corticospinal neuron activity associated with thalamocortical recruiting responses. Electroencephalogr Clin Neurophysiol 1961; 13:365–381.
18. Wilder BJ, Schmidt RP. Propagation of epileptic discharge from chronic neocortical foci in monkey. Epilepsia 1965; 6:296–309.
19. Mirski MA, Ferrendelli JA. Interruption of the mammillothalamic tracts prevents seizures in guinea pigs. Science 1984; 226:72–74.
20. Mirski MA, Ferrendelli JA. Selective metabolic activation of the mammillary bodies and their connections during ethosuximide-induced suppression of pentylenetrazol seizures. Epilepsia 1985; 51:194–203.
21. Mirski MA, Ferrendelli JA. Anterior thalamic mediation of generalized pentylenetrazol seizures. Brain Res 1986; 399:212–223.

22. Mirski MA, Ferrendelli JA. Interruption of the connections of the mammillary bodies protect against generalized pentylenetrazol seizures in guinea pigs. J Neurosci 1987; 7:662–670.

23. Mirski MA, Fisher RS. Electrical stimulation of the mammillary nuclei increases seizure threshold to pentylenetetrazol in rats. Epilepsia 1994; 35:309–316.

24. Mirski MA, Rossell LA, Terry JB, Fisher RS. Anticonvulsant effect of anterior thalamic high frequency electrical stimulation in the rat. Epilepsy Res 1997; 28:89–100.

25. Williams D. A study of thalamic and cortical rhythms in petit mal. Brain 1953; 76:50–69.

26. Prevett MC, Duncan JS, Jones T, Fish DR, Brooks DJ. Demonstration of thalamic activation during typical absence seizures using $H_2^{15}O$ and PET. Neurology 1995; 45:1396–1402.

27. Hajek M, Antonini A, Leenders KL, Wieser HG. Epilepsia partialis continua studied by PET. Epilepsy Res 1991; 9:44–48.

28. Detre JA, Alsop DC, Aguirre GK, Sperling MR. Coupling of cortical and thalamic ictal activity in human partial epilepsy: demonstration by functional magnetic resonance imaging. Epilepsia 1996; 37:657–661.

29. Velasco FM, Velasco M, Marquez I, Velasco G. Role of the centromedian thalamic nucleus in the genesis, propagation and arrest of epileptic activity. An electrophysiological study in man. Acta Neurochir Suppl 1993; 58:201–204.

30. Cooper IS, Upton AR, Amin I. Reversibility of chronic neurologic deficits. Some effects of electrical stimulation of the thalamus and internal capsule in man. Appl Neurophysiol 1980; 43:244–258.

31. Cooper IS, Upton AR. Therapeutic implications of modulation of metabolism and functional activity of cerebral cortex by chronic stimulation of cerebellum and thalamus. Biol Psychiatry 1985; 20:811–813.

32. Sussman NM, Goldman HW, Jackel RA, Kaplan L, Callanan M, Bergen J, Herner RN. Anterior thalamic stimulation in medically intractable epilepsy. Part II. Preliminary clinical results. Epilepsia 1988; 29:677.

33. Velasco F, Velasco M, Ogarrio C, Fanghanel G. Electrical stimulation of the centromedian thalamic nucleus in the treatment of convulsive seizures: a preliminary report. Epilepsia 1987; 28:421–430.

34. Fisher RS, Uematsu S, Krauss GL, Cysyk BJ, McPherson R, Lesser RP, Gordon B, Schwerdt P, Rise M. Placebo-controlled pilot study of centromedian thalamic stimulation in treatment of intractable seizures. Epilepsia 1992; 33:841–851.

35. Velasco F, Velasco M, Velasco AL, Jimenez F, Marquez I, Rise M. Electrical stimulation of the centromedian thalamic nucleus in control of seizures: long-term studies. Epilepsia 1995; 36:63–71.

36. Hodaie M, Wennberg RA, Dostrovsky JO, Lozano AM. Chronic anterior thalamus stimulation for intractable epilepsy. Epilepsia 2002; 42:603–608.

37. Velasco F, Velasco M, Jimenez F, Velasco AL, Brito F, Rise M, Carrillo-Ruiz JD. Predictors in the treatment of difficult-to-control seizures by electrical stimulation of the centromedian thalamic nucleus. Neurosurgery 2000; 47:295–304.

38. Tasker RR. Deep brain stimulation is preferable to thalamotomy for tremor suppression. Surg Neurol 1998; 49:145–153.

39. Gale K, Iadarola MJ. Seizure protection and increased nerve-terminal GABA: delayed effects of GABA transaminase inhibition. Science 1980; 208:288–291.

40. Iadarola MJ, Gale K. Substantia nigra: site of anticonvulsant activity mediated by gamma-aminobutyric acid. Science 1982; 218:1237–1240.

41. Chevalier G, Vacher S, Deniau JM, Desban M. Disinhibition as a basic process in the expression of striatal functions. I. The striato-nigral influence on tecto-spinal/tecto-diencephalic neurons. Brain Res 1985; 334:215–226.

42. Redgrave P, Simkins M, Overton P, Dean P. Anticonvulsant role of nigrotectal projection in the maximal electroshock model of epilepsy. I. Mapping of dorsal midbrain with bicuculline. Neuroscience 1992; 46:379–390.

43. Garant DS, Gale K. Lesions of substantia nigra protect against experimentally induced seizures. Brain Res 1983; 273:156–161.

44. McNamara JO, Galloway MT, Rigsbee LC, Shin C. Evidence implicating substantia nigra in regulation of kindled seizure threshold. J Neurosci 1984; 4:2410–2417.

45. Depaulis A, Snead OC, Marescaux C, Vergnes M. Suppressive effects of intranigral injection of muscimol in three models of generalized non-convulsive epilepsy induced by chemical agents. Brain Res 1989; 498:64–72.

46. Browning RA. Role of the brain-stem reticular formation in tonic-clonic seizures: lesion and pharmacological studies. Fed Proc 1985; 44:2425–2431.

47. Parent A, Hazrati LN. Functional anatomy of the basal ganglia. II. The place of subthalamic nucleus and external pallidum in basal ganglia circuitry. Brain Res Rev 1995; 20:91–127.

48. Veliskova J, Velsek L, Moshe SL. Subthalamic nucleur: a new anticonvulsant site in the brain. Neuroreport 1996; 7:1786–1788.

49. Le Gal LS, Kaijim M, Feldblum S. Abortive amygdaloid kindled seizures following microinjection of gamma-vinyl-GABA in the vicinity of substantia nigra in rats. Neurosci Lett 1983; 36:69.

50. Shin C, Silver JM, Bonhaus DW, McNamara JO. The role of substantia nigra in the development of kindling: pharmacologic and lesion studies. Brain Res 1987; 412:311–317.

51. De Sarro G, De Sarro A, Meldrum BS. Anticonvulsant action of 2-chloroadenosine injected focally into the inferior colliculus and substantia nigra. Eur J Pharmacol 1991; 194:145–152.

52. Garant DS, Iadarola MJ, Gale K. Substance P antagonists in substantia nigra are anticonvulsant. Brain Res 1986; 382:372–378.

53. Garant DS, Gale K. Infusion of opiates into substantia nigra protects against maximal electroshock seizures in rats. J Pharmacol Exp Ther 1985; 234:45–48.

54. Cavalheiro EA, Turski L. Intrastriatal N-methyl-D-aspartate prevents amygdala kindled seizures in rats. Brain Res 1986; 377:173–176.

55. Cavalheiro EA, Bortolotto ZA, Turski L. Microinjections of the gamma-aminobutyrate antagonist, bicuculline methiodide, into the caudate putamen prevent amygdala-kindled seizures in rats. Brain Res 1987; 411:370–372.

56. Turski L, Meldrum BS, Cavalheiro LA. Paradoxical anticonvulsant activity of the excitatory amino acid N-methyl-D-aspartate in the rat caudate putamen. Proc Natl Acad Sci USA 1987; 84:1689–1693.

57. Browning RA, Nelson DK, Mogharreban N, Jobe PC, Laird HE. Effect of midbrain and pontine tegmental lesions on audiogenic seizures in genetically epilepsy-prone rats. Epilepsia 1985; 26:175–183.

58. Dybdal D, Gale K. Postural and anticonvulsant effects of inhibition of the rat subthalamic nucleur. J Neurosci 2000; 20:6728–6733.

59. Deransart C, Riban V, Le BT, Hechler V, Marescaux C, Depaulis A. Evidence for the involvement of the pallidum in the modulation of seizures in a genetic model of absence epilepsy in the rat. Neurosci Lett 1999; 265:131–134.

60. Vercueil L, Benazzouz A, Deransart C, Bressand K, Marescaux C, Depaulis A, Benabid AL. High-frequency stimulation of the sub-thalamic nucleus suppresses absence seizures in the rat: comparison with neurotoxic lesions. Epilepsy Res 1998; 31:39–46.

61. Bressand K, Dermatteis M, Kahane P, Benazzouz A, Benabid AL. Involvement of the subthalamic nucleus in the control of temporal lobe epilepsy: study by high frequency stimulation in rats. Soc Neurosci 1999; 25:1656.

62. Benabid AL, Minotti L, Koudsie A, Saint Martin A, Hirsch E. Antiepileptic effect of high-frequency stimulation of the subthalamic nucleus (corpus luysi) in a case of medically intractable epilepsy caused by focal dysplasia: a 30-month follow-up: technical case report. Neurosurgery 2002; 50:1385–1392.

63. Loddenkemper T, Pan A, Neme Silvia, Baker KB, Rezai AR, Dinner DS, Montgomery EB, Luders HO. Deep brain stimulation in epilepsy. J Clin Neurophysiol 2001; 18:514–532.

64. Neme S, Montgomery E, Luders HO, Rezai A. Seizure outcome of deep brain stimulation of the subthalamic nucleus for intractable focal epilepsy. Epilepsia, 2001;42(suppl 2):124.(Abstract.)

65. Alaraj A, Comair Y, Mikati M, Wakim J, Louak E, Atweh S. Subthalamic nucleus deep brain stimulation: a novel method for the treatment of non-focal intractable epilepsy. Presented as a poster at Neuromodulation: Defining the Future, Cleveland, OH, June 8–10, 2001.

66. Benabid AL, Koudsie A, Pollak P, Kahane P, Chabardes S, Hirsch E, Marescaux C, Benazzouz A. Future prospects of brain stimulation. Neurol Res 2000; 22:237–246.

67. Benabid AL, Benazzouz A, Hoffmann D, Limousin P, Krack P, Pollak P. Long-term electrical inhibition of deep brain targets in movement disorders. Mov Disord 1998; 13(suppl 3):119–125.

68. Benabid AL, Pollak P, Gao D, Hoffmann D, Limousin P, Gay E, Payen I, Benazzouz A. Chronic electrical stimulation of the ventralis intermedius nucleus of the thalamus as a treatment of movement disorders. J Neurosurg 1996; 84:203–214.

69. Benazzouz A, Gao DM, Ni ZG, Piallat B, Bouali-Benazzouz R, Benabid AL. Effect of high-frequency stimulation of the subthalamic nucleus on the neuronal activities of the substantia nigra pars reticulata and ventrolateral nucleus of the thalamus in the rat. Neuroscience 2000; 99:289–295.

70. Beurrier C, Bioulac B, Audin J, Hammond C. High-frequency stimulation produces a transient blockade of voltage-gated currents in subthalamic neurons. J Neurophysiol 2001; 85:1351–1356.

71. Rezai AR, Lozano AM, Crawley AP, Joy ML, Davis KD, Kwan CL, Dostrovsky JO, Tasker RR, Mikulis DJ. Thalamic stimulation and functional magnetic resonance imaging: localization of cortical and subcortical activation with implanted electrodes. Technical note. J Neurosurg 1999; 90:583–590.

72. Kunzle H, Akert K. Efferent connections of cortical, area 8 (frontal eye field) in *Macaca fascicularis*. A reinvestigation using the autoradiographic technique. J Comp Neurol 1977; 173:147–164.

73. Carpenter MB, Carleton SC, Keller JT, Conte P. Connections of the subthalamic nucleus in the monkey. Brain Res 1981; 224:1–29.

74. Canteras NS, Shammah-Lagnado SJ, Silva BA, Ricardo JA. Afferent connections of the subthalamic nucleus: a combined retrograde and anterograde horseradish peroxidase study in the rat. Brain Res 1990; 513:43–59.

75. Maurice N, Deniau JM, Glowinski J, Thierry AM. Relationships between the prefrontal cortex and the basal ganglia in the rat: physiology of the corticosubthalamic circuits. J Neurosci 1998; 18:9539–9546.

76. Baker KB, Montgomery EB. Cortical evoked potentials from stimulation STN. Soc Neurosci Abstr 2000; 26:1226.

77. Iribe Y, Moore K, Pang KC, Tepper JM. Subthalamic stimulation-induced synaptic responses in substantia nigra pars compacta dopaminergic neurons in vitro. J Neurophysiol 1999; 82:925–933.

78. Engel J. Mesial temporal lobe epilepsy: what have we learned? Neuroscientist 2001; 7:340–352.

79. Weiss SRB, Li XL, Rosen JB, Li H, Heynen T, Post RM. Quenching: inhibition of development and expression of amygdala kindled seizures with low frequency stimulation. Neuroreport 1995; 4:2171–2176.

80. Berger ML, Lasmann H, Hornykoewicz O. Limbic seizures without brain damage after injection of low doses of kainic acid into the amygdala of freely moving rats. Brain Res 1989; 489:261–272.

81. Bragin ACL, Wilson CL, Engel J. Rate of interictal events and spontaneous seizures in epileptic rats after electrical stimulation of hippocampus and its afferents. Epilepsia 2002; 43(suppl 5):81–85.

82. Velasco M, Velsasco F, Velasco AL, Boleaga B, Jimenez F, Brito F, Marquez I. Subacute electrical stimulation of the hippocampus blocks intractable temporal lobe seizures and paroxysmal EEG activities. Epilepsia 2000; 41:158–169.

83. McDonough JH, Kesner RP. Amnesia produced by brief electrical stimulation of amygdala or dorsal hippocampus in cats. J Comp Physiol Psychol 1971; 77:171–178.

84. Lee GP, Loring DW, Smith JR, Flanigin JF. Material specific learning during electrical stimulation of the human hippocampus. Cortex 1990; 26:433–442.

85. Lee GP, Loring DW, Flanigin HF, Smith JR, Meador KJ. Electrical stimulation of the human hippocampus produces verbal intrusions during memory testing. Neuropsychologia 1988; 26:623–627.

23
Intraoperative Optical Imaging of Epileptiform and Functional Activity

Kenneth M. Little and Michael M. Haglund
Duke University Medical Center
Durham, North Carolina, U.S.A.

INTRODUCTION

Optical imaging (OI) has recently been introduced as an intraoperative technique for the localization of epileptic foci and eloquent cortex (1). OI detects variations in the scattering of incident light directed at the brain surface (2). These light-scattering variations, referred to as the intrinsic optical signal, are generated by multiple physiological processes associated with neuronal activity, including changes in blood oxygenation, blood volume, and extracellular volume (2). Current techniques such as electrocorticography (ECoG), electrical stimulation mapping (ESM), and functional imaging are limited in desired spatial and/or temporal resolution. With OI, however, it is possible to visualize epileptiform and functional activity over a broad range of spatial resolution from microscopic neuronal populations to macroscopic cortical regions with a temporal resolution of 200 msec. These benefits allow for greater accuracy in intraoperatively delineating Rolandic and language cortex, identifying interictal epileptiform discharges, pinpointing the onset of ictal events with precise localization, and directly observing the pathways by which seizure activity spreads. Because OI relies on physiological cortical activation rather than stimulation from external electrical currents, it can facilitate and enhance the intraoperative identification of cortical regions subserving cognitive functions. Though there are reports of OI in humans, it remains a research tool and will require further reliability testing and technical modifications before it can become feasible for routine clinical use.

OPTICAL IMAGING BACKGROUND STUDIES

Optical imaging has evolved from its beginnings into an intraoperative technique over the past several decades. In 1949, Hill and Keynes were the first to describe changes in the intrinsic light-scattering properties of neurons associated with electrical stimulation, referred to as the intrinsic optical signal (IOS) (3). Their observations were made using a photocell to record opacity changes in the crayfish nerve trunk without the use of voltage-sensitive dyes. The observed IOS was characterized by an increase in light transmission during stimulation (positive IOS) followed by a relatively prolonged decrease in light transmission after stimulation (negative IOS).

Over the past 20 years, a handful of investigators developed several applications for OI including the development and screening of voltage sensitive dyes (4–11). The technique was further advanced by Blasdel and Salama who employed a television camera (120 × 120) to improve the spatial resolution previously achieved with standard photodiode arrays (12 × 12) (12). Blasdel went on to apply OI toward in vivo functional mapping by augmenting the IOS with voltage-sensitive dyes to image ocular dominance columns and orientation preferences in nonhuman primate visual cortex. Grinvald and colleagues were later able to identify similar functional regions in the primate visual cortex without the use of voltage-sensitive dyes by directly imaging the IOS changes associated with cortical surface optical reflectance (7–9,13).

Several dynamic physiological processes have been identified as sources of the IOS including oxy- and deoxyhemoglobin concentrations, cytochrome oxygenation states, blood volume fluctuations, extracellular volume shifts, and neuronal and glial swelling (2,3,8,15). A correlation between the IOS and neuronal activity has more recently been established (16–18).

INTRAOPERATIVE OPTICAL IMAGING TECHNIQUE

Several sources of artifact can make the IOS difficult to discern; therefore, successful intraoperative OI requires minimizing patient movement, dampening physiologic brain pulsations, and uniform cortical surface illumination (Fig. 1). One of the most critical strategies during OI is to minimize movement. Brain pulsations associated with hemodynamic and respiratory patterns cause spatial shifts during image acquisition, making frame-to-frame IOS analysis difficult (19). This artifact can be overcome during image acquisition with mechanical dampening and during image analysis with image "warping" algorithms. Mechanical dampening is achieved by placing a glass plate ($4\,cm^2$, $9\,cm^2$, $16\,cm^2$, or $25\,cm^2$) over the cortical surface in the area of interest. The glass plate is mounted to an adjustable mechanical arm that is in turn mounted to a skull clamp. This rigid construct has become particularly important during awake craniotomies and during imaging of seizure activity when image acquisition is continuous over 1–2 min.

The brain surface is uniformly illuminated using a stable tungsten halogen light source. The incident light is filtered to the desired wavelength (typically 695-nm long-pass filter) with the operating theater darkened to minimize artifacts from ambient light sources. By selecting different wavelengths of light through filtration, specific

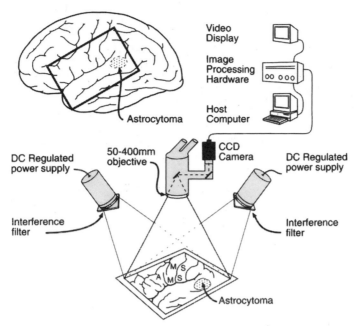

Figure 1. Schematic of intraoperative optical imaging setup. A CCD camera is attached to an operating microscope, with incident light source regulated by a DC power supply and filtered through a 695-nm filter. The cortex is stabilized from movement in the z-axis by a glass plate lowered onto the cortical surface. Percentage-difference images are calculated; image processing and data analysis performed with Imaging Technology, Inc. Imaging boards. (From Ref. 22.)

aspects of the IOS, and therefore specific physiological processes, may be emphasized. Imaging through a 610-nm or 695-nm filter, as reported in human studies, emphasizes changes in hemoglobin oxygenation (19–24).

A charge-coupled device (CCD) camera is mounted on the operating microscope and, to further minimize movement artifacts, the microscope is mounted to the operating table by a modified microscope base. Initially, a low-power objective is selected to allow for visualization of a relatively large cortical area ($25\,cm^2$). During seizure focus localization or functional mapping, images are collected at rate of ~50 Hz over a period of 1 min and using software developed by Daryl Hochman, image analysis can then be performed intraoperatively within 2 min. Images are analyzed by subtracting a baseline image (i.e., prior to cortical activation) from all subsequent images, yielding data that reflects frame-to-frame changes in the IOS. During analysis, statistical algorithms are applied to align successive images in order to compensate for residual microscopic movement artifacts. This is particularly important when images are acquired through a high-power objective, where small movements are magnified. Each series is viewed intraoperatively to evaluate epileptiform or functional activity. Despite efforts to minimize movement, ambient light, and thermal artifacts, a small amount of noise in the processed images is difficult to avoid (Fig. 2Ab).

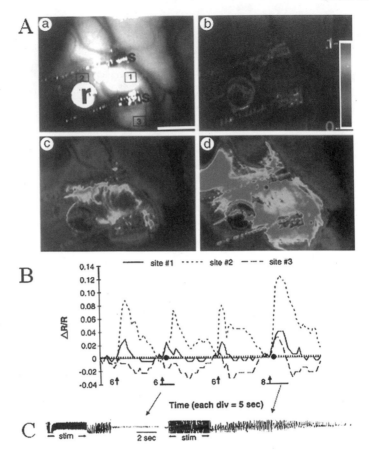

Figure 2. Images of human cortical surface demonstrating seizure activity evoked with four consecutive electrical bipolar stimulations, three at 6 mA and one at 8 mA. (*Aa*) Baseline image demonstrating positions of recording electrode (r), stimulating electrodes (s), and regions of interest where IOS changes were measured (1, 2, and 3). (*Ab*) Image demonstrating baseline noise created by subtracting one pre-stimulation image from another. Color bar on the right of Ab shows peak optical changes are indicated by orange and red. (*Ac, Ad*) Peak optical changes during a small (Ac) and larger (Ad) seizure corresponding to the short and long seizure episodes depicted in C, respectively. (*B*) Graphical representation of optical changes from A during stimulus-evoked seizures measured at sites 1 (solid line), 2 (short-dashed line), and 3 (long-dashed line). (*C*) Surface EEG recordings from s during two of the stimulus-evoked seizures. The first episode corresponds to the second stimulation (6 mA) depicted in B and Ac. The second episode corresponds to the fourth stimulation (8 mA) depicted in B and Ad. The peak optical changes are localized near the recording electrode at site 2, while a surrounding area at site 3 shows changes in the opposite direction. (From Ref. 1.)

OPTICAL IMAGING OF EPILEPTIFORM ACTIVITY

Optical imaging can be used intra-operatively to study seizure and interictal activity (1,24,25). Prior to imaging, surface EEG is used to roughly localize foci of epileptiform activity. Once localized, the ECoG electrodes are removed from the cortical surface, and a glass plate is placed over the site of interest together with an array of recording electrodes about the periphery and a pair of centrally located stimulating electrodes. In addition to imaging spontaneous activity, evoked interictal and seizure activity can be generated through bipolar stimulation at currents above the afterdischarge (AD) potential threshold. In five patients undergoing surgery for intractable epilepsy, Haglund et al. demonstrated that the IOS intensity, spread, and duration occurring during epileptiform activity evoked from bipolar stimulation correlated with the duration of electrical AD activity (Fig. 2) (1). The stimulus was delivered via electrodes separated by 1 cm (s in Fig. 2Aa) at an intensity just above the AD potential threshold and the IOS was compared to simultaneous surface EEG recordings (r in Fig. 2Aa). Each stimulation was followed by epileptiform AD activity of varying intensity and duration.

The spatial spread of the IOS was greatest when associated with long durations of AD activity (12–16 sec, lower right Fig. 2C) and less when associated with short durations of AD activity (<4 sec; lower left Fig. 2C). Figure 2 illustrates that the area of peak IOS intensity during the shorter seizure episode was more limited compared to the much greater spatial extent of IOS changes during the more intense seizure episode. Furthermore, the duration of IOS changes correlated with, but lasted longer than, the duration of electrical activity (Fig. 2A, B, and C).

In addition to a greater spatial extent and duration of IOS changes, longer seizure episodes were also associated with a greater magnitude (i.e., greater intensity) of IOS changes. The IOS changes at sites 1–3 (identified in Fig. 2Aa) during four successive stimulations are graphically depicted in Fig. 2B. Site 1 represents the area between the stimulating electrodes and shows the positive IOS changes during the four successive stimulations; the first three stimulations were at 6 mA and the last was at 8 mA. Electrical activity from only the first 6-mA stimulation is depicted in Fig. 2C; the second and third were of similar duration and intensity. Note that the magnitude of IOS change from site 2 (Fig. 2B) correlates with the intensity and duration of electrical changes recorded from r, with the largest positive IOS change occurring after the most prolonged episode of AD activity. Of interest, but still without a clear mechanism, are the negative IOS changes in the areas surrounding the focus of epileptiform discharges (measured at site 3). During each of the first three stimulations, the IOS changes at site 3 were in the negative direction, whereas during the fourth, most intense seizure episode, the change was initially positive before becoming negative. More detailed studies are needed to determine whether these negative IOS changes represent surround inhibition, shunting of extracellular fluid, shunting of blood volume toward active cortex, or changes in blood oxygenation.

Further analysis involving comparisons of IOS changes and surface EEG activity during different stages of seizure activity reveals that the magnitude and direction of IOS changes seem to correlate with changes in electrical activity. Figure 3 demonstrates IOS changes and surface electrode activity (R) measured simultaneously at baseline prior to stimulation (1), after stimulation during the seizure (2), during postseizure quiescence (3), and after return to baseline (4). During baseline activity, the region surrounding the recording electrode is black (neutral IOS), whereas during the seizure episode this area is clearly activated in the positive direction (white). During the postseizure period, when the electrical activity is quiescent compared to baseline (3), the area surrounding the recording electrode

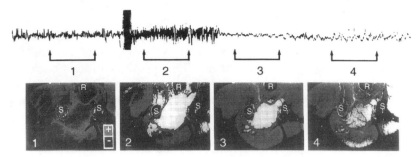

Figure 3. Upper trace demonstrates electrical activity recorded during bipolar stimulation (occurring between 1 and 2) and OI from the recording electrode labeled R in the lower panel. The images in the lower panel also depict sites of stimulation (S). The cortical surface area within each of the lower panels is $4\,cm^2$. The lower panel demonstrates the optical changes from baseline associated with the four different types of electrical activity recorded at R. The white areas represent increases in IOS, while the more light gray areas are below baseline (lower right-hand corner of image 1 of lower panel). During the peak of activation in 2, there is a large area of activation, while during the postictal phase in 3 the area around the recording electrode is primarily below baseline. (From Ref. 35.)

now shows a negative IOS (dark gray), which gradually returns to near baseline. These preliminary observations point toward a correlation between the direction of IOS changes and electrical activity where positive IOS changes closely correlate with increases in electrical activity and negative IOS changes correlate with below-baseline electrical activity.

OPTICAL IMAGING OF FUNCTIONAL CORTEX

Over the past decade, OI has been employed to study sensorimotor (1,19,20,26) and language (1,21,23) cortex as well as cortical regions subserving higher cognitive functions such as face matching and short-term memory (26).

Optical Imaging of Somatosensory Cortex

The ability to map somatosensory, motor, and language cortex using OI was first demonstrated by Haglund et al. in patients undergoing awake craniotomies for intractable epilepsy (1). Initially, tongue and palate sensory areas were identified with intraoperative ESM by evoking subjective tingling in those areas (sites 1 and 2; Fig. 4A1). Patients were then instructed to move their tongues from side to side within the closed mouth. During three trials with OI, tongue movements produced the greatest IOS changes within the tongue and palate somatosensory areas as identified by ESM. These IOS changes were similar to those associated with cortical activation after bipolar stimulation, indicating that they reflected somatosensory cortical activation most likely from sensory feedback associated with tongue movements. Motor cortex associated with face movements (as identified by ESM) demonstrated IOS changes in the negative direction during tongue movement. Similar shifts in the IOS of motor cortex have been observed during overt speech

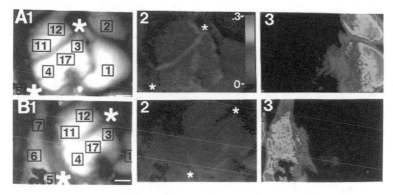

Figure 4. (*A1, B1*) Human Broca's area showing the inferior frontal gyrus at sites 5, 6, and 7; the lower portion of precentral gyrus at sites 3, 4, 11, 12, and 17; and the lower portions of the postcentral gyrus at sites 1 and 2. (*A2*) Baseline image prior to tongue movement; (*A3*) peak cortical activation with tongue movement; (*B2*) baseline image prior to naming; (*B3*) peak cortical activation with naming. Peak cortical activation associated with naming is distinctly different from that associated with tongue movement. (From Ref. 1.)

(26). It is tempting to suggest that these negative IOS changes represent decreased neuronal activity in face primary motor cortex during these simple movements. An alternative explanation is that the increased blood flow associated with somatosensory activation caused a shunting of blood flow away from primary motor cortex. We are currently investigating the relationship between blood volume and electrophysiological changes to determine which mechanism underlies this phenomenon (24).

More recently, others have corroborated the IOS changes seen with somatosensory activation (19,20). Cannestra et al. elicited somatosensory cortical activation with median nerve transcutaneous stimulation or 110-Hz finger vibration (20). There was a close spatial correlation between cortical evoked potentials and IOS changes. Similarly, Shoham and Grinvald elicited somatosensory cortical activation with electrical and tactile peripheral stimulation in 15 patients undergoing brain tumor or AVM resection under general anesthesia (19). Optical imaging was accompanied by surface-evoked potential recording. Owing to the presence of optical signal artifacts, they were unable to draw definitive conclusions. However, these authors were able to obtain reproducible high-resolution somatosensory IOS maps from the hand area in the nonhuman primate. The observed IOS changes associated with peripheral tactile stimulation correlated closely with single- and multiunit cortical recordings. These findings confirmed the association between positive IOS changes and somatosensory cortical activation.

Optical Imaging Identification of Language Cortex

Intraoperative ESM under local anesthesia during object naming is a safe, effective way to identify essential language cortex, particularly with the use of modern intravenous propofol anesthesia and local scalp anesthetic block (27). Stimulation mapping using other, infrequently tested language-related measures such as naming in another language (including American Sign Language), sentence reading, or recent verbal memory have demonstrated a dissociation in their cortical representation (28–30), and, under some circumstances, localizing and sparing these other language-related sites is important in avoiding postoperative deficits (30). However, mapping many different language functions, particularly when recent memory is included, is quite lengthy. Intraoperative OI may provide greater efficiency and detail during the functional localization of multiple cognitive and language functions (1,16,21,23,26).

Inferior Frontal Language Area

Haglund et al. performed OI in the inferior frontal language area (i.e., Broca's area) and somatosensory cortex (Fig. 4B1) of patients undergoing dominant hemisphere temporal lobe resections under local anesthesia (1). Optical imaging took place while patients silently viewed blank slides and while naming objects displayed on slides presented every 2 sec. Images obtained during naming showed activation of the premotor cortex (baseline, Fig. 4B2; naming, Fig. 4B3) while the ESM identified speech arrest (sites 3 and 4) and palate tingling (site 1) sites yielded IOS changes in the opposite direction (black areas, Fig. 4B3). The area that showed the greatest positive IOS changes during tongue movement was clearly different form the active area in the naming exercise (compare Figs. 4A3 and 4B3). The premotor cortical areas from which IOS changes occurred during the naming exercise were similar to those identified on positron emission tomography (PET) images obtained during single-word processing studies (31,32). The IOS changes were greatest in the anatomical area of cortex classically defined as Broca's area (the posterior portion of the inferior frontal gyrus; i.e., sites 5, 6, and 7 in Fig. 4B1) and not as expected in areas where electrical stimulation caused speech arrest (sites 3 and 4).

Further topographical definition of Broca's area was demonstrated by Cannestra et al. (21). Broca's area was defined by ESM in five patients undergoing craniotomies under local anesthesia for the resection of brain tumors and vascular malformations. After identification of Broca's area, OI was performed during object naming (n = 5), word discrimination (n = 4), auditory responsive naming (n = 4), and orofacial movement (n = 3) tasks. Two distinct subregions (anterior and posterior) within Broca's area were identified. Both auditory and visual object-naming paradigms were associated with increased IOS changes in both the anterior and posterior Broca's subregions. In contrast, word discrimination produced IOS changes only in the posterior subregion. They conclude that this functional heterogeneity may represent subspecialized cortical networks within Broca's area with anterior regions subserving semantic functions and posterior regions subserving phonological functions. Similar to the findings of Haglund et al. (1), there was incomplete agreement between ESM-identified language sites, and IOS changes, ESM, and IOS changes overlapped only in the posterior subregion of the OI defined Broca's area.

Perisylvian Language Areas

Optical imaging of posterior, perisylvian essential language sites (i.e., Wernicke's area) has demonstrated findings similar to those in Broca's area. Haglund et al. demonstrated that in posterior temporal cortex, IOS changes during object naming originated from the general region where ESM elicited naming errors (1). Similar to

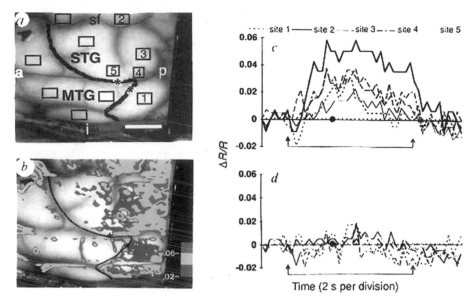

Figure 5. (*a*) Dominant temporal lobe with sites 1, 2, 3, 4, and 5 representing sites where speech was identified with either electrical stimulation (sites 1, 2, and 3) or when the resection (thick black line) came from anterior (a) to posterior (p) in the temporal lobe (sites 4 and 5). Open boxes represent areas where electrical stimulation had no effect on naming objects. (*b*) Peak optical changes above 2% with most of the changes localized in areas that were important for naming. (*c*) Optical changes during naming (arrows below the x-axis represent start and completion of naming) at sites important for language by electrical stimulation or from language being disrupted during the resection. (*d*) Postical changes during naming form sites not critical for naming as defined by ESM. (From Ref. 1.)

findings in Broca's area, the IOS changes covered a somewhat wider surrounding area compared to essential areas identified during ESM localization (Fig. 5). All IOS changes were observed in areas near sites where ESM altered naming. The IOS changes appeared within 2–5 sec of initiating naming, and disappeared over a slightly longer time following the termination of naming. Cannestra et al. demonstrated similar findings among six patients undergoing awake craniotomies for tumor or vascular lesion resection (21). IOS changes were observed from all ESM-defined perisylvian language areas as well as from adjacent cortex. As in Broca's area, they were able to identify subregions subserving different functions. Object-naming (n = 6) activated the central and anterior-inferior Wernicke subregions, whereas word discrimination (n = 5) preferentially activated the central and superior subregions, and auditory responsive naming preferentially activated the central, anterior-inferior, and superior regions. Additional task-specific activations were observed in the inferior-posterior subregion.

Implications for Cortical Resection

Optical imaging of inferior frontal and posterior perisylvian language areas has consistently shown that IOS changes are more diffuse than ESM identified regions. Cannestra et al. demonstrated that these surrounding regions may represent task-specific subregions (21). This more diffuse cortical language representation identified by optical imaging may account for the occurrence of deficits following resection of cortex within 1 cm of ESM identified essential language sites (33). In one case, we carried the temporal resection very close to an ESM-identified posterior temporal essential language site while testing language and stopped when naming errors occurred (see solid line in Fig. 5). As often occurs under similar circumstances, the patient's language returned to baseline soon after surgery. Interestingly, the resection extended to the margin of the region of IOS changes, suggesting that OI can provide the reliable localizing information needed to plan safe cortical resections.

Optical Imaging of Cognitive Function

In over 20 patients undergoing temporal lobe resections for intractable epilepsy, we studied dominant and nondominant temporal lobe neocortical IOS activation associated with several cognitive tasks (26). During dominant hemisphere resections, we found that IOS changes associated with short-term memory tasks localized to the posterior superior temporal gyrus (STG). In these patients, IOS changes associated with object-naming overlapped with ESM identified essential language sites. The IOS changes associated specifically with the memory task, however, were immediately anterior to the essential language site. Furthermore, activation with memory input occupied a discrete region that was immediately surrounded by positive IOS changes associated with memory retrieval. In a subset of patients undergoing nondominant hemisphere temporal lobe resections, we performed OI during face-matching, complex figure-matching, and facial expression interpretation tasks [paradigm described in detail by Ojemann et al. (34)]. Consistently, we identified negative IOS changes in the posterior MTG and STG during the tasks.

Our initial experiences with OI of language and higher cognitive functions indicate that OI will become a valuable means of ultimately mapping and precisely pinpointing the cortical representation of higher cognitive processes and assessing the temporospatial relationships associated with cortical processing during cognitive tasks. To date, mapping these functions with ESM has been difficult at best, and is often limited to functional imaging methods that often prove to be associated with localization errors.

CONCLUSION

Intraoperative OI has become a valuable tool that remains limited to research applications. Before OI can become a routine clinical method of functional mapping and epileptic focus identification, the physiologic mechanisms underlying optical changes at different wavelengths of light must be further explained, the clinical significance of OI identified functional cortex must be described, and the ease of setup must be improved. Furthermore, one should always be mindful of the inherent difficulty in obtaining hard human data using such techniques. A greater awareness of OI's limitations, particularly as it applies to defining an epileptogenic zone, compared to other functional mapping techniques such as fMRI, will become paramount in carefully designing and interpreting future clinical studies.

REFERENCES

1. Haglund MM, Ojemann GA, Hochman DW. Optical imaging of epileptiform and functional activity from human cortex. Nature 1992; 358:668–671.
2. Hochman DW. Intrinsic optical changes in neuronal tissue: basic mechanisms. Neurosurg Clin North Am 1997; 8(3):393–412.
3. Hill DK, Keynes RD. Opacity changes in stimulated nerve. J Physiol 1949; 1089:278–281.
4. Cohen LB, Salzberg BM. Optical measurement of membrane potential. Rev Physiol Biochem Pharmacol 1978; 83:33–88.
5. Cohen LB, Keynes RD, Landowne D. Changes in light scattering that accompany the action potential I squid giant axons: potential-dependent components. J Physiol (Lond) 1972; 224:701–725.
6. Cohen LB, Salzberg BM, Davila HV. Changes in axon fluorescence during activity: molecular probes of membrane potential. J Membr Biol 1974; 19:1–36.
7. Frostig RD, Lieke EE, Ts'o DY. Cortical functional architecture and local coupling between neuronal activity and the microcirculation revealed by in vivo high-resolution optical imaging of intrinsic signals. Proc Natl Acad Sci USA 1990; 87:6082–6086.
8. Grinvald A, Manker A, Segal M. Visualization of the spread of electrical activity in rat hippocampal slices by voltage-sensitive optical probes. J Physiol 1982; 333:269–291.
9. Grinvald A, Lieke EE, Frostig RD. Functional architecture of cortex revealed by optical imaging of intrinsic signals. Nature 1986; 324:361–364.
10. Orbach HS, Cohen LB, Grinvald A. Optical imaging of neuronal activity in the mammalian sensory cortex. J Neurosci 1985; 5:1886–1895.
11. Salzberg BM, Obaid AL, Gainer H. Large and rapid changes in light scattering accompany secretion by nerve terminals in the mammalian neurohypophysis. J Gen Physiol 1985; 86:395–411.
12. Blasdel GG, Salama G. Voltage-sensitive dyes reveal a modular organization in monkey striate cortex. Nature 1986; 321:579–585.
13. Ts'o DY, Frostig RD, Lieke EE. Functional organization of primate visual cortex revealed by high resolution optical imaging. Science 1990; 249:417–420.
14. Haglund MM, Blasdel GG. Optical imaging of acute epileptic foci in monkey visual cortex. Epilepsia, 1993; 34(suppl 6):21.
15. Haglund MM, Hochman DW, Meno J. Mechanisms underlying the intrinsic signal during optical imaging of rat somatosensory cortex. Soc Neurosci Abstr 1994; 20:1263.
16. Cannestra AF, Bookheimer SY, Martin NA. The characterization of language corticies utilizing intraoperative optical intrinsic signals. Neuroimage 1998; 7:52. (Abstract.)
17. Narayan SM, Santori EM, Toga AW. Mapping functional activity in rodent cortex using optical intrinsic signals. Cereb Cortex 1994; 4:195–204.
18. Toga AW, Cannestra AD, Black KL. The temporal/spatial evolution of optical signals in human cortex. Cereb Cortex 1995; 5:561–565.
19. Shoham D, Grinvald A. The cortical representation of the hand in *Macaque* and human area S-1: high resolution optical imaging. J Neurosci 2001; 21(17):6820–6835.
20. Cannestra AF, Pouratian N, Bookheimer SY, Martin NA, Becker DP, Toga AW. Temporal spatial differences observed by functional MRI and human intraoperative optical imaging. Cereb Cortex 2001; 11:773–782.
21. Cannestra AF, Bookheimer SY, Pouratian N, O'Farrell A, Sicotte N, Martin NA, Becker D, Rubino G, Toga AW. Temporal and topographical characterization of language corticies using intraoperative optical intrinsic signals. Neuroimage 2000; 12:41–54.
22. Haglund MM, Berger MS, Hochman DW. Enhanced optical imaging of human gliomas and tumor margins. Neurosurgery 1996; 38:308–316.

23. Pouratian N, Bookheimer SY, O'Farrell AM, Sicotte NL, Cannestra AF, Becker D, Toga AW. Optical imaging of bilingual cortical representations. J Neurosurg 2000; 93:676–681.

24. Hochman DW, Little KM, Haglund MM. Optical imaging of cortical epileptiform activity in primates. The American Epilepsy Society and The American Clinical Neurophysiology Society Joint Meeting, Philadelphia, 2001.

25. Schwartz TH, Bonohoeffer T. In vivo optical imaging of epileptic foci and surround inhibition in ferret cerebral cortex. Nat Med 2001; 7:1065–1067.

26. Hochman DW, Ojemann GA, Haglund MM. Optical imaging reveals alternating positive and negative changes during cognitive or sensory evoked cortical activity in awake humans. Soc Neurosci Abstr 1994; 20:5.

27. Silbergeld DL, Mueller WM, Ojemann GA. Use of propofol (Diprivan) for awake craniotomies: technical note. Surg Neurol 1992; 4:271.

28. Ojemann G, Whitaker H. Language localization and variability. Brain Lang 1978; 6:239–260.

29. Ojemann GA. Brain organization for language from the perspective of electrical stimulation mapping. Behav Brain Sci 1983; 6:189–206.

30. Ojemann GA, Dodrill CG. Intraoperative techniques for reducing language and memory deficits with left temporal lobectomy. Adv Epileptol 1987; 16:327–330.

31. Petersen SE, Fox PT, Posner ME, Mintum M, Raichle ME. Positron emission tomographic studies of the cortical anatomy of single word processing. Nature 1988; 331:585–589.

32. Frith CD, Friston KJ, Liddle PF, Frackowiak RS. A PET study of word finding. J Neuropsychol 1991; 29:1137–1148.

33. Haglund MM, Berger MS, Shamseldin MS. Cortical localization of temporal lobe language sites in patients with gliomas. Neurosurgery 1994; 34:567–576.

34. Ojemann JG, Ojemann GA, Lettich E. Neuronal activity related to faces and matching in human right nondominant temporal cortex. Brain 1992; 115:1–13.

35. Haglund MM. Intraoperative optical imaging of epileptiform and functional activity. Neurosurg Clin North Am 1997; 8(3):413–420.

24
Early Seizure Detection: Theoretical and Applied

Gregory K. Bergey, Piotr J. Franaszczuk, and Christophe Jouny
The Johns Hopkins University School of Medicine
Baltimore, Maryland, U.S.A.

WHAT IS SEIZURE DETECTION?

Epileptic seizures are episodic, rapidly evolving, temporary events, typically lasting less than a minute, characterized by increased network excitation with synchronous discharges from the involved neural networks and variable propagation. The clinical manifestations of a seizure reflect the regions of the brain involved, either initially at the seizure focus or subsequently, as there is seizure spread or secondary generalization. Some seizures, for instance those originating from frontal lobe regions, such as the orbital frontal regions, may have no clinical manifestations at the site of the initial focus, and only when they propagate to other areas do they produce clinical signs or symptoms.

One can think of the clinical manifestations as a type of seizure detection by the patient or observer. Indeed the concept of seizure "prediction" dogs is not the application of some complex canine nonlinear algorithm, but rather the recognition by the dog of the stereotyped clinical manifestations of the owner allowing the dog to reduce the risk of injury (1). These animals are therefore quite clearly seizure *detection* dogs, not seizure prediction dogs. In the context of ictal recordings of seizures, typically in long-term monitoring, the clinical signs of a seizure are correlated with the ictal EEG. The electroencephalographer examining ictal recordings will consider the earliest visually apparent changes as the ictal EEG onset. These EEG changes can occur before clinical manifestations if the seizure originates from a silent region. Conversely, if the recording array is remote from the seizure onset site, the clinical manifestations may occur before any visual EEG changes. Therefore early detection depends on appropriate placement recording arrays so that they are proximal to the site of seizure onset.

When a seizure occurs, there is increased abnormal synchronous firing. This may produce a variety of patterns during seizure initiation, involving few or many recording channels, and these patterns can vary depending on brain region and whether scalp or intracranial recording montages are being used. Common patterns of seizure initiation recorded from intracranial electrodes include low-voltage fast activity or periodic sharp activity. Scalp recordings may not reveal high-frequency, low-voltage activity. In addition, neocortical onset seizures may have broad regional electrodecremental changes, at times associated with low-voltage fast activity, making detection easy but localization difficult.

Any reliable seizure detection algorithm needs to recognize these dynamic ictal patterns. Often these patterns of seizure initiation are very different from the more organized rhythmic activity seen later in the seizure. Indeed, the onset and conclusion of seizures are typically characterized by relatively high complexity signals. If the goal is mere seizure detection, for instance in an epilepsy monitoring unit, then recognizing the prominent organized rhythmic activity (for instance the 6–8 Hz activity of a mesial temporal lobe–onset seizure) may be sufficient, even if this activity only occurs many seconds after seizure onset. If the desire is early seizure detection, for potential therapeutic intervention, then the challenges are considerably greater. Detection from intracranial electrodes is considerably easier than from scalp recordings, provided the recording array is near the area of seizure onset.

Fortunately, although ictal onset patterns can vary from patient to patient, in a given patient with a single seizure focus, the patterns of seizure initiation and early evolution are very stereotyped (Fig. 1). This is evident from visual analysis as well as detailed time-frequency decompositions of seizures. The benefit of stereotyped seizure dynamic patterns is that, particularly with intracranial recordings, detection algorithms, at times combining methods, can be tuned to be both sensitive and specific for the seizures of a given patient. Time-frequency analyses have also

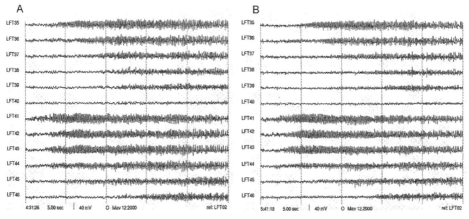

Figure 1. Similarity of epileptic seizures. The two panels illustrate two sequential frontal neocortical onset partial seizures, recorded from the same patient, separated by ~80 min. Selected channels near the region of seizure onset are shown; extensive subdural grid arrays were employed. Visual inspection indicates similar patterns of onset and evolution. This was further documented by time-frequency decompositions (not shown). The dotted time bars are 1 sec apart.

demonstrated that at seizure onset there is a dramatic change in signal complexity. Even if a given patient has seizures of varying length (due to secondary spread or generalization), the characteristics of the onset from a given focus are typically similar. This allows detection algorithms to be "tuned" for a given patient increasing specificity and sensitivity.

Early detection of seizures may be more important in real life than in the monitoring unit. For the purposes of presurgical evaluations, mere detection of seizures is sufficient. Sensitivity is desirable so seizures are not missed. Specificity is desirable so that staff members are not unnecessarily summoned for frequent false detections. Outside the monitoring unit, early detection becomes potentially much more important. Early seizure detection or prediction could allow the patient to take actions to avoid injury. Indeed, patients with reliable and prolonged auras can often remove themselves from potentially dangerous situations. As we begin to investigate devices for seizure detection, early detection is equally important so that intervention can be initiated early in the seizure. There is growing interest in the areas of early seizure detection so that devices can be implemented to either warn the patient or even intervene to terminate or prevent the seizure (see below).

THEORETICAL APPROACHES TO SEIZURE DETECTION

To develop a reliable method for detection of an event we need to have a good definition of this event in terms of some measurable properties. Most of the methods of seizure detection and prediction are based on analysis of measurements of electrical activity of the brain, i.e., scalp EEG or ECoG intracranially using subdural or depth electrodes in patients being evaluated for seizure surgery. There were also some attempts to use other measurements to detect seizure, most notably heart rate changes (2,3), but these methods also proved more reliable when combined with EEG (4).

Methods based on analysis of EEG recordings require digitized data and computerized methods of analysis. The detection of seizures using EEG recordings is possible due to the presence of clearly visible electrographic changes in the signal. It is relatively straightforward to define a seizure using these changes. There are many methods of efficient parameterization of these electrographic changes during seizures, and the computed parameters (sometimes called signal features) may be subsequently used to classify an epoch of the signal as a seizure.

To access the validity of the method we can use standard measures of sensitivity, i.e., the ratio of detected seizures (called true positives; TP) to all seizures in an analyzed record. The detection needs to be performed on a well-defined portion of the signal, i.e., the epoch (or window) of a given length. The binary detection method gives only two possible results: *detected* or *not detected*. For detection of a seizure as a single event, the window of detection needs to be large enough to contain the whole seizure, or the detector needs to skip a predefined portion of the signal after detection. The first solution (large window) is preferable because too small a window may cause the detector to miss the seizure after a false alarm. Unfortunately, this would prevent early detection of seizure because detection will occur after the end of the seizure.

One also needs an independent method (gold standard) to obtain the number of "true" seizures. Usually this is obtained by visual screening of EEG by a trained neurologist. By changing the parameters of the detection algorithm, the sensitivity can be tuned to obtain sensitivity as close to 100% as possible. Usually increasing the sensitivity leads to detection of some events (i.e., artifacts, normal sleep patterns, etc.), which are not seizures by the gold-standard definition. These detections are called false positives (FP) or false alarms (FA), and constitute the basis for definition of the specificity of the detection method.

In image analysis or in statistical signal processing, when statistical properties of the signal and noise could be defined, the performance of the detection can be quantified by constructing the receiver operating characteristics (ROC) (5). This is a plot of the probability of detection (i.e., sensitivity) versus the probability of a false alarm (i.e., specificity) for different values of the parameter of detection (threshold). The areas under the ROC curve provide a measure of performance of a detector. This area is equal to 1 for an ideal detector and ½ for random detection (i.e., deciding for each epoch randomly if there is a seizure or not).

In practice, seizures are a small portion of the monitored signal, so any usable algorithm is tuned to have very small proportion of false alarms in relation to the number of epochs used for detection. For these reason ROC curves have limited value in measuring performance of detection methods. Instead, in addition to sensitivity (defined as above), the rate of false positives per hour (FP/h) is used as a measure of specificity. Similarly as with the ROC curve, the designer of the algorithm needs to tune the parameters of detection to reach a compromise between sensitivity and specificity. This decision depends on the purpose of the detection. If the purpose is to assist a neurologist in reviewing the EEG for preoperative evaluation, missing a seizure—even a subclinical one—is undesirable. False alarms just increase the review time, which in any case will be shorter than reviewing all recorded data. In this case, detection parameters should be tuned to maximize sensitivity even if the false-alarm rate is relatively high.

On the other hand, when detection is for the purpose of intervention, and intervention is potentially harmful (e.g., administration of medication), missing some subclinical seizures may be acceptable, while too many false alarms may cause harm. In this case, parameters of detection should be tuned to decrease the rate of false alarms. This is also true if detection is for the purpose of notifying the occurrence of a seizure. Too many false alarms may lead to ignoring true detections.

DETECTION VERSUS PREDICTION: THE CONCEPT OF A PREICTAL STATE

There is considerable interest in predicting seizures. The concept of seizure prediction or anticipation is a provocative one. Since seizures are manifestations of increased network synchrony, it is a reasonable hypothesis that there are changes in activity, potentially embedded in the EEG signal that would reflect these synaptic or network changes before the actual seizure occurrence. Interestingly, examination of interictal spikes has not even convincingly shown that spike frequency increases prior to ictal initiation (6). Other investigators, however, feel that subclinical seizures, bursts, or "chirps" increase prior to clinical events (7).

The concept of these early changes, which conceivably could occur minutes or even hours before a clinical event is the concept of a *preictal state*. Where the controversy arises is when the preictal state ends and the ictal state begins and when "prediction" is really only early detection.

The above discussion is clearly applicable to detection of a seizure as it is occurring or even retrospectively for diagnostic purposes. Therapeutic applications need different approaches. The goal is to detect a seizure as early as possible to allow intervention to prevent it from developing into a clinical event or to warn a patient in advance. In this case, there is a need for a new definition of what constitutes a seizure and when it starts. Remembering that we are limiting our discussion to analysis of an EEG signal, we need to define the electrographic onset of the seizure. There are two possible extremes of the definition. The broadest one is to assume that any EEG changes detectable by any present or future method are different than the interictal baseline and are followed by a clinical seizure which is in fact a beginning of a seizure. This definition is an extension to the current practice followed by many neurologists performing visual analysis. They look at the EEG before the seizure for signal patterns that are distinct from that normally occurring during the interictal period. This definition does not allow for a separate definition of prediction of seizure; everything is early detection.

On the other hand, even this definition allows for the anticipation of a seizure, as the detection of electrographic changes which may indicate increased probability of seizure in the near future but not certainty. At one extreme there is the definition of the onset of the seizure as a pattern in EEG coincident with the clinical onset of the seizure. In this case, if a given method detects some changes in EEG before that, it could be called prediction if, after this change, a seizure always occurs. Strictly speaking, the prediction method should also include the time horizon of the prediction. If this time horizon is a range, it can also be associated with the probability of occurrence of the seizure in the given time interval. In this case the definition of prediction may overlap with the definition of anticipation. In the literature there was a tendency to use the term "prediction" starting with pioneering work of Viglione (8–10) and many publications related to nonlinear methods of analysis in the last decade (11–13), but recently the term "anticipation" is being more frequently used (14–16). Prediction is only possible if there is a preictal state. Litt and Lehnertz in a recent review (17) suggest that there is enough evidence to support existence of the preictal state. In this case, the prediction methods can be really treated as detection of preictal state. Litt et al. (7) identified prolonged bursts of epileptiform discharges as precursors to seizure activity. In this case, detection of such precursors will be synonymous with prediction or anticipation.

It is particularly important when applying means of seizure prediction that these applications not be corrupted by seizure clusters. A patient having seizures every 3 h may have residual changes in the postictal period that might be interpreted as "predicting" the next seizure, since a true baseline interictal period may not be reached during seizure clusters. Any objective test of accurate seizure prediction must be effective in predicting the first seizure of any seizure cluster.

SEIZURE DETECTION METHODOLOGY

Trained neurologists are able to detect electrographic signatures of the seizure by visual analysis of EEG recordings. This prompted the development of the expert systems of seizure detection (18–22). Expert systems attempt to extract from the signal the same features a trained neurologist uses in visual analysis. These features may include parameters of the shape of the EEG waveform, sometimes as simple as the length of the curve (23), relative amplitude, dominant frequency (24), amplitude, slope, curvature, rhythmicity, and frequency components (25). Most of these systems use various types of artificial neural network (ANN) algorithms to process the input features (18,20,25–28). In general, most of these algorithms require the training phase when parameters of the algorithm are tuned to obtain optimal detections in agreement with the analysis of the expert neurologist. These methods can be also described as pattern-matching techniques, where there is a certain pattern—defined by specific parameters—that is to be detected, and there is a procedure to train the system to learn how to recognize this pattern. Obviously, these methods can be successful in seizure detection if such patterns of early seizure onset can be defined with sufficient precision.

This different approach to detection has roots in general signal processing detection techniques. The main idea is to use a procedure that will yield a detection function. Values of the detection function in comparison with a certain threshold will indicate occurrence of the event subject to detection. The common characteristic of this approach is the use of the raw EEG signal as the input data, and to perform numerical computations on this signal to obtain the value of the detection function. It can be performed with every recorded channel of EEG separately, or it may involve multichannel methods to capture interactions between channels relevant for detection. For seizure detection, the signal processing methods can be classified as nonparametric methods without any clear assumptions about specific properties of the EEG signal or its generation, or about parametric methods where such assumptions are present. The most commonly applied nonparametric methods of EEG signal analysis include traditional spectral analysis using FFT (fast Fourier transforms) or, more recently, time-frequency or time-scale analyses (i.e., wavelet) (29–32) or matching pursuit decompositions (33). In application to detection, the multitude of parameters obtained from time-frequency methods is transformed into one synthetic measure. In the case of wavelet methods, it can be wavelet entropy. For matching pursuit it is Gabor atom density (GAD), measuring the complexity of the signal (Fig. 2). Parametric methods of signal processing utilize some assumption of the EEG signal or its generators. Typical examples of such methods would include single- and multichannel autoregressive models that assume that the background EEG signal is stochastic in nature.

These methods allow for computation of spectral properties of the EEG similarly to the nonparametric methods, but also allow for detection of portions of EEG which are less stochastic or fully deterministic. This is believed to be true for most epileptiform activity, so deviation from patterns predicted by AR models can be used as detectors of seizures. Another parametric approach to EEG analysis successfully applied to early seizure detection or even prediction is based on the assumption that EEG signal is not stochastic but deterministic all the time, only that the underlying process is nonlinear and chaotic. Recently, different nonlinear measures based on this assumption were applied to epileptic EEG signals. Iasemidis et al. introduced the idea of using nonlinear dynamical parameters, primarily Lyapunov exponents for characterizing EEG (34). Lehnertz et al. used nonlinear measures of EEG complexity such as correlation dimension to analyze preictal EEG (11,35). Le Van Quen et al. used another nonlinear measures—i.e., dynamical

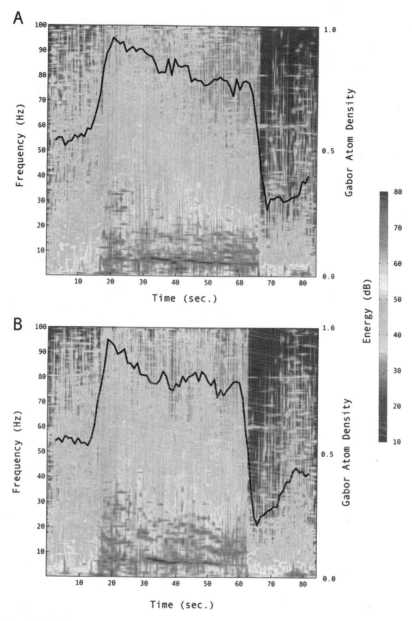

Figure 2. Similarity of epileptic seizures. Panel A represents the time-frequency analysis of a mesial temporal onset complex partial from a single channel, that closest to the seizure focus. The energy of each time-frequency component is color-coded (blue = low relative energy; red = high relative energy). The black trace represents the Gabor atom density (GAD) that quantifies the complexity of the underlying time-frequency decomposition. The changes in GAD can be used for early seizure detection. Panel B is the time-frequency analysis of another seizure from the same patient, occurring 3 ½ h after that shown in panel A. The time-frequency components and GAD pattern are similar. The high-theta frequency range activity that corresponds to the period of organized rhythmic activity is seen in both and has a similar frequency for both seizures with a similar monotonic decline.

similarity index (16,36). A recent discussion of different nonlinear approaches was published (17). Jerger et al. showed that for early seizure detection (i.e., short time prediction) linear methods based on classical frequency and phase measures can be as effective as nonlinear methods (37). In the future, with ever faster computer processors, seizure detection and prediction methods will probably use combinations of different methods, using linear or nonlinear signal analysis methods for advanced feature extraction and for further processing by artificial neural network systems.

APPLICATIONS OF SEIZURE DETECTION

EEG Monitoring

With the increased utilization of epilepsy monitoring units, means for seizure detection have become increasingly desirable. In these instances, however, as mentioned above, the most desirable detection algorithms are those that are very sensitive, so as not to miss seizures, and relatively specific to minimize false alarms. Early detection, although desirable so staff can respond to the patients, is not essential. And whether detection occurs after several or many seconds is certainly not critical. This allows these detection algorithms to be tuned to the organized rhythmic activity of a seizure rather that the more challenging ictal initiation patterns. The similarity of ictal patterns for a given patient allows modification of detection algorithms for the individual patient.

Seizure Localization

Seizure localization, often in the setting of an epilepsy monitoring unit, is a type of early seizure detection. One of the essential goals of the presurgical evaluation of patients is the localization of sequential seizures. Localization is the identification of the earliest ictal onset from the electrode(s) in the recording array being employed. Early seizure detection here, in most monitoring units, employs visual analysis of the multichannel recordings to determine time and location of seizure onset. Obviously, if the recording arrays are not optimally placed with electrodes near the seizure focus, early seizure detection cannot be accomplished since seizures are detected only after regional propagation. This is important for surgical planning, but suboptimally placed electrode arrays can also compromise the assessment of the proposed detection methods discussed above. Although preictal changes may potentially occur at sites distinct and even remote from the ictal focal onset (as has been postulated by some), assessment of these changes in relation to the ictal onset requires that recording electrodes also be near the actual seizure focus for comparison.

A number of seizure types can present challenges for seizure localization (and by extension, early detection). Neocortical seizures, particularly those originating from frontal neocortex, but also those from other areas, can propagate extremely rapidly and may involve many channels early in the seizure. Seizures originating from foci in orbitofrontal regions or intrahemispheric regions (e.g., supplementary motor area, cingulated gyrus) may not be apparent on scalp recordings or even intracranial recordings, unless electrodes are appropriately placed. While the pattern of evolution of mesial temporal onset seizures is often quite characteristic, the deep location of these structures of seizure origin may make detection of ictal onset elusive to scalp or surface electrodes. Indeed, even depth or basal temporal subdural strips,

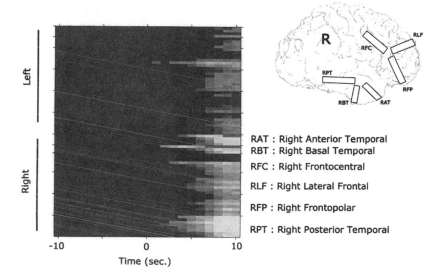

RAT : Right Anterior Temporal
RBT : Right Basal Temporal
RFC : Right Frontocentral
RLF : Right Lateral Frontal
RFP : Right Frontopolar
RPT : Right Posterior Temporal

Figure 3. Color-coded sequential multichannel GAD averaged over six seizures from the same patient. The color scale is red for high relative energy and blue for low relative energy. Time 0 is the GAD determined onset of the seizures and is used to synchronize the seizures. The earliest and highest increases in GAD are seen in the electrode contacts closest to the focus, the most mesial contacts of the right basal temporal strip.

if not close to the focus, can sometimes provide misleading information. For the purposes of presurgical evaluations, basal temporal subdural strips are as good for localizing mesial temporal onset seizures as depth electrodes, but well-positioned depth electrode arrays will usually reveal slightly earlier ictal changes than strip arrays in most patients.

Better methods (than mere visual inspection) are needed for seizure localization in those seizures (e.g., those of neocortical onset) that may be difficult to localize, even with optimally placed intracranial arrays. As discussed above, the Gabor atom density method may permit identification of early changes in seizure complexity, beginning first in the channels of seizure onset (Fig. 3). Other methods of seizure detection, particularly if they are able to be readily applied online, could assist in seizure localization by providing early detection of changes in contacts or channels nearest the seizure focus.

Application of Early Seizure Detection Devices to Treatment of Epilepsy

Possibly the most exciting area involving early seizure detection, or even earlier seizure prediction, is the promise for new methods of seizure therapy. Investigations to date have utilized recordings from intracranial electrodes; indeed, it appears that application of these modalities will require chronic intracranial electrodes if these applications are to truly have maximum sensitivity and specificity. With routine utilization of deep brain stimulation (DBS) for movement disorders, there is a growing body of information indicating that such chronically implanted devices can be safe, effective, and well tolerated.

The goal of these devices is to link early seizure detection to therapeutic intervention. To provide meaningful benefit, this would require an automated system with rapid response. Ideally, the intervention would reduce seizure duration so that alteration of consciousness or secondary generalization did not occur. Obviously, if such intervention, regardless of specificity, only results in a 50-sec complex partial seizure being reduced to a 45-sec complex partial seizure, there will be no real benefit to the patient. If seizure prediction algorithms allow identification of a preictal state change minutes (or longer) before a seizure, then the window and options for intervention are considerably greater than with early detection devices.

Automated Focal Drug Delivery Systems

The potential exists for early seizure detection devices to be coupled with drug delivery systems. Using such a device in rats, computerized detection of ictal onset triggered application of diazepam to experimental seizure foci. The application could be administered quickly enough (<5 sec after seizure onset) to produce a 64% reduction in seizure duration (38,39). Perhaps if such a device could be coupled with a seizure prediction algorithm, greater seizure reduction or even prevention could result. Rapid cooling has also been linked with early seizure detection devices (40).

Responsive Brain Stimulation Devices

To date, brain stimulation for the treatment of epilepsy has used chronic stimulation paradigms designed theoretically to modulate brain activity, potentially affect background synchronization, and reduce seizure frequency. The only FDA-approved device, the vagus nerve stimulator (VNS; see Chapter 15 in this volume by Naritoku) (41,42) acts on a polysynaptic pathway and utilizes chronic intermittent stimulation. Anterior thalamic stimulation (43,44), currently under investigation, also utilizes chronic stimulus paradigms. Neither the vagus nerve stimulator nor the anterior thalamic stimulator relies on seizure detection; stimulus parameters of these devices are largely independent of seizure activity, although the VNS has the option of magnet activation by the patient or observer. No good controlled studies exist to indicate whether such activation affects seizure duration. While the VNS has been shown to be well tolerated and produce responder rates (>50% seizure reduction) of 40–50% in highly refractory patient populations, utilization of the VNS rarely (<5–10%) makes patients seizure-free, and the anterior thalamic stimulator is unlikely to significantly improve upon these seizure-free rates.

Responsive brain stimulation employs potentially therapeutic stimulation that is triggered by a detected event. This could be early detection of an epileptic seizure or detection of some preictal event. Animal studies and simulations have employed closed-loop electrical stimulation (45,46). At present, studies are under way investigating external responsive neurostimulators in humans undergoing presurgical evaluations. The first preliminary report of these applications was recently published (47).

The concept behind the application of the responsive neurostimulation is that seizure detection algorithms can be applied to intracranial recordings of seizures that are sensitive and specific. The detected event would then trigger a responsive

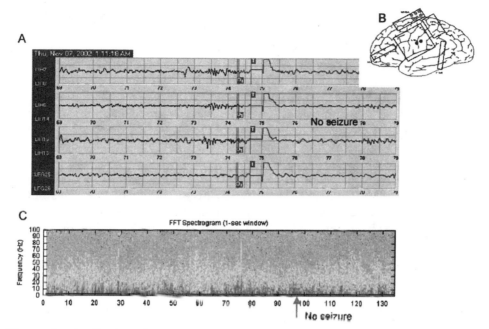

Figure 4. Application of external responsive neurostimulation. The recordings shown in panel A were from a patient who had completed her presurgical evaluation (subdural arrays as shown in B). Panel A revealed seizure onset (from interhemispheric contacts) that was detected and triggered responsive stimulation (stimulation artifact). There was no further seizure evolution after stimulation. The FFT spectrum (panel C, different time scale from panel A) confirms the absence of increased synchronous activity that was seen in fully evolved seizures. The red contacts (B) were the anodal contacts for stimulation; the black contacts (B) were the cathodal contacts. (Courtesy of NeuroPace, Inc.)

stimulation of the brain with the goal of seizure termination (Fig. 4). The idea of delivering excitatory stimuli to disrupt abnormal rhythms as a concept for the treatment of epileptic seizures is relatively novel, since one typically thinks of an epileptic seizure as a state of hyperexcitability and treatments to date have focused on reducing this hyperexcitability either intrinsically (e.g., reduced voltage-dependent sodium conductances) or by increasing inhibition. Model neural networks have shown that external excitatory stimuli can interrupt recurrent bursting if delivered at appropriate times (48,49). Interestingly, network inhibition is not necessary for burst termination in these models. It appears that, when successful, the excitatory stimuli disrupt the seizure dynamics, resulting in premature seizure termination. In contrast to the heart, where a strong depolarizing stimulus is needed to stop ventricular arrhythmias, in the brain, only small currents seem to be needed to produce burst termination. Direct application of currents to human after-discharges produced by cortical stimulation (for presurgical mapping) can terminate some discharges, but these methods have not utilized detection algorithms, relying instead on visual identification of the afterdischarges (50,51).

The ideal responsive stimulator would accurately detect seizures and be effective in terminating seizures early, preferably after several seconds, before either subclinical or simple partial seizures become complex partial or secondarily generalized seizures. As mentioned, a recent report of application of an external device to 12 patients undergoing presurgical evaluations with intracranial recording electrodes has demonstrated that seizure detection can be extremely reliable in most patients, stimulation is well tolerated (no sensation to patient) and, in these limited uncontrolled trials, appears to result in early seizure termination in a number of the patients. Because these applications are within the normal period of presurgical evaluations, opportunities for activation of the external system may be limited (e.g., those patients with few seizures).

The technology exists and is being applied to manufacture an implantable device (placed within the thickness of the skull) that can chronically deliver, via intracranial electrodes, stimuli after early seizure detection (Fig. 5). This device, which contains a microprocessor, battery, stimulator, and data storage capability, is amenable to subsequent modification of either seizure detection or stimulus parameters after implantation. To date, the optimal stimulus parameters have not been established. It is also not known whether stimulation must occur early in the seizure or close to the seizure focus if the most effective termination is to occur.

The question is often asked how one knows that activity prompting a responsive stimulation would have evolved into a seizure. The answer would require extensive blinded, randomized stimulation paradigms. But, if indeed the stimuli are benign, it may not matter whether additional stimuli are delivered. Potentially such stimuli, if applied to what would be brief subclinical electrical seizures, could still reduce the chance of clinical events.

The application of responsive devices that utilize preictal events is further from clinical application. A similar implantable device could be employed with

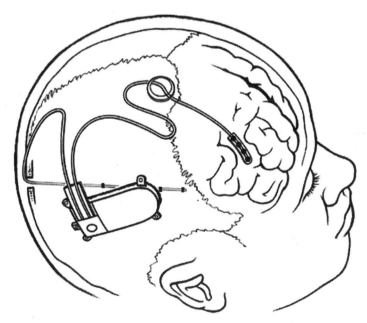

Figure 5. Schematic showing illustration of Responsive NeuroStimulator (RNS) implant with two lead configuration. (Illustration courtesy of Neuropace, Inc.)

intracranial electrodes. At the very least, such a preictal warning could be transmitted to the patient, hopefully minutes (or more) before the seizure, so that the patient could move to safety, avoid at-risk behavior, or perhaps take or activate medical treatment. It is more difficult to postulate what stimulation parameters would be effective in the preictal period to prevent seizure occurrence.

CONCLUSION

Early seizure detection is attracting considerable attention. Instead of merely applying these methods in epilepsy-monitoring units, there is growing interest in linking detection devices to therapeutic interventions. Indeed, the application of such interventions is now technically feasible, and holds promise for automated drug delivery or brain stimulation. The concept of responsive brain stimulation requires accurate seizure detection, and for this to benefit the patient, this must also represent early seizure detection. The methodology to apply these methods exists; further investigations are necessary to identify the best stimulus parameters. Responsive brain stimulation holds the promise to be a more specific, targeted and potentially more effective treatment modality than the chronic stimulation treatments currently employed that do not utilize seizure detection.

Seizure prediction depends on the identification of a true preictal state, not merely the early detection of clear ictal changes. Which sophisticated methods will ultimately prove to be the best at seizure prediction is not known at present. Clearly, the ability to predict seizures increases the time for potential therapeutic intervention. What intervention will be best also remains to be determined.

REFERENCES

1. Strong V, Brown SW, Walker R. Seizure-alert dogs—fact or fiction? Eur J Epilepsy 1999; 8:62–65.
2. O'Donovan CA, Burgess RC, Luders HO, Turnbull JP. Computerized seizure detection based on heart-rate changes. Epilepsia 1995; 36:115–115.
3. Burgess RC, Turnbull JP, Bartolo A, O'Donovan C. Heart rate signal artifact identification improves tachycardiograph seizure detection. Epilepsia 1996; 37(suppl 5):63.
4. Burgess RC, Turnbull JP, Bartolo A, Rekhson MS. Combined EEG and EKG detection algorithms improve computerized seizure identification. Epilepsia 1997; 38(suppl 3):155.
5. Kay SM. Fundamentals of Statistical Signal Processing: Detection Theory. Upper Saddle River, NJ: Prentice-Hall PTR, 1998.
6. Katz A, Marks DA, McCarthy G, Spencer SS. Does interictal spiking change prior to seizures? Electroencephalogr Clin Neurophysiol 1991; 79:153–156.
7. Litt B, Esteller R, Echauz J, D'Alessandro M, Shor R, Henry T. Epileptic seizures may begin hours in advance of clinical onset: a report of five patients. Neuron 2001; 30:51–64.
8. Viglione SS, Walsh GO. Epileptic seizure prediction. Electroencephalogr Clin Neurophysiol 1976; 41:649–650.
9. Yeager CL, Spire JP, Fischer A, Viglione SS. Selection and evaluation of cases for epileptic seizure prediction program. Electroencephalogr Clin Neurophysiol 1976; 41:650–650.

10. Viglione SS, Walsh GO, Yeager CL, Spire JP. EEG analysis and epileptic seizure prediction. Epilepsia 1977; 18:289–289.

11. Elger CE, Lehnertz K. Seizure prediction by non-linear time series analysis of brain electrical activity. Eur J Neurosci 1998; 10:786–789.

12. Litt B, Echauz J. Prediction of epileptic seizures. Lancet 2002; 1:22–30.

13. Salant Y, Gath I, Henriksen O. Prediction of epileptic seizures from two-channel EEG. Med Biol Eng Comput 1998; 36:549–556.

14. Navarro V, Martinerie J, Le Van Quyen M, Clemenceau S, Adam C, Baulac M. Seizure anticipation in human neocortical partial epilepsy. Brain 2002; 125:640–655.

15. Widman G, Bingmann D, Lehnertz K, Elger CE. Reduced signal complexity of intracellular recordings: a precursor for epileptiform activity? Brain Res 1999; 836:156–163.

16. Le Van Quyen M, Martinerie J, Baulac M, Varela F. Anticipating epileptic seizures in real time by a non-linear analysis of similarity between EEG recordings. Neuroreport 1999; 10:2149–2155.

17. Litt B, Lehnertz K. Seizure prediction and the preseizure period. Curr Opin Neurol 2002; 15:173–177.

18. Liu HS, Zhang T, Yang FS. A multistage, multimethod approach for automatic detection and classification of epileptiform EEG. IEEE Trans Biomed Eng 2002; 49:1557–1566.

19. Osorio I, Frei MG, Wilkinson SB. Real-time automated detection and quantitative analysis of seizures and short-term prediction of clinical onset. Epilepsia 1998; 39:615–627.

20. Pradhan N, Sadasivan PK, Arunodaya GR. Detection of seizure activity in EEG by an artificial neural network: a preliminary study. Comput Biomed Res 1996; 29:303–313.

21. Si Y, Gotman J, Pasupathy A, Flanagan D, Rosenblatt B, Gottesman R. An expert system for EEG monitoring in the pediatric intensive care unit. Electroencephalogr Clin Neurophysiol 1998; 106:488–500.

22. Weng W, Khorasani K. An adaptive structure neural networks with application to EEG automatic seizure detection. Neural Networks 1996; 9:1223–1240.

23. Esteller R, Echauz J, Tcheng T, Litt B, Pless B. Line length: an efficient feature for seizure onset detection. In: IEEE International Conference on Engineering in Medicine and Biology, Istanbul, Turkey, 2001.

24. Murro AM, King DW, Smith JR, Gallagher BB, Flanigin HF, Meador K. Computerized seizure detection of complex partial seizures. Electroencephalogr Clin Neurophysiol 1991; 79:330–333.

25. Webber WRS, Lesser RP, Richardson RT, Wilson K. An approach to seizure detection using an artificial neural network (ANN). Electroencephalogr Clin Neurophysiol 1996; 98:250–272.

26. Gabor AJ, Leach RR, Dowla FU. Automated seizure detection using a self-organizing neural network. Electroencephalogr Clin Neurophysiol 1996; 99:257–266.

27. Gabor AJ. Seizure detection using a self-organizing neural network: validation and comparison with other detection strategies. Electroencephalogr Clin Neurophysiol 1998; 107:27–32.

28. Petrosian A, Prokhorov D, Homan R, Dasheiff R, Wunsch D. Recurrent neural network based prediction of epileptic seizures in intra- and extracranial EEG. Neurocomputing 2000; 30:201–218.

29. Geva AB, Kerem DH. Forecasting generalized epileptic seizures from the EEG signal by wavelet analysis and dynamic unsupervised fuzzy clustering. IEEE Trans Biomed Eng 1998; 45:1205–1216.

30. Sartoretto F, Ermani M. Automatic detection of epileptiform activity by single-level wavelet analysis. Clin Neurophysiol 1999; 110:239–249.

31. Schiff SJ, Milton J, Heller J, Weinstein SL. Wavelet transforms and surrogate data for electroencephalographic spike and seizure localization. Optical Eng 1994; 33:2162–2169.

32. Senhadji L, Wendling F. Epileptic transient detection: wavelets and time-frequency approaches. Neurophysiol Clin 2002; 32:175–192.

33. Jouny CC, Franaszczuk PJ, Bergey GK. Characterization of epileptic seizure dynamics using Gabor atom density. Clin Neurophysiol 2003; 114:426–437.

34. Iasemidis LD, Sackellares JC, Zaveri HP, Williams WJ. Phase space topography and the Lyapunov exponent of electrocorticograms in partial seizures. Brain Topogr 1990; 2:187–201.

35. Lehnertz K. Non-linear time series analysis of intracranial EEG recordings in patients with epilepsy—an overview. Int J Psychophysiol 1999; 34:45–52.

36. Le van Quyen M, Adam C, Baulac M, Martinerie J, Varela FJ. Nonlinear interdependencies of EEG signals in human intracranially recorded temporal lobe seizures. Brain Res 1998; 792:24–40.

37. Jerger KK, Netoff TI, Francis JT, Sauer T, Pecora L, Weinstein SL. Early seizure detection. J Clin Neurophysiol 2001; 18:259–268.

38. Fisher RS, Ho J. Potential new methods for anticpileptic drug delivery. CNS Drugs 2002; 16:579–593.

39. Stein AG, Eder HG, Blum DE, Drachev A, Fisher RS. An automated drug delivery system for focal epilepsy. Epilepsy Res 2000; 39:103–114.

40. Yang XF, Duffy DW, Morley RE, Rothman SM. Neocortical seizure termination by focal cooling: temperature dependence and automated seizure detection. Epilepsia 2002; 43:240–245.

41. Labar D, Murphy J, Tecoma E. Vagus nerve stimulation for medication-resistant generalized epilepsy. E04 VNS Study Group. Neurology 1999; 52:1510–1512.

42. Morris GL, Mueller WM. Long-term treatment with vagus nerve stimulation in patients with refractory epilepsy. The Vagus Nerve Stimulation Study Group E01-E05. Neurology 1999; 53:1731–1735.

43. Velasco M, Velasco F, Velasco AL, Jimenez F, Brito F, Marquez I. Acute and chronic electrical stimulation of the centromedian thalamic nucleus: modulation of reticulo-cortical systems and predictor factors for generalized seizure control. Arch Med Res 2000; 31:304–315.

44. Velasco F, Velasco M, Velasco AL, Jimenez F, Marquez I, Rise M. Electrical stimulation of the centromedian thalamic nucleus in control of seizures: long-term studies. Epilepsia 1995; 36:63–71.

45. Osorio I, Frei MG, Manly BFJ, Sunderam S, Bhavaraju NC, Wilkinson SB. An introduction to contingent (closed-loop) brain electrical stimulation for seizure blockage, to ultra-short-term clinical trials, and to multidimensional statistical analysis of therapeutic efficacy. J Clin Neurophysiol 2001; 18:533–544.

46. Peters TE, Bhavaraju NC, Frei MG, Osorio I. Network system for automated seizure detection and contingent delivery of therapy. J Clin Neurophysiol 2001; 18:545–549.

47. Bergey GK, Britton JW, Cascino GD, Choi H-M, Kossoff E. Implementation of an external responsive neurostimulator system (eRNS) in patients with intractable epilepsy undergoing intracranial seizure monitoring. Epilepsia 2002 (in press).

48. Franaszczuk PJ, Kudela P, Bergey GK. External excitatory stimuli can terminate bursting in neural network models. Epilepsy Res 2003; 53:65–80.

49. Kudela P, Franaszczuk PJ, Bergey GK. External termination of recurrent bursting in a model of connected local neural sub-networks. Neurocomputing 2002; 44:897–905.

50. Karceski SC, Morrell MJ, Emerson R, Thompson T. Termination of afterdischarges with electrical stimulation during cortical mapping. Epilepsia 2000; 41(suppl 7):202.
51. Lesser RP, Kim SH, Beyderman L, Miglioretti DL, Webber WR, Bare M. Brief bursts of pulse stimulation terminate afterdischarges caused by cortical stimulation. Neurology 1999; 53:2073–2081.

25
Arresting Epileptogenesis: The Current Challenge

Philip A. Schwartzkroin
University of California, Davis
Davis, California, U.S.A.

INTRODUCTION: WHAT IS EPILEPTOGENESIS?

The Goal of Antiepileptogenesis Is Epilepsy *Prevention*

While we have long sought treatments that fall under the rubric of antiepileptic (or anticonvulsant), our attention to the concept of antiepileptogenesis is relatively recent. In large measure, the neglect has been due to a general lack of understanding about the processes of epileptogenesis, and thus a practical inability to develop measures that would be effective antiepileptogenic treatments. Why, now, should we shift our attention to epileptogenesis—*the processes by which a relatively "normal" brain becomes capable of generating spontaneous, repeated seizures*—i.e., becomes epileptic? The rationale lies in our current, more ambitious clinical goals—to utilize treatments that will not only prevent seizure occurrence, but produce a "cure"—so that the individual being treated no longer has an epileptic condition. As is the case for many medical conditions, the most effect treatment/cure may lie in *prevention*. We as "epileptologists" would really like to put ourselves out of business by developing procedures that stop the epileptogenic process before it becomes a chronic disease state. Antiepileptogenesis is thus not just a conceptual endpoint, but rather a real and important clinical goal.

Abbreviations: AMPA, α-amino-3-hydroxy-5-methyl-4-isoxazoleproprionic acid; GABA, γ-amino-butyric acid; NMDA, N-methyl-D-aspartate.

Epileptogenesis is a *Process*, Not a State

Unlike the epileptic state, epileptogenesis is a *process*—or more likely, a complex set of processes. Epileptogenesis is probably different for different epilepsy endpoints, perhaps different for different individuals, and undoubtedly different depending on the etiological origins of the process. Thus, to think about antiepileptogenesis is to consider hitting not one but several moving targets. Currently, we are significantly worse at dealing with epileptogenesis than we are at treating epilepsy (which, although it comes in multiple forms, is at least a relatively stationary target). In our attempts to "cure" epilepsy, we have developed a set of rather effective surgical approaches. But antiepileptogenesis requires a different mindset. Would we recognize an antiepileptogenic treatment if we stumbled over it? For example, is the ketogenic diet—at least on occasion—antiepileptogenic?

Although somewhat intimidating, it is certainly worthwhile considering the complexity of epileptogenic processes. To be sure, we could proceed along the same lines that have worked in developing antiepileptic treatments—empirical trial and error, often arising from a serendipitous finding that serves as a basis for developing potential treatments. Surely elucidation of at least some of the processes underlying epileptogenesis would provide a significantly more effective method for developing antiepileptogenic treatments. In addition, it seems likely that such research could uncover multiple mechanisms involved in any given epileptogenic process, suggesting several points of intervention. One simple way to view this scenario is to consider the flow diagram in Figure 1. Here, the solid arrows linking the boxes represent epileptogenic processes that lead to Seizures/Epilepsy. In the paragraphs below, I'll outline at least a few of the candidate processes that should receive attention. But as we consider these possibilities, it is important to ask about each of them:

1. Why? What stimuli trigger these changes, and do these changes actually represent potential epileptogenic precursors?
2. When? When do these processes come into play, both with respect to the initiating stimuli (e.g., what is the latent period) and with respect to developmental programs (i.e., how do epileptogenic processes interact with the brain's developmental programs)?
3. Where? Where in the brain do these changes take place, and what types of cells are affected?

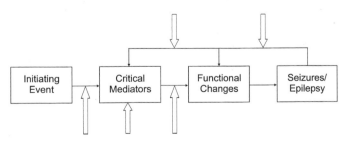

Figure 1. Aspects of the epileptogenic process. Solid arrows indicate likely epileptogenic pathways. Open arrows signify opportunities for intervention—i.e., for therapies that might interrupt epileptogenesis.

4. How much? At what level/magnitude do these changes constitute an epileptogenic threat (is there a "threshold")?
5. Alone or in concert? How do these changes interact with each other and with normal elements of the affected brain?
6. Are they necessary and/or sufficient to cause epilepsy?

Ideally, antiepileptogenesis involves the identification of potential epilepsy patients before they develop a chronic seizure disorder. A major goal of anti-epileptogenesis is to treat "at risk" patients *before* a chronic epileptic state is established. This goal is a bit tricky, since epileptologists normally don't see their patients until seizures have become a fact of life—often a chronic disorder that has been in place for years. There are two important factors to consider in dealing with this problem: First, epileptogenesis may well be a "progressive" process, so that even interfering with apparently established epileptic activity will have antiepileptogenic efficacy (especially in the young brain). Second, and perhaps most obvious, we need to be able to identify the at-risk populations in which treatment will decrease the likelihood of future epilepsy. Thus, in approaching antiepileptogenesis, we are not only talking about developing new treatments (directed against "new" mechanisms), but are also concerned with developing a science of *prediction*. Although there are a number of epidemiological studies that provide a starting point for this effort (1,2), this predictive effort is still in its infancy.

Effective antiepileptogenic treatment and clinical management require an emphasis on education for family practitioners, pediatricians, and general neurologists. A large part of any effective antiepileptogenic treatment program will be out of the hands of clinical epileptologists. Certainly, in current practice, the epilepsy specialist (often a physician in a tertiary care medical center) does not see his/her patient until that patient has a chronic (and difficult-to-control) epileptic condition. The health care providers that are key to prediction—and thus play such a critical role in antiepileptogenesis—are the family practitioners, pediatricians, and general neurologists who first see the "at-risk" patient. These patients often consult their family doctors in response to the "precipitating event" that puts them at risk, and it is the referral and/or treatment by these physicians that will determine (and limit) the pathway(s) of treatment for these individuals. Thus, a major aspect of any antiepileptogenic effort is to provide these primary care physicians with information and education—about factors that put their patients at risk, as well as about treatments that will decrease the risk of epilepsy.

FACTORS THAT CONTRIBUTE TO EPILEPTOGENESIS

Although somewhat simplistic in approach, the factors that determine the likelihood of chronic seizures developing from a precipitating event (or baseline condition) can be grouped into three broad categories. It is important to note at the outset that these categories are not clearly separate, and that interactions across categories make the search for underlying factors very complicated. Nevertheless, it is useful to consider these general factors, since they are likely to influence virtually every epileptogenic process.

Genetics

It's now very clear that some epilepsies are genetically based. Recent investigations have revealed a number of relatively rare epilepsies that are attributable to single gene mutations, most frequently (but not consistently) involving voltage-gated ion channels or ligand-gated receptor subunits (3–6). Further, we know that a number of genes responsible for developmental brain abnormalities—such as lissencephaly or tuberous sclerosis—are associated (in a high percentage of cases) with early-onset epilepsies (7,8). Finally, we now have rather good evidence that some of the more common epilepsies—e.g., juvenile myoclonic epilepsy (JME)—are due to multigenic interactions of a complex nature (9). It is important to note, however, even in those cases in which genes have been clearly implicated, that not all individuals with the relevant genetic defect exhibit an epilepsy phenotype.

Increasingly, genetic complement is seen as a "predisposing" factor in the appearance of epileptic seizures. This concept, suggesting that the genetic pattern of an individual (or family) provides a baseline state of more or less seizure susceptibility, is strongly supported by studies of animal models (10). Our recent experiments involving different mouse strains—none of which are spontaneously epileptic—show that the strain background determines several seizure-related features, including seizure threshold, seizure severity, seizure-induced pathology, and seizure-related mortality; indeed, these factors appear to be independently regulated, perhaps by separate sets of genes (59).

Genetic determinants of epileptogenesis have not been examined, but it would be truly surprising if genetic complement did not play a significant role in the epileptogenic process. Indeed, without this genetic influence, it is difficult to explain why a given traumatic insult delivered to a population of different individuals (or mice) results in such variable seizure-related endpoints. Exactly what genes might be involved—perhaps genes other than those that we already know influence seizure threshold/susceptibility—remain to be determined. Increased understanding of such genes is a critical step in identifying at-risk individuals.

Brain Developmental Programs

As indicated above, developmental brain abnormalities are often linked to epileptic syndromes, although we have an only vague idea about why/how such structural abnormalities result in epilepsy. This question is particularly difficult given that not all similar abnormalities result in the same seizure state. Nevertheless, aberrant brain structure appears to be a definite risk factor. The difficult questions now revolve around some of the basic questions posed above. What are the effects of aberrations at different times during brain development? How do abnormalities in different brain regions affect the likelihood of epileptogenesis? Does the size of the structural abnormality determine the level of risk? And so forth. In dealing with epileptogenesis, these questions involve a rather subtle understanding of underlying processes, for the baseline state may well appear relatively normal. In addition, one must factor into this analysis the ongoing developmental processes—those aspects of brain development that, when normal, yield a nonepileptic neuronal system. Slight changes in these dynamic systems could interact with, and support, epileptogenic processes without producing a clear structurally abnormal phenotype.

Environmental Influences

When we think about epileptogenesis, we usually think about the processes associated with such insults as head trauma, stroke, infection, or even seizures (e.g., those associated with febrile illnesses). These events appear to initiate a set of processes that can—sometimes—result in a chronic seizure state. What we don't know, however, is what features of these insults are truly epileptogenic. Do all head injuries put an individual at risk? Are only some individuals (determined by genetics) or only individuals at some ages (e.g., the young in whom developmental programs are still robust) likely to respond to such trauma with epileptogenic processes? These precipitating events have already received attention from those interested in epileptogenesis (because we can see them and "quantitate" them), but better feature analysis of epileptogenic stimuli is still an important experimental goal. Most ideas about antiepileptogenic treatments revolve around the mechanisms observed in response to environmental trauma. Undoubtedly, as we become more sophisticated in elucidating epileptogenic features of these events, we will begin to appreciate the critical nature of their interactions with baseline genetic and developmental programs.

POTENTIAL MECHANISMS OF EPILEPTOGENESIS: GENERAL THEMES AND ISSUES

Epileptogenesis May Involve Different Mechanisms from Those We've Identified as Important in Seizure Genesis/Initiation and/or in Maintenance of the Epileptic State

The vast majority of research into the underlying mechanisms of the epilepsies has focused on processes of seizure initiation. Within this context, it has become commonplace to point to the balance between excitatory and inhibitory processes as the key to understanding (11). This emphasis, in turn, has led to a considerable preoccupation with mechanisms of inhibitory control and possible compromises in inhibitory status (e.g., loss of inhibitory interneurons, disinhibition, changes in the subunit composition of GABA-A receptors, etc.) (12–14), as well as a growing interest in possible changes in glutamate-mediated excitatory events (changes in the AMPA/NMDA balance, calcium entry through glutamate-gated channels, etc.) (15). These mechanisms undoubtedly have relevance to seizure initiation (there is good evidence that a decrease in inhibition does foreshadow the onset of seizure discharge) (16,17), and may also be important for the maintenance of an underlying epileptic state (fragility of inhibition, for example, may characterize some forms of epilepsy) (18–20). However, there is little evidence to suggest that these mechanisms are key to epileptogenic processes. Indeed, these seizure-supporting features may be the *consequences* of other changes associated with epileptogenesis. While epileptogenic mechanisms have yet to be identified, we should not be biased by our history of studying seizure mechanisms. Especially in light of the explosion in molecular biology, we have an amazing assortment of potential mechanisms to explore.

Epileptogenic Processes are Initiated by Some Event or Abnormal Condition (e.g., From Areas of Damage/Lesion and/or Structural Abnormality)

We generally think about epileptogenesis having a relatively specific initiation time and site, often associated with a specific brain insult. As such, these changes in brain structure, chemistry, metabolism, and function represent "reactive" processes. What might such processes be? Among the most obvious of changes associated with brain damage are the reactive glial processes. While investigators have remarked on reactive gliosis for many years, it is difficult to identify exactly what constitutes a reactive glial cell (is it simply a change in its GFAP (glial fibrillary acidic protein) expression? Are reactive glia simply responding to a change in their environment, or do they actively shape the damaged brain region? Investigators have recently identified interesting differences between reactive glia in epileptic brain and normal astrocytes (21); it is unclear whether these differences are cause or effect.

Another, related area of reactivity concerns the infiltration of microglia into traumatized brain regions, and their involvement in phagocytosing damaged neurons. There is now evidence that microglial cells release powerful factors (e.g., cytokines) that may further influence the viability (and likely functional properties) of surrounding cells (neurons and astrocytes) (22). Glial cells, as well as neurons, may also release a variety of growth factors that influence the patterns of process regeneration and/or the generation of new synaptic contacts, and/or support the survival of surrounding cell types (23,24). Finally, the reactive process may involve a "reversion" of cells to immature phenotypes, including the facilitation of neurogenesis (25). While this latter mechanism may add cells to affected circuits, it is still unclear (especially in the mature CNS) if (or how) such newly generated cells (glia and neurons) are (or should be) integrated into existing networks.

Although there may be a specific lesion or insult that initiates a set of plastic processes, one may argue that some epileptogenic pathways are "hard-wired." That is, they may simply reflect an intrinsic abnormality (i.e., an aberrant gene) that will eventually give rise to a seizure state, irrespective of changes in structure or of ongoing activity. Should we view such a condition as a "process," or rather as a state (similar to an epileptic state) that requires its own special treatment? Finally, we know that injury/lesion triggers all kinds of brain changes. What kinds of changes ("plasticity") are appropriately adaptive and what types are epileptogenic?

Are Epileptogenic Processes Progressive? Self-Sustaining? Activity-Dependent?

There is considerable interest in the concept that epileptogenesis is a progressive process; that is, it involves a positive feedback mechanism through which a small amount of abnormal activity/function exacerbates the original pathology, leading to more severe abnormal activity/function, and so on (26). Such a progressive change is thought to occur during "kindling," which has served as the prototypical model of a progressive epileptogenic process (27,28). Whether a kindlinglike mechanism underlies human epilepsies is still controversial. Reports of the development of secondary, or mirror, foci support this idea of progressive abnormality (26). If some epilepsies are progressive, there are several important implications:

1.   It is important to identify and stop/interrupt even the subclinical processes that are initiated by potentially epileptogenic stimuli, since continuing subclinical activity may lead to progressive pathology and, sooner or later, *chronic* seizures. The usual formulation of this view assumes that the progressive process involves some form of electrical discharge—for example, that subthreshold discharge activity occurring in the hippocampus and related structures causes more and more cell death. This version of "activity dependency" suggests that one way of interfering with the progressive process is to block ongoing electrical discharge. However, "activity" may take other forms, perhaps at the molecular level (e.g., gene transcription, protein translation, and related functional changes, which then activate a new cycle of gene transcription, etc.). These different forms of "activity" would require rather different interventional approaches.

2.   The progressive activity is self-sustaining; that is, it does not require any external boost once the process has been initiated. Thus, once a pathway toward abnormality has been initiated, the pathology that is initially induced is sufficient to generate the ultimate epileptic state. If that is the case, intervention possibilities are significantly more limited than if these processes require continuing interaction with external stimulation. However, if one could identify an (the?) underlying process, then its interruption could conceivably constitute a "cure."

OPPORTUNITIES FOR INTERVENTION

Once we characterize the epileptogenic process, what can we do with this information? The goal for treatment of epileptogenesis is early intervention—to prevent the establishment of the epileptic state before it becomes a stable, and difficult-to-control abnormality.

Early Detection

Ideally, an important goal is to detect an epileptogenic process in an early stage. Identification of these processes would allow us to be more specific in our treatment approaches than to treat all at-risk patients in the same way. Development of *markers* of epileptogenesis is therefore crucial. Currently, the most feasible approach to early diagnosis appears to be the detection and prevention of early seizures and/or abnormal electrical brain activity. The therapeutic value of blocking early seizure activity is based on the assumption that epileptogenesis is a progressive process which involves subclinical and/or early discharges. The more difficult goal of "normalizing" aberrant EEG activity is based on the idea that such EEG is a reflection of an underlying brain state that supports the epileptogenic process. In either case, such intervention will depend critically on the further development of techniques to characterize EEG, and to detect and predict seizure occurrence (29,30). Especially if seizures participate in a progressive process, early seizure detection might allow one to abort oncoming events and thus interfere with the positive feedback process (Fig. 1).

Disruption of early/initial electrical abnormalities may be effected through stimulation protocols that are now being developed as anticonvulsant treatment (31).

Especially if repeated discharge acts to strengthen abnormal circuits (e.g., potentiation, kindling) (32) and/or establish population synchrony, interfering with such activity could have antiepileptogenic results. Along with increasing sophistication in detecting abnormal electrical discharge, techniques are being developed to alter current gradients, to deliver pulsed electrical (and pharmacological) stimuli, and to use electrical stimulation to release endogenous modulatory agents (33,34). The parameters of such antiepileptogenic stimuli have still to be developed, and the technology for delivering these signals—to disrupt abnormal subclinical activities—is in its infancy.

It is worth noting that non-electrical markers may be more easily obtained and/ or constitute more reliable predictors of epileptogenesis. For example, some markers of cell death may provide precisely the kind of early information that is needed (35).

Pharmacological Approaches

There are no drugs yet identified with an antiepileptogenic mechanism. Indeed, all of the current AEDs are essentially "anticonvulsant" (not even antiepileptic). Given the possibility—indeed, the likelihood—that epileptogenesis depends on processes different from those involved in seizure generation, there is clearly a need for a new antiepileptogenic pharmacopeia. What mechanisms should new antiepileptogenic drugs target?

If one critical epileptogenic process is ongoing electrical activity, then it may be important to block such activity even if it doesn't take the form of overt seizures. Our current AEDs are quite good at antagonizing dramatic paroxysmal events, but their use in antagonizing more subtle abnormalities (or for "normalizing" background discharge) has been poorly explored. In drug trials to explore the efficacy of phenytoin and valproate as prophylactic agents against epileptogenesis following traumatic head injury, these mainstream AEDs have not proved to be effective (36,37). Whether that means that the key underlying processes are not "electrical" or that these drugs do not control subclinical electrical abnormalities, remains to be determined. Further, it may be that once the abnormal electrical activity is established, it is "too late"—and that we should be targeting earlier changes—e.g., at the level of receptors, to prevent receptor subunit reorganization (14).

Another major target for new antiepileptogenic therapy is cell *protection*. Many studies have suggested that neuronal cell death can be an epileptogenic stimulus, and that the relevant cells die over a long period of time. Thus, pharmacological agents that block this cell death process—e.g., calcium channel blockers or NMDA-type glutamate receptor antagonists—might reduce the likelihood of epileptogenesis. In considering this strategy, however, it is important to determine whether the "rescued" cells behave normally or they have abnormal properties that might contribute to an epileptogenic process.

There are many reports to show that epileptic brain/foci are characterized by significant reorganization of neuronal connections—i.e., there is not only cell loss/ damage, but also robust growth (38,39). While it's still unclear how or to what degree this "sprouting" contributes to epileptogenesis, investigators are already targeting antagonists of growth-promoting molecules (e.g., neurotrophic factors) as potentially antiepileptogenic (40). In addition, recent studies have suggested that neuronal (and glial) proliferation occurs in the epileptic brain (25). Again, the contribution of such proliferative processes to the seizure state has not been determined; however, prevention of neuronal (or glial) proliferation may constitute an important antiepileptogenic therapy.

A somewhat neglected target in epilepsy therapy, and one that should not be overlooked in searching for antiepileptogenic treatments, is the brain glia—particularly the astrocytes and microglia. Normal astrocyte function is critical for regulation of the extraneuronal environment, and astrocyte dysfunction has significant effects on neural excitability (41). Many epileptogenic stimuli alter glial properties, either causing significant glial cell death or producing "reactive" astrocytes. The functional properties of the latter are not well understood; preventing such reactivity may be important in antiepileptogeneis. Similarly, preventing the invasion of microglia, and the release of microglia-associated agents (e.g., cytokines), may be a significant pharmacological strategy.

Finally, there is accumulating evidence that epileptogenic stimuli cause alterations in cell properties, in part by activating gene transcription programs that are reminiscent of immature/developing neurons (42). Again, interference with such programs may have effective antiepileptogenic consequences. However, these changes (i.e., reversion to immature states) may have functional importance (e.g., increasing the plastic capacity of injured brain). Thus, it will be important to balance antiepileptogenic treatments with potential enhancement of functional restoration.

Surgery and/or Repair

To date, epilepsy surgery is the only existing "antiepileptic" treatment we have. Whether surgery can be antiepileptogenic remains to be determined. With the use of appropriate markers to identify tissue that is (or will become) epileptic, there are a number of surgical strategies that may effectively interfere with the epileptogenic process. One approach is simply to remove "bad brain." If abnormal brain generates activity that can "kindle" surrounding tissue, or if it releases "epileptogenic" substances (e.g., grow factors) that affect normal neighbors, then removal of this tissue makes good sense. The efficacy of such a program will undoubtedly depend on the integrity of the remaining brain tissue. Currently, such a surgical approach is limited to mechanical resections that are relatively gross with respect the target abnormal cells/circuits. New techniques for removal or inactivation may provide a more selective approach. For example, "noninvasive lesions" may be made radiologically with impressive accuracy (43). Or, as we learn more about what constitutes abnormality in neurons that generate the epileptic state, we may be able to label and kill such cells selectively.

In some cases, the insult that leads to the epileptic state itself removes critical cell types that are essential to the control of brain excitability—e.g., inhibitory interneurons, or glia. In such cases, it may be feasible to "add" appropriate cell types via transplantation techniques (44) and to direct them to become appropriately integrated within the affected circuitry. New culture, gene expression, and transplantation technologies may allow us to "repair" injured brain tissue before the epileptogenic process begins.

Finally, for many epilepsies, there is no grossly identifiable cell/tissue abnormality to be removed or replaced. Recent studies have identified gene abnormalties in many forms of epilepsy (3–6), and these genes lead—in a developmental sequence—to epileptic function. In these cases, "gene therapy" becomes an option worth considering (45). Indeed, for familial epilepsies in which offspring are at considerable risk, such therapies may be initiated in utero, so that the epileptogenic process is completely short-circuited.

Other Approaches

Given our current knowledge about causes of the epilepsies (i.e., those processes that are involved in generating an epileptic condition), there are a number of potentially useful therapeutic strategies that deserve additional research attention:

    1.   Immunological therapies. Some forms of early onset epilepsies (e.g., Rasmussen's encephalitis) have been linked to autoimmune processes which can result in altered structure and/or function (46). For other epilepsies, infection is viewed as the likely initiating insult (47). In such cases, early treatment with agents that antagonize antibody-mediated effects may have antiepileptic efficacy.

    2.   Treatment with antioxidants. Many precipitating injuries—e.g., stroke— are due to excitotoxicity-mediated processes that damage cells in epilepsy-sensitive brain regions (48). Protection against cell death and/or injury (e.g., using agents that block the production or action of free radicals) is a rather general therapeutic strategy (49,50) that may have important consequences for the development of a chronic epileptic state.

    3.   Development of dietary treatments. It is already clear that some epilepsies are a result of vitamin (or other dietary) insufficiency, and that restoration of the missing element "cures" the seizure disorder (51). Still unclear is whether more subtle deficiencies might underlie some epilepsies (e.g., critical amino acids) (52). Also still to be explored is whether some dietary regimens, such as the ketogenic diet, might not only be antiepileptic, but also antiepileptogenic (53).

    4.   Hormonal therapies. The observations that steroid treatment (e.g., ACTH) is sometimes effective in the treatment of infantile spasms (54) and that gonadal hormones have powerful epileptic (estrogen) and antiepileptic (progesterone) effects (55,56), suggest that some epilepsies may develop as a result of hormone imbalance. Further, an excessive stress hormone level has been linked to cell death (57), so that antagonism of this action in critical brain regions (such as hippocampus) could have antiepileptogenic consequences.

CONCLUSIONS: THE FUTURE FOR RESEARCH IN ANTIEPILEPTOGENESIS

There are a host of challenges—*and opportunities*—for those hoping to treat epilepsy by preventing its occurrence. What are the immediate issues and achievable goals that challenge us at this early stage of research development?

    1.   Identify "at-risk" patients. We need not only insightful epidemiological studies, but also predictive biological markers of epileptogenic processes.

    2.   Develop treatments that target molecular changes that *precede* seizure appearance. Ideally, we don't want to wait for the appearance of seizures before we start treatment. At the current time, one useful approach may be to work toward

preventing cell death and/or cell damage/reactivity. We already have a number of pharmacological and molecular tools for enhancing neuronal survival.

3. Stop early seizures and try to normalize baseline brain electrical activity. It's unclear whether current AEDs work on this level, but our pharmacological armamentarium is rich, and new techniques are now available for electrical stimulation to interfere with subclinical hyperexcitability/abnormal discharge.

4. Evaluate and treat trauma-induced plasticity. For many types of epilepsy, the development of new connections appears to be a salient hallmark. Will blockade of these new/aberrant circuits (even those at the molecular level) disrupt the epileptogenic process? How might such blockade affect normal brain function?

5. Finally, there is a need for a reorientation with respect to the goal of treatment. Why is antiepileptogenesis so critical? We think its important because chronic seizure activity, especially in young brains (in which epileptogenesis is most likely to occur) has significant effects on long-term function and maturation. Thus, the real focus of our work is on the *consequences* of seizures (e.g., developmental delay, etc.)—not the seizures themselves (58). It is prevention of those consequences that must guide our research and our choice of antiepileptogenic treatments.

ACKNOWLEDGMENTS

I am grateful to Drs. Daniel H. Lowenstein, Jong M. Rho, W. Donald Shields, and Edie E. Zusman for thought-provoking discussions.

REFERENCES

1. Annegers JF, Rocca WA, Hauser WA. Causes of epilepsy: contributions of the Rochester epidemiology project. Mayo Clin Proc 1996; 71:570–575.
2. Hesdorffer DC, Verlty CM. Risk factors. In: Engel J Jr, Pedley TA, eds. Epilepsy: A Comprehensive Textbook. Philadelphia: Lippincott-Raven, 1997:59–67.
3. Noebels JL. Single-gene models of epilepsy. Adv Neurol 1999; 79:227–238.
4. Scheffer IE, SF Berkovic SF. Genetics of the epilepsies. Curr Opin Pediatr 12:536–542.
5. Stafstrom CE, Tempel BL. Epilepsy genes: the link between molecular dysfunction and pathophysiology. Ment Retard Dev Disabil Res Rev 2000; 6:281–292.
6. Steinlein OK. Genes and mutations in idiopathic epilepsy. Am J Med Genet 2001; 106:139 145.
7. Schwartzkroin PA, Walsh CA. Cortical malformations and epilepsy. Ment Retard Dev Disabil Res Rev 2000; 6:268–280.
8. Guerrini R, Andermann E, Avoli M, Dobyns WB. Cortical dysplasias, genetics, and epileptogenesis. Adv Neurol 1999; 79:95–121.
9. Delgado-Escueta AV, Ganesh S, Yamakawa K. Advances in the genetics of progressive myoclonus epilepsy. Am J Med Genet 2001; 106:129–138.
10. Loscher W, Cramer S, Ebert U. Differences in kindling development in seven outbred and inbred rat strains. Exp Neurol 1998; 154:551–559.
11. Lothman EW. Basic mechanisms of seizure expression. Epilepsy Res Suppl 1996; 11:9–16.
12. Buckmaster PS, Jongen-Relo AL. Highly specific neuron loss preserves lateral inhibitory circuits in the dentate gyrus of kainate-induced epileptic rats. J Neurosci 1999; 19:9519–9529.

13. Bouilleret V, Loup F, Kiener T, Marescaux C, Fritschy JM. Early loss of interneurons and delayed subunit-specific changes in GABA(A)-receptor expression in a mouse model of mesial temporal lobe epilepsy. Hippocampus 2000; 10:305–324.

14. Coulter DA. Epilepsy-associated plasticity in gamma-aminobutyric acid receptor expression, function, and inhibitory synaptic properties. Int Rev Neurobiol 2001; 45:237–252.

15. Mody I, MacDonald JF. NMDA receptor-dependent excitotoxicity: the role of intracellular Ca^{2+} release. Trends Pharmacol Sci 1995; 16:356–359.

16. Faingold CL, Anderson CA. Loss of intensity-induced inhibition in inferior colliculus neurons leads to audiogenic seizure susceptibility in behaving genetically epilepsy-prone rats. Exp Neurol 1991; 113:354–363.

17. Min MY, Melyan Z, Kullmann DM. Synaptically released glutamate reduces gamma-aminobutyric acid (GABA)ergic inhibition in the hippocampus via kainate receptors. Proc Natl Acad Sci USA 1999; 96:9932–9937.

18. Cronin J, Obenaus A, Houser CR, Dudek FE. Electrophysiology of dentate granule cells after kainate-induced synaptic reorganization of the mossy fibers. Brain Res 1992; 573:305–310.

19. Franck JE, Pokorny J, Kunkel DD, Schwartzkroin PA. Physiologic and morphologic characteristics of granule cell circuitry in human epileptic hippocampus. Epilepsia 1995; 36:543–558.

20. Coulter DA. Mossy fiber zinc and temporal lobe epilepsy: pathological assocation with altered "epileptic" gamma-aminobutyric acid A receptors in dentate granule cells. Epilepsia 2000; 41(suppl 6):S96–S99.

21. Bordey A, Sontheimer H. Properties of human glial cells associated with epileptic seizure foci. Epilepsy Res 1998; 32:286–303.

22. Vezzani A, Moneta D, Conti M, Richichi C, Ravizza T, DeLuigi A, DeSimoni MG, Sperk G, Andell-Jonsson S, Lundkvist J, Iverfeldt K, Bartfai T. Powerful anticonvulsant action of IL-1 receptor antagonist on intracerebral injection and astrocytic over-expression in mice. Proc Natl Acad Sci USA 2000; 97:11534–11539.

23. Patel MN, McNamara JO. Selective enhancement of axonal branching of cultured dentate gyrus neurons by neurotrophic factors. Neuroscience 1995; 69:763–770.

24. Collin C, Vicario-Abejon C, Rubio ME, Wenthold RJ, McKay RD, Segal M. Neurotrophins act at presynaptic terminals to activate synapses among cultured hippocampal neurons. Eur J Neurosci 2001; 13:1273–1282.

25. Parent JM, Yu TW, Leibowitz RT, Geschwind DH, Sloviter RS, Lowenstein DH. Dentate granule cell neurogenesis is increased by seizures and contributes to aberrant network reorganization in the adult rat hippocampus. J Neurosci 1997; 17:3727–3738.

26. Engel J Jr. Clinical evidence for the progressive nature of epilepsy. Epilepsy Res Suppl 1996; 12:9–20.

27. Sutula TP. Secondary epileptogenesis, kindling, and intractable epilepsy: a reappraisal from the perspective of neural plasticity. Int Rev Neurobiol 2001; 45:355–386.

28. Cavazos JE, Das I, Sutula TP. Neuronal loss induced in limbic pathways by kindling: evidence for induction of hippocampal sclerosis by repeated brief seizures. J Neurosci 1994; 14:3106–3121.

29. Lehnertz K, Andrzejak RG, Arnhold J, Kreuz T, Mormann F, Rieke C, Widman G, Elger CE. Nonlinear EEG analysis in epilepsy: its possible use for interictal focus localization, seizure anticipation, and prevention. J Clin Neurophysiol 2001; 18:209–222.

30. Litt B, Esteller R, Echauz J, D'Alessandro M, Shor R, Henry T, Pennell P, Epstein C, Bakay R, Dichter M, Vachtsevanos G. Epileptic seizures may begin hours in advance of clinical onset: a report of five patients. Neuron 2001; 30:51–64.

31. Gluckman BJ, Nguyen H, Weinstein SL, Schiff SJ. Adaptive electric field control of epileptic seizures. J Neurosci 2001; 21:590–600.

32. Teyler TJ, Morgan SL, Russell RN, Woodside BL. Synaptic plasticity and secondary epileptogenesis. Int Rev Neurobiol 2001; 45:253–267.

33. Mazarati AM, Hohmann JG, Bacon A, Liu H, Sankar R, Steiner RA, Wynick D, Wasterlain CG. Modulation of hippocampal excitability and seizures by galanin. J Neurosci 2000; 20:6276–6281.

34. Vezzani A, Rizzi M, Conti M, Samanin R. Modulatory role of neuropeptides in seizures induced in rats by stimulation of glutamate receptors. J Nutr 2000; 130(4S suppl): 1046S–1048S.

35. Sankar R, Shin DH, Wasterlain CG. Serum neuron-specific enolase is a marker for neuronal damage following status epilepticus in the rat. Epilepsy Res 1997; 28:129–136.

36. Temkin NR, Dikmen SS, Wilensky AJ, Keihm J, Chabal S, Winn HR. A randomized, couble-blind study of phenytoin for the prevention of post-traumatic seizures. N Engl J Med 1990; 323:497–502.

37. Temkin NR, Dikmen SS, Anderson GD, Wilensky AJ, Holmes MD, Cohen W, Newell DW, Nelson P, Awan A, Winn HR. Valproate therapy for prevention of posttraumatic seizures: a randomized trial. J Neurosurg 1999; 91:593–600.

38. Prince DA, Salin P, Tseng GF, Hoffman S, Parada J Axonal sprouting and epileptogenesis. Adv Neurol 1997; 72:1–8.

39. Wenzel HJ, Woolley CS, Robbins CA, Schwartzkroin PA. Kainic acid–induced mossy fiber sprouting and synapse formation in the dentate gyrus of rats. Hippocampus 2000; 10:244–260.

40. Binder DK, Routbort MJ, Ryan TE, Yancopoulos GD, McNamara JO. Selective inhibition of kindling development by intraventricular administration of TrkB receptor body. J Neurosci 1999; 19:1424–1436.

41. Emmi A, Wenzel HJ, Schwartzkroin PA, Taglialatela M, Castaldo P, Bianchi L, Nerbonne J, Robertson GA, Janigro D. Do glia have heart? Expression and functional role for ether-a-go-go currents in hippocampal astrocytes. J Neurosci 2000; 20:3915–3925.

42. Elliott RC, Khademi S, Pleasure SJ, Parent JM, Lowenstein DH. Differential regulation of basic helix loop-helix mRNAs in the dentate gyrus following status epilepticus. Neuroscience 2001; 106:79–88.

43. Regis J, Bartolomei F, Rey M, Hayashi M, Chauvel P, Peragut JC. Gamma knife surgery for mesial temporal lobe epilepsy. J Neursurg 2000; 93(suppl 3):141–146.

44. Zaman V, Shetty AK. Fetal hippocampal CA3 cell grafts transplanted to lesioned CA3 region of the adult hippocampus exhibit long-term survival in a rat model of temporal lobe epilepsy. Neurobiol Dis 2001; 8:942–952.

45. Yenari MA, Fink SL, Sun GH, Chang LK, Patel MK, Kunis DM, Onley D, Ho DY, Sapolsky RM, Steinberg GK. Gene therapy with HSP72 is neuroprotective in rat models of stroke and epilepsy. Ann Neurol 1998; 44:584–591.

46. McNamara JO, Whitney KD, Andrews PI, He XP, Janumpalli S, Patel MN. Evidence for glutamate receptor autoimmunity in the pathogenesis of Rasmussen encephalitis. Adv Neurol 1999; 79:543–550.

47. Garg RK. HIV infection and seizures. Postgrad Med J 1999; 75:387–390.

48. Culmsee C, Condada S, Mattson MP. Hippocampal neurons of mice deficient in DNA-dependent protein kinase exhibit increased vulnerability to DNA damage, oxidative stress and excitotoxicity. Brain Res Mol Brain Res 2001; 87:257–262.

49. Bozzi Y, Vallone D, Borrelli E. Neuroprotective role of dopamine against hippocampal cell death. J Neurosci 2000; 20:8643–8649.

50. Morrison RS, Wenzel HJ, Kinoshita Y, Robbins CA, Donehower LA, Schwartzkroin PA. Loss of the p53 tumor suppressor gene protects neurons from kainate-induced cell death. J Neurosci 1996; 16:1337–1345.

51. Gospe SM Jr. Current perspectives on pyridoxine-dependent seizures. J Pediatr 1998; 132:919–923.

52. Gietzen DW, Dixon KD, Truong BG, Jones AC, Barrett JA, Washburn DS. Indispensable amino acid deficiency and increased seizure susceptibility in rats. Am J Physiol 1996; 271:R18–R24.

53. Todorova MT, Tandon P, Madore RA, Stafstrom CE, Seyfried TN. The ketogenic diet inhibits epileptogenesis in EL mice: a genetic model for idiopathic epilepsy. Epilepsia 2000; 41:933–940.

54. Snead OC 3rd. How does ACTH work against infantile spasms? Bedside to bench. Ann Neurol 2001; 49:288–289.

55. Woolley CS, Schwartzkroin PA. Hormonal effects on the brain. Epilepsia 1998; 39(suppl 8):S2–S8.

56. Reddy DS, Rogawski MA. Enhanced anticonvulsant activity of neuroactive steroids in a rat model of catamenial epilepsy. Epilepsia 2001; 42:337–344.

57. Yusim A, Ajilore O, Bliss T, Sapolsky R. Glucocorticoids exacerbate insult-induced declines in metabolism in slelctively vulnerable hippocampal cell fields. Brain Res 2000; 870:109–117.

58. Shields WD. Catastrophic epilepsy in childhood. Epilepsia 2000; 41(suppl 2):S2–S6.

59. McKhann GM 2nd, Welzel HJ, Robbins CA, Sosunov AA, Schwartzkroin PA. Mouse strain differences in kainic acid sensitivity, seizure behavior, mortality, and hippocampal pathology. Neuroscience 2003; 122:551–561.

Index

ISBN 0-8247-5043-8

90000